AIDS

IMMUNOLOGY SERIES

1. Mechanisms in Allergy: Reagin-Mediated Hypersensitivity
   Edited by Lawrence Goodfriend, Alec Sehon and Robert P. Orange
2. Immunopathology: Methods and Techniques
   Edited by Theodore P. Zacharia and Sidney S. Breese, Jr.
3. Immunity and Cancer in Man: An Introduction
   Edited by Arnold E. Reif
4. *Bordetella pertussis:* Immunological and Other Biological Activities
   J.J. Munoz and R.K. Bergman
5. The Lymphocyte: Structure and Function (in two parts)
   Edited by John J. Marchalonis
6. Immunology of Receptors
   Edited by B. Cinader
7. Immediate Hypersensitivity: Modern Concepts and Development
   Edited by Michael K. Bach
8. Theoretical Immunology
   Edited by George I. Bell, Alan S. Perelson, and George H. Pimbley, Jr.
9. Immunodiagnosis of Cancer (in two parts)
   Edited by Ronald B. Herberman and K. Robert McIntire
10. Immunologically Mediated Renal Diseases: Criteria for Diagnosis and Treatment
    Edited by Robert T. McCluskey and Giuseppe A. Andres
11. Clinical Immunotherapy
    Edited by Albert F. LoBuglio
12. Mechanisms of Immunity to Virus-Induced Tumors
    Edited by John W. Blasecki
13. Manual of Macrophage Methodology: Collection, Characterization, and Function
    Edited by Herbert B. Herscowitz, Howard T. Holden, Joseph A. Bellanti, and Abdul Ghaffar
14. Suppressor Cells in Human Disease
    Edited by James S. Goodwin
15. Immunological Aspects of Aging
    Edited by Diego Segre and Lester Smith
16. Cellular and Molecular Mechanisms of Immunologic Tolerance
    Edited by Tomáš Hraba and Milan Hašek

17. Immune Regulation: Evolution and Biological Significance
    Edited by Laurens N. Ruben and M. Eric Gershwin
18. Tumor Immunity in Prognosis: The Role of Mononuclear Cell Infiltration
    Edited by Stephen Haskill
19. Immunopharmacology and the Regulation of Leukocyte Function
    Edited by David R. Webb
20. Pathogenesis and Immunology of Treponemal Infection
    Edited by Ronald F. Schell and Daniel M. Musher
21. Macrophage-Mediated Antibody-Dependent Cellular Cytotoxicity
    Edited by Hillel S. Koren
22. Molecular Immunology: A Textbook
    Edited by M. Zouhair Atassi, Carel J. van Oss, and Darryl R. Absolom
23. Monoclonal Antibodies and Cancer
    Edited by George L. Wright, Jr.
24. Stress, Immunity, and Aging
    Edited by Edwin L. Cooper
25. Immune Modulation Agents and Their Mechanisms
    Edited by Richard L. Fenichel and Michael A. Chirigos
26. Mononuclear Phagocyte Biology
    Edited by Alvin Volkman
27. The Lactoperoxidase System: Chemistry and Biological Significance
    Edited by Kenneth M. Pruitt and Jorma O. Tenovuo
28. Introduction to Medical Immunology
    Edited by Gabriel Virella, Jean-Michel Goust, H. Hugh Fudenberg, and Christian C. Patrick
29. Handbook of Food Allergies
    Edited by James C. Breneman
30. Human Hybridomas: Diagnostic and Therapeutic Applications
    Edited by Anthony J. Strelkauskas
31. Aging and the Immune Response: Cellular and Humoral Aspects
    Edited by Edmond A. Goidl
32. Complications of Organ Transplantation
    Edited by Luis H. Toledo-Pereyra
33. Monoclonal Antibody Production Techniques and Applications
    Edited by Lawrence B. Schook
34. Fundamentals of Receptor Molecular Biology
    Donald F. H. Wallach
35. Recombinant Lymphokines and Their Receptors
    Edited by Steven Gillis
36. Immunology of the Male Reproductive Organs
    Edited by Pierre Luigi Bigazzi

37. The Lymphocyte: Structure and Function
Edited by John J. Marchalonis

38. Differentiation Antigens in Lymphohemopoietic Tissues
Edited by Masayuki Miyasaka and Zdenek Trnka

39. Cancer Diagnosis In Vitro Using Monoclonal Antibodies
Edited by Herbert Z. Kupchik

40. Biological Response Modifiers and Cancer Therapy
Edited by J. W. Chiao

41. Cellular Oncogene Activation
Edited by George Klein

42. Interferon and Nonviral Pathogens
Edited by Gerald I. Byrne and Jenifer Turco

43. Human Immunogenetics: Basic Principles and Clinical Relevance
Edited by Stephen D. Litwin, with David W. Scott, Lorraine Flaherty, Ralph A. Reisfeld, and Donald M. Marcus

44. AIDS: Pathogenesis and Treatment
Edited by Jay A. Levy

Additional Volumes in Preparation

AIDS

PATHOGENESIS AND TREATMENT

Edited by

JAY A. LEVY

School of Medicine
University of California
San Francisco, California

Marcel Dekker, Inc. **New York and Basel**

Cover: **"The Cell." Painting by George Habergritz (dedicated to Maya). Photograph by Jose Picaya.**

LIBRARY OF CONGRESS
Library of Congress Cataloging-in-Publication Data

AIDS, pathogenesis and treatment / edited by Jay A. Levy.
p. cm. -- (Immunology series ; 44)
Includes index.
ISBN 0-8247-7684-4
1. AIDS (Disease)--Pathogenesis. 2. AIDS (Disease)--Treatment.
I. Levy, Jay A. II. Series: Immunology series ; v. 44.
[DNLM: 1. Acquired Immunodeficiency Syndrome—etiology.
2. Acquired Immunodeficiency Syndrome—therapy. W1 IM53K v. 44 /
WD 308 A288375]
RC607.A26A34857 1989
616.97'92--dc19
DNLM/DLC 8-23795
for Library of Congress CIP

MARCEL DEKKER, INC.
270 Madison Avenue, New York, New York 10016

Current printing (last digit):
10 9 8 7 6 5 4 3 2 1

PRINTED IN THE UNITED STATES OF AMERICA

To Sharon

Series Introduction

History has given us many examples of new diseases that have burst on the scene with devastating consequences. The epidemics of plague and syphilis are cogent examples. Initially, hundreds of thousands—perhaps millions—died during the first years after a new outbreak. Eventually, the disease waned in prevalence and severity. Sometimes the most susceptible members of the population are eliminated; sometimes the etiological agent surrenders its most destructive properties in order to enter a more stable host-parasite equilibrium.

The acquired immunodeficiency syndrome (AIDS) is a current, dramatic example of a newly evolved disease. Its origins are still uncertain, but, in its present form, AIDS has been with us for less than a decade. Yet the extent of its spread and the degree of its pathogenicity match those of the great epidemics of the past. The virulence is due to several unique attributes of the AIDS virus. It is transmitted by intimate contact, affording little exposure to neutralizing antibodies. As a retrovirus, it is genetically highly variable in antigenicity because it lacks the remediation intrinsic to DNA replication. It integrates into the host cell genome, perhaps for the life of the host. It seems to circumvent an effective cytotoxic T-cell response. Among its major targets are the cell populations responsible for initiating and maintaining an immune response—the macrophage and helper/inducer lymphocyte.

In ancient times, it was learned that those who survive an epidemic disease can safely nurse its victims. From that observation grew the term "immunity" and the concept of immunology. Perhaps from the long-term survivors of AIDS will spring the newer knowledge needed to deal with this latest scourge.

In the present volume, Dr. Levy and his coauthors have given us up-to-date information about the pathogenesis of AIDS. Treatment is still in its infancy but will surely improve rapidly. The ultimate goal of prevention is still a distant dream. Every day, however, that goal comes closer as we better understand how the immune system operates and how it can be manipulated.

Noel R. Rose
Department of Immunology
and Infectious Diseases
The Johns Hopkins University
School of Hygiene and Public Health
Baltimore, Maryland

Foreword

The advent of AIDS and the discovery of its causative agent have had a profound and dramatic effect on science as well as society. We might well ask: "What might have been our fate if the spread of the human immunodeficiency virus [HIV] had occurred before the development of molecular biology and of the scientific talent and armamentarium needed to deal with it!" Even in its richness and variety, the relevant scientific community has as yet not been able to halt the spread of this virus. We must assume that, in time, it will be possible to arrest the virus and the deteriorating effect it has on the immune system, although it challenges to the extreme the ingenuity of the scientists and physicians now marshaled to counter a threat that, in some parts of the world, is not far from genocidal.

As this volume shows, a vast body of new knowledge has accumulated with unprecedented rapidity. When one appreciates the relative sizes of the target of our foe and of the brainpower and technology we possess to avoid this microbe, we are like Gulliver trying to escape the Lilliputians. It is not for lack of will on our part that the virus of AIDS has not yet been countered successfully. What are the reasons, when other infectious agents have yielded to far less sophisticated scientific and technical capabilities? Only when a way has been found to bring AIDS under control will the reasons become clear. For this to occur, HIV may well have to yield therapeutically and/or prophylactically. Thus far, precedents have provided negative rather than positive clues, thus challenging theoreticians as well as experimentalists called on to conceive new ideas and devise experiments that might point the way to effective intervention.

At this stage of transition between laboratory research and human experimentation, I will venture the guess that we may be on the threshold of insights that will soon provide a glimmer of light. This is a safe speculation since, as this book shows so well, we seem to be dealing not only with a paradoxical and complex virus but with a syndrome whose immunological, clinical, and epidemiological manifestations have not as yet been fully revealed. It appears altogether likely that multiple strategies—rather than any single one—will be required to bring about the control of this virus in the individual and in the community.

For the infected individual, there is need for some form of therapy; for those not yet infected, some form of prophylaxis. To prevent infection, some form of immunoprophylaxis will be required. While therapy might be accomplished chemically, it is conceivable that it may be possible to develop some form of immunotherapy. Herein lies the challenge and the need for devising not one but multiple strategies from which to choose. Given the nature of the host-parasite relationship, how might any of this be done? For a virus disease like influenza, all that is required is to induce and maintain levels of antibody high enough to prevent infection of the susceptible cells at the portal of entry of the respiratory tract, which is also the site of pathology, and to do so for the changing spectrum of strains and types. For poliomyelitis all that is required is to induce immunological memory just sufficient for an anamnestic-type antibody response to block CNS invasion by the three immunological types of poliovirus. For HIV, however, the answer is not as simple. Only in the most general way do experiences in the immunological control of other virus diseases help point the way to what needs to be done to control HIV infection, which involves intracellular parasitism with the agent integrated into the genetic substance of the infected cell itself. Therefore, the nature of the challenge is far more complex, requiring knowledge as well as methods pertinent to autoimmune and neoplastic diseases as well.

This book provides much food for thought in the form of the knowledge it summarizes as well as the speculations made that need to be tested experimentally. In the course of experimentation, and especially that to be undertaken in human subjects, the relevant answers will be found. If morbidity and mortality are to be reduced as soon as possible, more clinical investigation will be required, both immunotherapeutic as well as chemotherapeutic, in asymptomatic as well as symptomatic HIV-infected individuals. However, studies for the development of some form of immunoprophylaxis for uninfected individuals will be far slower and more difficult to carry out, as will field studies required for demonstrating efficacy.

The story continues to unfold. This book will be a helpful source of ideas and directions to explore for those who desire to enter the contest.

Jonas Salk
The Salk Institute
La Jolla, California

Preface

After the initial recognition in 1981 of an increased incidence of *Pneumocystis carinii* pneumonia and Kaposi's sarcoma in young homosexual men, efforts were made to uncover the mystery of the new disease called acquired immunodeficiency syndrome (AIDS). Starting with the involvement of a relatively small number of investigators working in epidemiology, immunology, and virology, the challenge of AIDS has since called forth the efforts of several thousand researchers and clinicians throughout the world. When first identified in the United States and Europe, this disease was found to be already present in Africa; it is now recognized in almost all countries of the world. Its origin, despite frequent finger-pointing, is not clear. AIDS has had devastating effects, particularly in Haiti and regions of Africa where the cofactors of venereal disease and malnutrition contribute to the severity and spread of the disease. And recently, in certain parts of the African continent, a new subtype (HIV-2) of the AIDS virus (HIV-1) has emerged to further complicate the problems for the control of this spreading epidemic.

The purpose of this book is to review the historic events leading to the recognition of AIDS and its causative agents, and to discuss the many facets of this disease complex. The transmission and varied expression of AIDS in many parts of the world and in different population groups are described in several chapters. The pathogenesis of HIV and cofactors involved in the development of AIDS are also considered in detail. The chapters on immunology and virology are dedicated particularly to the basic characteristics of HIV-induced disease that affect many tissues of the body. These areas of study bear directly on the problems faced in antiviral therapies and the development of a vaccine.

The contributors to this volume, all experts in the field, describe the prominent features of the different opportunistic infections, neurological illnesses, and cancers associated with AIDS, and the existing treatments for these diseases. Moreover, one chapter highlights and describes the initial efforts at San Francisco General Hospital to establish an AIDS medical unit. This clinical service has since become a model for similar AIDS treatment centers throughout the world. All the sections have been updated through the beginning of this year to include the most recent relevant references to the topic. Finally, the introduction and conclusions to the book are written by two pioneer vaccinologists: Dr. Jonas Salk and Dr. Maurice Hilleman. They describe the problems encountered in developing vaccines against other human viruses and provide insights into approaches that could be considered to conquer the human immunodeficiency virus.

The large number of figures, many in color, help to illustrate the multifaceted nature of AIDS and its infectious agent. Thus, the reader can observe the clinical manifestations of AIDS with its related diseases as they appear to the practicing physician. Most important, each chapter presents basic information first, and then discusses approaches by which problems can be solved or therapies instituted.

I trust that this book will answer many of the questions about AIDS posed by researchers and clinicians, and will serve as background information to incoming students in the field. These latter participants are greatly needed for the ongoing struggle with AIDS. They will help write the next chapters in what we hope will be a short history of this new and challenging human disease.

Jay A. Levy

Contents

Contributors

Donald I. Abrams, M.D. Assistant Clinical Professor, Cancer Research Institute, School of Medicine, University of California, and Assistant Director, AIDS Activities Division, San Francisco General Hospital, San Francisco, California

Arthur J. Ammann, M.D. Director, Collaborative Medical Research, Genentech, Inc., South San Francisco, California

Jay H. Beckstead, M.D. Associate Professor, Department of Pathology, School of Medicine, University of California, San Francisco, California

Dale E. Bredesen, M.D. Assistant Adjunct Professor, Department of Neurology, School of Medicine, University of California, San Francisco, California

Nathan Clumeck, M.D. Associate Professor and Chief, Infectious Diseases, Department of Internal Medicine, St. Pierre Hospital and Free University of Brussels, Brussels, Belgium

Judith B. Cohen, Ph.D. Program Director, Project AWARE, San Francisco General Hospital, and Associate Research Epidemiologist, Department of Medicine, School of Medicine, University of California, San Francisco, California

Michael B. Cohen, M.D.* Chief Resident, Department of Pathology, School of Medicine, University of California, San Francisco, California

Morton J. Cowan, M.D. Associate Professor, Department of Pediatrics, School of Medicine, University of California, San Francisco, California

Richard L. Davis, M.D. Professor of Pathology, Departments of Neurological Surgery, Neurology, and Pathology, School of Medicine, University of California, San Francisco, California

W. Lawrence Drew, M.D., Ph.D. Director, Clinical Microbiology and Infectious Diseases, Department of Pathology and Laboratory Medicine, Mount Zion Hospital and Medical Center, San Francisco, California

Kim S. Erlich, M.D. Post-Doctoral Fellow in Infectious Diseases, Department of Internal Medicine, School of Medicine, University of California, San Francisco, California

Stephen E. Follansbee, M.D. Assistant Clinical Professor, Department of Medicine and Family Practice, School of Medicine, University of California, San Francisco, California

Gayling Gee, R.N., M.S.[†] Administrative Nurse, Ward 86, AIDS/Oncology Clinic, AIDS Activities Division, School of Medicine, University of California, and San Francisco General Hospital, San Francisco, California

Jeffrey A. Golden, M.D. Associate Professor, Department of Medicine, School of Medicine, University of California, San Francisco, California

---

Current affiliations

*Assistant Professor, Department of Pathology, College of Physicians and Surgeons of Columbia University, New York, New York.

†Director, Outpatient Nursing, Division of Outpatient and Community Services, San Francisco General Hospital, and Assistant Clinical Professor, Department of Physiological Nursing, School of Nursing, University of California, San Francisco, California.

Deborah Greenspan, B.D.S. Associate Clinical Professor, Division of Oral Medicine, School of Dentistry, University of California, San Francisco, California

John S. Greenspan, B.Sc., B.D.S., Ph.D., F.R.C.Path. Professor and Chair, Division of Oral Biology, School of Dentistry, and Professor, Department of Pathology, School of Medicine, University of California, San Francisco, California

Maurice R. Hilleman, Ph.D., D.Sc. Director, Merck Institute for Therapeutic Research, West Point, Pennsylvania

Warren D. Johnson, Jr., M.D. Professor and Chief, Division of International Medicine, Department of Medicine, Cornell University Medical College, New York, New York

Marion A. Koerper, M.D. Associate Clinical Professor, Department of Pediatrics, School of Medicine, University of California, San Francisco, California

John F. Krowka, Ph.D. Assistant Research Immunologist, Department of Laboratory Medicine, School of Medicine, University of California, San Francisco, California

Evelyne T. Lennette, Ph.D. Co-Director, Virolab, Inc., Berkeley, California

Jay A. Levy, M.D. Professor of Medicine and Research Associate, Cancer Research Institute, Department of Medicine, School of Medicine, University of California, San Francisco, California

Robert M. Levy, M.D., Ph.D. Assistant Professor, Departments of Surgery (Neurosurgery) and Physiology, Northwestern University Medical School, Chicago, Illinois

John Mills, M.D. Professor of Medicine, Microbiology, and Laboratory Medicine, Department of Medicine, School of Medicine, University of California, and Chief, Division of Infectious Diseases, San Francisco General Hospital, San Francisco, California

Dewey J. Moody, Ph.D.* Visiting Scientist, Department of Laboratory Medicine, School of Medicine, University of California, San Francisco, California

Jean W. Pape, M.D. Assistant Professor, Division of International Medicine, Department of Medicine, Cornell University Medical College, New York, New York, and Faculté de Medecine, Université d'Etat d'Haiti, Port-au-Prince, Haiti

Herbert A. Perkins, M.D. Executive and Scientific Director, Irwin Memorial Blood Bank of the San Francisco Medical Society, and Clinical Professor, Department of Medicine, School of Medicine, University of California, San Francisco, California

Arnold B. Rabson, M.D. Senior Staff Fellow, Laboratory of Molecular Microbiology, National Institute of Allergy and Infectious Diseases, National Institutes of Health, Bethesda, Maryland

Mark L. Rosenblum, M.D. Professor, Department of Neurological Surgery, School of Medicine, University of California, San Francisco, California

George W. Rutherford, M.D. Medical Director, AIDS Office, San Francisco Department of Public Health, and Assistant Clinical Professor, Department of Pediatrics and Department of Epidemiology and International Health, School of Medicine, University of California, San Francisco, California

Daniel P. Stites, M.D. Professor; Vice-Chairman; and Director, Immunology Laboratory; Department of Laboratory Medicine, School of Medicine, University of California, San Francisco, California

Paul A. Volberding, M.D. Associate Professor, Department of Medicine, School of Medicine, University of California, and Director, AIDS Activities Division, San Francisco General Hospital, San Francisco, California

---

Current affiliation

*Senior Scientist, Department of Immunobiology, Applied ImmuneSciences, Menlo Park, California.

Girish N. Vyas, Ph.D. Professor and Director, Transfusion Research Program, Department of Laboratory Medicine, School of Medicine, University of California, San Francisco, California

David Werdegar, M.D., M.P.H. Director of Health, San Francisco Department of Public Health, and Professor, Department of Community and Family Medicine and Department of Medicine, School of Medicine, University of California, San Francisco, California

Constance B. Wofsy, M.D. Co-Director, AIDS Activities Division, San Francisco General Hospital, and Associate Clinical Professor, Department of Medicine, School of Medicine, University of California, San Francisco, California

John L. Ziegler, M.D. Associate Chief of Staff/Education, Veterans Administration Medical Center; Director, AIDS Clinical Research Center, and Professor, Department of Medicine, School of Medicine, University of California, San Francisco, California

AIDS

1

The Epidemiology of Acquired Immunodeficiency Syndrome

George W. Rutherford and David Werdegar
San Francisco Department of Public Health
and School of Medicine
University of California
San Francisco, California

I. Introduction

The epidemiologies of acquired immunodeficiency syndrome (AIDS) and of its causative agent, human immunodeficiency virus (HIV), have been well described in the seven years since AIDS was first recognized (1). During this period, over 70,000 cases have been reported worldwide, and it is likely that several million people have been infected with HIV and are at risk of developing AIDS (171,172). This chapter reviews the current and future epidemiology of AIDS and HIV infection and examines possible future trends of this pandemic.

II. Historical Background

In June 1981, the Centers for Disease Control (CDC) reported a cluster of five previously healthy homosexual men from Los Angeles with *Pneumocystis carinii* pneumonia and candidiasis (1). Three of these patients had in vitro abnormalities of cell-mediated immunity, and the report concluded that the cluster suggested "the possibility of a cellular immune dysfunction

Table 1 HIV Transmission and CDC Transmission Categories

Route	Transmission category
Sexual	Homosexual and bisexual men
	Heterosexual contacts
	Haitians
Parenteral	Intravenous drug users
	Blood transfusion recipients
	Hemophiliacs
	Health care workers
Perinatal	Infants of mothers at high risk for AIDS
Sexual or parenteral	Homosexual and bisexual men with histories of intravenous drug use
Unknown	Undetermined

related to a common exposure that predisposes individuals to opportunistic infections such as pneumocystosis and candidiasis'' (1).

By August 1981, 111 unusual cases of *Pneumocystis carinii* pneumonia as well as Kaposi's sarcoma had been reported to the CDC, and national surveillance and a national case-control study had been organized (2). The epidemiology of this new disorder was striking—99% of the patients were male, 95% were 25-49 years old, 94% were homosexual or bisexual, 77% were white, and, most important, 40% were dead (2).

These and other early reports (3-8) heralded the beginning of the AIDS epidemic. Subsequently, AIDS was described in intravenous drug users (5, 9), Haitians (10), hemophiliacs (11,12), blood transfusion recipients (13), infants of mothers at increased risk for AIDS (14), and female sexual partners of men with AIDS (15,16). These patient groups are now known to reflect different patterns of HIV transmission with homosexual and bisexual men, heterosexual partners, and Haitians primarily having acquired HIV sexually; intravenous drug users, blood transfusion recipients, and hemophiliacs having acquired HIV parenterally; and infants of mothers with AIDS or at risk for AIDS having acquired HIV perinatally (Table 1).

III. Definitions

A. AIDS

The disorder AIDS is a clinical syndrome characterized by diseases, which are at least moderately predictive of abnormal cell-mediated immunity, in a person with no known underlying cause for cellular immunodeficiency (17). For purposes of AIDS reporting and surveillance, a case definition of AIDS

Table 2 CDC Surveillance Case Definition of AIDS (22a)

I. Without laboratory evidence for HIV infection

If laboratory tests for HIV were not performed or gave inconclusive results and the patient had no other cause of immunodeficiency listed in Section I.A below, then any disease listed in Section I.B indicates AIDS if it was diagnosed by a definitive method.

A. Cause of immunodeficiency that disqualify diseases as indicators of AIDS in the absence of laboratory evidence for HIV infection
   1. High-dose or long-term systemic corticosteroid therapy or other immunosuppressive/cytotoxic therapy ⩽3 months before the onset of the indicator diseases
   2. Any of the following diseases diagnosed ⩽3 months after diagnosis of the indicator disease: Hodgkin's disease, non-Hodgkin's lymphoma (other than primary brain lymphoma), lymphocytic leukemia, multiple myeloma, any other cancer of lymphoreticular or histiocytic tissue, or angioimmunoblastic lymphadenopathy
   3. A genetic (congenital) immunodeficiency syndrome or an acquired immunodeficiency syndrome atypical of HIV infection, such as one involving hypogammaglobulinemia

B. Indicator diseases diagnosed definitively
   1. Candidiasis of the esophagus, trachea, bronchi, or lungs
   2. Cryptococcosis, extrapulmonary
   3. Cryptosporidiosis with diarrhea persisting ⩾1 month
   4. Cytomegalovirus disease of an organ other than liver, spleen, or lymph nodes in a patient ⩾1 month of age
   5. Herpes simplex virus infection causing a mucocutaneous ulcer that persists longer than 1 month; or bronchitis, pneumonitis, or esophagitis for any duration affecting a patient ⩾1 month of age
   6. Kaposi's sarcoma affecting a patient ⩽60 years of age
   7. Lymphoma of the brain (primary) affecting a patient ⩽60 years of age
   8. Lymphoid interstitial pneumonia and/or pulmonary lymphoid hyperplasia (LIP/PLH complex) affecting a child ⩽12 years of age
   9. *Mycobacterium avium* complex or *M. kansasii* disease, disseminated (at a site other than or in addition to lungs, skin, or cervical or hilar lymph nodes)
   10. *Pneumocystis carinii* pneumonia
   11. Progressive multifocal leukoencephalopathy
   12. Toxoplasmosis of the brain affecting a patient ⩾1 month of age

II. With laboratory evidence for HIV infection

Regardless of the presence of other causes of immunodeficiency (I.A), in the presence of laboratory evidence of HIV infection, any disease listed above (I.B) or below (II.A or II.B) indicates a diagnosis of AIDS.

Table 2 (continued)

A. Indicator diseases diagnosed definitively
   1. Bacterial infections, multiple or recurrent (any combination of at least two within a 2-year period), of the following types affecting a child ≤13 years of age:
      Septicemia, pneumonia, meningitis, bone or joint infection, or abcess of an internal organ or body cavity (excluding otitis media or superficial skin or mucosal abscesses), caused by Haemophilus, Streptococcus (including pneumococcus), or other pyogenic bacteria
   2. Coccidioidomycosis, disseminated (at a site other than or in addition to lungs or cervical or hilar lymph nodes)
   3. HIV encephalopathy (also called "HIV dementia," "AIDS dementia," or "subacute encephalitis due to HIV")
   4. Histoplasmosis, disseminated (at a site other than or in addition to lungs or cervical or hilar lymph nodes)
   5. Isosporiasis with diarrhea persisting ≥1 month
   6. Kaposi's sarcoma at any age
   7. Lymphoma of the brain (primary) at any age
   8. Other non-Hodgkin's lymphoma of B-cell or unknown immunological phenotype and the following histologic types:
      a. Small noncleaved lymphoma (either Burkitt or non-Burkitt type)
      b. Immunoblastic sarcoma (equivalent to any of the following, although not necessarily all in combination: immunoblastic lymphoma, large-cell lymphoma, diffuse histiocytic lymphoma, diffuse undifferentiated lymphoma, or high-grade lymphoma)
         Note: Lymphomas are not included here if they are of T-cell immunological phenotype or their histologic type is not described as "lymphocytic," "lymphoblastic," "small cleaved," or "plasmacytoid lymphocytic"
   9. Any mycobacterial disease caused by mycobacteria other than *M. tuberculosis*, disseminated (at a site other than or in addition to lungs, skin, or cervical or hilar lymph nodes)
   10. Disease caused by *M. tuberculosis*, extrapulmonary (involving at least one site outside the lungs, regardless of whether there is concurrent pulmonary involvement)
   11. Salmonella (nontyphoid) septicemia, recurrent
   12. HIV wasting syndrome (emaciation, "slim disease")

B. Indicator diseases diagnosed presumptively
   Note: Given the seriousness of diseases indicative of AIDS, it is generally important to diagnose them definitively, especially when therapy that would be used may have serious side effects or when definitive diagnosis is needed for eligibility for antiretroviral therapy. Nonetheless, in some situations, a patient's condition will not permit the performance of definitive tests. In other situations, accepted clinical practice may be to diagnose presumptively based on the presence of characteristic clinical and laboratory abnormalities.

Table 2 (continued)

1. Candidiasis of the esophagus
2. Cytomegalovirus retinitis with loss of vision
3. Kaposi's sarcoma
4. Lymphoid interstitial pneumonia and/or pulmonary lymphoid hyperplasia (LIP/PLH complex) affecting a child ≤13 years of age
5. Mycobacterial disease (acid-fast bacilli with species not identified by culture), disseminated (involving at least one site other than or in addition to lungs, skin, or cervical or hilar lymph nodes)
6. *Pneumocystis carinii* pneumonia
7. Toxoplasmosis of the brain affecting a patient ≥1 month of age

III. With laboratory evidence against HIV infection

With laboratory test results negative for HIV infection, a diagnosis of AIDS for surveillance purposes is ruled out unless:

A. All the other causes of immunodeficiency listed above in Section I.A are excluded *and*
B. The patient has had either:
   1. *Pneumocystis carinii* pneumonia diagnosed by a definitive method *or*
   2. a. Any of the other diseases indicative of AIDS listed above in Section I.B. diagnosed by a definitive method *and*
      b. A T-helper/inducer (CD4) lymphocyte count ≤400/mm3

A case of AIDS is defined as a reliably diagnosed opportunistic disease in an adolescent or an adult at least moderately indicative of underlying cellular immunodeficiency and with no other known cause of underlying cellular immunodeficiency or any other reduced resistance reported to be associated with an opportunistic disease, including secondary immunodeficiencies associated with immunosuppressive therapy, lymphoreticular malignancy, or starvation.
Source: Ref. 173.

was first published in 1982 (17) and successively modified to increase its specificity and sensitivity (18-22,173). The current national surveillance definition of AIDS is shown in Table 2 (173).

Because of a slightly different clinical spectrum of AIDS and a variety of congenital immunodeficiency syndromes that must be excluded before a diagnosis is established, CDC published a separate definition for surveillance of AIDS in children under 13 years of age in 1984 (21) (see Chapter 6). The current surveillance definition of pediatric AIDS is shown in Table 2 (173).

B. HIV Infection

The other clinical manifestations of HIV infection, including AIDS-related complex, progressive generalized lymphadenopathy, slim disease, and others, have until recently been less rigidly defined. Three classification systems for HIV infection in adult patients have been published (23-25), each describing

Table 3 Summary of CDC Classification System for Human Immunodeficiency Virus Infection

Group I.	Acute infection
Group II.	Asymptomatic infection[a]
Group III.	Persistent generalized lymphadenopathy[a]
Group IV.	Other disease
Subgroup A.	Constitutional disease
Subgroup B.	Neurologic disease
Subgroup C.	Secondary infectious diseases
Category C-1	Specified secondary infectious diseases listed in the CDC surveillance definition for AIDS[b]
Category C-2	Other specified secondary infectious diseases
Subgroup D.	Secondary cancers[b]
Subgroup E.	Other conditions

[a]Patients in groups II and III may be subclassified on the basis of a laboratory evaluation.
[b]Includes those patients whose clinical presentation fulfills the definition of AIDS used by CDC for national reporting.
Source: Ref. 25.

a spectrum of clinical disease ranging from asymptomatic infection to frank AIDS. The current CDC definition for clinical HIV infection is shown in Table 3 (25). Recently, a somewhat similar classification scheme for HIV infection in children has also been described (26).

IV. Natural History of HIV Infection

A. Prevalence of HIV Infection

The prevalence of HIV infection in the United States is not known (174,175). Among blood donors and military recruits, groups that have been widely used as surrogates for the population at large, the prevalence has ranged from 0.04% among blood donors (27) to 0.15% among military recruits (28). In both these groups the prevalence among men (0.07% in blood donors and 0.16% in military recruits) has been greater than among women (0.006% and 0.06%, respectively). Additionally, prevalence has varied by race among military recruits with infection found in 0.09% of whites, 0.39% of blacks, and 0.26% of others (Hispanics, Asians, and American Indians) (28).

The prevalence of HIV infection among selected risk groups can be somewhat more easily estimated. Studies of homosexual and bisexual men living in large cities in the United States and Europe have found seroprevalences of 32-42% in Seattle (29), 42% in Los Angeles (30), 21-45% in Manhattan (31-33), 17% in London (34), 31% in Amsterdam (35), 10% in Zurich (36), 8% in Denmark (32), and 33-73% in San Francisco (37-43). From these

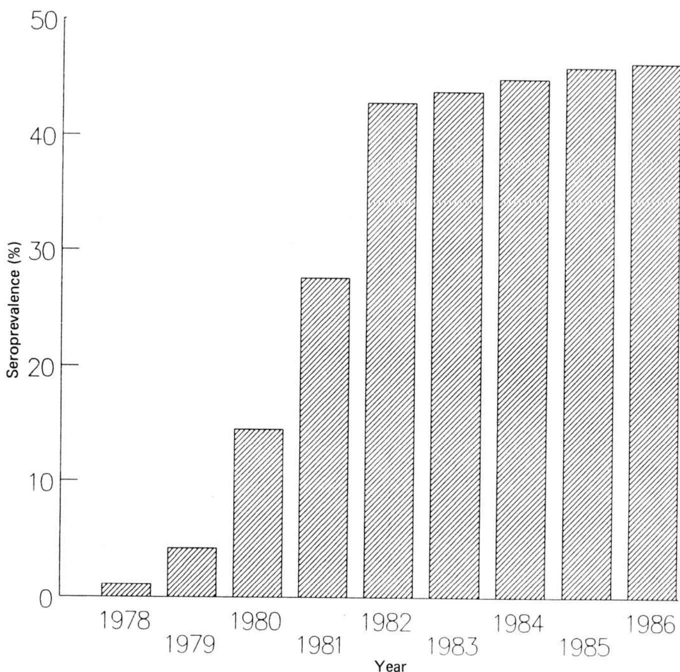

Figure 1 Cumulative prevalence of HIV infection in a cohort of homosexual and bisexual men who participated in the Hepatitis B Vaccine Trials at the San Francisco City Clinic. The prevalence of infection rose from 1% in 1978 to 46% in 1986. Note the relative leveling after 1982. (From Ref. 176.)

studies it can be shown that the first cases of HIV infection in this population occurred in the late 1970s and that new cases are continuing to occur, albeit at a much slower rate (Figure 1; 39,40,42,43,176,177).

Among intravenous drug users the prevalence of HIV infection has been reported to range from 2% in California (44) to 50% in New Jersey (45,174) to 72% in New York City (45,46,178,179). In Europe, the prevalence among intravenous drug users has been reported to be as high as 51%, 52-60%, 51%, and 50%, in Edinburgh, Italy, southern France, and Spain, respectively (47-51). Among hemophiliacs in the United States, between 40% and 88% are now estimated to be infected (52-54,180).

B. Incidence of HIV Infection

Data on the annual incidence—that is, new cases per year—of HIV infection are limited. In three cohorts of homosexual and bisexual men from San

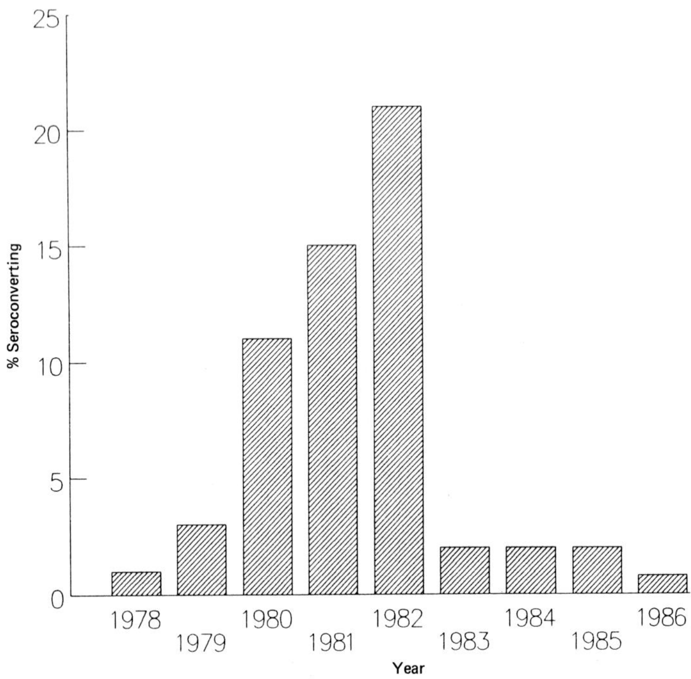

Figure 2 Percentage of previously uninfected homosexual and bisexual men (Hepatitis B Vaccine Trial participants, San Francisco City Clinic Cohort Study) newly infected with HIV by year. Note the rapid rise between 1978 and 1982 and the decline in 1983 and subsequent years. (From Ref. 176.)

Francisco, the annual incidence between 1985 and 1986 was 3-5% (41-43, 176,177). When compared, however, with previous years, this incidence was quite low, paralleling a similar decline in the incidence of gonorrheal proctitis among men in San Francisco (Figure 2; 43,176).

The annual incidence among intravenous drug users has been estimated from serial seroprevalence surveys of methadone and detoxification clients. In a one-year period between 1985 and 1986, the prevalence of infection in a San Francisco methadone clinic rose from 10% to 14% (55; R.E. Chaisson, personal communication), whereas during a two-year period, 1984-1986, the prevalence rose from 5% to 20% and to 64% among treatment populations in Edinburgh (47). These and similar data from New York, New Jersey, and Italy demonstrate the potential for rapid spread of HIV infection among intravenous drug users (179).

C. Persistence of HIV Infection

As with other mammalian retroviral diseases, HIV infection can persist for several years (56). Persistent viremia for up to 69 months has been documented in homosexual men (57), and seropositivity has been clearly correlated with viremia in between 67% and 85% of symptomatic and asymptomatic individuals (57-62). Because of this close association between seropositivity and viremia, seropositivity should be considered presumptive evidence of HIV infection and infectibility (56).

D. Outcome of HIV Infection

Human immunodeficiency virus can cause a broad spectrum of clinically apparent diseases ranging from an acute mononucleosislike syndrome (63) (see Chapter 8) to frank AIDS (23-25). Cohort studies of homosexual men (41,64-69,181), intravenous drug users (70,71), and hemophiliacs (72,73, 182) using survival analysis have predicted that between 8% and 36% of infected patients will develop AIDS over periods of time ranging from 36 to 88 months (69,74,75,183).

In a study of 63 homosexual and bisexual men whose date of seroconversion was known, all of whom had seroconverted before October 1983, 30% had developed AIDS, 48% had developed other definable HIV-related symptoms, and 22% had remained asymptomatic over an average followup of 76 months after infection (69; Table 4). Additionally, using survival analysis, it could be estimated that 36% (95% confidence interval, 26-46%) would develop AIDS within 88 months of infection (69; Figure 3). In this cohort, the mean incubation period between infection and diagnosis of AIDS was 55 months (69).

Among transfusion recipients with AIDS, patients whose date of infection is known, the mean incubation period observed to date is 29 months for

Table 4 Clinical Outcomes of 63 Men with Long-Term HIV Infection: San Francisco City Clinic Cohort Study

Condition	Cases (*n*)	%	95% confidence interval
AIDS	19	30	19-41
HIV-related conditions			
Generalized lymphadenopathy	17	27	16-38
Other signs or symptoms[a]	13	21	11-31
Asymptomatic	14	22	

[a]Oral candidiasis, weight loss, or persistent idiopathic fever or diarrhea. Nine participants had coincident generalized lymphadenopathy.

Followup was an average of 76 months.

Source: Ref. 69.

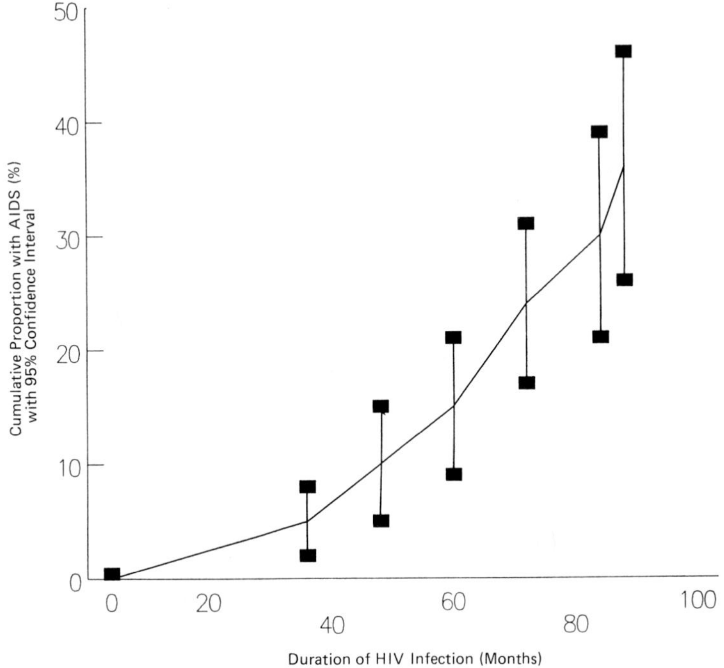

Figure 3 Cumulative percentage of men (San Francisco Clinic Cohort Study) developing AIDS as a function of the duration of HIV infection. This Kaplan-Meier graph shows the cumulative risk of AIDS increases as duration of infection increases and appears to accelerate after 5 years. (From Ref. 69.)

adults and 14 months for infants (76,77). Among infants with perinatally transmitted HIV infection, the mean age at diagnosis of AIDS is 12 months, which represents the minimal incubation period for perinatally acquired AIDS (78). However, these estimates are likely underestimates of the true incubation period because cases with a longer incubation period may not yet have been diagnosed (79).

E. Risk Factors for the Development of Clinical Disease

With the development of an effective HIV antibody test, cofactors for the development of clinical disease, as opposed to those associated with seroconversion, could be studied separately. Preliminary data from case-control studies suggested that volatile alkyl nitrites, substances known to be in vitro immunosuppressants and widely used by homosexual men (80), were possibly a cofactor in the development of Kaposi's sarcoma (81-86). Other studies, however, have not confirmed this finding (68,87-89). The most consistent cofactors that have been demonstrated to date are duration of infection (69, 74,87,181), degree of immunological dysfunction (41,90,181), and, possibly, age (91), none of which can be effectively modified at the present time.

V. AIDS in the United States

A. Descriptive Epidemiology

As of March 28, 1988, 57,575 cases of AIDS and 32,190 (56%) deaths from AIDS had been reported in the United States. The incidence of AIDS is cur-

Table 5 AIDS Cases by Transmission Category and Sex: United States[a]

	Males		Females		Total	
Group[b]	*n*	(%)	*n*	(%)	*n*	(%)
Adults/adolescents						
Homosexual/bisexual male	36,234	(69)			36,234	(64)
Intravenous (IV) drug user	7971	(15)	2221	(51)	10,192	(18)
Homosexual/bisexual male and IV drug user	4226	(8)			4226	(7)
Hemophilia/coagulation disorder	548	(1)	23	(1)	571	(1)
Heterosexual cases[c]	1034	(2)	1251	(29)	2285	(4)
Transfusion, blood/components	896	(2)	479	(11)	1375	(2)
Undetermined[d]	1404	(3)	375	(9)	1779	(3)
Subtotal [% of all cases]	52,313	[92]	4349	[8]	56,662	[100]
Children[e]						
Hemophilia/coagulation disorder	48	(10)	2	(0)	50	(5)
Parent with/at risk of AIDS[f]	352	(71)	350	(83)	702	(77)
Transfusion, blood/components	74	(15)	51	(12)	125	(14)
Undetermined[d]	19	(4)	17	(4)	36	(4)
Subtotal [% of all cases]	493	[54]	420	[46]	913	[100]
Total [% of all cases]	52,806	[92]	4769	[8]	57,575	[100]

[a]These data are provisional to March 28, 1988.

[b]Cases with more than one risk factor other than the combinations listed in the tables or footnotes are tabulated only in the category listed first.

[c]Includes 1338 persons (293 men, 1045 women) who have had heterosexual contact with a person with AIDS or at risk for AIDS and 947 persons (741 men, 206 women) without other identified risks who were born in countries in which heterosexual transmission is believed to play a major role although precise means of transmission have not yet been defined.

[d]Includes patients on whom risk information is incomplete (due to death, refusal to be interviewed, or loss to followup), patients still under investigation, men reported only to have had heterosexual contact with a prostitute, and interviewed patients for whom no specific risk was identified.

[e]Includes all patients under 13 years of age at time of diagnosis.

[f]Epidemiological data suggest transmission from an infected mother to her fetus or infant during the perinatal period.

Table 6 AIDS Cases and Incidence by Standard Metropolitan Statistical Areas: United States[a]

	Cases	Population[b]	Incidence[b]
New York	13,210	9.12	1448.5
San Francisco	5100	3.25	1569.2
Los Angeles	4559	7.48	609.5
Houston	1887	2.91	648.5
Washington (District of Columbia)	1753	3.06	572.9
Newark (New Jersey)	1669	1.97	847.2
Miami	1457	1.63	893.9
Chicago	1416	7.10	199.4
Dallas	1195	2.97	402.3
Philadelphia	1160	4.72	245.8
Atlanta	911	2.03	448.8
Boston	851	2.76	308.3
San Diego	753	1.86	404.8
Fort Lauderdale	737	1.02	722.5
Jersey City (New Jersey)	706	0.56	1260.7
Nassau-Suffolk (New York)	651	2.61	249.4

[a]Provisional data to March 28, 1988.
[b]In millions. Incidence, cases per million population.
Source: Centers for Disease Control.

rently 243.5 cases per million population. Of these 57,575 patients, 52,313 (91%) were adult and adolescent men, 4349 (8%) were adult and adolescent women and 913 (1%) were children (Table 5). Fifty-nine percent of patients were white, 26% black, 14% Hispanic, 1% Asian and Pacific Islander, and less than 1% American Indians or Alaskan Natives. Cases have been now reported from all 50 states, the District of Columbia, Puerto Rico, the Virgin Islands, Guam, and the Trust Territory of the Pacific but tend to be clustered in major metropolitan areas (Table 6).

Sixty-four percent of adult and adolescent cases involve homosexual or bisexual men, 18% heterosexual intravenous drug users, 7% homosexual or bisexual male intravenous drug users, 4% heterosexual partners of persons with AIDS or at risk for AIDS or heterosexuals from tropical countries where heterosexual transmission is the predominant mode of transmission, 2% blood transfusion recipients, 1% hemophiliacs, and 3% persons with undetermined risk (Table 6). Among children less than 13 years old, 77% were children of parents with or at risk for AIDS, 14% blood transfusion recipients, 5% hemophiliacs, and 4% persons with undetermined risk (Table 5). Blacks and Hispanics compose 80% of heterosexual intravenous drug users with AIDS, 82% of heterosexually transmitted cases, and 85% of infants with perinatally transmitted infection.

Table 7 AIDS Cases and Deaths by Initial Opportunistic Disease: United States

Initial opportunistic disease	Cases		Deaths	
	n	%	*n*	%
Pneumocystis carinii pneumonia	35,705	(62)	20,235	(57)
Other opportunistic diseases	15,863	(28)	9,112	(57)
Kaposi's sarcoma	6,007	(10)	2,843	(47)
Total	57,575	(100)	32,190	(56)

[a]Provisional data to March 28, 1988.
Source: Centers for Disease Control.

Table 8 AIDS Cases by 10 Most Frequent Opportunistic Infections and Malignancies: United States[a]

	AIDS Patients (%)
Pneumocystis carinii pneumonia	64
Kaposi's sarcoma	21
Esophageal candidiasis	11
Cryptococcosis	7
Cytomegalovirus disease	5
Dissemination *Mycobacterium avium* complex	4
Chronic mucocutaneous *herpes simplex*	4
Chronic enteric cryptosporidiosis	3
Toxoplasmosis of the brain	3
Immunoblastic sarcoma	1

[a]Through February 9, 1987.
Source: Ref. 184.

Sixty-two percent of AIDS patients present with *Pneumocystis carinii* pneumonia, 10% with Kaposi's sarcoma, and 28% with other opportunistic infections and malignancies (Tables 7 and 8). Kaposi's sarcoma tends to be a malignancy almost exclusively of homosexual and bisexual men (92,184), and patients who present with Kaposi's sarcoma tend to live longer than patients presenting with other diseases (93,185). However, its incidence appears to be decreasing recently (92,185,186).

Trends

The number of cases of AIDS diagnosed in the United States will continue to increase over the next several years (94). Projections of the number of cases in the United States have been made by fitting quadratic equations to the present epidemic curve (94). This model predicts that there will be a total of 270,000 cases reported by the end of 1991 and that there will be 74,000 cases diagnosed in 1991 alone (94). Using a 1988 estimate of the overall prevalence of HIV infection in the United States of between 1,000,000 and 1,500,000 people (174) and assuming that no further transmission occurs, this model predicts that 18-27% of people infected with HIV will develop AIDS by 1991. This estimate is consistent with observed AIDS morbidity from cohort studies (69,74).

Quadratic modeling also has been used to predict changes in transmission category, geographic distribution, age, race, and sex. Major trends that were predicted included increasing numbers of transfusion-associated and heterosexual contact cases to 2.5% and 5.0% of the 1991 cases, respectively. Moreover, a redistribution of cases away from New York City, San Francisco, and Florida was considered with 76.9% of cases in 1991 diagnosed outside of these areas as opposed to 52.6% in 1986 (94). Emergence of new transmission patterns, such as bidirectional heterosexual transmission among adolescents or low-income populations, or effective therapeutic interventions to prevent infection, such as vaccination, will affect these estimates. Furthermore, efforts to limit the progression of clinical disease among persons with asymptomatic or mildly symptomatic HIV infection will markedly change both the overall projections and projections by age, sex, race, geographic distribution, and transmission category.

B. Epidemiology by Type of Transmission

Sexual Transmission

Sixty-eight percent of adult and adolescent AIDS patients acquired HIV infection sexually. This means of HIV transmission was the first one recognized. Early case-control studies of AIDS in homosexual and bisexual men demonstrated a correlation between sexual activity, as measured by numbers of sexual partners and histories of certain sexually transmitted diseases, and the development of AIDS (95-97). The risk of sexually acquiring HIV infection depends on two variables: the probability of exposure to an infected partner and the probability of transmission from an infected partner (98). As the prevalence of HIV infection increases in a population, the probability of a randomly chosen sexual partner being infected increases so that, for instance, the risk of exposure per contact now is substantially higher for a homosexual man than it was in 1980. The second variable, the risk of actual transmission, depends on the body fluid to which the uninfected partner is exposed, the anatomical site that is exposed, and the titer of HIV in the infected partner's body fluids (98). More recent studies of HIV seroconversion among homosexual men have demonstrated that sexual activities in which the rectal mucosa of the uninfected partner is traumatized, such as receptive anal intercourse, douching, and fisting (99,100), or is ulcerated (187,188) are correlated with infection and have suggested that the risk of infection per partner with whom receptive anal intercourse is practiced (as a marker of risk per episode of intercourse) is 9% (101). Further studies are under way to delineate the relative risk of other sexual activities, such as insertive anal intercourse and oral intercourse, which appears extremely low (42), and the protective effect of condoms.

Among women, the number of sexual contacts with an infected man has been associated with seroconversion (102,103,189). The prevalence of HIV infection among steady female sexual partners of infected men has ranged from 9.5% to 71% (103-107). Additionally, receptive anal intercourse has also been associated with transmission (103). However, transmission both from male to female and from female to male can and does occur, although at lower frequency, in the absence of anal intercourse (103-110) (see Chapters 7 and 8).

Homosexual and bisexual men: Sixty-four percent of adult and adolescent AIDS cases involve homosexual and bisexual men who acquired HIV infection sexually. It was in this population that AIDS was first described, and AIDS is the leading cause of death among homosexual and bisexual men. In some cohort studies of homosexual and bisexual men, the overall AIDS-specific morbidity exceeds 7% and the AIDS-specific mortality 4% (69). Homosexual and bisexual men with AIDS are predominantly white, 30-49 years old, and from major urban areas, including New York City, San Francisco, Los Angeles, and Houston. It is expected that AIDS will continue to be principally a disease of homosexual/bisexual men, with 70% of cases in 1991 involving this risk group, 8% of whom will also have histories of intravenous drug use (94).

Homosexual and bisexual male intravenous drug users: Seven percent of adult and adolescent cases of AIDS involve homosexual or bisexual men with histories of intravenous drug use. These men may have been infected sexually or parenterally by sharing needles contaminated with infected blood. In addition to possible needle exposure, behavioral studies have demonstrated a correlation between alcohol and drug use and high-risk sexual activities. These observations suggest an indirect disinhibitory role for alcohol and drugs in HIV transmission (111).

Heterosexuals: Four percent of adult and adolescent AIDS cases involve persons who acquired HIV infection through heterosexual contact. Of these 2285 patients, 1338 (59%), including 293 men and 1045 women, were sexual contacts of a person with AIDS or at risk for AIDS, and 947 (41%) of this group, 741 men and 206 women, were born in Haiti or Central Africa and had no other identifiable risk factors. Patients who were sexual contacts of persons with or at risk for AIDS were primarily contacts of intravenous drug users, black and Hispanic, and from the urban Northeast. It is expected that in 1991 5% of all AIDS cases will be in this category (94). Given the high incidence of sexually transmitted diseases in this population and potential bidirectional transmission, the possibility for multiple-generation transmission from intravenous drug users to their communities certainly exists.

Haitian immigrants in southern Florida and New York City compose the large majority of patients from tropical countries with endemic sexually transmitted HIV infection. Many of these patients acquired HIV infection early in the epidemic either sexually or through infected transfusions or needles in Haiti prior to emigrating to the United States (112), and for this reason, cases among Haitians are expected to decrease to 0.3% of the total in 1991 (94) (see also Chapter 3).

In addition, transmission has also been described as the result of infected donor semen during artificial insemination (113). Although the method of inoculation of semen may influence infectivity, universal screening of sperm donors for HIV antibody has been recommended (114).

Parenteral Transmission

Currently, 29% of adult and adolescent AIDS cases and 19% of pediatric AIDS cases involve persons who acquired HIV infection parenterally, that is, from blood contact. This number includes 18% of the adult and adolescent patients who are heterosexual intravenous drug users, 7% who are homosexual or bisexual male intravenous drug users, 1% who are hemophiliacs or have coagulation disorders, and 3% who are blood or blood component transfusion recipients. In addition, in this category are 5% of the pediatric patients who are hemophiliacs and 14% who are blood transfusion recipients. As with sexual transmission, the risk of parenteral transmission is determined by the risk of exposure and the probability of transmission occurring during that exposure. Since the body fluid in parenteral transmission is by definition blood, the probability of transmission is presumably dependent on the volume of blood, that is, there is a minimal infecting dose. For instance, a patient who received multiple infected units of blood has a higher probability of acquiring HIV infection than a health care worker who sustained a single needle stick injury from an infected patient (56,115,117). Among intravenous drug users, the risk of transmission appears to be related to the frequency of needle sharing (45,116,118,178), presumably reflecting both an increased risk of exposure (46,118) and the relative efficiency of HIV transmission through drug paraphernalia. Transmission is likely facilitated by the practice of "booting," or aspirating blood into the syringe; this procedure leaves larger amounts of residual blood in the syringe and needle together than is possible in only a needle stick injury. Among hemophiliacs,

HIV transmission was clearly related to the use of factor VIII before factor VIII became routinely heat-treated to inactivate HIV (119-121). Patients with greater factor VIII dependency had higher rates of infection than those with less severe disease (122).

Intravenous drug users: Heterosexual intravenous drug users currently account for 18% of all adolescent and adult AIDS cases. Among these 10,192 patients are 2221 (22%) women and 8184 (80%) nonwhites. Fifty-one percent of all cases of women with AIDS and 36% of all adult and adolescent nonwhites with AIDS are heterosexual intravenous drug users. They tend to cluster predominantly in the large urban centers of the Northeast, with relatively few cases yet in California. However, cases in San Francisco have recently doubled during one six-month period, thereby suggesting that the exponential phase of the epidemic in this group is now beginning on the West Coast (123). Nationally, in 1991, heterosexual intravenous drug users are expected to compose 16.4% of adult cases (94).

Heterosexual intravenous drug users also are the major source of secondary spread of HIV infection, both sexually and perinatally. Currently, more than two-thirds of the female heterosexual contact cases and one-half of the perinatally transmitted cases can be ascribed to intravenous drug users (124-126). Additionally, the disinhibitory influences of drugs may contribute to sexual transmission of HIV among intravenous drug users in high-prevalence areas, as has been described for homosexual and bisexual men (111).

Transfusion recipients: Recipients of infected blood or blood products currently account for 3% of all adult and adolescent AIDS cases, 14% of all pediatric AIDS cases, and 3% of overall AIDS cases (see Chapter 5). Compared with other AIDS cases, transfusion-associated cases tend to be in older patients with a median age range of 50-59 years (94). Among adult and adolescent patients, 75% are white, but among pediatric patients 54% are white; the reason for this disparity is unknown. Human immunodeficiency virus has been transmitted in whole blood, red cells, plasma, and platelets (13,76,77,127), and also in transplanted kidneys (128). There is no laboratory or epidemiological evidence of HIV in immune serum globulin (129) or hepatitis B vaccine (130). National screening of all donated blood, plasma, and organs was initiated in April 1985 to prevent further transfusion-associated transmission (114), but, because of the long incubation period of AIDS, cases will continue to occur over the next several yeas. In 1991, 2.5% of all adolescent and adult AIDS cases are expected to be transfusion-associated (94).

Hemophiliacs: Currently, 1% of all adolescent and adult AIDS cases, 5% of all pediatric AIDS cases, and 1% of overall AIDS cases are in hemophiliacs

(190) (see Chapter 4). Because hemophilia A, the major coagulation disorder requiring pooled plasma products for treatment, is a sex-linked disease, 97% of these cases are in males. Clotting factor concentrates and cryoprecipitate have been implicated in HIV transmission (11,72,73,119,131,132). Use of heat-treated factor VIII and other clotting factor concentrates to inactivate HIV was initiated in 1985 (121,133); again, because of the long incubation, cases are expected to continue to occur, with 1.4% of cases in 1991 involving hemophiliacs (94).

Health care workers: The transmission of HIV from infected patients to health care workers after needle stick injury has been reported (117,134-136,191). However, the risk of HIV transmission after needle stick injury from a known infected patient is believed to be very low, on the order of less than 0.5% (115,117), and certainly much lower than the risk of hepatitis B transmission (137). Additionally, there are case reports of a mother who provided extended nursing care for her child with transfusion-associated AIDS and seroconverted after prolonged and repeated mucous membrane exposure to AIDS blood (138), a nurse with severe dermatitis who provided home care for an AIDS patient and seroconverted and developed AIDS after prolonged and repeated percutaneous exposure to blood (139), a laboratory worker who seroconverted following prolonged nonparenteral exposure to high concentrations of HIV (192), and three health care workers who seroconverted following significant blood exposure to abraded skin or mucous membranes (193). Prevention of transmission to health care workers has focused on minimizing needle sticks and percutaneous and mucous membrane exposure to blood (115,140-144,194).

Perinatal Transmission

Perinatally transmitted cases currently compose 99% of all pediatric AIDS cases (see Chapter 6). Perinatal transmission can occur from mother to child in the prepartum, intrapartum, or immediate postpartum periods (78). Although transmission presumably occurs transplacentally or as the placenta separates from the uterine wall at birth, a single case of postnatal transmission presumably through breast milk has been described (145), and HIV has been isolated from milk (146). The risk of transmission from an infected mother varies between 20% and 65% in various series (113,147,148), but is generally believed to be around 50%. Because of passively transfused maternal antibody, many infants will be seropositive for several months after birth (78); a small number may also be viremic and seronegative (195).

Seventy percent of perinatally transmitted AIDS cases have been in children born to a parent with a history of intravenous drug use, 17% have been in children born to Haitian parents, and 13% have been in children born to parents with other risk factors for AIDS (94). The median age for diagnosis of AIDS in these patients is 12 months (78), and the male:female ratio is approximately 1:1. Eighty-six percent of these children are nonwhite, and 88% of all pediatric AIDS cases among blacks and 80% of cases among Hispanics are perinatally transmitted. Because of the correlations between intravenous drug use and Haitian ancestry and perinatal transmission, these cases cluster in New York, New Jersey, and southern Florida (78). However, as the geographic distribution of intravenous drug use-associated HIV infection changes, the distribution of perinatally transmitted cases will change as well.

Other Routes of Transmission

Currently, no clear route of transmission has been described for 3% of adolescent and adult AIDS cases and for 4% of pediatric AIDS cases. Patients in this "undetermined" category include those whose risk information is incomplete because of death, refused to be interviewed, or were lost to followup; those still under investigation; men reported to have had sexual contact with a female prostitute; and those who were interviewed and for whom no specific risk could be determined (149,196). Approximately one-half of this heterogeneous group includes people on whom risk information is incomplete, and some proportion probably represents non-AIDS-related cases of Kaposi's sarcoma (149,196). Although 63% of these patients are nonwhite, the proportion of the total cases falling into this category has remained stable over time (102).

None of the identified cases of HIV infection in the United States is known to have been transmitted in school, daycare, or foster care settings or through casual person-to-person contact (150). Other than sexual partners of HIV-infected patients, infants born to infected mothers, or two cases involving apparent percutaneous transmission of HIV to persons providing extended nursing care (138,139), none of the family members of AIDS patients reported to CDC have developed AIDS or HIV infection (150). Studies from the United States (104,151-160), Europe (197), and Africa (161) have failed to demonstrate HIV transmission to adults who were not sexual contacts of the infected patients or to children who were not already infected perinatally (198). In addition to evidence against casual household transmission, case-control studies of the seroprevalence of a variety of arboviruses in HIV-infected persons and controls have failed to demonstrate evidence of vector-borne transmission (162,199).

VI. AIDS Outside the United States (Excluding Haiti and Africa)

A. AIDS in Europe

As of January 6, 1988, 8775 cases of adult and pediatric AIDS had been reported to the World Health Organization (WHO) from 26 of the 27 countries

Table 9 AIDS Cases and Incidence: Europe[a]

Country	Cases (n)	Population[b]	Incidence[b]
Austria	120	7.58	15.8
Belgium	280	9.87	28.4
Bulgaria	3	8.97	0.3
Czechoslovakia	7	15.47	0.5
Denmark	202	5.11	39.5
Federal Republic of Germany	1588	61.39	25.9
Finland	22	4.87	4.5
France	2523	54.87	46.0
German Democratic Republic	4	16.72	0.2
Greece	78	9.88	7.9
Hungary	6	10.68	0.6
Iceland	4	0.24	16.7
Ireland	25	3.58	7.0
Italy	1104	57.00	19.4
Luxembourg	8	0.37	21.6
Malta	7	0.36	19.4
Netherlands	370	14.44	25.6
Norway	64	4.15	15.4
Poland	3	36.89	0.1
Portugal	81	10.05	8.1
Romania	2	22.68	0.9
Spain	624	38.44	16.2
Sweden	156	8.34	18.7
Switzerland	299	6.50	46.0
Union of Soviet Socialist Republics	4	272.50	<0.1
United Kingdom	1170	56.02	20.9
Yugoslavia	21	23.00	0.9
Total	8775	763.01	11.5

[a]Provisional data to January 6, 1988.
[b]Population in millions. Incidence per 1,000,000 population. Population total includes all European countries including USSR.
Source: Ref. 163.

in Europe (163). The largest numbers of cases were reported from France (2523, 29%), the Federal Republic of Germany (1558, 18%), the United Kingdom (1170, 13%), Italy (1104, 13%), Spain (624, 7%), the Netherlands (370, 4%), and Switzerland (299, 3%). No cases were reported from Albania. The incidence of AIDS was highest in Switzerland (46.0 cases per million population), France (46.0), and Denmark (39.5) (163; Table 9).

Of the 3281 adult cases reported through June 30, 1986, 2948 (90%) were in Europeans and 333 (10%) were in non-Europeans, including 186

(56%) Africans and 131 (39%) from the Americas (163,200). Ninety percent were male and 63% were between 20 and 39 years of age (163). Seventy-three percent of adult patients were homosexual or bisexual men, 12% were heterosexual intravenous drug users, 3% were homosexual or bisexual men with histories of intravenous drug use, 2% were transfusion recipients, 4% were hemophiliacs, and 2% were not in these risk groups (163). Of the 352 patients not in risk groups, 204 (58%) were of non-European origin and represented 66% of the total cases among non-Europeans. These patients were principally Africans and Haitians who presumably acquired HIV infection in their native countries. The majority of these patients were diagnosed in Belgium, France, Greece, and Switzerland (164).

Homosexual and bisexual men accounted for 60-100% of cases in all countries except Belgium, Greece, Italy, and Spain, where they accounted for less than 50% of cases (164). In Belgium and Greece, a majority of patients were cases from Africa, whereas in Italy and Spain, intravenous drug users compose the largest patient group. In Italy in 1985, 37% of all AIDS cases were in heterosexual intravenous drug users; in Spain, 42%. Overall in 1986, 73% of all cases among intravenous drug users were reported from Spain and Italy (163). Additionally, in the Mediterranean region of France, there is a disproportionate number of cases among intravenous drug users (R. de Andres, Centro National de Microbiologia, Virologia e Inmunologia Sanitarias, Madrid, personal communication).

B. AIDS in the Americas

As of January 6, 1988, 7201 adult and pediatric cases of AIDS had been reported in the Americas excluding the United States (see also Chapter 3). The largest numbers of cases were from Brazil (2325, 32%), Canada (1423, 20%), Haiti (912, 13%), Mexico (713, 10%), and the Dominican Republic (352, 5%). No cases had been reported from Greenland, Montserrat, or the Netherlands Antilles. The overall incidence in non-Latin (non-Spanish-speaking) Caribbean, Central American, and South American countries, 130.8 cases per million, was substantially higher than in Latin America, 11.2 cases per million. The incidence of AIDS was highest in Bermuda (1500.0 cases per million population), French Guiana (1328.6), the Bahamas (708.7), and Turks and Caicos (400.0) (Table 10).

The distribution of cases among risk groups can vary markedly by country. For instance, in Brazil 85% of the cases involve homosexual or bisexual men and less than 2% involve intravenous drug users, whereas in the Bahamas the reverse is true (165). Unlike in Europe, there has not yet been universal testing of blood for HIV, and, in addition to increases in sexually transmitted HIV infection, transfusion-associated infection should be expected to continue into the near future.

Table 10 AIDS Cases and Incidence: the Americas[a]

Subregion and country	Cases	Population[b]	Incidence[b]
North America			
Bermuda	75	0.05	1500.0
Canada	1423	25.14	56.6
Mexico	713	77.66	9.2
United States of America	57,575	236.41	243.5
Subtotal	59,786	339.36	176.2
Caribbean			
Anguilla	2	0.05	200.0
Antigua and Barbuda	3	0.08	37.5
Bahamas	163	0.23	708.7
Barbados	52	0.25	208.0
Cayman Islands	2	0.02	100.0
Cuba	6	10.00	0.6
Dominica	5	0.07	71.4
Dominican Republic	352	6.42	54.8
Grenada	7	0.11	63.6
Guadeloupe, St. Martin, and St. Barthélemy	51	0.31	164.5
Haiti	912	5.08	179.5
Jamaica	30	2.39	12.6
Martinique	27	0.33	81.8
St. Christopher and Nevis	1	0.04	25.0
St. Lucia	6	0.12	50.0
St. Vincent and the Grenadines	7	0.14	50.0
Trinidad and Tobago	206	1.17	176.1
Turks and Caicos	4	0.01	400.0
Subtotal	1836	27.08	67.8
Central America			
Belize	4	0.14	28.6
Costa Rica	39	2.69	14.5
El Salvador	16	5.10	3.1
Guatemala	30	7.96	3.8
Honduras	51	4.42	11.5
Nicaragua	19	2.91	6.5
Panama	22	2.10	10.5
Subtotal	181	25.18	7.2
South America			
Argentina	120	30.10	4.0
Bolivia	4	6.04	0.7
Brazil	2325	134.38	17.3

Table 10 (Continued)

Subregion and country	Cases	Population[b]	Incidence[b]
Chile	56	11.66	4.8
Colombia	153	28.25	5.4
Ecuador	52	9.09	5.7
French Guiana	93	0.07	1328.6
Guyana	5	0.90	5.6
Paraguay	14	3.62	3.9
Peru	44	19.16	2.3
Suriname	6	0.35	17.1
Uruguay	14	2.93	4.8
Venezuela	101	18.55	5.4
Subtotal	2973	265.10	11.2

[a]Through January 6, 1988, except the United States (through March 28, 1988).
[b]Population in millions. Incidence per 1,000,000 population. Population total includes all countries; Caribbean subtotals exclude Puerto Rico and U.S. Virgin Islands (included in U.S. total).
Source: Pan American Health Organization.

C. AIDS in Asia and Oceania

To date, very few cases of AIDS have been reported from Asian countries to WHO. As of January 6, 1988, there had been a total of 215 cases reported, with the largest number in Japan (59, 27%; incidence, 0.5 cases per million) and Israel (43, 20%; incidence, 8.8) (WHO, unpublished data; Table 11).

In contrast, 681 cases have been reported from Australia, and 59 have been reported from New Zealand (WHO, unpublished data). Cases from Australia and New Zealand have involved primarily homosexual and bisexual men and seem to have originally been imported from the United States.

VI. Conclusions

HIV has spread rapidly throughout the world since the initial description of AIDS in 1981 and the disease is now, with over 70,000 cases reported, considered pandemic. In the absence of effective antiviral therapy, cases of AIDS should be expected to continue to increase well into the future even if HIV transmission could be interrupted today. Certain types of HIV transmission, such as transfusion- or hemophilia-associated transmission, can be interrupted with careful screening of donated blood and heat treatment of clotting-factors as has been done in North America, Australia, Europe, and parts of Asia and Oceania, but the other modes of transmission will require unprecedented health education efforts to be even slowed (166-169,201). It is likely that definitive prevention will be dependent on the development of

Table 11 AIDS Cases and Incidence: Asia and Oceania[a]

Continent and country	Cases	Population[b]	Incidence[b]
Asia			
China	2	1034.91	<0.1
Cyprus	3	0.66	4.5
Hong Kong	6	5.29	1.1
India	9	746.39	<0.1
Indonesia	1	169.44	<0.1
Israel	43	4.90	8.8
Japan	59	119.90	0.5
Korea	1	42.00	<0.1
Jordan	3	2.69	1.1
Lebanon	3	2.60	1.2
Malaysia	1	15.33	0.1
Philippines	10	55.53	0.2
Sri Lanka	2	15.93	0.1
Singapore	2	2.53	0.8
Taiwan	1	19.12	<0.1
Thailand	12	51.73	0.2
Turkey	21	50.21	0.4
Subtotal	251	2775.58	0.1
Oceania			
Australia	681	15.46	44.0
French Polynesia	1	0.15	6.7
New Zealand	59	3.24	18.2
Tonga	1	0.11	9.1
Subtotal	742	23.93	31.0

[a]Provisional data through January 6, 1988. Countries with no cases are not listed.
[b]Population in millions. Incidence per 1,000,000 population. Population total includes all Asian countries and territories includes 36 cases from Eastern Mediterranean region except USSR and all Oceania countries and territories.
Source: World Health Organization.

a safe, effective, and inexpensive vaccine. However, given the magnitude of the AIDS pandemic, it is unacceptable to wait for a vaccine, and governments throughout the world need to reach out and educate their citizens frankly about sexuality, drug use, and other factors involved in the prevention of AIDS.

References

1. Centers for Disease Control. *Pneumocystis* pneumonia—Los Angeles. MMWR 1981; 30:250-2.

2. Centers for Disease Control. Follow-up on Kaposi's sarcoma and *Pneumocystis* pneumonia. MMWR 1981; 30:409-10.
3. Centers for Disease Control. Kaposi's sarcoma and *Pneumocystis* pneumonia among homosexual men—New York City and California. MMWR 1981; 30: 305-8.
4. Hymes KB, Cheung T, Greene JB, et al. Kaposi's sarcoma in homosexual men—a report of eight cases. Lancet 1981; 2:598-600.
5. Gottlieb M, Schroff R, Schauber H, et al. *Pneumocystis carinii* pneumonia and mucosal candidiasis in previously healthy homosexual men. N Engl J Med 1981; 305:1425-31.
6. Masur H, Michelis MA, Greene JB, et al. An outbreak of community-acquired *Pneumocystis carinii* pneumonia: initial manifestation of cellular immune dysfunction. N Engl J Med 1981; 305:1431-8.
7. Siegal FP, Lopez C, Hammer GS, et al. Severe acquired immunodeficiency in male homosexuals, manifested by chronic perianal ulcerative Herpes simplex lesions. N Engl J Med 1981; 305:1439-44.
8. Durack DT. Opportunistic infections and Kaposi's sarcoma in homosexual men [editorial]. N Engl J Med 1981; 305:1465-7.
9. Centers for Disease Control. Update on Kaposi's sarcoma and opportunistic infections in previously healthy persons—United States. MMWR 1982; 31:294, 300-1.
10. Centers for Disease Control. Opportunistic infections and Kaposi's sarcoma among Haitians in the United States. MMWR 1982; 31:353-4, 360-1.
11. Centers for Disease Control. *Pneumocystis carinii* pneumonia among persons with hemophilia A. MMWR 1982; 31:365-7.
12. Centers for Disease Control. Update on acquired immunodeficiency syndrome (AIDS) among patients with hemophilia A. MMWR 1982; 31:644-6, 652.
13. Centers for Disease Control. Possible transfusion-associated acquired immune deficiency syndrome (AIDS)—California. MMWR 1982; 31:652-4.
14. Centers for Disease Control. Unexplained immunodeficiency and opportunistic infections in infants—New York, New Jersey, California. MMWR 1982; 31: 665-7.
15. Masur H, Michelis MA, Wormser GP, et al. Opportunistic infection in previously healthy women: initial manifestations of a community-acquired cellular immunodeficiency. Ann Intern Med 1982; 97:533-9.
16. Centers for Disease Control. Immunodeficiency among female sexual partners of males with acquired immunodeficiency syndrome. MMWR 1983; 31:697-8.
17. Centers for Disease Control. Update on acquired immune deficiency syndrome (AIDS)—United States. MMWR 1982; 31:507-8, 513-4.
18. Jaffe HW, Bregman DJ, Selik RM. Acquired immune deficiency syndrome in the United States: the first 1,000 cases. J Infect Dis 1983; 148:339-45.
19. Jaffe HW, Selik RM. Acquired immune deficiency syndrome: is disseminated aspergillosis predictive of underlying cellular deficiency? [letter]. J Infect Dis 1984; 149:829.
20. Selik RM, Haverkos HW, Curran JW. Acquired immune deficiency syndrome (AIDS) trends in the United States, 1979-1982. Am J Med 1984; 76:493-500.

21. Centers for Disease Control. Update: acquired immunodeficiency syndrome (AIDS)—United States. MMWR 1984; 32:688-91.
22. Centers for Disease Control. Revision of the case definition of acquired immunodeficiency syndrome for national reporting—United States. MMWR 1985; 43:373-5.
23. Haverkos HW, Gottlieb MS, Killen JY, Edelman R. Classification of HTLV-III/LAV-related diseases [letter]. J Infect Dis 1985; 152:1095.
24. Redfield RR, Wright DC, Tramont EC. The Walter Reed staging classification for HTLV-III/LAV infection. N Engl J Med 1986; 314:131-2.
25. Centers for Disease Control. Classification system for human T-lymphotropic virus type-III/lymphadenopathy-associated virus infections. MMWR 1986; 35: 334-9.
26. Centers for Disease Control. Classification system for human immunodeficiency virus (HIV) infection in children under 13 years of age. MMWR 1987; 36: 225-30, 235-6.
27. Schorr JB, Berkowitz A, Cumming PD, Katz AJ, Sandler SG. Prevalence of HTLV-III antibody in American blood donors [letter]. N Engl J Med 1985; 313: 384-5.
28. Centers for Disease Control. Human T-lymphotropic virus type III/lymphadenopathy-associated virus antibody prevalence in U.S. military recruit applicants. MMWR 1986; 35:421-4.
29. Collier AC, Barnes RC, Handsfield HH. Prevalence of antibody to LAV/HTLV-III among homosexual men in Seattle. Am J Public Health 1986; 76:564-5.
30. Schwartz K, Vischer BR, Detels R, Taylor J, Nishanian P, Fahey JL. Immunological changes in lymphadenopathy virus positive and negative symptomless male homosexuals: two years of observation [letter]. Lancet 1985; 2:831-2.
31. Safai B, Sarngadharan MG, Groopman JE, et al. Seroepidemiological studies of human T-lymphotropic retrovirus type III in acquired immunodeficiency syndrome. Lancet 1984; 1:1438-40.
32. Blattner WA, Biggar RJ, Weiss SH, et al. 3-year AIDS incidence after HTLV-III: 5 cohorts and cofactor analysis. International Conference on AIDS, Paris, France, June 1986.
33. Stevens CE, Taylor PE, Rodriquez de Cordoba S, Rubinstein P. AIDS virus infection in homosexual men and volunteer blood donors in New York City. International Conference on AIDS, Paris, France, June 1986.
34. Cheingsong-Popov R, Weiss RA, Dalgleish A, et al. Prevalence of antibody to human T-lymphotropic virus type III in AIDS and AIDS-risk patients in Britain. Lancet 1984; 2:477-80.
35. VanGriensven GJP, Tielman RAP, Goudsmit J, Van der Noordaa J, DeWolf F, deContingho RA. Prevalence of LAV/HTLV-III antibodies in relation to lifestyle characteristics in homosexual men in the Netherlands. International Conference on AIDS, Paris, France, June 1986.
36. Schupback J, Haller O, Vogt M, et al. Antibodies to HTLV-III in Swiss patients with AIDS and pre-AIDS and in groups at risk for AIDS. N Engl J Med 1985; 312:265-70.
37. Anderson RE, Levy JA. Prevalence of antibody to AIDS-associated retrovirus in single men in San Francisco [letter]. Lancet 1985; 1:250.

38. Moss AR, Osmond D, Bacchetti P, Chermann J-C, Barre-Sinoussi F, Carlson J. Risk factors for AIDS and HIV seropositivity in homosexual men. Am J Epidemiol 1987; 125:1035-47.
39. Jaffe HW, Darrow WW, Echenberg DF, et al. The acquired immunodeficiency syndrome in a cohort of homosexual males: a 6-year follow-up study. Ann Intern Med 1985; 103:210-4.
40. Centers for Disease Control. Update: acquired immunodeficiency syndrome in the San Francisco Cohort Study. MMWR 1985; 34:573-5.
41. Moss AR, Bacchetti P, Osmond D, et al. Seropositivity for HIV and the development of AIDS or AIDS related condition: three year follow-up of the San Francisco General Hospital cohort. Br Med J 1988; 296:745-50.
42. Winkelstein W Jr, Samuel M, Padian N, et al. The San Francisco Men's Health Study. III. Reduction in human immunodeficiency virus transmission among homosexual/bisexual men in San Francisco, 1982-1986. Am J Pub Health 1987; 76:685-9.
43. Echenberg DF, Rutherford GW, Darrow WW, O'Malley PM, Bodecker T, Jaffe HW. The incidence and prevalence of LAV/HTLV-III infection in the San Francisco City Clinic Cohort Study, 1985 [poster]. International Conference on AIDS, Paris, France, June 1986.
44. Levy N, Carlson CR, Hinrichs S, Lerche N, Schenker M, Gardner MB. The prevalence of HTLV-III/LAV antibodies among intravenous drug users attending treatment programs in California: a preliminary report [letter]. N Engl J Med 1986; 314:446.
45. Weiss SH, Ginzburg HM, Goeddert JJ, et al. Risk for HTLV-III exposure and AIDS among parenteral drug abusers in New Jersey. International Conference on Acquired Immunodeficiency Syndrome (AIDS), Atlanta, Georgia, April 1985.
46. Spira TJ, Des Jarlais DC, Bokos D, et al. HTLV-III/LAV antibodies in intravenous (IV) drug abusers—comparison of high and low risk areas for AIDS. International Conference on Acquired Immunodeficiency Syndrome (AIDS), Atlanta, Georgia, April 1985.
47. Robertson JR, Bucknall ABV, Wiggins P. Regional variations in HIV antibody seropositivity in British intravenous drug users [letter]. Lancet 1986; 1:1435-6.
48. Angarano G, Pastore G, Monno L, Santantonio T, Luchena N, Schiraldi O. Rapid spread of HTLV-III infection among drug addicts in Italy [letter]. Lancet 1985; 2:1302.
49. Lazzarin A, Crocchiolo P, Galli M, Uberti Foppa C, Re T, Moroni M. Milan as a possible starting point of LAV/HTLV-III infection among Italian drug addicts. International Conference on AIDS, Paris, France, June 1986.
50. Federlin M, Smilovici W, Montalegre A, Watrigant MP, Ducos J, Armengaud M. LAV/HTLV-III virus endemic among a population of 431 former drug users. International Conference on AIDS, Paris, France, June 1986.
51. Rodrigo JM, Serra MA, Aguilar E, Del Olmo JA, Gimeno V, Aparisi L. HTLV-III antibodies in drug addicts in Spain [letter]. Lancet 1985; 2:156-7.
52. Ragni MV, Tegtmeier GE, Levy JA, et al. AIDS retrovirus antibodies in hemophiliacs treated with Factor VIII or Factor IX concentrates, cryoprecipitate, or fresh frozen plasma: prevalence, seroconversion rate, and clinical correlations. Blood 1986; 67:592-5.

53. Jason J, McDougal JS, Holman RC, et al. Human T-lymphotropic retrovirus type III/lymphadenopathy-associated virus antibody. Association with hemophiliacs' immune status and blood component usage. JAMA 1985; 253:3409-15.
54. Goedert JJ, Sarngadharan MG, Eyster ME, et al. Antibodies reactive with human T-cell leukemia viruses in the serum of hemophiliacs receiving factor VIII concentrate. Blood 1985; 65:492-5.
55. Chaisson RE, Moss AR, Oniski R, Osmond D, Carlson JR. Human immunodeficiency virus infection in heterosexual intravenous drug users in San Francisco. Am J Public Health 1987; 77:169-72.
56. Curran JW, Morgan WM, Hardy AM, Jaffe HW, Darrow WW, Dowdle WR. The epidemiology of AIDS: current status and future prospects. Science 1985; 229:1352-7.
57. Jaffe HW, Feorino PM, Darrow WW, et al. Isolation of a T-lymphotropic virus type III/lymphadenopathy-associated virus in apparently healthy homosexual men. Ann Intern Med 1985; 102:627-8.
58. Barre-Simoussi F, Cherman J-C, Rey F, et al. Isolation of a T-lymphotropic retrovirus from a patient at risk for acquired immune deficiency syndrome (AIDS). Science 1983; 220:868-71.
59. Gallo RC, Salahuddin SZ, Popovic M, et al. Frequent detection and isolation of cytopathic retroviruses (HTLV-III) from patients with AIDS and at risk for AIDS. Science 1984; 224:500-3.
60. Levy JA, Hoffman AD, Kramer AD, et al. Isolation of lymphocytopathic retrovirus from San Francisco patients with AIDS. Science 1984; 225:840-2.
61. Feorino PM, Jaffe HW, Palmer E, et al. Transfusion-associated acquired immunodeficiency syndrome: evidence for persistent infection in blood donors. N Engl J Med 1985; 312:1293-6.
62. McCormick JB, Krebs JW, Mitchell SW, et al. Isolation of human immunodeficiency virus from African AIDS patients and persons without AIDS or IgG antibody to human immune deficiency virus. Am J Trop Med Hyg 1987; 36:102-6.
63. Cooper DA, Gold J, Maclean P, et al. Acute AIDS retrovirus infection: definition of a clinical illness associated with seroconversion. Lancet 1985; 1:537-40.
64. Goedert JJ, Sarngadharan JG, Biggar RJ, et al. Determinants of retrovirus (HTLV-III) antibody and immunodeficiency conditions in homosexual men. Lancet 1984; 2:711-6.
65. Melbye M, Biggar RJ, Ebbesen P, et al. Seroepidemiology of HTLV-III antibody in Danish homosexual men: prevalence, transmission, and disease outcome. Br Med J 1984; 289:573-5.
66. Goedert JJ, Biggar RJ, Winn DM, et al. Decreased helper T-lymphocytes in homosexual men: I. Sexual contact in high-incidence areas for the acquired immunodeficiency syndrome. Am J Epidemiol 1985; 121:629-36.
67. Goedert JJ, Biggar RJ, Winn DM, et al. Decreased helper T-lymphocytes in homosexual men: II. Sexual practices. Am J Epidemiol 1985; 121:637-44.
68. Biggar JR, Melbye M, Ebbesen P, et al. T-lymphocyte ratios in homosexual men: epidemiologic evidence for a transmissable agent. JAMA 1984; 251:1441-6.
69. Hessol NA, Rutherford GW, O'Malley PM, et al. The natural history of human immunodeficiency virus (HIV) infection: a 7-year prospective study. III International Conference on AIDS, Washington, D.C., June 1987.

70. Orangio GR, Pitlick SD, della Latta P, et al. Soft tissue infections in parenteral drug abusers. Ann Surg 1984; 199:97-100.
71. Orangio GR, della Latta P, Mario C, et al. Infections in parenteral drug abusers: further immunologic studies. Am J Surg 1983; 146:738-41.
72. Eyster E, Goedert JJ, Sarngadhavan MG, et al. Development and early natural history of HTLV-III antibodies in persons with hemophilia. JAMA 1985; 253: 2219-23.
73. Goedert JJ, Sarngadhavan MG, Eyster ME, et al. Antibodies reactive with human T-cell leukemia virus (HTLV-III) in the sera of hemophiliacs receiving factor VIII concentrate. Blood 1985; 65:492-5.
74. Goedert JJ, Biggar RJ, Ebbesen P, et al. Three-year incidence of AIDS in five cohorts of HTLV-III-infected risk group members. Science 1986; 231:992-5.
75. Melbye M. The natural history of human T-lymphotropic virus-III infection: the cause of AIDS. Br Med J 1986; 292:5-12.
76. Curran JW, Lawrence DN, Jaffe HW, et al. Acquired immunodeficiency syndrome (AIDS) associated with transfusion. N Engl J Med 1984; 310:69-75.
77. Lui KJ, Lawrence DN, Morgan WM, et al. A model-based approach for estimating the mean incubation period of transfusion-associated acquired immunodeficiency syndrome. Proc Natl Acad Sci USA 1986; 83:3051-5.
78. Rogers MF. AIDS in children: a review of the clinical, epidemiologic and public health aspects. Pediatr Infect Dis 1985; 4:230-6.
79. Peterman TA, Drotman DP, Curran JW. Epidemiology of the acquired immunodeficiency syndrome (AIDS). Epidemiol Rev 1985; 7:1-21.
80. Newell GR, Adams SC, Mansell PWA, Hersh EM. Toxicity immunosuppressive effects and carcinogenic potential of volatile nitrites: possible relationship to Kaposi's sarcoma. Pharmacotherapy 1984; 4:284-91.
81. Marmor M, Friedman-Klein AE, Laubenstein L, et al. Risk factors for Kaposi's sarcoma in homosexual men. Lancet 1982; 1:1083-7.
82. Haverkos HW, Pinsky PF, Drotman DP, et al. Disease manifestations among homosexual men with acquired immunodeficiency syndrome (AIDS): a possible role of nitrites in Kaposi's sarcoma. Sex Transm Dis 1985; 12:203-8.
83. Goedert JJ, Newland CY, Wallen WC, et al. Amyl nitrite may alter T-lymphocytes in homosexual men. Lancet 1982; 1:412-6.
84. Mathur-Wagh U, Enlow RW, Spigland I, et al. Longitudinal study of persistent generalized lymphadenopathy in homosexual men: relation to acquired immunodeficiency syndrome. Lancet 1984; 1:1033-8.
85. Mathur-Wagh U, Mildvan D, Senie RT. Follow-up at 4-1/2 years on homosexual men with generalized lymphadenopathy [letter]. N Engl J Med 1985; 313: 1542-3.
86. Osmond D, Moss AR, Bachetti P, Volberding P, Barre-Sinoussi F, Cherman J-C. A case-control study of risk factors for AIDS in San Francisco. International Conference on Acquired Immunodeficiency Syndrome (AIDS), Atlanta, Georgia, April 1985.
87. Darrow WW, Byers RH, Jaffe HW, O'Malley P, Rutherford GW, Echenberg DF. Cofactors in the development of AIDS and AIDS-related conditions. International Conference on AIDS, Paris, France, June 1986.

88. CDC Task Force on Kaposi's Sarcoma and Opportunistic Infections. Epidemeologic aspects of the current outbreak of Kaposi's sarcoma and opportunistic infections. N Engl J Med 1982; 306:248-52.
89. Marmor M, Friedman-Klein AE, Zolla-Pazner S, et al. Kaposi's sarcoma in homosexual men: a seroepidemiologic case-control study. Ann Intern Med 1984; 100:809-15.
90. Goedert JJ, Biggar RJ, Melbye M, et al. Effect of T4 count and co-factors on the incidence of AIDS in homosexual men infected with human immunodeficiency virus. JAMA 1987; 257:331-4.
91. Wiley JA, Rutherford GW, Moss AR, Winkelstein W Jr. Age and cumulative incidence of AIDS among seropositive homosexual men in high incidence areas of San Francisco. III International Conference on AIDS, Washington, D.C., June 1987.
92. Rutherford GW, Echenberg DF, Rauch KJ, et al. The epidemiology of AIDS-related Kaposi's sarcoma in San Francisco: evidence for decreasing incidence. International Conference on AIDS, Paris, France, June 1986.
93. Lemp GF, Barnhart JL, Rutherford GW, Temelso T, Werdegar D. Predictors of survival for AIDS cases in San Francisco. American Public Health Association 115th Annual Meeting, New Orleans, Louisiana, October 1987.
94. Morgan WM, Curran JW. Acquired immunodeficiency syndrome: current and future trends. Public Health Rep 1986; 101:459-65.
95. Jaffe HW, Choy K, Thomas PA, et al. National case-control study of Kaposi's sarcoma and *Pneumocystis carinii* pneumonia in homosexual men: I. Epidemiologic results. Ann Intern Med 1983; 99:145-51.
96. Goedert JJ, Sarngadharan MG, Biggar RJ, et al. Determinants of retrovirus (HTLV-III) antibody and immunodeficiency conditions in homosexual men. Lancet 1984; 2:711-6.
97. Marmor M, Friedman-Klein AE, Zolla-Pazner S, et al. Kaposi's sarcoma in homosexual men: a seroepidemiologic case-control study. Ann Intern Med 1984; 100:809-15.
98. Peterman TA, Curran JW. Sexual transmission of human immunodeficiency virus. JAMA 1986; 256:2222-6.
99. Darrow WW, Echenberg DF, Jaffe HW, et al. Risk factors for human immunodeficiency virus (HIV) infection in homosexual men. Am J Public Health 1987; 77:479-83.
100. Winkelstein W Jr, Lyman DM, Padian N, et al. Sexual practices and risk of infection by the human immunodeficiency virus: The San Francisco Men's Health Study. JAMA 1987; 257:321-5.
101. Grant RM, Wiley JA, Winkelstein W. Infectivity of the human immunodeficiency virus: estimates from a prospective study of homosexual men. J Infect Dis 1987; 156:189-93.
102. Centers for Disease Control. Update: acquired immunodeficiency syndrome (AIDS)—United States. MMWR 1987; 36:522-6.
103. Padian N, Marquis L, Francis DP, et al. Male-to-female transmission of human immunodeficiency virus. JAMA 1987; 258:788-90.
104. Peterman TA, Stoneburner RL, Allen JR. Risk of HTLV-III/LAV transmission to household contacts of persons with transfusion-associated AIDS. International Conference on AIDS, Paris, France, June 1986.

105. Kreiss JK, Kitchen LW, Prince HE, et al. Antibody to human T-lymphotropic virus type III in wives of hemophiliacs: evidence for heterosexual transmission. Ann Intern Med 1985; 102:623-6.
106. Jason J, McDougal JS, Dixon G, et al. HTLV-III/LAV antibody and immune status of household contacts and sexual partners of persons with hemophilia. JAMA 1986; 255:212-5.
107. Redfield RR, Markham PD, Salahuddin SZ, et al. Frequent transmission of HTLV-III among spouses of patients with AIDS-related complex and AIDS. JAMA 1985; 253:1571-3.
108. Kreiss JK, Koech D, Plummer FA, et al. AIDS virus infection in Nairobi prostitutes. N Engl J Med 1986; 31:414-8.
109. Hira SK, Perine PL, Redfield RR, et al. The epidemiology and clinical manifestations of the acquired immune deficiency syndrome (AIDS) and its related complex (ARC) in Zambia. International Conference on AIDS, Paris, France, June 1986.
110. Mann JM, Quinn T, Francis H, et al. Sexual practices associated with LAV/ HTLV-III seropositivity among female prostitutes in Kinshasa, Zaire. International Conference on AIDS, Paris, France, June 1986.
111. Stall R, McKusick L, Wiley J, Coates TJ, Wiley J. Alcohol and drug use during sexual activity and compliance with safe sex guidelines for AIDS: The AIDS Behavioral Research Project. Health Educ Q 1986; 13:359-71.
112. Pitchenik AE, Fishl MA, Dickinson, et al. Opportunistic infection and Kaposi's sarcoma among Haitians: evidence of a new acquired immunodeficiency state. Ann Intern Med 1983; 98:277-84.
113. Stewart GJ, Tylor JPP, Cunningham AL, et al. Transmission of human lymphotropic virus type III (HTLV-III) by artificial insemination by donor. Lancet 1985; 2:581-5.
114. Centers for Disease Control. Provisional Public Health Service inter-agency recommendations for screening donated blood and plasma for antibody to the virus causing acquired immunodeficiency syndrome. MMWR 1985; 34:1-5.
115. Sande MA. Transmission of AIDS: the case against casual contagion [editorial]. N Engl J Med 1986; 314:380-2.
116. Robertson JR, Bucknall ABV, Welsby PD, et al. Epidemic of AIDS-related virus (HTLV-III/LAV) infection among intravenous drug abusers. Br Med J 1986; 292:527-9.
117. Gerberding JL, Bryant-LeBlanc CE, Nelson K, et al. Risk of transmitting the human immunodeficiency virus, cytomegalovirus, and hepatitis B virus to health care workers exposed to patients with AIDS and AIDS-related conditions. J Infect Dis 1987; 156:1-8.
118. Friedland GH, Harris C, Butkus-Small C, et al. Intravenous drug abusers and the acquired immunodeficiency syndrome (AIDS): demographic, drug use, and needle-sharing patterns. Arch Intern Med 1985; 8:1413-37.
119. Evatt BL, Gomperts ED, McDougal JS, et al. Coincidental appearance of LAV/HTLV-III in hemophiliacs and the onset of the AIDS epidemic. N Engl J Med 1985; 312:483-6.
120. Evatt BL, Ramsey RB, Lawrence DN, et al. The acquired immunodeficiency syndrome in patients with hemophilia. Ann Intern Med 1984; 100:499-504.

121. Centers for Disease Control. Update: acquired immunodeficiency syndrome in persons with hemophilia. MMWR 1984; 33:589-91.
122. Ramsey RB, Palmer EL, McDougal JS, et al. Antibody to lymphadenopathy-associated virus in hemophiliacs with and without AIDS [letter]. Lancet 1984; 2:397-8.
123. San Francisco Department of Public Health. AIDS among intravenous drug users—San Francisco. San Francisco Epidemiologic Bulletin 1986, 2(6):1-3.
124. Centers for Disease Control. Heterosexual transmission of human T-lymphotropic virus type III/lymphadenopathy-associated virus. MMWR 1985; 34:561-3.
125. Guinan ME, Hardy A. Epidemiology of AIDS in women in the United States. JAMA 1987; 257:2039-42.
126. Schwarcz SK, Rutherford GW. Acquired immunodeficiency syndrome in infants, children, and adolescents. J Drug Issues (in press).
127. Curran JW, Lawrence DL, Jaffe H, et al. Acquired immunodeficiency syndrome (AIDS) associated with transfusions. N Engl J Med 1984; 310:69-75.
128. Prompt CA, Reis MM, Grillo FM, et al. Transmission of AIDS virus at renal transplantation. Lancet 1985; 2:672.
129. Food and Drug Administration. Safety of immune globulins in relation to HTLV-III. FDA Drug Bull 1986; 16:3.
130. Centers for Disease Control. Hepatitis B vaccine: evidence confirming lack of AIDS transmission. MMWR 1984; 33:685-7.
131. Centers for Disease Control. Changing patterns of acquired immunodeficiency syndrome in hemophilia patients—United States. MMWR 1985; 34:241-3.
132. Gjerset GF, McGrady G, Counts RB, et al. Lymphadenopathy-associated virus antibodies and T cells in hemophiliacs treated with cryoprecipitate or concentrate. Blood 1985; 66:718-20.
133. Centers for Disease Control. Survey of non-U.S. hemophilia treatment centers for HIV seroconversions following therapy with heat-treated factor concentrates. MMWR 1987; 36:121-4.
134. Centers for Disease Control. Update: evaluation of human T-lymphotropic virus type III/lymphadenopathy-associated virus infection in health-care personnel—United States. MMWR 1985; 34:575-8.
135. Lancet. Needlestick transmission of HTLV-III from a patient infected in Africa. Lancet 1984; 2:1376-7.
136. Stricoff RL, Morse DL. HTLV-III/LAV seroconversion following a deep intramuscular needle stick injury (letter). N Engl J Med 1986; 314:1115.
137. Gerberding JL, Hopewell PC, Kamingley LS, Sande MA. Transmission of hepatitis B without transmission of AIDS by accidental needlestick [letter]. N Engl J Med 1985; 312:56.
138. Centers for Disease Control. Apparent transmission of human T-lymphotropic virus type III/lymphadenopathy-associated virus from a child to a mother providing health care. MMWR 1986; 35:76-9.
139. Grint P, McEvoy M. Two associated cases of the acquired immune deficiency syndrome (AIDS). Commun Dis Rep 1985; 42:4.
140. Centers for Disease Control. Acquired immunodeficiency syndrome (AIDS): precautions for clinical and laboratory staffs. MMWR 1982; 31:577-80.

141. Centers for Disease Control. Acquired immunodeficiency syndrome (AIDS): precautions for health-care workers and allied professionals. MMWR 1983; 32:450-1.
142. Centers for Disease Control. Recommendations for preventing transmission of infection with human T-lymphotropic virus type III/lymphadenopathy-associated virus in the workplace. MMWR 1985; 34:682-6, 691-5.
143. Centers for Disease Control. Recommendations for preventing transmission of infection with human T-lymphotropic virus type III/lymphadenopathy-associated virus during invasive procedures. MMWR 1986; 35:221-3.
144. Centers for Disease Control. Human T-lymphotropic virus type III/lymphadenopathy-associated virus: agent summary statement. MMWR 1986; 35:540-2.
145. Ziegler JB, Cooper DA, Johnson RO, Gold J. Postnatal transmission of AIDS-associated retrovirus from mother to infant. Lancet 1985; 1:896-8.
146. Thiry L, Sprecher-Goldberger S, Jonckheer T, et al. Isolation of AIDS virus from cell-free breast milk of three healthy virus carriers [letter]. Lancet 1985; 2:891-2.
147. Scott GB, Fischl MA, Klimas N, et al. Mothers of infants with the acquired immunodeficiency syndrome: evidence for both symptomatic and asymptomatic carriers. JAMA 1985; 235:363-6.
148. Scott GB, Fischl MA, Klimas N, Fletcher M, Dickinson G, Parks W. Mothers of infants with the acquired immunodeficiency syndrome: outcome of subsequent pregnancies. International Conference on Acquired Immunodeficiency Syndrome (AIDS), Atlanta, Georgia, April 1985.
149. Centers for Disease Control. Heterosexual transmission of human T-lymphotropic virus type III/lymphadenopathy-associated virus. MMWR 1985; 34:561-3.
150. Centers for Disease Control. Education and foster care of children infected with human T-lymphotropic virus type III/lymphadenopathy-associated virus. MMWR 1985; 34:517-21.
151. Fishl MA, Dickinson GM, Scott GB, et al. Evaluation of heterosexual partners, children, and household contacts of adults with AIDS. JAMA 1987; 257: 640-4.
152. Friedland GH, Saltzman BR, Rogers MF, et al. Lack of transmission of HTLV-III/LAV infection to household contacts of patients with AIDS or AIDS-related complex with oral candidiasis. N Engl J Med 1986; 314:344-9.
153. Jason JM, McDougal JS, Lawrence DN, Kennedy DS, Hilgartner M, Evatt BL. Lymphadenopathy-associated virus (LAV) antibody and immune status of household contacts and sexual partners of persons with hemophilia. JAMA 1986; 255:212-5.
154. Kaplan JE, Oleske JM, Getchell JP, et al. Evidence against transmission of HTLV-III/LAV in families of children with AIDS. Pediatr Infect Dis 1985; 4: 468-71.
155. Lawrence DN, Jason JM, Bouhasin JD, et al. HTLV-III/LAV antibody status of spouses and household contacts assisting in home infusion of hemophilia patients. Blood 1985; 66:703.
156. Lewin EB, Zack R, Ayodele A. Communicability of AIDS in a foster care setting. International Conference on Acquired Immunodeficiency Syndrome (AIDS), Atlanta, Georgia, April 1985.

157. Redfield RR, Markham PD, Salahuddin SZ, et al. Frequent transmission of HTLV-III among spouses of patients with acquired immunodeficiency syndrome (AIDS) or AIDS-related complex: a family study. JAMA 1985; 253: 1571-3.
158. Rogers MF, White CR, Sanders R, et al. Can children transmit human T-lymphotropic virus type III/lymphadenopathy-associated virus (HTLV-III/LAV)? International Conference on AIDS, Paris, France, June 1986.
159. Saltzman BR, Friedland GH, Rogers MF, et al. Lack of household transmission of HTLV-III/LAV infection. International Conference on AIDS, Paris, France, June 1986.
160. Thomas PA, Lubia K, Enlow RW, et al. Comparison of HTLV-III serology. T-cell levels, and general health status of children whose mothers have AIDS with children of healthy inner city mothers in New York. International Conference on Acquired Immunodeficiency Syndrome (AIDS), Atlanta, Georgia, April 1985.
161. Mann JM, Quinn T, Francis H, et al. Prevalence of HTLV-III/LAV in household contacts of patients with controls in Kinshasa, Zaire. JAMA 1986; 256: 721-4.
162. Centers for Disease Control. Update: AIDS—Palm Beach County, Florida. MMWR 1986; 35:609-12.
163. World Health Organization. Acquired immunodeficiency syndrome (AIDS)—situation in the WHO European Region as of 30 June 1986. Weekly Epidemiology Record 1986; 61:93.
164. Centers for Disease Control. Update: AIDS—Europe. MMWR 1985; 34:589-9.
165. Pan American Health Organization. AIDS surveillance in the Americas: report through 31 December 1985. Epidemiology Bulletin 1986; 9(2):7-8.
166. Office of the Assistant Secretary for Health. Surgeon General's Report on Acquired Immunodeficiency Syndrome. Washington, DC: Public Health Service, 1986.
167. MacDonald DI. Coolfont report: a PHS plan for prevention and control of AIDS and the AIDS virus. Public Health Rep 1986; 101:341-8.
168. Acheson ED. AIDS: a challenge for the public health. Lancet 1986; 1:622-6.
169. Francis DP, Chin J. The prevention of AIDS in the United States: an objective strategy for medicine, public health, business, and the community. JAMA 1987; 257:1357-66.
170. Selik RM, Starcher ET, Curran JW. Opportunistic diseases reported in AIDS patients: Frequencies, associations, and trends. AIDS 1987; 1:175-82.
171. Piot P, Plummer FA, Mhalu FS, Lamboray J-L, Chin J, Mann JM. AIDS: an international perspective. Science 1988; 239:573-9.
172. Curran JW, Jaffe HW, Hardy AM, Morgan WM, Selik RM, Dondero TJ. Epidemiology of HIV infection and AIDS in the United States. Science 1988; 239:610-6.
173. Centers for Disease Control. Revision of the CDC surveillance case definition for acquired immunodeficiency syndrome. MMWR 1987; 36(suppl 1):1S-15S.
174. Centers for Disease Control. Human immunodeficiency virus infection in the United States: a review of current knowledge. MMWR 1987; 36(suppl 5-6): 1-48.

175. Centers for Disease Control. Quarterly report to the Domestic Policy Council on the prevalence and rate of spread of HIV and AIDS in the United States. MMWR 1988; 37:223-6.
176. Hessol NA, O'Malley PM, Rutherford GW, et al. Sexual transmission of human immunodeficiency virus infection in a cohort of homosexual and bisexual men who participated in hepatitis B vaccine trials. Society for Epidemiologic Research 20th Annual Meeting. Amherst, Massachusetts, June 1987.
177. Greenblatt RM, Samuel M, Osmond D, et al. Risk factors for seroconversion with human immunodeficiency virus among homosexual men in San Francisco, 1983-1987. III International Conference on AIDS, Washington, D.C., June 1987.
178. Marmor M, Des Jarlais DC, Cohen H, et al. Risk factors for infection with human immunodeficiency virus among intravenous drug abusers in New York City. AIDS 1987; 1:39-44.
179. Lange RW, Snyder FR, Lozovsky D, et al. Geographic distribution of human immunodeficiency virus markers in parenteral drug abusers. Am J Pub Health 1988; 78:443-6.
180. Ragni MV, Winkelstein A, Kingsley L, Spero JA, Lewis LH. 1986 update of HIV seroprevalence, seroconversion, AIDS incidence, and immunologic correlates of HIV infection in patients with hemophilia A and B. Blood 1987; 70: 786-90.
181. Polk BF, Fox R, Brookmeyer R, et al. Predictors of the acquired immunodeficiency syndrome developing in a cohort of serpositive men. N Engl J Med 1987; 316:61-6.
182. Eyster ME, Gail MH, Ballard JO, et al. Natural history of immunodeficiency virus infection in hemophiliacs: effects of T-cell subsets, platelet counts and age. Ann Intern Med 1987; 107:1.
183. Piot P, Colebunders R. Clinical manifestations and the natural history of HIV infection in adults. West J Med 1987; 147:709-12.
184. Selik RM, Starcher ET, Curran JW. Opportunistic diseases reported in AIDS patients: frequencies, associations, and trends. AIDS 1987; 1:175-82.
185. Rotherberg R, Woelfel M, Stoneburner R, Milberg J, Parker R, Truman B. Survival with the acquired immunodeficiency syndrome: experience with 5833 cases in New York City. N Engl J Med 1987; 317:1297-302.
186. Drew WL, Mills J, Hauer LB, Miner RC, Rutherford GW. Declining prevalence of Kaposi's sarcoma in homosexual AIDS patients paralleled by fall in cytomegalovirus transmission (letter). Lancet 1988; 1:66.
187. Greenblatt RM, Lukehart SA, Plummer FA, et al. Genital ulceration as a risk factor for human immunodeficiency virus infection. AIDS 1988; 2:47-50.
188. Handsfield HH, Ashley RL, Rompalo AM, Stamm WE, Wood RW, Corey L. Association of anogenital ulcer diseases with human immunodeficiency virus infection in homosexual men. III International Conference on AIDS, Washington, D.C., June 1987.
189. Padian NS. Heterosexual transmission of acquired immunodeficiency syndrome: international perspectives and national projections. Rev Infect Dis 1987; 9:947-60.

190. Stehr-Green JK, Holman RC, Jason JM, Evatt BL. Hemophilia-associated AIDS in the United States, 1981 to September 1987. Am J Pub Health 1988; 78:439-42.
191. Weiss SH, Saxinger C, Rechtman D, et al. HTLV-III infection among health care workers: association with needle-stick injuries. JAMA 1985; 254:2089-93.
192. Weiss SH, Goedert JJ, Gartner S, et al. Risk of human immunodeficiency virus (HIV-1) infection among laboratory workers. Science 1988; 239:68-71.
193. Centers for Disease Control. Update: human immunodeficiency virus infections in health-care workers exposed to blood of infected patients. MMWR 1987; 36:285-9.
194. Centers for Disease Control. Recommendations for prevention of HIV transmission in health-care settings. MMWR 1987; 36(suppl 2S):3S-18S.
195. Goetz DW, Hall SE, Harbison RW, Reid MJ. Pediatric acquired immunodeficiency virus antibody response by enzyme-linked immunosorbent assay and Western blot. Pediatrics 1988; 81:356-9.
196. Castro KG, Lifson AR, White CR, et al. Investigations of AIDS patients with no previously identified risk factors. JAMA 1988; 259:1338-42.
197. Berthier A, Chamaret S, Fauchet R, et al. Transmissibility of human immunodeficiency virus in haemophiliac and non-haemophiliac children living in a private school in France. Lancet 1986; 2:598-601.
198. Lifson AR. Do alternate modes for transmission of human immunodeficiency virus exist: a review. JAMA 1988; 259:1353-6.
199. Castro KG, Lieb S, Jaffe HW, et al. Transmission of HIV in Belle Glade, Florida: lessons for other communities in the United States. Science 1988; 239: 193-6.
200. Downs AM, Ancelle RA, Jager HJC, Brunet JH-B. AIDS in Europe: current trends and short-term predictions estimated from surveillance data, January 1981-June 1986. AIDS 1987; 1:53-7.
201. Mann JM. The World Health Organization's global strategy for the prevention and control of AIDS. West J Med 1987; 147:732-4.

2
AIDS in Africa

Nathan Clumeck
St. Pierre Hospital
Free University of Brussels
Brussels, Belgium

I. Introduction

Acquired immunodeficiency syndrome (AIDS) has been recognized in Africa since the early 1980s. From that time, the disease has been spreading at a rapid rate, but because of the lack of official reports, little is presently known about the extent of the epidemic in Africa. Retrospective serological data suggest that the AIDS virus, human immunodeficiency virus (HIV), or a related virus has been present in central Africa at least since 1959 (1a). Its prevalence today could have resulted from transmission by blood donation, scarification, and unsterilized, shared needles. The sudden appearance of the disease, however, is unexplained and current epidemiological studies favor predominant heterosexual transmission of the virus in Africa. Transcontinental spread of the epidemic by sexually active heterosexual man and women ("free women," prostitutes) is thus likely to occur. These possibilities need to be better defined by future studies.

Whereas the natural history of AIDS virus infection in Africa appears similar to that observed in Western countries, the clinical patterns vary in Africans. Thus, for Africa, a newly adapted case definition is needed which considers that endemic Kaposi's sarcoma (KS) is unrelated to AIDS virus infection. It is also important to understand, sociological, and political consequences of AIDS in Africa in order to propose realistic preventive measures to control the epidemic there. Educational campaigns about sexually transmitted diseases, compulsory screening of blood donors, and the use of sterilized material for medical procedures are strategic approaches that need to be applied rapidly. Only an international mobilization of resources can eventually help to realize even such a minimal program. This chapter will review our knowledge of the epidemiology and the clinical and pathogenic features of AIDS in Africans.

II. Epidemiology

A. History

AIDS among Africans was first recognized in late 1982 when men and women, either resident in, or referred to, Belgium were examined for diagnosis (2). Later it became apparent from retrospective case reports that the disease could have been present in central Africa in the 1970s before it was observed in America (1,3-5). Initial observations of 23 African patients with AIDS showed that the disease was equally distributed among men and women without any known risk factors for AIDS. This finding suggested heterosexual transmission of the disease (6). African patients originating mostly from central/equatorial Africa were seen mainly in Belgium (7) and France (8), but also in Switzerland, the United Kingdom, Greece, and Czechoslovakia (9). Africans from 22 different countries accounted for 10% of cases reported in Europe as of September 30, 1985. Nevertheless, by March 1986, only four African nations (Zambia, Tanzania, Kenya, and Sudan) officially reported the presence of small numbers of AIDS cases to the World Health Organization. This underreporting is in sharp contrast to the results of investigations in Rwanda (10), Zaire (11), Zambia (12), and Uganda (13). This difference may result from the difficulty in making an accurate diagnosis of AIDS in countries with limited health care systems, but it is more likely linked to political considerations (14). Because AIDS most commonly occurs among American homosexual men and intravenous (IV) drug users, this identification has given a social stigma to the disease. Homosexuality is taboo in equatorial Africa. In spite of epidemiological evidence that argues against homosexuality as a risk factor in these regions, many African people are still reluctant to admit the existence of AIDS in their countries. In addition, because the present evidence suggests that AIDS probably started in central Africa, fear of being designated as a scapegoat, as well as fears of racism and its possible consequences have surfaced. Discrimination campaigns and the loss of foreign currency and tourism are other reasons that make many African governments minimize the extent of the problem.

A. What Is the Extent of AIDS and AIDS-Related Disease in Africa?

The first reported AIDS cases in Africa were readily found in late 1983 in Rwanda and Zaire; these countries were the source of many of the initial African patients referred to Belgium. During a 4-week period, 26 patients were diagnosed in Kigali, Rwanda, giving an annual incidence of AIDS for the city of about 80 per 100,000 (10). During the same period 38 patients were identified in Kinshasa, Zaire, and the annual case rate for Kinshasa was estimated in 1982 to be at least 17 per 100,000 (11). However, city-wide, hospital-based surveillance for AIDS in Kinshasa revealed 190 new cases during the period from July to November 1984. This number gave a higher annual incidence rate of at least 30 cases per 100,000 inhabitants (15). During the same period (by December 1984), the rates in New York and San Francisco were respectively 28 and 25 per 100,000 (16). These African AIDS cases, also diagnosed in Zambia as aggressive Kaposi's sarcoma (12), or in Uganda as "slim disease" (13), represent only the visible part of HIV infection which is endemic in most central African countries.

The results of limited seroprevalence studies performed in various parts of Africa are summarized in Table 1. Most of the people tested were controls for case control studies and were principally healthy adults of both sexes. Some were seen during a routine medical examination as out- or inpatients for problems apparently unrelated to AIDS. The rate of seropositivity reported from the central African countries, Zaire, Rwanda, and Uganda, varies between 1.5% and 20.0% in the population of adults who characteristically do not have homo- or bisexuality or IV drug abuse as life-style risk factors. However, among healthy female prostitutes and their customers seroprevalence was higher, 84% and 30%, respectively (21).

In Rwanda, a higher prevalence of HIV seropositivity was actually noted in young adults living in urban centers than in adults living in rural areas or in infants. These findings differ from other surveys of anti-HIV antibodies in a remote rural area of eastern Zaire or in some parts of Kenya (19,27). It could be that the sera from rural Rwanda were all taken by chance from uninfected subjects within endemic regions, but gross sampling errors seem unlikely. This fact has raised the question of whether African sera tend to give spuriously positive results with certain antiglobulin enzyme-linked immunosorbent assays (ELISA) for anti-HIV, particularly among malaria patients with circulating immune complexes (33). In addition, when tested by Western blotting technique, most positive bands from these discordant studies were generally weak, raising doubt about the specificity of antibodies detected (34,35).

The other possibility is that the seropositivity noted is due to cross-reactivity of antibodies against yet unrecognized antigens, or a related virus endemic

Table 1 HIV Seroepidemiological Studies from Various Parts of Africa (1980-1985)

Country	Population studies	Year of sera collection	Number studied	Methods[a]	HIV seropositivity (%)	Reference
Central Africa						
Zaire	Healthy mothers	1980	100	EIA/RIPA	5	17
Kinshasa	Hospitalized patients (noninfectious)	1983	100	EIA/RIPA	7	
	Healthy adults	1985	254	EIA	7	18
Rural eastern	Adults	1984	233	EIA	12.6	19
	Children		17	WB	35.6	
Rwanda	Healthy adults	1985	581	EIA	17.7	20-22
Kigali	Adolescent	1985	62	EIA	1.5	
Rural area	Healthy adults	1985	273	EIA	3.6	
	Infants (3-8 months)	1985	242	EIA	4.5	
Butare	Healthy prostitutes	1983/84	84	EIA/WB	80	
	Male STD clinic patients	1984	25	EIA	28	
Southern Africa						
Zambia	Healthy adults	1985	158	RIA	2	23
(Copper belt) Border with Zaire	Healthy adults	1985	62	EIA-comp.	22.5	24

Malawi	Healthy adults	1985	661	EIA and IFA	18	25, 26
	Healthy adults	1985	87	EIA and IFA	24	
Zimbabwe	Healthy adults	1985	500	EIA and IFA	0.8	25, 26
South Africa	Black blood donors	1985	1740	EIA and IFA	0.3	25, 26
Nambia	Adults	1985	143	EIA and IFA	0	25, 26
East and West Africa						
Kenya	Out patients	1984	110	EIA	10.9	27
	Healthy prostitutes	1985	90	EIA	55	
Nairobi	Healthy adults	1985	42	EIA/WB	2	28
	Male STD clinic patients	1985	40	EIA/WB	8	
Ethiopia	Migrants to Israel	1985	55	RIA	0	29
Nigeria	Blood donors	1982	124	EIA	6.4	30
	Schoolchildren	1982	52	EIA	0	
Senegal	Prostitutes	1985	289	EIA/WB	0.01	31
	Adults, surgical patients	1985	122	EIA/WB		
Uganda	Healthy adults	1985	51	RIA	20	23
	Not provided	1985	340	RIA	23	32

[a]Abbreviations: EIA, direct ELISA; EIA-comp., competitive ELISA; IFA, indirect immunofluorescence technique; RIA, competitive radioimmunoassay; RIPA, radioimmunoprecipitation assay; WB, Western blot technique.

in these regions. In this respect, the recent finding of antibodies against an HIV-related human retrovirus with antigens similar to the simian immunodeficiency virus (SIV) among residents of Senegal, without a history of AIDS or AIDS-related illness, is noteworthy (31,36). Whether this virus is nonpathogenic awaits further longitudinal studies. Moreover, the isolation of an AIDS virus, LAV-2 (37), from West Africa indicates the possible existence of pathogenic HIV variants, resembling SIV, coming from various parts of Africa (38). A comparison of different isolates in the world as well as the clinical status of the infected host should help define any important changes that are or have been occurring in the AIDS virus. Although some genomic heterogeneity has been seen among AIDS retroviral isolates from North America and Zaire, to date the differences observed have not been correlated to differences in immunopathogenicity (26). The West African isolate, now considered sufficiently different to be called HIV-2, appear to have emerged recently in this part of the world and have only just been recovered in Europe. Monitoring their spread should provide more information on the transmission and cofactors involved in AIDS.

Limited surveys have pointed to the central African belt as an important focus of HIV infection among heterosexual populations. The virus is not, at present, endemic in the southern (39) and northern part of Africa (40). It is new to Kenya, as shown by the rising prevalence of HIV antibodies in Nairobi from 1980 to 1984 (41). It likely has been present in Zaire for a longer time (1,42).

So far, five retrospective studies on stored African sera have been performed (41-45). The oldest specimens tested for HIV seropositivity are from Nahmias et al. (1a) who assayed 672 sera obtained originally in 1959 from the Belgian Congo (Zaire), from Rwanda-Urundi (Rwanda, Burundi), and from Southern Sudan by ELISA, indirect immunofluorescence techniques, and Western blot. Only one serum from Leopoldville (Kinshasa) was positive and suggested that a virus related to HIV may have been present in Zaire in 1959 at a very low prevalence (0.2%). In another study of 677 sera obtained primarily from Uganda from 1964 to 1975, no positive sera were found. Many of the sera came from patients with Burkitt's lymphoma or endemic Kaposi's sarcoma (45). In a study comparing 805 sera obtained from Kinshasa mothers in 1970 with 498 sera collected in 1980, Desmyter et al. (42) showed two sera positive in 1970 and 15 in 1980 by both competitive ELISA and immunofluorescent techniques. Thus in this small series an increase of about 10-fold (0.25-3%) of HIV seropositivity.

Finally, in a recent study conducted on sera collected in a remote village in Zaire, no difference in seroprevalence was noted in a 10-year period. Blood specimens obtained in 1976 for a Lassa fever study showed 0.76% of the population infected by HIV. Subsequent serum samples collected in 1986 showed the same level of HIV infection (91).

These data show that if HIV infection existed in central Africa in the

1960s or early 1970s, it was only in sporadic cases; conceivably the virus was present without expression of disease. In spite of the lack of clinical record keeping, this assumption fits well with the clinical experience of physicians who have practiced in central Africa for several decades. They have only recently noted an increased incidence and a changing pattern of diseases such as cryptococcosis (46) and aggressive Kaposi's sarcoma (12). Furthermore, a retrospective review of case records since 1970 at St. Pierre University Hospital, Brussels, a referring hospital for many wealthy Zairians, revealed only one case of an illness suggesting AIDS. This unique case was diagnosed in 1978 in a young male Zairian originating from Kinshasa. The patient died from generalized Kaposi's sarcoma together with cerebral toxoplasmosis and generalized cryptococcosis. This case seemed so extraordinary to the physicians that they published it as a "curiosity" in 1980 (5). Since that time, the number of African AIDS cases in Belgium has followed an epidemic curve; six patients were identified by the end of 1981, seven cases in 1982, 27 in 1983, and 46 in 1984.

If HIV and AIDS were already sporadically present in equatorial Africa a few decades ago, one can ask why the epidemic did not occur until recently. The answer probably lies in the modes of transmission of the virus in Africa and the socioeconomical background of African tropical countries during the past three decades. Due to the low amount of virus present in the vaginal secretions, heterosexual transmission of HIV is likely to be less efficient than homosexual transmission (47,48). It is then conceivable that it took many years to develop an epidemic from a few sporadic cases. In addition, many sociological factors may have recently encouraged the transmission of HIV in central Africa. These include:

1. Uncontrolled growth of urban centers
2. Disruption of family units
3. Urban immigration of male workforce
4. Movements of various armies
5. Increase in female prostitution
6. Breakdown of the health services
7. Increased use by local doctors of drugs intramuscularly or intravenously

All of these trends have developed commonly during the last three decades in most African equatorial countries.

III. Human Immunodeficiency Virus Type 2

HIV isolates from central Africa are quite similar to American or European isolates in their biological and serological properties, although African isolates exhibit a larger polymorphism indicating that they may be evolving for a longer period (26). In 1985, Kanki and colleagues isolated from a macaque monkey a retrovirus they called simian T lymphotropic virus type III (STLV-III, now known as SIV) (93). It was subsequently found that 30 to 70% of African green monkeys were naturally infected with SIV without any clinical manifestation (94). In contrast, only captive macaque monkeys showed infection by SIV and they did develop an immunodeficiency syndrome similar to human AIDS (93). This finding that macaque monkeys in the wild do not show evidence of SIV infection suggests that this virus infected these monkeys in captivity from an as yet unknown source. Molecular studies showed that SIV had 50-60% homology to HIV-1 (95).

These observations on SIV were followed by the finding that 20 healthy prostitutes from Senegal showed a greater immune response against SIV than against HIV (31). These data led to the recovery of a virus from one of these individuals (36). Termed HLTV-IV, this virus had limited cytopathology in vitro and was not found associated with AIDS or its related disorders. Subsequent studies showed the seroprevalence of HTLV-IV in six Western African countries (96,97); up to 65% of healthy sexually active adults in some regions were infected. In Guinea Bissau, Burkina Faso, and the Ivory Coast, the highest prevalence of antibodies to HTLV-IV were found (97,98). These results strongly suggested that the major transmission for the virus was by heterosexual contact as it is for HIV-1 in Africa (1).

In 1985, Clavel et al. also identified a new virus (initially designated as LAV-2) among patients with AIDS or ARC coming from Guinea Bissau and the Cape Verde Islands (37). This virus also showed envelope and genomic similarity with SIV and seemed evolutionarily more closely related to the monkey virus than HIV-1. The overall organization of LAV-2, however, was similar to that of HIV-1, as shown by subsequent molecular studies (99). The LAV-2 isolate has now been termed HIV-2 because its genetic sequence differs from HIV-1 by over 50% (99,100). One difference between LAV-2 and HTLV-IV was the association of the former virus with patients with disease (100-102). These variations in pathogenicity could be due to varied subtypes of HIV-2 or susceptibility of the population studied. Moreover, recent evidence has now indicated that HTLV-IV is an SIV contaminant of the cell line used for the isolation of virus from the seropositive Senegalese woman (103-105). Thus, some of the differences in its unusual biological and serologic properties can be explained by this fact. Nevertheless, further studies need to be conducted before any conclusions can be drawn on the relative pathogenicity of the HIV-2 strain.

In the past two years, other HIV-2 strains have been described, including SBL-6669 (106) and HIV-2_{UC-1} (107). These viruses have many characteristics similar to those of the initial LAV-2 strain of HIV; the UC-1 isolate, however, is unusual in its lack of cytopathic properties (see Chapter 8). The HIV-2 subtype is very prominent in Guinea Bissau and the Gambia, where the most AIDS cases have been found (100,102,109,110). The virus is rare in central African countries (97,102). Nevertheless, in the Ivory Coast, individuals have shown evidence of infection by both subtypes of HIV (98). In vitro, HIV-2 also shows a selective infection for CD4+ cells (108) (see further discussion on these two HIV subtypes in Chapter 8).

IV. Modes of Transmission of HIV in Africa

A. Heterosexual Contact

African AIDS is characteristically a disease of young-to-middle age, sexually active men and women. It also affects children less than 5 years old. The ratio of males to females is nearly equal in contrast to the 14:1 ratio in the United States, Europe, and Australia. The risk factors of homosexuality and IV drug abuse are not found in African patients. Homosexuality is taboo in African society and thus it may be that an accurate perception of this risk factor is not possible. However, if it exists in Africa, this mode of transmission is only marginal; otherwise, one would very quickly expect an imbalance there in the sex ratio of infected persons. A past history of sexually transmitted disease (urethritis or genital ulceration) and heterosexual promiscuity are constant findings in most Africans with AIDS. Indeed, in the study of Odio, 67% of the women were prostitutes (so-called "free women" in Zaire) and 68% of the men admitted to having multiple extramarital sexual contacts (49). In fact, if male AIDS patients admit to heterosexual promiscuity, the group of women with AIDS could be subdivided into those who consider themselves "free women" (mostly young, single women with a mean age of 24 years) and those who are the nonpromiscuous spouse of a promiscuous man (married women, mean age: 35 years) (author's personal observation). A history of medical injections is elicited in 38-78% of the cases (49,50) but there is no difference between cases and controls with regard to this potential risk factor (11). However, it is not yet clear that the prevalence of HIV reflects infection in certain locations as measured in sexually transmitted disease (STD) clinics where many of the sexually active individuals go for treatment. It must be noted, however, that a previous history of medical injections with reused needles was not found among Belgian AIDS patients working in Zaire or Rwanda and among African AIDS cases evaluated in Brussels who were from the affluent stratum of African society (6).

Although in the United States, sexual transmission of HIV from female to male is less evident than sexual transmission from male to female, epidemiological data show an efficient bidirectional transmission of the virus in Africa. Indeed, a case-control study of heterosexual African men with AIDS or related conditions in Belgium and Rwanda showed a significant association of HIV infection with a history of contact with prostitutes and with an increased number of female partners per year (51). Furthermore, the finding of very high seropositivity among female prostitutes in Rwanda (21) and in Nairobi (32) demonstrates that female prostitutes are a high-risk group for AIDS as well as other STDs, and also are a likely reservoir for HIV as suggested by the existence of healthy seropositive prostitutes (21).

Epidemiological studies in the United States and Europe have shown that receptive anal intercourse is highly associated with the risk of infection with AIDS virus among homosexual men (52). The factors that predispose to heterosexual transmission of HIV in Africa are far less well known. There are thus sharp discrepancies between the epidemiology of AIDS in developing countries and that in the United States and Europe. Some myths concerning the possible modes of transmission of HIV in equatorial Africa have been stated (Table 2). The heterosexual versus needle transmission as discussed above is an important question which often arouses debates (53,54). This question is not an academic one. The "needle hypothesis" is reassuring for the developed countries where the problem of sharing of unsterilized medical needles remains confined to the IV drug users. If shared use of dirty needles is the main mode of transmission in Africa, one would conclude that heterosexual spread of HIV will remain low in more-developed countries. However, if HIV is mainly a sexually transmitted disease, spreading more or less easily among the heterosexual population, the African epidemic could represent a vision of America's and Europe's future. Obviously, there is an urgent need to clarify the factors that could favor heterosexual transmission. One must take adequate measures aimed to avoiding future extension of HIV infection from limited groups of bisexual people or heterosexual IV drug users to the general population. It remains unclear, however, whether be-

Table 2 Myths About Transmission of HIV in Central Africa

Myths	Why it is untrue
1. Due to infubulation, vaginal intercourse is chronically associated with bleeding.	Infubulation is a ritual traditional practice limited to some African tribes. It is not applied in urban areas.
2. Anal intercourse is a common route of transmission for heterosexual African partners.	This practice is taboo in Africa.
3. Ritual scarification and blood letting practices are a common feature of the people of central Africa.	Ritual scarification is mainly practiced in childhood with heated instruments.
4. Homosexuality is a taboo subject. Many male Africans engage in homosexual relationships for material profit.	The male/female ratio of AIDS cases in Africa argues against homosexuality as a risk factor.
5. As with Ebola fever, HIV is transmitted by unsterilized needles used for treating gonorrhea or syphilis or when collecting blood.	AIDS virus could be transmitted in this manner. Data obtained from wealthy Africans, who do not use unsterilized needles, clearly favor heterosexual transmission.
6. As with arboviruses, mosquitoes are efficient vectors of HIV.	All epidemiological studies argue against this mode of transmission.

havioral or biological factors or both could favor heterosexual transmission in Africa. Coexistence of other heterosexually transmitted diseases (herpes, gonorrhea, syphilis, pelvic inflammatory disease, etc.), vaginal contacts during menses, trauma during sex, anal intercourse, and abrasions to the lining of the vagina or penile urethra are all likely to play a role which has not been clearly investigated so far. Finally, the recent finding of HIV in vaginal secretions of women with antibodies to the virus strengthens the notion that the AIDS virus could infect males through normal vaginal intercourse (47,48).

B. Other Modes of Transmission

Vertical transmission from mother to child also occurs in Africa. Although there is a lack of epidemiological information, one can roughly estimate that children account for 15-25% of AIDS cases in central Africa. In Rwanda, where, as of December 1985, 319 cases of AIDS have been disclosed, 86 of the AIDS patients are children under 15 years of age. In Africa, AIDS among children is likely to become a major problem in the future since most of the African women infected by HIV are in their reproductive years. In addition, the virus has recently been isolated from maternal milk (55) which is the main nutritional source for children aged 0-2 years in Africa.

The role of transfusions as another route of transmission of the AIDS virus in Africa has until now not been assessed. In a study of 181 patients in Kinshasa, only three cases, including two children with sickle cell disease, had a history of multiple transfusions during previous years (49). These patients are likely to be the counterpart of the hemophiliac patients in Western countries. In our experience of 103 African patients seen in Brussels, we found nine cases of previous blood transfusions and a case record clearly linked to blood donation has been reported from Rwanda (57). Due to the high level of seropositivity among the general population of urban centers (17,20), one can expect to find the same level of seroprevalence among blood donors (22). In this respect the initiation of relatively easy control measures and compulsory screening of blood donors will probably come up at least against economic difficulties. The lack of public health measures related to blood donors in central Africa will certainly contribute to the AIDS epidemic in the future. The possible role of cultural practices in transmission of HIV needs to be appreciated in some regions of Africa (92).

Concerning the possible role of mosquitoes or other insects as vectors of the AIDS virus, all the present epidemiological data argue strongly against this hypothesis.

V. Clinical Aspects

A. Endemic Kaposi's Sarcoma

It is difficult to delineate with certainty the different clinical patterns of AIDS or AIDS-related conditions in Africa. This fact is due not only to the lack of diagnostic procedures in most African countries, but also to the potential confusion which could exist between some common African diseases such as chronic diarrhea, generalized lymphadenopathy, or chronic endemic Kaposi's sarcoma, and those due to the immunodeficiency state. The unique and troublesome existence of Kaposi's sarcoma in central Africa has led some to argue a possible relationship between African Kaposi's sarcoma and homosexuality (58) or to claim that endemic Kaposi's sarcoma was evidence against the concept of AIDS as a new disease in Africa (59). It is now clear that endemic Kaposi's sarcoma is not related to HIV infection. In fact, the natural history of AIDS virus infection in Africa is in many ways similar to that in the more developed countries (see above).

B. Clinical Manifestations of HIV Infection in African Patients

As observed with American or European patients infected with HIV, the clinical spectrum presented by African patients is wide. To date there are only few reports on the clinical manifestations of AIDS virus infection in Africa (10,11,49). Primary infection could include a mononucleosis-like syndrome (33) and unexplained lymphocytic meningitis (60). Healthy asympto-

Table 3 Clinical Classification of HIV Infection Among African Patients

Stage I: Healthy asymptomatic seropositive

These people are sexual partners of patients with AIDS or AIDS-related conditions. They have no complaints and no signs or symptoms of HIV infection. Their physical examination is normal.

Stage II: Persistent generalized lymphadenopathy (PGL)

Patients have at least two extrainguinal sites of lymphadenopathy lasting for at least 3 months in the absence of any constitutional signs or symptoms.

Stage III: AIDS-related complex (ARC)

Patients in this group have any two (or more) of the following signs and symptoms lasting for 3 months or longer and unexplained.

- Lymphadenopathy in more than two noninguinal sites
- Weight loss > 10% normal body weight
- Fever ⩾ 37 °C
- Intermittent or continuous diarrhea
- Pruritic rash

Stage IV: AIDS according to the definition of the CDC/WHO (63)

matic African carriers of HIV have also been detected from index cases with AIDS or AIDS-related complex (ARC) (51). However, only few data are presently available on the relative importance of asymptomatic seropositive people among the group of seropositives as a whole. They account for 82% of the seropositive people detected in Kinshasa, Zaire (62).

African patients seeking European countries for care could provide a unique opportunity to study the mode of presentation and the natural progression of AIDS virus infection in Africa. So far, during a 4-year period we saw, in Brussels, 117 HIV seropositive central African heterosexual patients identified by ELISA and Western blot techniques as previously reported (22). Some 68% of the patients originated from Zaire; the others were from Rwanda, Burundi, Tchad, Angola, and Ghana. All people were examined at approximately a 3-month period for a mean duration of 16 months. According to their clinical status, they were classified into four groups as defined in Table 3.

Immunological studies from this cohort (Table 4) showed that there was a linear decrease in the cellular immunity from healthy asymptomatic individuals to AIDS patients. Healthy asymptomatic people had a normal lymphocytosis with an inversed T4/T8 ratio and a normal lymphocyte response to phytohemagglutinin. Absence of immunosuppression in healthy Zairians who were positive for HIV antibodies has previously been reported (64). This adds further evidence to a similar natural history of AIDS virus infection in central Africa and in developed countries.

Patients with lymphadenopathy (stage II) had a slight decrease in their cellular immunity with the characteristic pattern of nonspecific follicular hyperplasia in pathological studies of lymph node biopsies (111). There are, however, many causes of persistent generalized lymphadenopathy (PGL) in Africa, and cohort prospective studies of seropositive Africans and seronegative controls are needed to assess the importance of extrainguinal adenopathy as a major clinical sign of AIDS virus infection in equatorial Africa.

C. Progression to AIDS

During a study period of 16 months in a cohort of African individuals observed by our group, no healthy seropositive subjects developed signs or symptoms of HIV infection. Three of 36 patients (8.3%) with PGL developed AIDS after a mean evolution of 33 months (range: 23-41 months). When converted to an annual basis. 1.1% of our cohort progressed from PGL to AIDS each year. This rate of progression was higher in the cohort of patients with ARC. Indeed, 12 of 38 individuals (32%) with ARC developed AIDS after a mean time of 7 months (range: 1-23 months) which gives an annual rate of progression to AIDS of 20.7% each year. In the study, 21 of 36 patients with AIDS died after a mean evolution of 5 months (range: 1-7 months).

Table 4 Immunological Parameters of 117 African Patients at Various Stages of AIDS Virus Infection

Immunologic values (mean ± SD)	Normal values	Clinical status (stage)[a]				p value
		HAS I n = 7	PGL II n = 36	ARC III n = 38	AIDS IV n = 36	
Lymphocytosis (cell/mm³)	1330-4500	1225 ± 512	1762 ± 841	1361 ± 909	1032 ± 844	NS except II vs. III and II vs. IV; $p < 0.05$
OKT4 cells (%)	27-65	24 ± 12	19 ± 9	13 ± 9	9 ± 8	II vs. III; $p < 0.005$ III vs. IV; $p < 0.05$
OKT8 cells (%)	12-40	47 ± 9	53 ± 12	58 ± 11	57 ± 17	NS
OKT4/OKT8 ratio	1.12-2.25	0.55 ± 0.32	0.42 ± 0.31	0.23 ± 0.18	0.16 ± 0.18	II vs. III and II vs. IV $p < 0.005$
In vitro lymphocyte response to PHA (% of normal control)	62-200	80 ± 23	61 ± 28	33 ± 25	18 ± 17	II vs. III; $p < 0.005$ III vs. IV; $p < 0.05$

[a]Abbreviations: HAS, healthy asymptomatic; PGL, lymphadenopathy; NS, nonsignificance; see Table 3 for definition.

The rates of progression to AIDS documented at Brussels and Kinshasa among African heterosexual patients and at San Francisco, New York, or Denmark among lymphadenopathic homosexuals or bisexuals are strikingly similar (62,66-71). One can then conclude that Africans are probably not experiencing a more aggressive clinical evolution of infection from the AIDS virus compared with patients from developed countries. They probably differ in exposure to cofactors which promote progression from asymptomatic or less symptomatic stages to AIDS-related conditions and AIDS. Differences in environmental factors are also likely to explain variations in the type of opportunistic pathogens to which Africans are prone.

D. Opportunistic Infections

As far as opportunistic infections are concerned, there are striking differences between patients in United States and those in Africa. Among African patients seen in Europe, *Pneumocystis carinii* pneumonia is not the leading clinical infection (6,8). In spite of an extensive search, *P. carinii* was isolated from only 12% of the patients seen in Brussels (author's personal observation). In contrast, cerebral toxoplasmosis and cryptococcal infection are, together with gastrointestinal candidiasis and mucocutaneous herpes simplex infection, the most frequent clinical presentation of immunodeficiency among African patients (6-8). Similar clinical discrepancies which reflect the different spectrum of latent infections in developing countries have also been noted among Haitian patients with AIDS (72). One can then expect to find, in the future, descriptions of other pathogens common in a tropical setting.

In addition to the opportunistic pathogens listed in the Centers for Disease Control/World Health Organization (CDC/WHO) case definition for acquired immunodeficiency syndrome (63), there is evidence that pulmonary or extrapulmonary tuberculosis, atypical herpes zoster, or salmonella infections could be indicative in developing countries of HIV infection or AIDS (73,74). In our experience, tuberculosis (pulmonary or extrapulmonary) preceded the opportunistic infections in 15% of the cases. A similar figure has been noted with herpes zoster, which characteristically involved more than two dermatomes and was of longer duration, painful, and with scars [Figure 1 (see Plate I, facing page 356)]. This observation suggests that in equatorial Africa, physicians who are specifically oriented toward identifying signs and symptoms suggestive of AIDS virus infection would consider these clinical manifestations as at least indicative of a possible HIV infection.

E. Slim Disease

Recently, a syndrome called "slim disease" characterized by weight loss, chronic diarrhea, itchy maculopapular rash, prolonged fever, and oral candidiasis has been reported from Uganda (13) among seropositive patients.

In a prospective study of 23 such patients (S. Lucas, personal communication), stool examinations have shown Cryptosporidium in 43% and *Isospora belli* in 13%. These findings link slim disease to the enteropathic form of AIDS found in patients in United States. In some cases, HIV itself may be the causative agent (see Chapter 8).

F. Staging of AIDS

In a recent Zairian study, 181 patients with AIDS (50% died during the study period) seen in Kinshasa were reported to fit into three main clinical presentations:

1. "SIDA humide" (wet AIDS) characterized by profound weight loss and diarrhea which accounted for 80% of patients
2. "SIDA chaud" (hot AIDS) characterized by weight loss and fever which accounted for 14% of the cohort
3. Disseminated Kaposi's sarcoma (6% of the cohort) (49).

All these facts stress the need of a new, appropriate case definition designed for a situation peculiar to Africa since laboratory and technical supports are generally not available. In addition, Kaposi's sarcoma, which is a diagnostic criterion for AIDS, has to be distinguished in central Africa between the endemic chronic form and the rapidly aggressive one. Only the aggressive form has been linked to AIDS virus infection (23). A clinical definition of AIDS in adults was proposed at the WHO Conference on AIDS held in Bangui, Central African Republic, October 1985 (63). The usefulness of this definition, which classified the signs and symptoms as major and minor, is being evaluated (65).

VI. AIDS in African Children

To date, there are no published clinical reports on the clinical manifestation of AIDS among African children. A clinical study performed on 16 children seen in Brussels showed that the manifestations of HIV infection in African children vary, as in adults, from an asymptomatic carrier state to frank AIDS (75). In these series, the early onset of clinical manifestation was associated with the most severe manifestation of the disease. The children were classified into three groups. The first group included five infants who died before the age of 1 year from an illness comparable to the one described in American children with AIDS. The second group of eight children had a mild or moderately severe chronic illness, with fatal outcome in one of them. These children were older than those in the first group when they became symptomatic. Most of the clinical manifestations observed in these patients could be linked to lymphoid hyperplasia which was found in the lung, parotid gland, liver, and lymph nodes. The third group included three asymptomatic children. One of them had virus isolation in the absence of antibodies to

HIV. Another prospective study performed in Rwanda has shown that 49 children with AIDS or ARC presented with weight loss, failure to thrive, persistent generalized lymphadenopathy, chronic diarrhea, and chronic fever. In 10 cases of AIDS, Cryptosporidium was the most common pathogen isolated (50%) (76). This fact underlines among children, too, the importance of enteropathic AIDS as a major clinical presentation in central Africa.

VII. Endemic and Epidemic Kaposi's Sarcoma in Africa

The patterns of the two forms of Kaposi's sarcoma (KS) that actually coexist in central Africa are summarized in Table 5. In equatorial Africa, KS is an extremely common tumor [Figure 2 (see Plate I, facing page 356)], and accounts for 12.8% of all malignant tumors in Zaire, 4.5% in Tanzania, 4.2% in Uganda, and 2.9% in Kenya (58). In adults, the disease, as defined during the 1960s and 1970s (77), was mainly cutaneous nodular on feet or hands with a benign clinical course. Some patients had more aggressive disease, usually several years after an indolent course, with extensive cutaneous lesions on one or more extremities and generally associated with involvement of adjacent bone. Cutaneous lesions in the florid group are exophytic tumor, whereas in the infiltrative group, deep lesions associated with dense fibrosis predominated. Florid KS responded promptly to actinomycin D and vincristine in over 90% of patients. Relapses after 2 to 3 years were uncommon but responded to treatment with the same or alternative cytotoxic drug (12). Among these patients, prospective studies, performed in the area of endemicity (East Zaire or Zambia) failed to demonstrate any significant impairment of cellular immunity or presence of antibodies to HIV (78).

The changing pattern of KS was first reported in 1983, in Lusaka, Zambia (12). The "new" pattern of KS among African patients consists of gen-

Table 5 Differences Between Classical and AIDS-Associated Kaposi's Sarcoma in Central Africa

	"Classical" form	Associated with AIDS
Sex ratio, M:F[a]	15:1	2:1
Geographical distribution	East Zaire Rwanda Uganda	Not restricted
Clinical form	Cutaneous localized, lower extremities	Cutaneous localized; organ involvement
Evolution	Chronic, indolent	Rapidly fatal
Cellular immunity	Grossly normal	Severely impaired
AIDS virus infection	No	Yes

[a]Abbreviations: F, female; M, male.

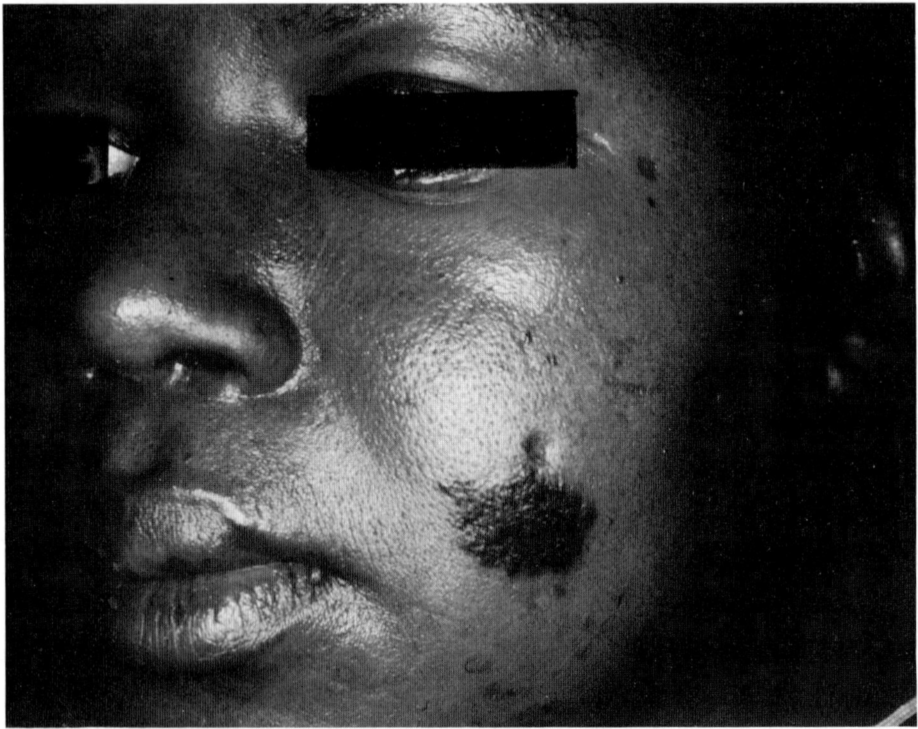

Figure 3 Aggressive form of Kaposi's sarcoma on the face.

eralized systemic lymphadenopathy, oral, gastrointestinal or bronchial lesions, together with cutaneous infiltrative plaques on the trunk, the genital organs, the face (Figure 3), or more rarely the limbs [Figure 4 (see Plate I, facing page 356)]. When associated with opportunistic infection, the evolution is rapidly fatal. Response to therapy with high doses of recombinant α-interferon or vinblastine/vincristine occurs at the same range as the one noted with American or European homosexual patients (author's personal observation).

The prevalence of aggressive KS among African heterosexual patients seems to be lower than among homosexuals or bisexuals from Western countries. A prevalence rate of 6-15% has been noted in comparison with 25-30% among homosexuals (7,10,11,49). A similarly lower rate of KS has been noted among IV drug users in United States (79). This finding suggests that homosexuals or bisexuals in contrast with heterosexuals (whether African or IV drug user) are more susceptible to KS because of cofactors in them that have not yet been identified.

VIII. Cofactors of AIDS in Africa

The possible cofactors involved in African AIDS are summarized in Table 6. Mostly due to environmental conditions, African people are prone to develop various infectious diseases. Overcrowding, poor hygiene, microbial contamination of drinking water and food, and malnutrition, together with a lack of control of natural reservoirs of various pathogens, are all factors that could explain why infection remains the one leading cause of death in many African countries.

Parasitic diseases and malnutrition are two possible causes of immunodepression in Africa. A wide range of prevalent protozoal and helminthic infections have been reported to induce immunodeficiency. In malaria, the number of T lymphocytes is reduced (80) but cell-mediated immunity, except for a transient inversion of the T helper/T suppressor ratio (81), seems to be unaffected, and only humoral immunity is impaired (82). African trypanosomiasis has been shown to be associated with several T-cell dysfunctions (83). Diffuse cutaneous leischmaniasis is known to induce immunosuppression, but it is restricted to parasite-specific antigens (84). Schistosomiasis and filariasis are also able to impair the immune responses to parasite-related antigens (85). On the basis of repeated examinations of blood and stool specimens, as well as serological tests, active parasitic infestation was not noted among African patients with AIDS seen in Brussels. Past malarial infections were reported by 55% of patients—a figure similar to that observed among African patients without AIDS virus infection (author's personal data). This fact, however, does not preclude the possible role of parasitic diseases as cofactors in the development of AIDS, by means of polyclonal B-cell activation or other immune dysfunctions (86).

Since the AIDS virus seems mostly transmitted by heterosexual contacts in Africa, it may be that other venereal diseases are important in enhancing its transmission. There is clearly a high prevalence of STD in Africa (87) and a seroepidemiological study of HIV, *Trepomena pallidum*, *Chlamydia trachomatis*, and hepatitis B virus among African prostitutes, their male customers, and male and female controls showed a significant association between HIV seropositivity and positive test for the other venereal diseases

Table 6 Possible Cofactors of AIDS in Africa

1. Environmental
   - Potential immunosuppressive infections
     - Malaria
     - Other parasitic infections
     - Hepatitis B, cytomegalovirus, Epstein-Barr virus
     - Sexually transmitted diseases
   - Malnutrition
2. Genetic

(88). Coexistence of STDs, particularly those "tropical" ones that cause genital ulcers, such as chancroid or lymphogranuloma venereum, could conceivably facilitate access to the blood stream for the AIDS virus through damaged skin or mucosa. Moreover, copious inflammatory secretions would bring more infected cells and free virus into genital secretions. Finally, from studies performed in Trinidad, it has been claimed that black people from African origin could be more susceptible to AIDS virus infection (89).

IX. Perspectives and Strategic Approaches for Control of AIDS in Africa

It is likely that AIDS, which is now epidemic and spreading transcontinentally in tropical Africa, will emerge as a major public health problem for most central African countries. It threatens to spread throughout the African continent. Due to fear and anxiety, the AIDS epidemic has also raised, in Africa as in United States, sociopolitical issues. With the elaboration of a new case definition more adapted to the tropical setting, it should technically be possible to confirm and to report the AIDS cases on-site in Africa. There remains, however, a tremendous need in the field for diagnostic procedures and treatment of AIDS virus infection, its associated illnesses, and cancer. The spread of AIDS in Africa heterosexually is the result of the role of socioeconomic factors (90). It is likely that mobile "free women" or prostitutes constitute a reservoir of the AIDS virus. They contribute, together with promiscuous men, who contaminate their nonpromiscuous secondary contacts (usually their spouses), to the interregional spread of HIV. This fact indicates that the control of the epidemic will be very difficult unless extensive education and eventually mass vaccination against the AIDS virus can be conducted. The heterogeneity of the African retroviruses may also lead to further difficulties in the realization of a vaccine (36,38). The strategic approaches for the control of AIDS in Africa that immediately need to be initiated are summarized in Table 7. Due to the lack of resources of African countries, which have to deal with many other public health problems, only an international mobilization of such efforts could eventually help to realize such a minimal program.

Table 7 Strategic Approaches for the Control of AIDS in Africa

1. Surveillance system at the state level
    a. Clinical: AIDS and AIDS-related conditions
    b. Serological: healthy asymptomatic groups at risk
2. Compulsory screening of blood donors
3. Risk-reduction program for unsterilized materials
4. Mass education campaigns about sexually transmitted diseases

References

1. Quinn TC, Mann JM, Curran JW, Piot P. AIDS in Africa: An epidemiologic paradigm. Science 1986; 234:955-63.

1a. Nahmias AJ, Weiss J, Yao X, Lee F, Kodsi R, Schandfield M, Matthews T, Bolognesi D, Durack D, Motulsky A, Kanki P, Essex M. Evidence for human infection with an HTLV-III/LAV-like virus in Central Africa, 1959. Lancet 1986; i:1279-80.

2. Clumeck N, Mascart-Lemone F, De Maubeuge J, Brenez D, Marcelis L. Acquired immune deficiency syndrome in black Africans. Lancet 1983; i:642.

3. Vandepitte J, Verwilghen R, Zachee P. AIDS and cryptococcosis (Zaire, 1977). Lancet 1983; i:925-6.

4. Bygjerg IC. AIDS in a Danish surgeon (Zaire, 1976). Lancet 1983; i:925.

5. Rutsaert J, Melot C, Ectors M, Cornil A, DePrez C, Flament J. Complications infectieuses pulmonaires et neurologiques d'un sarcome de Kaposi. Ann Anat Pathol 1980; 25:125-38.

6. Clumeck N, Sonnet J, Taelman H, Mascart-Lemone F, De Bruyére M, Van de Perre P, Dasnoy J, Marcelis L, Lamy M, Jonas C, Eyckmans L, Noel H, Vanhaeverbeek M, Butlzer JP. Acquired immunodeficiency syndrome in African patients. New Engl J Med 1984; 310:492-7.

7. Clumeck N, Sonnet J, Taelman H, Cran S, Henrivaux P. Acquired immune deficiency syndrome in Belgium and its relation to Central Africa. Ann NY Acad Sci 1984; 437:264-9.

8. Katlama C, Leport C, Matheron S, Brun-Vezinet F, Rouzioux C, Vittecoq D, Lambolez T, Lebras P, Petitprez P, Offenstadt G, Vachon F, Vilde JL, Coulaud JP, Saimot AG. Acquired immunodeficiency syndrome (AIDS) in Africans. Ann Soc Belg Med Trop 1984; 64:379-89.

9. Leads from the MMWR. JAMA 1986; 255:717-25.

10. Van de Perre P, Rouvroy D, Lepage P, Bogaerts J, Kestelyn P, Kayhigi J, Hekker AC, Butzler JP, Clumeck N. Acquired immunodeficiency syndrome in Rwanda. Lancet 1984; ii:62-5.

11. Piot P, Quinn TC, Taelman H, Feinsod FM, Minlangu KG, Wobin O, Mbendi N, Mazebo P, Ndangi K, Stevens W, Kalambayi K, Mitchell S, Bridts C, McCormick JB. Acquired immunodeficiency syndrome in a heterosexual population in Zaire. Lancet 1984; ii:65-9.

12. Bayley AC. Aggressive Kaposi's sarcoma in Zambia, 1983. Lancet 1984; i:1318-20.

13. Serwadda D, Mugerwa RD, Sewankambo NK, Lwegaba AL, Carswell JW, Kirya GB, Bayley AC, Downing RG, Tedder RS, Clayden SA, Weiss RA, Dalgleish AG. Slim disease: a new disease in Uganda and its association with HTLV-III infection. Lancet 1985; ii:849-52.

14. Norman C. Politics and science clash in African AIDS. Science 1985; 230:1140-1.

15. Mann JM, Francis H, Quinn T, Asila PK, Bosenge N, Nzilambi N, Bila K, Tamfum M, Ruti K, McCormick J, Curran JW. Surveillance for acquired immunodeficiency syndrome in a central African city: Kinshasa, Zaire. JAMA 1986; 255:3255-9.

16. Brunet JB, Ancelle RA. The international occurrence of the acquired immunodeficiency syndrome. Ann Intern Med 1985; 103:670-4.
17. Brun-Vezinet F, Rouzioux C, Montagnier L, Chamaret S, Gruest J, Barré-Sinoussi F, Geroldi D, Chermann JC, McCormick J, Mitchell S, Piot P, Taelman H, Mirlangu KB, Wobin O, Mbendi N, Mazebo P, Kayembe K, Bridts C, Desmyter J, Feinsod FM, Quinn TC. Prevalence of antibodies to lymphadenopathy-associated retrovirus in African patients with AIDS. Science 1984; 226: 453-6.
18. Kayembe K, Mann JM, Francis H, Lurhuma Z, Muyembe T, Piot P, et al. LAV/HTLV-III seroprevalence among patients without AIDS or AIDS-related complex hospitalized at the University hospital, Kinshasa, Zaire. International Conference on Acquired Immunodeficiency Syndrome (AIDS), Paris, France. 1986: 129.
19. Biggar RJ, Melbye M, Kestens L, de Feyter M, Saxinger C, Bodner AJ, Paluko L, Blattner WA, Gigase PL. Seroepidemiology of HTLV-III antibodies in a remote population of eastern Zaire. Br Med 1985; 290:808-10.
20. Van de Perre P, Kanyamupira JB, Carael M, Bogaerts J, Akingeneye E, Demol P, Sibomana J, Le Pollain B, Nzabihimana E, Kayihigi J, Clumeck N. HTLV-III/LAV infection in Central Africa. International Symposium on African AIDS, Brussels, Belgium. 1985:04/I.
21. Van de Perre P, Clumeck N, Carael M, Nzabihimana E, Robert-Guroff M, Demol P, Freyens P, Butzler JP, Gallo RC, Kanyamupira JB. Female prostitutes: a risk group for infection with human T-cell lymphotropic virus type III. Lancet 1985; ii:524-6.
22. Clumeck N, Robert-Guroff M, Van de Perre P, Jennings A, Sibomana J, Demol P, Cran S, Gallo RC. Seroepidemiological studies of HTLV-III antibody prevalence among selected groups of heterosexual Africans. JAMA 1985; 254: 2599-602.
23. Bayley AC, Downing RG, Cheingsong-Popov R, Tedder RS, Dalgleish AG, Weiss RA. HTLV-III serology distinguishes atypical and endemic Kaposi's sarcoma in Africa. Lancet 1985; i:359-61.
24. Buchanan DJ, Downing RG, Tedder RS. HTLV-III antibody positivity in Zambian copper belt. Lancet 1986; i:155.
25. Sher R. Seroepidemiological studies of HTLV-III/LAV infections in Southern African countries. International Symposium on African AIDS, Brussels, Belgium. 1985:06/I.
26. Benn S, Rutledge R, Folks T, Gold J, Baker G, McCormich J, Feorino P, Piot P, Quinn T, Martin M. Genomic heterogeneity of AIDS retroviral isolates from North America and Zaire. Science 1985; 230:949-51.
27. Biggar RJ, Johnson BK, Oster C, Sarin PS, Ocheng D, Tukei P, Nsanze H, Siongok TA, Gallo RC, Blattner WA. Regional variation in prevalence of antibody against human T-lymphotropic virus types I and III in Kenya. Int J Cancer 1985; 35:764-7.
28. Kreiss JK, Koech D, Plummer FA, Holmes KK, Lightfoote M, Piot P, Ronald AR, Ndinya-Achola JO, D'Costa LJ, Roberts P, Ngugi EN, Quinn TC. AIDS virus infection in Nairobi prostitutes. N Engl J Med 1986; 314:414-8.

29. Karpas A, Maayan S, Raz R. Lack of antibodies to adult T-cell leukaemia virus and to AIDS virus in Israeli Falashas. Nature 1986; 319:794.
30. Williams CKO. AIDS and cancer in Nigerians. Lancet 1986; i:36-7.
31. Barin F, M'Boup S, Denis F, Kanki P, Allan JS, Lee TH. Serological evidence for virus related to simian T lymphotropic retrovirus III in residents of West Africa. Lancet 1985; ii:1387-9.
32. Serwadda D, Downing R, Carswell W, Bayley AC, Tedder RS, Levin A, Rubinstein E, Dalgleish AG, Weiss RA. HTLV-III/LAV serology in Africa and correlation with disease states. International Symposium on African AIDS, Brussels, Belgium. 1985:P06.
33. Biggar RJ, Gigase PL, Melbye M, Kestens L, Sarin PS, Bodner AJ, Demedts P, Stevens W, Paluku L, Delacolette C, Blattner WA. ELISA HTLV retrovirus antibody reactivity associated with malaria and immune complexes in healthy Africans. lancet 1985; ii:520-23.
34. Hunsmann G, Schneider J, Wendler I, Fleming AF. HTLV positivity in Africans. Lancet 1985; ii:952-3.
35. Biggar RJ. The AIDS problem in Africa. Lancet 1986; i:79-82.
36. Kanki PJ, Barin F, M'Boup S, Allan JS, Romet-Lemonne JL, Marlinck R, McLane MF, Lee TH, Arbeille B, Denis F, Essex M. New human T-lymphotropic retrovirus related to simian T-lymphotropic virus type III (STLV-III AGM). Science 1986; 232:238-43.
37. Clavel F, Guetard D, Brun-Vezinet F, Chamaret S, Rey M-A, Santos-Ferreira S, Laurent AG, Dauguet C, Katlama C, Rouzioux C, Klatzmann D, Champalimaud JL, Montagnier L. Isolation of a new human retrovirus from West African patients with AIDS. Science 1986; 233:343-6.
38. Quinn TC, Mann JM, Curran JW, Piot P. AIDS in Africa: an epidemiologic paradigm. Science 1986; 234:955-63.
39. Lyons SF, Shoub BD, McGillivray GM, Sher R, Dos Santos L. Lack of evidence of HTLV-III endemicity in Southern Africa. New Engl J Med 1985; 312: 1257-8.
40. Benslimane A, Benchemsi N, de Thé GB, Carraz M. Prevalence des Human T cell leukemia lymphoma virus (HTLV-I et HTLV-III) au Maroc. International Symposium on African AIDS, Brussels, Belgium. 1985:P08.
41. Piot P, Plummer FA, Rey M, Ngugi EN, Rouzioux C, Ndinya-Achola JO, D'Costa LJ, Vercauteren G, et al. Retrospective seroepidemiology of AIDS virus infection in Nairobi populations. International Conference on Acquired Immunodeficiency Syndrome (AIDS), Paris, France. 1986:101.
42. Desmyter J, Goubau P, Chamaret S, Montagnier L. Anti-LAV/HTLV-III in Kinshasa mothers in 1970 and 1980. International Conference on Acquired Immunodeficiency Syndrome, Paris, France. 1986:106.
43. Saxinger WC, Levine PH, Dean AG, de Thé GB, Lange-Wantzin G, Moghissi J, Laurent F, Hoh M, Sarngadharan MG, Gallo RC. Evidence for exposure to HTLV-III in Uganda before 1973. Science 1985; 227:1036-8.
44. Epstein JS, Moffitt AL, Mayner RE, Phelan MA, Meyer BC, Quinnan GV, Meyer HM. Antibodies reactive with HTLV-III found in freezer-banked sera from children in West Africa. 25th Interscience Conference on Antimicrobial Agents and Chemotherapy, Minneapolis. 1985: nb 217, 130.

45. Levy JA, Pan L-Z, Beth-Giraldo B, Kaminsky L, Henle G, Henle W, Giraldo G. Absence of antibodies to the human immunodeficiency virus in sera from Africa prior to 1975. Proc Natl Acad Sci USA 1986; 83:7935-7.
46. Lamey B, Melameka N. Aspects cliniques et épidémiologiques de la cryptococcose à Kinshasa. A propos de 15 cas personnels. Med Trop 1982; 42:507-11.
47. Vogt MW, Witt DJ, Craven DE, Byington R, Crawford DF, Schooley RT, Hirsh MS. Isolation of HTLV-III/LAV from cervical secretions of women at risk for AIDS. Lancet 1986; i:525-7.
48. Wofsy CB, Cohen JB, Hauer LB, Padian NS, Michaelis BA, Evans LA, Levy JA. Isolation of AIDS-associated retrovirus from genital secretions of women with antibodies to the virus. Lancet 1986; i:527-9.
49. Odio W, Kapita B, Mbendi N, Kayembe K, Ndangi K, Muyembe T, Mazebo P, Izzia K, Lurhuma Z, Sansa A, Declercq D, Henry MC, Mbongo M, McCormick JB, Taelman H, Piot P. Le syndrome d'immunodéficience acquise (SIDA) à Kinshasa, Zaire: observations cliniques et épidémiologiques. Ann Soc Belg Med Trop 1985; 65:357-61.
50. Mann JM, Ruti R, Francis H, Kapita B, Quinn T, Curran JW. AIDS surveillance in a central African city: Kinshasa, Zaire. International Conference on Acquired Immunodeficiency Syndrome (AIDS), Atlanta. 1985:37.
51. Clumeck N, Van de Perre P, Carael M, Rouvroy D, Nzaramba D. Heterosexual promiscuity among African patients with AIDS. N Engl J Med 1985; 312:182.
52. Winkelstein W, Jr, Lyman DM, Padian N, Grant R, Samuel M, Wiley JA, Anderson RE, Lang W, Riggs J, Levy JA. Sexual practices and risk of infection by the human immunodeficiency virus: the San Francisco Men's Health Study. JAMA 1987; 257:321-5.
53. Dagleish AG. Sexual transmission of AIDS. Br J Hosp Med 1985; 319:314.
54. Seale J. Sexual transmission of AIDS virus (editorial). Br J Hosp Med 1985; 319:71.
55. Thiry L, Sprecher-Goldberger S, Jonkheer T, Levy J, Van de Perre P, Henrivaux P, Cogniaux-Leclercq J, Clumeck N. Isolation of AIDS virus from cell-free breast milk of three healthy virus carriers. Lancet 1985; ii:891-2.
56. Izzia KW, Lepira B, Kayambe K, Odio W. Syndrome d'immunodéficience acquise et trepanocytose homozygote. Ann Soc Med Trop 1984; 64:391-6.
57. Van de Perre P, Munyambuga D, Zissis G, Butzler JP, Nzaramba D, Clumeck N. Antibody to HTLV-III in blood donors in central Africa. Lancet 1985; i: 336-7.
58. Weber J. Is AIDS an epidemic form of African Kaposi's sarcoma?: discussion paper. J R Soc Med 1984; 77:572-6.
59. De Cock KM. AIDS: an old disease from Africa? Br Med J 1984; 289:306-8.
60. De Wit S, Hermans P, Zissis G, Clumeck N. HTLV-III/LAV as a likely causative agent of unexplained lymphocytic meningitis in AIDS. International Conference on Acquired Immunodeficiency Syndrome (AIDS), Paris, France. 1986: 57.
61. Clumeck N, Sprecher S, De Wit S, De Caluwe JP, Taelman H, Cogniaux J. HTLV-III/LAV antigen prevalence among homosexual and heterosexual patients with HTLV-III/LAV antibodies. International Conference on Acquired

Immunodeficiency Syndrome (AIDS), Paris, France. 1986:150.
62. Mann JM, Bila K, Colebunders RL, Kalemba K, Khonde N, Bosenge N, Nzilambi N, Malonga M, Jansegers L, Francis H, McCormick JB, Piot P, Quinn TC, Curran JW. Natural history of human immunodeficiency virus infection in Zaire. Lancet 1986; ii:707-9.
63. WHO, ed. Acquired immunodeficiency syndrome (AIDS). Weekly Epidemiol Rec 1986; 10:69-72.
64. Kestens L, Biggar RJ, Melbye M, Bodner AJ, De Feyter M, Gigase PL. Absence of immunosuppression in healthy subjects from eastern Zaire who are positive for HTLV-III antibody. N Engl J Med 1985; 312:1517-8.
65. Colebunders R, Mann JM, Francis H et al. Evaluation of a clinical case-definition of acquired immunodeficiency syndrome in Africa. Lancet 1987; i:492-494.
66. Jaffe HW, Darrow WW, Echenberg DF, et al. The acquired immunodeficiency syndrome in a cohort of homosexual men: a six-year follow-up study. Ann Intern Med 1985; 103:210-4.
67. Goedert JJ, Biggar RJ, Quinn DM, Greene MH, Gallo RC, Sarngadharan MG, Weiss SH, Grossman RJ, Bodner AJ, Strong DM, Blattner WA. Determinants of retrovirus (HTLV-III) antibody and immunodeficiency conditions in homosexual men. Lancet 1984; ii:711-6.
68. Feorino PM, Jaffe HW, Palmer EE, Peterman TA, Francis GP, Kalyanaraman VS, Weinstein RA, Stoneburner RL, Curran JW. Tranfusion-associated acquired immunodeficiency syndrome. N Engl J Med 1985; 312:1293-6.
69. Melbye M, Biggar RJ, Ebbeson P, Sarngadharan MG, Weiss SH, Gallo RC, Blattner WA. Seroepidemiology of HTLV-III antibody in Danish homosexual men: prevalence, transmission and disease outcome. Br Med J 1984; 289:573-5.
70. Mathur-Wagh U, Mildvan D, Senie RT. Follow-up at 4 years on homosexual men with generalized lymphadenopathy. N Engl J Med 1985; 313:1542-3.
71. Clumeck N, Hermans P, De Wit S. Disease outcome among heterosexual Africans with HTLV-III/LAV infection. 26th Interscience Conference on Antimicrobial Agents and Chemotherapy, New Orleans. 1986:283.
72. Pape JW, Liautaud B, Thomas F, Mathurin JR, St Amand MMA, Boncy M, Pean V, Pamphile M, Laroche AC, Dehovitz J, Johnson WD. The acquired immunodeficiency syndrome in Haiti. Ann Intern Med 1985; 103:674-8.
73. Pitchenik AE, Cole C, Russel BW, MAFischl, Spira TJ, Snider DE Jr. Tuberculosis, atypical mycobacteriosis, and the acquired immunodeficiency syndrome among Haitian and non-Haitian patients in South Florida. Ann Intern Med 1984; 101:641-5.
74. Van de Perre P, Akingeneye E, Clumeck N. Atypical presentation of herpes zoster infection in young African adults: an early manifestation of HTLV-III infection? International Symposium on African AIDS, Brussels, Belgium. 1985: 28.
75. Jonckheer T, Levy J, Van de Perre P, Thiry L, Henrivaux P, Sacré JP, Schepens G, Mees N, Dab I, Taelman H, Mascart-Lemone F, Zissis G. Clumeck N, Butzler JP, Sprecher-Goldberger S. LAV/HTLV-III infection in children of African origin: experience in Belgium. Eur J Paediatr 1986, in press.

76. Lepage P. Clinical, immunological and serological findings in HTLV-III/LAV-infected children and their families. International Symposium on African AIDS, Brussels, Belgium. 1985:05/II.
77. Taylor JI, Templeton AC, Vogel CL, Ziegler JL, Kyalwazi SK. Kaposi's sarcoma in Uganda: a clinico-pathological study. Int J Cancer 1971; 8:122-35.
78. Biggar RJ, Melbye M, Kestems L, et al. Kaposi's sarcoma in Zaire is not associated with HTLV-III infection. N Engl J Med 1984; 16:1051.
79. Safai B, Johnson KG, Myskowski PL, Koziner B, Yang SY, Cunningham-Rundles S, Godbold JH, Dupont B. The natural history of Kaposi's sarcoma in the acquired immunodeficiency syndrome. Ann Intern Med 1985; 103:744-50.
80. Wiler DJ. Peripheral lymphocyte subpopulations in human *P. falciparum* malaria. Clin Exp Immunol 1976; 23:471-6.
81. Whittle HC, Brown J, Marsh K, Greenwood BM, Seidelin P, Tighe H, Wedderburn L. T-cell control of Epstein-Barr virus infected B cells is lost during *P. falciparum* malaria. Nature 1984; 312:447-50.
82. Clayton CE. Immunosuppression in trypanosomiasis and malaria. In: The role of the spleen in the immunology of parasitic diseases. Basel: Schwabe, 1979: 97-115.
83. Askonas BA, Corsini AC, Clayton CE, Ogilvie BM. Functional depletion of T- and B-memory cells and other lymphoid cell subpopulations during trypanosomiasis. Immunology 1979; 36:313-21.
84. Petersen EA, Neva FA, Oster CN, Diaz HB. Specific inhibition of lymphocyte-proliferation responses by adherent suppressor cells in diffuse cutaneous leishmaniasis. N Engl J Med 1982; 306:387-92.
85. Wilkins HA, Brown J. *Schistosoma haematobium* in a Gambian community: II. Impaired cell-mediated immunity and other immunological abnormalities. Ann Trop Med Parasitol 1977; 71:59-66.
86. Levy JA, Ziegler JL. Acquired immunodeficiency syndrome is an opportunistic infection and Kaposi's sarcoma results from secondary immune stimulation. Lancet 1983; ii:78-80.
87. Aral SO, Holmes KK. Epidemiology of sexually transmitted diseases. In: Holmes KK, Mardh PA, Sparling PF, Wiesner PJ, eds. Sexually transmitted diseases. New York: McGraw Hill, 1984:126-41.
88. Van de Perre P, Clumeck N, Steens M, Zissis G, Carael M, Lagasse R, Nzabihimana E, De Wit S, Lafontaine T, Demol P, Butzler JP. Seroepidemiological study on sexually transmitted diseases and hepatitis B in African promiscuous heterosexuals in relation to HTLV-III infection. 1986 (submitted).
89. Bartholomew C, Charles W, Saxinger C, Blattner W, Robert-Guroff M, Raju C, Ratan P, Ince W, Quamina D, Basdeo-Maharaj K, Gallo RC. Racial and other characteristics of human T cell leukemia/lymphoma (HTLV-I) and AIDS (HTLV-III) in Trinidad. Br Med J 1985; 290:1243-6.
90. Carael M, Van de Perre P, Akingeneye E, Kanyamupira JB, Butzler JP, Clumeck N. Socio-cultural factors in relation to HTLV-III/LAV transmission in urban areas in Central Africa. International Symposium on African AIDS, Brussels, Belgium. 1985:05.I.
91. Nzilambi N, DeCock KM, Forthal DN, et al. The prevalence of infection with

human immunodeficiency virus over a 10-year period in rural Zaire. N Engl J Med 1988; 318:276-9.

92. Hrdy DB. Cultural practices contributing to the transmission of human immunodeficiency virus in Africa. Rev Infect Dis 1987; 9:1109-19.
93. Kanki PJ, MacLane MF, King NW, et al. Serologic identification and characterization of macaque T-lymphotropic retrovirus closely related to human T-lymphotropic retroviruses (HTLV) type III. Science 1985; 228:1199-201.
94. Kanki PJ, Kurth R, Becker W, et al. Antibodies to simian T-lymphotropic virus type III in African green monkeys and recognition of STLV-III viral proteins by AIDS and related sera. Lancet 1985; i:1330-2.
95. Franchini G, Gurgo C, Guo HG, et al. Sequence of the simian immunodeficiency virus and its relationship to the human immunodeficiency viruses. Nature 1987; 328:539-43.
96. Kanki PJ, M'Boup S, Ricard D, et al. Human T lymphotropic virus type 4 and the human immunodeficiency virus in West Africa. Science 1987; 236:827-31.
97. Kanki PJ. West African human retroviruses related to STLV-III. AIDS 1987; 1:141-5.
98. Denis F, Barin F, Gershy-Damet G, et al. Prevalence of human T-lymphotropic retroviruses type III (HIV) and type IV in Ivory Coast. Lancet 1987; i:408-11.
99. Guyader M, Emerman M, Sonigo P, et al. Genome organization and transactivation of the human immunodeficiency virus type 2. Nature 1987; 326:662-9.
100. Clavel F, Mansinho K, Chamaret S, et al. Human immunodeficiency virus type 2 infection associated with AIDS in West Africa. N Engl J Med 1987; 316:1180-5.
101. Brun-Vézinet F, Rey MA, Katlama C, et al. Lymphadenopathy-associated virus type 2 in AIDS and AIDS-related complex. Lancet 1987; i:128-32.
102. Clavel F. HIV-2, the West African AIDS virus. AIDS 1987; 1:135-40.
103. Kornfeld H, Riedl N, Viglianti GA, et al. Cloning of HTLV-IV and its relation to simian and human immunodeficiency viruses. Nature 1987; 326:610-3.
104. Hahn BH, Kong LI, Lee S-W, et al. Relation of HTLV-4 to simian and human immunodeficiency-associated viruses. Nature 1987; 330:184-6.
105. Kestler HW, III, Li Y, Naidu YM, et al. Comparison of simian immunodeficiency virus isolates. Nature 1988; 331:619-22.
106. Albert J, Bredberg U, Chiodi F, et al. A new human retrovirus isolate of West African origin (SBL-6669) and its relationship to HTLV-IV, LAV-II, and HTLV-IIIB. AIDS Res Retroviruses 1987; 3:3-8.
107. Evans LA, Moreau J, Odehouri K, et al. Characterization of a non-cytopathic HIV-2 strain with unusual effects on CD4 antigen expression. Science 1988; in press.
108. Sattentau Q, Beverley PCL, Halabi FA, et al. A comparison of the interaction of HIV1 and HIV2 with the CD4 antigen. III International Conference on AIDS, Washington 1987; Abstract TH.9.6.:160.
109. Mabey DCW, Tedder RS, Hughes ASB, et al. Human retroviral infections in The Gambia: prevalence and clinical features. British Med J 1988; 296:83-6.
110. Clavel F. HIV-2, the West African AIDS virus. AIDS 1987; 1:135-40.
111. Piot P, Plummer FA, Mhalu FS, et al. AIDS: An international perspective. Science 1988; 239:573-9.

3

AIDS in Haiti

Warren D. Johnson, Jr.
Cornell University Medical College
New York, New York

Jean W. Pape
Cornell University Medical College
New York, New York
and Faculté de Medecine
Université d'Etat d'Haiti
Port-au-Prince, Haiti

I. Introduction

Cases of the acquired immunodeficiency syndrome (AIDS) were first recognized in Haiti in 1979 and reported in 1983 (1,2). Since that time, the Haitian Study Group on Kaposi's Sarcoma and Opportunistic Infections (GHESKIO) has evaluated and treated 554 AIDS patients with documented opportunistic infections or Kaposi's sarcoma (KS) in Port-au-Prince, Haiti (Table 1). The first patient with Kaposi's sarcoma was diagnosed in June 1979, and the first patient with an opportunistic infection was seen in February 1980. In 1983 we surveyed the 21 practicing dermatologists and pathologists in Haiti about their experience in that country with Kaposi's sarcoma. Before 1979,

Table 1 AIDS Cases Diagnosed by the Haitian Study Group on Kaposi's Sarcoma and Opportunistic Infection (GHESKIO)

Year	Kaposi's sarcoma	Opportunistic infection	Total
1979	2	0	2
1980	2	5	7
1981	7	9	16
1982	5	35	40
1983	8	53	61
1984	11	103	114
1985	8	136	144
1986	10	160	170
1987[a]	8	159	167
Total	61	660	721

[a]Selective enrollment of cases after July 1987.

the only case recognized by these physicians occurred in a 54-year-old man with Kaposi's sarcoma documented by biopsy in 1972. The course of his illness is not known. A review of records of cancer biopsies from three private hospitals in Port-au-Prince, with a combined total of 180 beds, revealed that no cases of Kaposi's sarcoma were recorded during the period from 1968 to 1983. A similar review of the records of over 1000 cancer biopsies at the Albert Schweitzer Hospital in Deschapelles, Haiti, revealed that no cases of Kaposi's sarcoma were recorded during the same period. This hospital serves a rural population of 115,000 persons (3). A review of its autopsy records from 1978 to July 1982 also failed to reveal any cases of Kaposi's sarcoma. Hospital records did include those of a previously healthy 20-year-old-man who had generalized seizures in July 1978 and died 2 weeks later. At autopsy he was found to have central nervous system toxoplasmosis without evidence of underlying cancer. He had not received immunosuppressive therapy. He is the earliest patient with possible AIDS in Haiti known to our group (1).

We also have had the opportunity to test for HIV in the sera of 191 adults bled in Haiti during a 1977-1979 outbreak of dengue (4). The mean age of the group was 27 years. Sera were tested utilizing an ELISA (whole virus) and a radioimmunoprecipitation assay (RIPA) for antibody to the p25 and gp 120 HIV antigens (see Chapter 8). None of the sera were confirmed positive. These findings and the aforementioned epidemiological data have led us to conclude that AIDS did not exist in Haiti prior to 1978-1979. This period coincides with the earliest reports of AIDS in the United States and is over 20 years after an HIV seropositive person was identified in Africa (5). In addition, we have not identified any Haitians with AIDS who have history of previous travel to Africa. In contrast, 10-15% of Haitian AIDS patients seen by us had been to either the United States or Europe during the 5 years prior to the onset of their illness. Haiti also has been popular among French- and English-speaking tourists, including homosexuals. These data and studies from Africa (6) are consistent with hypothesis that HIV most likely originated in that continent, came to the United States and Europe, and subsequently was introduced into Haiti by either tourists or returning Haitians.

II. Prevalence of HIV in Haiti

The prevalance of AIDS in Haiti is not known. There is neither a national reporting system nor a data base similar to that collated by the United States Centers for Disease Control. Table 1 indicates the number of AIDS cases annually diagnosed by our group in Port-au-Prince since 1979. It is of note that 57% of the 554 cases were diagnosed in 1985-1986. These data cannot be used to estimate the rate of increase in AIDS cases in the country as a whole because our patients are primarily from Port-au-Prince and increased numbers of patients may have sought care or been referred to us as our interest in AIDS became known.

We have undertaken studies of the seroprevalence of HIV within Haiti utilizing the ELISA (whole virus) and RIPA (p25, gp 120) (7). As part of a case-control study to determine risk factors for transmission of HIV, we evauated 384 AIDS patients, 174 of their heterosexual sex partners, and 224 of their siblings and friends in 1984-1985 (Table 2). The seroprevalence rate for the 278 male and 106 female AIDS patients was identical: 96%. Among the group of 136 sex-matched siblings, 17% were seropositive—19% of the males and 14% of females. None of the siblings were bisexual or had been transfused. The seroprevalence of HIV was 19% in the 108 sex-matched friends with no sexual relationship to the patient. This seropositivity was limited to males—26% of male friends were seropositive, whereas all of the women were seronegative. Bisexuality was reported by only 5% of the male friends (all seropositive). Two percent of the male and 3% of the female friends had received blood transfusions during the preceding 5 years but none was HIV-seropositive. Finally, 55% of the serum samples from 174 regular sex partners or spouses of the AIDS patients were positive for HIV antibody. The seroprevalence rate was comparable for male and female sex partners: 61% and 54%, respectively. Only 3% and 6% of male and female spouses, respectively, had received a transfusion, and neither bisexuality nor IV drug abuse was reported by either group.

Sera from a number of Haitian population groups unrelated to our case-control study sample were also analyzed for antibody to HIV. Sera were obtained from urban and rural groups. In two groups of apparently healthy urban adults—hotel and factory workers (Table 3)—seroprevalence was 12%

Table 2 Prevalence of HIV Antibody in AIDS Patients, Family Members, Friends, and Sex Partners/Spouses in 1984-85

Group	Males			Females			Total HIV antibody (%)
	n	Mean age (yrs)	HIV antibody (%)	*n*	Mean age (yrs)	HIV antibody (%)	
AIDS patients	278	34	96	106	31	96	369/384 (96)
Siblings[a]	86	29	19	50	29	14	23/136 (17)
Friends[b]	82	30	26	26	29	0	21/108 (19)
Sex partners/spouses[c]	38	36	61	136	30	54	96/174 (55)

[a]Same-sex siblings of AIDS patients, matched for age within 5 years.
[b]Same-sex friends of AIDS patients, with no sexual relationship to the patient, matched for age within 5 years.
[c]Heterosexual sex partners of AIDS patients included 38 male sex partners who were spouses of female AIDS patients and 136 sex partners who were spouses of male AIDS patients.

Table 3 HIV Seroprevalence in Haiti in 1986

Groups[a]	*n*	Mean age (yrs)	HIV (%)
Medical workers	57	40	0
College graduates	54	35	0
Blood donors			
Rural	245	32	4
Factory workers	84	30	5
Leprosy patients	157	40	4
Lab specimens			
Lab A	353	38	6
Lab B	188	37	8
Lab C	496	36	9
Total	1037	37	8
Other adults[b]			
Urban	190	33	13
Rural	191	29	1
Hotel workers	25	45	12
Mothers of sick infants			
Urban	502	29	12
Rural	97	25	3
Tuberculosis patients			
Urban	129	32	45
Rural	112	34	15
Prostitutes	139	24	53

[a]All persons lived in Port-au-Prince unless identified as "rural." Rural subjects were bled in either hospitals or clinics ≥ 75 miles from Port-au-Prince. "Urban" refers to Port-au-Prince.
[b]Low socioeconomic group.

and 5%, respectively. Rates were comparable for men and women. In a group of 502 mothers of children hospitalized with diarrhea and in a group of 190 urban adults with a comparable socioeconomic background, the seroprevalence rates were 12% and 13%, respectively. As reported in numerous other studies, of a sample of 57 health workers involved in the care of AIDS patients, all were seronegative. Overall, 10% of 912 healthy urban adults (medical workers, college graduates, factory and hotel workers, mothers of sick infants, and other adults) were seropositive to HIV. In contrast, the seroprevalence rate was 3% in rural areas. The seroprevalence rate in 97 mothers of children hospitalized with dehydration was 3%; 4% of 245 unscreened rural blood donors had antibody to HIV. In an area even more distant from urban centers 1% of 191 adults who came for immunizations were seropositive. Koenig et al. reported a HIV seroprevalence rate of 10% in 250 healthy Haitian sugarcane cutters working in the Dominican Republic and 2-4% in urban heterosexual Dominicans (8). Their results suggested that HIV infection was more prevalent in Haiti than in the Dominican Republic, which shares the same island of Hispaniola.

Eight percent of sera obtained from 1037 adults bled during the first 6 months of 1986 by three commercial laboratories in Port-au-Prince were also positive for HIV antibody (Table 3) (4). The sera were not obtained for the purpose of HIV testing but rather for other tests and were "left over" after the recommended tests were performed. The health status of these persons was not known, but since none of the three laboratories perform HIV serologic tests, persons were not being bled for that purpose. These sera represent about 10% of the total number of persons bled for serum by the three laboratories during that period. Finally, we determined that 31% of 241 patients with active tuberculosis were HIV-seropositive, with higher rates in the urban patients (45%) than in the rural patients (15%) (Table 3). The seroprevalence in leprosy patients was lower (5%) than that in the normal adult population. The highest rates observed were in the Haitian prostitutes (53%). Collectively, these data indicate that HIV infection is widespread and more prevalent in urban areas and in lower socioeconomic groups.

III Modes of Transmission

In the United States, over 95% of non-Haitian AIDS patients report either homosexuality, transfusions, or IV drug abuse. In contrast, these risk factors have been reported in less than 15% of both Haitian-American and African patients. The initial observations in Haiti were largely retrospective and identified these factors in less than 20% of AIDS patients seen prior to 1983 (1). Prospective studies in 1983 identified potential risk factors in 74% of patients (Table 4) (9). We have subsequently documented a progressive *decrease* in the percentage of patients reporting bisexuality and blood transfusions, and an *increase* in those reporting a spouse with antecedent AIDS, a history of prostitution, or none of the aforementioned activities. In 1986, only 11% of the 170 male and female AIDS patients reported either bisexuality, blood transfusions, or IV drug abuse. Heterosexual transmission is assumed in the 16% of patients who were prostitutes or had a spouse with AIDS and is the most probable source of the infection in the patients reporting none of the aforementioned. Additional evidence for heterosexual transmission of HIV is the finding that 53% of 139 Haitian prostitutes in the Port-au-

Table 4 Risk Factors in Haitian AIDS Patients (%)[a]

	Year of AIDS diagnosis				
	1983	1984	1985	1986	Total
Bisexual	50	27	8	4	16
Transfusion	23	12	8	7	10
IVDA	<1	1	1	0	1
Heterosexual[b]	5	6	14	16	12
Undetermined	21	54	69	73	61

[a]The number of AIDS cases with complete risk factor data available by year: 1983, 53 patients; 1984, 103 patients; 1985, 131 patients; 1986, 170 patients.
[b]The category "heterosexual" includes persons who accepted money for sex (prostitutes) and persons whose spouse had a diagnosis of AIDS prior to the onset of their illness.

Prince area were seropositive. Prostitute contact among males was common and reported by 61% of the AIDS patients and 40% of their siblings and friends. Of the male sex partners of female AIDS patients, 50% also reported contact with prostitutes.

Another potential mode of transmission of HIV is through the use of contaminated needles. It is a common practice in Haiti for persons to obtain intramuscular injections when they are "not feeling well." The injections are frequently given for nonspecific symptoms (fatigue, malaise, and myalgias) without a specific etiological diagnosis. The injections may be given by either medical personnel or *piquristes* (injection givers). Disposable needles and syringes are not readily available in Haiti, so both may be reused without sterilization. During the 5-year period before the onset of AIDS symptoms, intramuscular medications were received by 83% of male and 88% of female AIDS patients (10). Injections were reported by 66% of male and 69% of female siblings and friends ($p < 0.001$ for the difference between AIDS patients and their siblings and friends). Despite the comparable injection rates, the seroprevalence of HIV was much lower in the female siblings and friends (9% versus 22%, Table 2), suggesting that factors other than intramuscular injections were responsible for HIV transmission. One of these may be the number of opposite sex partners. The female siblings and friends had a mean of 1 ± 1 sex partners per year during the preceding 5 years and an HIV seroprevalence rate of 9%, while the male siblings and friends had six or seven opposite sex partners annually and a seroprevalence of 22%. These conclusions are tentative, and further assessment of the role of injections in HIV transmission is needed.

Mosquitoes have been suggested as another potential mode of HIV transmission. *P. falciparum* infection is endemic in Haiti, with prevalence rates of 5 to 40% in some areas. We examined the relationships between the presence of antibody to HIV and *P. falciparum* in 154 persons: 112 were HIV seropositive and 22 were definitely positive by IFA for antibodies to *P. falciparum* (11). There was no correlation between the presence of antibody to HIV and malaria. We also have found that within the families of AIDS patients, children aged 5-13 years are almost invariably HIV-seronegative despite frequent transmission of dengue and malaria in the environment. These epidemiological and serologic data, together with the recent detailed studies by the CDC in Florida (12), provide no evidence for an arthropod vector of HIV.

IV. Clinical Features and Treatment

The physical appearance of an AIDS patients in Haiti is sufficiently characteristic that the term *maladi mor* has been applied—literally, "illness of death." This designation connotes the prognosis as well as the physical appearance, unlike the African description "slim disease" (see Chapter 2).

Most of the patients referred to our AIDS clinic for evaluation have little or no prior medical workup. Nonetheless, the syndrome is so easily recognized that only 16% of patients are subsequently found to be HIV-seronegative and to have conditions that appear to be unrelated to AIDS. We have devised a classification that has been useful in defining the spectrum of HIV infection in Haiti (13). Table 5 shows the classification of 339 patients referred to our AIDS clinic from July 1983 to June 1985 and their condition 1 year later. AIDS was previously diagnosed or was evident (lesions of Kaposi's sarcoma) in 11% of patients at their initial evaluation. All other patients

Table 5 Classification of HIV Infection in Haiti

	Number of patients (%)			
Groups	Initial evaluation		1-yr evaluation	
1. Asymptomatic	7	(2)	3	(1)
2. Prurigo	29	(9)	7	(2)
3. Adenopathy	7	(2)	1	(<1)
4. Oral thrush[a]	48	(14)	36	(11)
5. Weight loss and either fever or diarrhea[b]	209	(62)	27	(8)
6. AIDS	39	(11)	211	(62)
Dead	—	—	54	(16)

[a]Alone or with tuberculosis, salmonellosis, or *Herpes zoster* infection.
[b]For more than 2 months.

were placed in six groups based on their major symptoms or findings. The subjects in group 1 were asymptomatic and referred because of known exposure to HIV. Group 2 patients had intensely pruritic skin lesions (prurigo) alone, and those in group 3 had lymphadenopathy in at least two noncontiguous sites. Group 4 had oropharyngeal candidiasis, alone [21]* or with tuberculosis [18], salmonellosis [5], or *Herpes zoster* infection [4]. Weight loss in excess of 10% of body weight was the common finding in the patients in group 5 and was associated with either fever of diarrhea for ≥ 2 months. The principal difference between this classification and the provisional WHO clinical case definition is the inclusion of prurigo, diffuse lymphadenopathy, and oropharyngeal candidiasis as major signs that alone suggest AIDS in the absence of other know causes of immunosuppression (14). The validity of the classification is evident in the status of these patients when recategorized 1 year later. At the initial evaluation, 62% of the patients were in group 5 (weight loss and either fever or diarrhea), 14% had oropharyngeal candidiasis alone or with other infections, 11% had AIDS, and 11% had either prurigo or adenopathy. During the following year, 16% died, 62% had AIDS, and only 21% remained in the other groups.

The availability of HIV serologic testing futher refines this classification. There were only 66 patients referred to us during this period (July 1983 to June 1985) who were HIV-seronegative and had other diagnoses established: pulmonary tuberculosis [30], extrapulmonary tuberculosis [3], typhoid fever [4], hepatitis [2], giardiasis [2], ameobiasis [2], irritable bowel disease [4], pseudomembranous colitis [2], lichen planus [2], and 15 asymptomatic individuals. Twenty-five were either lost [14] or not followed [11].

The prevalence of the different opportunistic infections in AIDS patients in Haiti differs considerably from that seen in the United States. The frequency of infectious agents in Haitian AIDS patients is contrasted with the experience in the New York Hospital-Cornell Medical Center's first 80 AIDS patients (Table 6). Oroesophageal candidiasis (68%) and cryptosporidiosis (48%) were most common in Haiti, while *Pneumocystis carinii* pneumonia (71%) and cytomegalovirus infection (40%) were most common in New York.

Mycobacterial infections were common in both groups, but in New York they were predominately *M. avium-intracellulare* while in Haiti they were almost exclusively due to *M. tuberculosis.* The Haitians had either pulmonary tuberculosis (43%), miliary disease (23%), or tuberculous lymphadenitis (34%). Tuberculosis preceded full-blown AIDS in 25% of cases and occurred during the course of AIDS in 72%; only 3% of patients developed active tuberculosis after the diagnosis of AIDS was established. There was a difference in the type of tuberculosis depending on whether tuberculosis preceded AIDS or was diagnosed at the same time (within 2 months) of the diagnosis

---

*Brackets indicate number of patients.

Table 6 AIDS: Opportunistic Pathogens (%)[a]

Agents	Haiti	New York[b]
Candida	68	21
Cryptosporidium	48	11
Mycobacterium	31	25
Herpes virus	16	29
Isospora	16	<1
Cytomegalovirus	8	40
Toxoplasma	7	5
Pneumocystis	7	71
Salmonella	5	5
Cryptococcus	5	8
Aspergillus	2	6

[a]Data from 131 Haitian AIDS patients (1983-1984) and from 80 New York AIDS patients (1981-1983).
[b]Data from Ref. 17.

of AIDS. When tuberculosis preceded AIDS, 52% of cases had tuberculous lymphadenitis and 48% had pulmonary tuberculosis; there were no cases of disseminated tuberculosis. In contrast, when tuberculosis occurred at the same time as AIDS, 27% of cases had tuberculous lymphadenitis, 42% pulmonary tuberculosis, and 31% disseminated tuberculosis. This high percentage of tuberculous lymphadenitis seen in our patients, particularly when tuberculosis preceded AIDS (52%), is in marked contrast to the percentage of HIV-antibody-negative adult patients evaluated in a major tuberculosis clinic in Port-au-Prince (5%). Hence, Haitian adults with tuberculosis, particularly those with tuberculous lymphadenitis, should be investigated for HIV infection. A similar conclusion has been made for these patients in Africa (Chapter 2).

Over 95% of *M. tuberculosis* strains were sensitive to all antituberculous drugs including isoniazid (INH), and AIDS patients responded to therapy as promptly as did non-AIDS patients. Two drugs (INH and either rifampin or ethambutol) were as effective as all three drugs together. However, relapse following therapy in AIDS patients did occur, and the length of optimal therapy of tuberculosis in AIDS patients is unknown. Six of nine patients who had completed a 12-month course of treatment with either isoniazid and rifampin [4] or isoniazid, rifampin, and ethambutol [2] had recurrence of fever and night sweats within 2 months of stopping therapy. In two of six patients, tuberculosis was documented by liver biopsy; in all patients disappearance of fever was noted within 1 month of resuming treatment with the same antituberculous drugs.

Coccidial infections of the gastrointestinal tract occurred in 64% of Haitian AIDS patients (15). Cryptosporidia (48%) and *Isospora belli* (16%) were found only in patients with diarrhea and were not detected in the spouses and siblings of AIDS patients (14). The reservoir for these organisms and the modes of transmission are unknown. In all patients with isosporiasis, diarrhea stopped within 2 days of initiating treatment with oral trimethoprim-sulfamethoxazole. Recurrent symptomatic isosporiasis developed in 50% of the patients, but it also responded promptly to therapy with trimethoprim-sulfamethoxazole. We believe that an initial short course (1 to 2 weeks) of therapy, followed by prophylaxis for an indefinite period with either daily doses of trimethoprim-sulfamethoxazole or weekly doses of pyrimethamine-sulfadoxine may represent optimal management. Unlike isosporiasis, cryptosporidiosis did not respond to any of the therapeutic regimens employed.

Salmonella bacteremia occurred in 5% of Haitian AIDS patients. Surprisingly, all patients had *S. enteriditis* (91% group D, 9% group B); no strains of *S. typhi* were isolated. Salmonellosis was the first infection diagnosed in 61% of cases. *S. enteriditis* was the most common organism isolated from blood (92%) in AIDS and ARC patients presenting with fever, followed by *Escherichia coli* (8%). *S. enteriditis* was isolated six times more frequently during the dry season of the year when potable water is scarce. All isolates were sensitive to chloramphenicol, ampicillin, and Bactrim. All patients had resolution of fever within 48 hours of initiating therapy. There were no recurrences of bacteremia during a mean follow-up period of 6 months in patients who completed a 2-week course of either chloramphenicol, ampicillin, or Bactrim.

Another clinical manifestation of AIDS that is different in Haiti compared to the United States and Europe is the occurrence of intensely pruritic skin lesions (prurigo) for which neither specific etiological nor categorical diagnoses can be established (1,16) (Figure 1). Prurigo occurred in 50% of patients and was characterized by multiple, erythematous, round macules or papules 2 to 8 mm in diameter, which usually first appeared on the exterior surface of the arms but subsequently involved the legs, trunk, and face. The scalp, palms, and soles were not involved. These lesions were not present in the family members of AIDS patients unless they were also infected with HIV. Prurigo resembled insect bites but was unresponsive to all therapeutic regimens (antihistamines, phenothiazine, topical steroids, lindane) and usually persisted throughout the entire AIDS illness. Histologically, the usual pathological diagnosis was "dermal hypersensitivity reaction." There was no correlation between the occurrence of prurigo and either eosinophilia or serum IgE levels. An association with an unknown environmental factor was suggested by the disappearance of prurigo in three patients within 2 weeks of traveling to the United States. The prevalence of prurigo

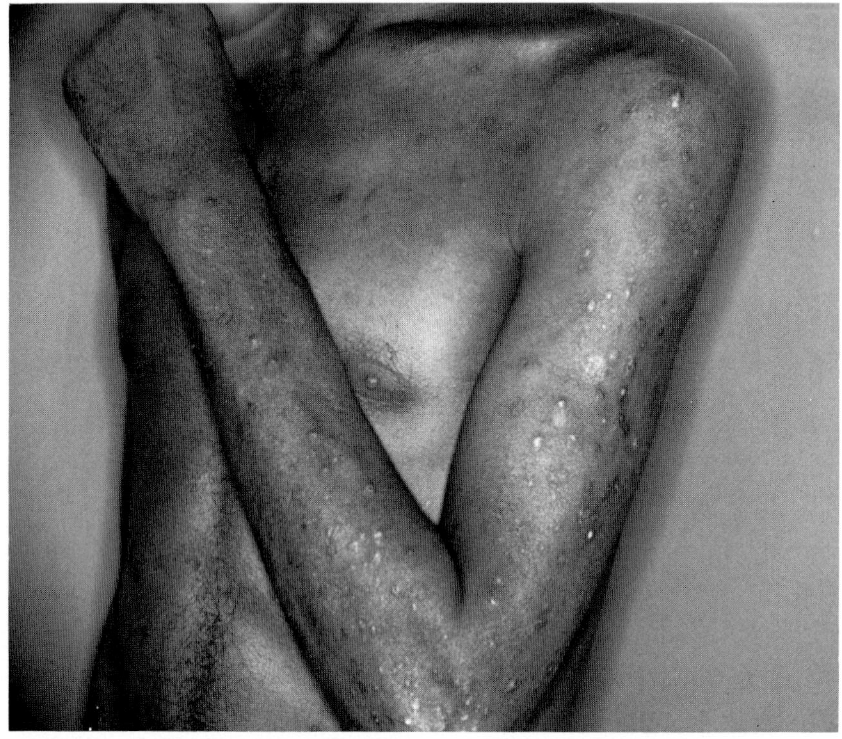

Figure 1 Haitian patient with prurigo.

was also much higher in patients living in tropical regions of Haiti (50%), as opposed to residents of temperature mountainous areas (6%). This condition is also often recognized in Africa (Chapter 2).

V. Summary

The first cases of AIDS in Haiti were recognized in 1978-1979, a period that coincides with the earliest reports of AIDS in the United States. Current data are consistent with the hypothesis that AIDS originated in Africa, came to the United States and Europe, and subsequently was introduced into Haiti by either tourists or returning Haitians. The seroprevalence of HIV among healthy sexually active adults in Port-au-Prince, Haiti, is approximately 10%. This rate of HIV infection is threefold that observed in rural areas. The highest prevalence rates were observed in female prostitutes (53%) and in the male and female spouses of AIDS patients (55%).

The types of opportunistic infections and the clinical course in Haitians with AIDS were similar in many respects to those in patients with AIDS in the United States. Important differences were noted in the prevalence of specific opportunistic pathogens in Haiti. It resembled observations on these infections in Africa.

During the past 4 years, there has been a progressive decrease in the percent of patients reporting bisexuality and blood transfusions, and an increase in those reporting either a spouse with antecedent AIDS, prostitution, or none of the aforementioned activities. In 1986, heterosexual transmission probably accounted for over 70% of AIDS cases.

Acknowledgment

This work was supported by grant AI 22624 from the U.S. Public Health Service.

References

1. Pape JW, Liautaud B, Thomas F, Mathurin JR, St. Amand MM, Boncy M, Pean V, Pamphile M, Laroche AC, Johnson WD Jr. Characteristics of the acquired immunodeficiency syndrome (AIDS) in Haiti. N Engl J Med 1983; 309:945-50.
2. Malebranche R, Arnoux E, Guerin JM, Pierre GD, Laroche AC, Pean-Guichard C, Elie R, Morisset PH, Spira T, Mandeville R, Drotman P, Seemayer T, Dupuy J-M. Acquired immunodeficiency syndrome with severe gastrointestinal manifestations in Haiti. Lancet 1983; 2:873-8.
3. Berggren WL, Ewbank DC, Berggren GG. Reduction of mortality in rural Haiti through a primary-health-care program. N Engl J Med 1981; 304:1324-30.

4. Pape JW, Stanback ME, Pamphile M, Verdier RI, Deschamps MM, Johnson WD Jr. Pattern of HIV infection in Haiti 1977-1986. III International Conference on Acquired Immunodeficiency Syndrome (AIDS), Washington, D.C., 1987.
5. Nahmias AJ, Weiss J, Yao X, Lee F, Kodsi R, Schanfield M, Matthews T, Bolognesi D, Durack D, Motulsky A, Kanki P, Essex M. Evidence for human infection with an HTLV III/LAV-like virus in Central Africa, 1959. Lancet 1986; 1:1279.
6. Quinn TC, Mann JM, Curran JW, Piot D. AIDS in Africa: an epidemiologic paradigm. Science 1986; 234:955-63.
7. Pape JW, Stanback M, Pamphile M, Boncy M, Deschamps MM, DeHovitz JA, Verdier R, Beaulieu ME, Lasseque A, Blattner W, Johnson WD Jr. Seroepidemiology of HIV in Haiti. Clin Res 1987: 35:329A.
8. Koenig RE, Pittaluga J, Bogart M, Castro M, Nunez F, Vilorio I, Delvillar L, Calzada M, Levy JA. Prevalence of antibodies to the human immunodeficiency virus in Dominicans and Haitians in the Dominican Republic. JAMA 1987; 257: 631-4.
9. Pape JW, Liautaud B, Thomas F, DeHovitz J, Deschamps MM, Verdier RI, Stanback ME, Johnson WD Jr. Changing patterns of AIDS epidemiology. Clin Res 1986; 34:528A.
10. Pape JW, Liautaud B, Thomas F, Mathurin JR, St. Amand MM, Boncy M, Pean V, Pamphile M, Laroche AC, DeHovitz J, Johnson WD Jr. The acquired immunodeficiency syndrome in Haiti. Ann Intern Med 1985; 103:674.
11. Johnson WD Jr, Stanback M, Howard R, Quakyi I, Pape JW. Malaria and HIV infection in Haiti. 27th Interscience Conference on Antimicrobial Agents and Chemotherapy, N.Y., 1987.
12. CDC. Acquired immunodeficiency syndrome (AIDS) in Western Palm Beach County, Florida. MMWR 1986; 35:609-12.
13. Pape JW, Deschamps MM, Kellie S, Verdier RI, Johnson WD Jr. Classification of HIV infection in the Third World (abstract). III International Conference on Acquired Immunodeficiency Syndrome (AIDS), Washington, D.C., 1987, p. 67.
14. CDC. Revision of the CDC surveillance case definition for acquired immunodeficiency syndrome. MMWR 1987; 36:15-155.
15. DeHovitz JA, Pape JW, Boncy M, Johnson WD Jr. Clinical manifestations and therapy of *Isospora belli* infection in patients with the acquired immunodeficiency syndrome. N Engl J Med 1986; 315:87-90.
16. Liautaud B, Pape JW, DeHovitz JA, Verdier RI, Deschamps MM, Johnson WD Jr. Malignant prurigo of AIDS (abstract). III International Conference on Acquired Immunodeficiency Syndrome (AIDS), Washington, D.C., 1987, p. 67.
17. Roberts RB, Murray HW, Rubin BY, Masur H. Opportunistic infections and impaired cell-mediated immune responses in patients with the acquired immune deficiency syndrome. Am Clin Climat Assoc 1983; 95:40-51.

4

AIDS and Hemophilia

Marion A. Koerper
School of Medicine
University of California
San Francisco, California

I. Introduction

Individuals with hemophilia require ongoing treatment with blood products throughout their lives; therefore they are exposed to the largest numbers of blood donors. Hemophiliacs have long been at risk for developing hepatitis B and non-A, non-B hepatitis, and thus it was no coincidence that the first cases of transfusion-associated acquired immunodeficiency syndrome (AIDS) were reported in hemophiliac patients.

Hemophilia is an inherited disorder of the clotting system which affects 20,000 individuals in the United States and 2 million people worldwide. Two main types are recognized. Hemophilia A, or classic hemophilia, in which factor VIII is the clotting protein that is missing or defective, accounts for 80% of all cases. Hemophilia B, or Christmas disease, in which factor IX is the missing or defective clotting protein, accounts for the remaining 20%. Both the genes for factor VIII and factor IX reside on the X chromosome; thus, 99% of all cases are male. The heterozygous female rarely may show a bleeding tendency. Three levels of severity are recognized based on clinical symptoms and the level of clotting factor in the blood: 1) Severely affected individuals have less than 1% of normal factor VIII or IX activity (normal

50-150%) and have bleeding into their joints or muscles once or twice weekly. 2) Moderately affected individuals have factor VIII or IX levels of 1-5% and bleed less often, perhaps once a month. 3) Mildly affected individuals have factor VIII or IX levels between 5 and 30% of normal and bleed infrequently, at most once or twice a year after severe trauma or surgery. The only way to stop or prevent these bleeding episodes is to transfuse the hemophiliac with blood or a blood product containing the missing clotting factor protein. Obviously the more severely affected patients require the largest quantities of this blood product.

II. Clotting Factors

Prior to 1965, hemophiliacs were transfused with whole blood or plasma in an attempt to stop bleeding. These products were not very effective because they contained the same amount of factor VIII or IX as found in normal plasma. The volume needed to raise the clotting factor level to normal was too large to give without risking heart failure from fluid overload. In 1965, *cryoprecipitate*, a preparation of factor VIII made from single volunteer donations of plasma by a quick freezing and slow-thawing procedure, was developed (1). These preparations, which contain five to six times the amount of factor VIII in plasma, were beneficial to individual patients to stop bleeding (2). Shortly thereafter, this technique was adapted to produce lyophilized factor VIII and IX *concentrates* commercially from large pools of plasma. These readily available concentrates containing 25 times the level of factor VIII or IX in normal plasma greatly helped to normalize the hemophiliac's coagulation system, stop or prevent bleeding, and prolong life (3,4).

In the first five years of concentrate usage, however, large numbers of hemophiliacs developed evidence of serum hepatitis. At one center, 38% of hemophilia A patients and 77% of hemophilia B patients had elevated serum transaminases, and 60% of hemophilia A patients and 70% of hemophilia B patients had antibodies to the hepatitis B virus surface antigen (HBsAb) (5). Statistics from another center documented a marked increase in the incidence of hepatitis B in hemophiliacs in 1973-1974, the years that commercial concentrates came into general use, and a 3% incidence of hepatitis B surface antigen (HBsAg) in their blood (6,7).

The explanation for this sudden increase in hepatitis B lies in the difference in numbers and types of plasma donations used to make cryoprecipitate and factor concentrates. Cryoprecipitate is made from volunteer donors; one donor unit of whole blood results in one bag (unit) of cryoprecipitate, and one treatment consists of 2-12 bags of cryoprecipitate. In contrast, commercial concentrates are prepared from plasma obtained from paid donors who often have no other source of income. These donors include a large number of intravenous (IV) drug users who are chronic carriers of hepatitis B. Each lot of concentrate is prepared from 1000-5000 or more of these paid plasma donations. In 1975 the U.S. Food and Drug Administration began to require the pharmaceutical companies to screen all donors for hepatitis B surface antigen and to reject plasma units that were found to be positive. With this procedure, the incidence of *acute* hepatitis B infection declined substantially. However, virtually all patients treated with commercial concentrates still developed antibodies to both hepatitis B surface antigen and core antigen (8). This observation indicated the continued presence of hepatitis B virus in the concentrates even though the donors tested negative for HBsAg. Presumably some HBsAg-negative donors are antihepatitis B *core* antigen positive and thus capable of transmitting the infectious virus.

III. Hepatitis in Hemophiliacs

The introduction of hepatitis B vaccine in 1982 has eliminated the risk of post-transfusion infection with this form of hepatitis. However, non-A, non-B hepatitis is also transmitted by lyophilized factor concentrates (9, 20), so that the possible development of chronic liver disease remains a threat for hemophiliacs. In a recent study of hemophiliacs infused with concentrate for the first time, 76% developed non-A, non-B hepatitis as evidenced by a more than 2.5-fold increase in aspartate aminotransferase (AST) and alanine aminotransferase (ALT) levels after six exposure-days (8). Moreover, non-A, non-B infection causes persistent elevation of these liver enzymes, suggesting continuous liver destruction. One hemophilia center has followed 78 patients every six months and performed percutaneous liver biopsies on 34 of 56 that had elevated AST and ALT values for more than 6 months. Of the 34, four had cirrhosis. Ten others with chronic persistent or chronic active hepatitis were rebiopsied two to eight years later; five more had progressed to cirrhosis and two of the other five to chronic active hepatitis (11). Thus, 72% developed non-A, non-B hepatitis, and 11% progressed to cirrhosis in eight years; another 6% had persistently abnormal biopsies, some with progression from chronic persistent to chronic active hepatitis. These findings indicate that non-A, non-B hepatitis is not the benign disease it was once thought to be when studied in individuals with single exposures. Repeated exposure in hemophiliacs to the causative agent(s) appears to result in progressive destruction of hepatocytes and eventually end-stage liver disease (11).

IV. Development of AIDS

The occurrence of AIDS in hemophiliacs was the first indication that, like hepatitis B and non-A, non-B hepatitis, the etiological agent could be transmitted via blood transfusions and blood products. The first three hemophiliacs with AIDS were reported by the Centers for Disease Control (CDC) in July 1982 (12). Now, five and one half years later, 552 hemophiliacs have developed the disease, and 326 have died. Of these 552, 281 have no risk

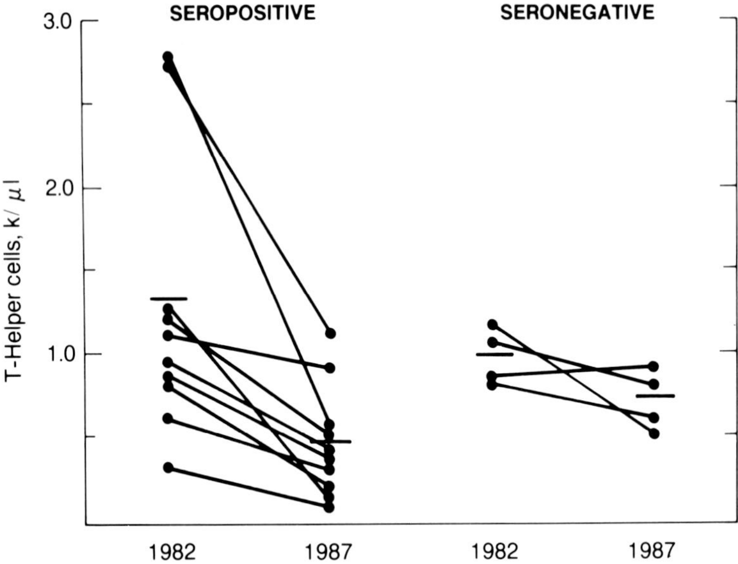

Figure 1 Changes in absolute T-helper cell counts in 10 HIV-positive hemophiliacs from 1982 to 1987, compared with 4 seronegative hemophiliacs.

factors other than the receipt of commercially prepared clotting factor concentrates. Of those remaining, 223 received blood transfusions, 31 are homosexual, 12 are IV drug abusers, and 5 have had heterosexual contact with a person in a high-risk group (13,79). Ninety-five percent have hemophilia A.

The age range of hemophiliacs with AIDS is 3-81 years, with a median age of 34 years. Compared with a median age of 25 for all hemophiliacs (14), this observation indicates that older hemophiliacs are more susceptible to the disease. This fact may reflect lifetime exposure to a greater number of units of concentrate, higher incidence of inflammatory joint disease, greater incidence of chronic hepatitis, and immunological attrition with advancing age.

At least 43 states of residence have been reported for hemophiliacs with AIDS. In fact, the first occurrence of AIDS cases in many of these states was in hemophiliacs (15). This observation supports the conclusion that the mode of spread of the disease in hemophiliacs is via the factor concentrates, which are manufactured in a few locations in the country and then distributed nationwide. It is not primarily through sexual encounters, blood transfusions, or intravenous drug abuse.

The disease is particularly virulent in hemophiliacs, with the vast majority having either *Pneumocystis carinii* pneumonia (69%) or other opportunistic infections (25%). Only five hemophiliacs have had Kaposi's sarcoma, and 15 have had lymphoma. The interval from diagnosis of AIDS to death is quite short, with a median of one month (16). This time period is one of the shortest for known populations at risk for developing AIDS (see Chapter 1).

In Europe, as of September 30, 1985, there were 52 cases of AIDS among hemophiliacs living in West Germany (21 cases), Spain (12), Great Britian (9), France (3), Sweden (2), Austria (1), Denmark (1), Greece (1), Italy (1), and Norway (1). One German hemophiliac with AIDS was also homosexual and an IV drug abuser. The majority of these patients had received factor VIII and IX concentrates manufactured in the United States (17).

V. Prevalence of Anti-HIV Antibodies and Infectious Virus

The development of a test to measure the presence of antibody to the AIDS retrovirus occurred in 1984, after the human immunodeficiency virus (HIV) had been isolated and identified (18-20). We have been regularly surveying our hemophiliac population for the presence of antibodies to HIV by a sensitive immunofluorescence assay (21). We found that, in 1982, 80% of our heavily treated patients were seropositive, and that by 1984, 100% were positive (Table 1). These results indicated that most patients had already been infected by HIV by the time the first cases of AIDS in hemophiliacs were being reported (22). Other investigators with serum repositories extending back to 1978 have shown that the majority of seroconversions in hemophiliacs occurred between 1980 and 1982 (23-25). Patients treated with factor IX concentrates showed a lag time in acquisition of infection; the majority occurred between 1982 and 1984 (25). This finding may explain the relatively fewer cases of AIDS in hemophilia B patients compared to hemophilia A patients. Alternatively, there may be differences in processing techniques that eliminate HIV from the factor IX products. Also, patients with hemophilia B

Table 1 Prevalence of Antibody to Human Immunodeficiency Virus (HIV) in Hemophiliacs Treated at UCSF

		No. anti-HIV positive/total tested				
Blood product	Units/kg/ year	1982	1984	1985	1986	1987
Factor VIII	>300	12/15	28/28	37/37	43/43	43/43
concentrate	<300	0/2	2/4	2/4	2/4	2/6
Factor IX	>300	0/0	6/8	7/10	8/11	9/12
concentrate	<300	0/3	3/13	3/15	3/15	3/17
Cryoprecipitate	>300	0/2	4/7			
	<300	0/3	0/10			

Prevalence of antibody to HIV in patients with hemophilia treated with large or small amounts of factor VIII and IX concentrates and cryoprecipitate. In October 1984, all patients were switched to heat-treated factor VIII and IX concentrates (60° or 68° for 72-77 hours).

have milder disease than those with hemophilia A and are therefore exposed to less blood product.

In European countries, varying prevalences of seropositivity were reported depending on whether patients were treated with factor concentrates manufactured in the United States or from locally obtained plasma. Seropositivity rates for countries using American products include Denmark 64% (26), Germany 53% (27), France 67-79% (28), England 54% (29), Spain 68-73.5% (30,31). Some of these centers reported a lower rate of seropositivity for hemophilia B patients using American concentrate: United Kingdom 6.3% (32) or Spain 50% (31). In comparison, countries that produce their own factor have lower prevalences of seropositivity: Belgium 6.5% (28) and Scotland 15.6% (33).*

The presence of antibodies to HIV in hemophiliacs' blood does not necessarily indicate that these individuals have received infectious virus from factor concentrates. It is possible that they have merely been exposed to inactive viral particles that were antigenic; therefore, they could have been immunized rather than infected. This possibility is being examined by following antibody titers over time in this risk group. If no infection has occurred, the antibody titer should decrease, and no virus should be present in the blood.

We have cultured peripheral blood mononuclear cells (PMC) from 35 individuals including 32 with hemophilia A or B, two wives, and one child of a hemophiliac. Infectious virus was recovered from 55% of our asymptomatic, HIV antibody-positive patients. This observation suggests that transmission of infectious virus has occurred readily via the factor concentrates (34). Other groups have also reported the ability to recover HIV from peripheral blood mononuclear cells of hemophiliacs with AIDS (19,35). Gomperts et al. (36) in 1985 recovered HIV from 6 of 19 (32%) seropositive children with hemophilia, five of whom had lymphadenopathy. Andrews et al. (81) cultured virus from 16 of 66 (24%) seropositive hemophiliacs; three of 16 culture-positive patients developed AIDS and two ARC within 18 months.

VI. Immunological Abnormalities in Hemophilia

Immunological abnormalities are not part of the inherited disorder of hemophilia. Prior to the July 1982 report of the occurrence of AIDS in three persons with hemophilia (12), no detailed observations of immunodeficiency in this population were published. However, at least one multicenter cooperative study from 1975 to 1979 of 1551 hemophiliacs documented that 9.3% had lymphocytopenia and 5.0% had thrombocytopenia on entry, well before the disease AIDS had been recognized in any patient group. These ab-

*In South Africa, two of 39 children with hemophilia were found to be seropositive, for a low overall rate of 5.4% (80); however, the two seropositive children had received imported concentrate, whereas 35 of 36 seronegative children had received only locally prepared concentrate.

normalities were found to be correlated with the degree of liver disease in these patients (37).

After the recognition of AIDS, numerous studies have documented immunologic abnormalities in otherwise healthy, asymptomatic, potentially HIV-seropositive hemophiliacs. These disorders include decreased total T-cell number, decreased T-helper cells, increased T-suppressor cells, and decreased helper/suppressor ratio (38-40). These abnormalities are more pronounced in patients treated with lyophilized factor concentrates than in those treated with cryoprecipitate (41-45). In a study of 10 HIV-positive hemophiliacs followed by us for five years, marked decreases in T-cell number was observed over time (Figure 1).

In one study the differences in T-cells were also more pronounced in patients receiving higher compared with lower amounts of lyophilized concentrates (46). Other investigators, however, did not find such a difference (42, 45, 48). All these observations most likely reflect relative exposure to HIV.

Other immunological abnormalities reported in presumed HIV-seropositive hemophiliacs include increased immunoglobulins (39, 40, 42, 46, 49), decreased concanavalin A response (41, 49), and decreased pokeweed mitogen response (46, 49). These results are also more pronounced in the groups treated with concentrate as compared with cryoprecipitate (41). In contrast, the mixed lymphocyte culture response was normal in all patient groups studied regardless of the type of therapy (44-45). Additional immune disorders included increased β_2-microglobulin serum levels (49) and decreased PMC response to interleukin 2 (50). Kessler et al. (49) also reported an inverse relationship between serum thymosin α_1 level and the helper/suppressor ratio.

Two studies have shown results of serial immunological studies in patients. Goldsmith et al. (40) found no significant change in helper cells, suppressor cells, or helper/suppressor ratio in 30 of 35 patients restudied 8-14 months after initial evaluation. In contrast, de Shazo et al. (51) found a significant increase in the helper/suppressor ratio on followup examination. It was due to a decrease in suppressor cells in the clinically symptomatic group. In all other groups there was no change in helper cells, suppressor cells, or helper/suppressor ratio. All 30 patients showed lower responses to phytohemagglutinin on repeat testing 6-12 months later (51).

Ludlam et al. (52) in Scotland followed a group of 33 patients with hemophilia A treated with the same lot of concentrate prepared from Scottish donors in 1983, when there were no reported cases of AIDS in Scotland. Fifteen of the patients seroconverted, whereas the other 18 did not. Those individuals who seroconverted had lower T-helper cells and helper/suppressor ratios prior to exposure to the implicated lot of concentrate and also used more vials of the infected lot as well as more total units of factor VIII per year (52). This finding suggested that the hemophiliacs who became infected were those who already had an altered immune system due to receipt of large quantities of factor VIII concentrate alone. The exposure to blood products *per se* appeared to induce an immunological abnormality in these patients that could have made them susceptible to infection with the AIDS virus. However, the hepatitis status of these patients was not discussed. Of note, 10 additional patients received factor IX concentrate made from the same plasma source and none of them seroconverted. This finding suggests that the infectious virus was retained in the cryoprecipitate from which the factor VIII concentrate was made. An alternative explanation is that the hemophilia B patients, who had normal T-helper cells prior to exposure to the infected lot, used fewer vials of that lot and fewer total vials per year.

VII. HIV Transmission to Other Individuals

A. Sexual Partners

Individuals with hemophilia also provided early evidence that the AIDS virus can be spread by heterosexual contact. At least 16 wives with AIDS have been reported (53,54,79). Three sexual partners with generalized lymphadenopathy and decreased helper/suppressor ratio have also been observed (54-56). Moreover, two surveys of large numbers of HIV antibody-positive hemophiliacs and their wives or sexual partners have demonstrated a seroconversion rate in the spouses and sexual partners of 9.5% (54, 57). Several groups have looked at the helper/suppressor ratios of spouses and sexual partners of hemophiliacs (48, 58-60). They have found depressed T-helper/suppressor ratios in none to 16.7% of spouses. When only the spouses of hemophiliacs with depressed ratios were considered, 0-25% had depressed ratios.

One group reported the transient presence of HIV-antibody and mildly decreased T-helper cells in the wife of an HIV antibody-positive hemophiliac with lymphadenopathy syndrome (61). The month after discovery of their antibody positivity, the hemophiliac developed AIDS, and sexual activity between the couple ceased. The following month the wife was HIV antibody negative, and her T-helper cell number was normal. Six months later she was still antibody negative with a normal level of T-helper cells (61). The inference is that discontinuance of exposure to semen allowed her to eliminate the virus and return to a normal status. Whether she was exposed only to HIV antigen was not determined. This phenomenon has not been documented in other sexual partners.

B. Children

Children of hemophiliacs are at risk of becoming infected with HIV in utero or perinatally if the wives are HIV-seropositive. Hilgartner (62) conducted a survey of American hemophilia centers regarding children born to wives of hemophiliacs between 1979 and 1985. Of 530 such children reported, two had AIDS, one had ARC, one had failure to thrive, and two had leukemia. Thus only 0.6% had symptoms of HIV infection, a much lower rate than one would predict. The explanation may lie in the relatively low incidence of seropositivity in wives of hemophiliacs (see above). Nevertheless, the number with leukemia is greater than one would predict (incidence = 1 in 2800 in the general population). Whether this phenomenon is another manifestation of HIV infection is unknown, as these children were not tested for antibody to HIV.

In separate reports, two HIV antibody-negative children of HIV-positive hemophiliacs have been identified: one child with AIDS (63) and the other with AIDS-related complex (ARC) (34). In both cases the mother was also HIV antibody positive, and both children became symptomatic within the first year of life. This observation suggests transmission from the infected mother at a time when the immune system of the fetus had not developed. Another child has been reported who was seropositive and had lymphadenopathy syndrome and recurrent infections beginning at four months of age (64,82). Both his hemophiliac father, who had ARC, and his mother, who had lymphadenopathy syndrome, were also seropositive. In this same study, two siblings born to seropositive asymptomatic parents were seronegative, as were five other children born to seronegative wives of seropositive hemophiliacs (64). These findings confirm observations in other risk groups that maternal transmission of HIV does not occur 100% of the time.

C. Household Contacts

Other reports have documented only antibody-negative children born to mothers of seropositive hemophiliacs (54,65). Siblings, parents, and grandparents residing in the household of HIV-positive hemophiliacs have not been found to be HIV antibody-positive, even when these individuals have helped the hemophiliac with home infusion of factor concentrates (54,58, 65). Children residing in a boarding school in France with seropositive hemophiliacs have not seroconverted to HIV over a 3-year period of observation (83). These findings imply that casual household contact is not a route of transmission of HIV infection.

VIII. Protection with Heat-Treated Products

In December 1982, Dolana and associates (66) of Hyland Laboratories reported that heat treatment of factor VIII concentrate greatly reduced the risk of hepatitis B and non-A, non-B infection. While their method did not entirely eradicate hepatitis infection, it did suggest a method for eliminating HIV infection from concentrates. In 1984, Levy, working in conjunction with Mozen and Mitra of Cutter Laboratories, reported on the effect of heat on a mouse type C retrovirus (67). The mouse virus was added to pooled plasma in a concentration of 10^8 infectious particles (IP)/ml. Preparation of cryoprecipitate from the plasma reduced the viral titer to $10^{7.2}$ IP/ml. Two different methods of heating were then employed. In the first, the liquid containing virus was heated at 56 °C for 12 h and sampled hourly for presence of virus. After less than 1 h, no infectious virus could be detected; this observation indicated the sensitivity of retroviruses to heating in the liquid state. In the second procedure, the cryoprecipitated factor VIII was lyophilized, reducing the viral titer to $10^{4.8}$ IP/ml. The lyophilized concentrate plus virus was then heated at 68°C for 96 h, with aliquots removed for assay as 12-h intervals. Infectious virus was still detectable in decreasing amounts up to 72 h. This finding indicated the extent of resistance to heating of retroviruses in the lyophilized state (67).

In subsequent studies (68), the same group added HIV to plasma in a concentration of 10^4 IP/ml, and the cryoprecipitate was made. An aliquot was heated in the liquid state at 60 °C for 10 h, and no infectious virus could be recovered. The remaining cryoprecipitate was concentrated, lyophilized, and heated in the dry state at 68 °C for 72 h, with aliquots removed at 10-12-h intervals to assay for presence of the virus. Infectious viral particles were detected through 34 h of heating but were no longer detected after 48 h (Table 2) (68). These studies on both the mouse and human retroviruses indicated the resistance of this family of viruses to inactivation by clotting factor concentration and their relative resistance to inactivation by heating. Other workers also reported on the efficacy of heating HIV in the wet and dry state as a method of inactivating the virus (69-72).

In the United States, the four principal manufacturers of factor VIII and IX concentrates each chose a different time and temperature for heating their products (Table 3). One company, Alpha Therapeutic Co., claimed to use a "wet" heating process that required only a short time for viral inactivation (see above). In reality, their product was lyophilized and then aerosolized in the liquid detergent Heptene during heating; the virus was therefore not in a true liquid state during the heating process. As can be seen by comparing Table 2 with Table 3, only one company, Cutter Biological, heats at the same temperature and for the same length of time as was shown to be effective in the experiments with retroviruses (67, 68). It is unknown, therefore, if some infectious virus might still remain when a lower temperature (60°C) and heating for shorter periods of time (20-30 h) are employed. There have now been reports of seroconversions in patients receiving the products of Armour Pharmaceutical Co. (73, 74) and Alpha Therapeutic Co. (75). In addition, three other seroconversions in pediatric patients using three different products have been reported, but the manufacturers were not identified (76). Armour Pharmaceutical Co. has recently released a product that is heated at 60 °C for 10 h in the true liquid state (pasteurized) (77). This product, as expected, has not transmitted HIV. Cutter Biological has also released a product pasteurized in the same manner.

Table 2 Heat Inactivation of HIV:Recovery of HIV After Addition to Plasma and Subsequent Production of Lyophilized Concentrate

	Infectious particles/ml
Plasma + HIV	10^4
Concentrate solution (liquid)	10^4
Heat 60°	
10 h	No virus
Lyophilized concentrate (dry)	$10^{2.8}$
Heat 68°	
24 h	$10^{0.3}$
34 h	$10^{0.1}$
48 h	No virus

Source: Ref. 68.

Heat-treated products were first made generally available by the manufacturers between 1983 and 1985; however, these first heated products were made from plasma that had not been pretested for antibodies to HIV. Compulsory testing of all plasma collected for concentrate preparation began in May 1985. Since the time from collection to finished product may take up to one year, the above reported seroconversions could be explained by patients receiving less than optimally heated products made from plasma not pretested for HIV antibody. Recently, there have been no reported cases of seroconversion in patients receiving only antibody-tested, heat-treated product (76).

In the near future, more highly purified factor VIII and IX products will become available. These include products separated on column using a monoclonal antibody as well as recombinant DNA-productd factor VIII and IX. The latter should totally eliminate the transmission of any viral illnesses via commercial clotting factor concentrates.

Table 3 Conditions Under Which Each American Manufacturer Heats Its Factor VIII and Factor IX Concentrate Products

Manufacturer	Process	Temperature (°C)	Time (h)
Alpha	Wet	60	20
Armour	Dry	60	30
Hyland	Dry	60	72
Cutter	Dry	68	72-77

Table 4 Prevalence of Antibody to HIV in Hemophiliacs: Lack of Seroconversion in Hemophiliacs Treated Exclusively with Heat-Treated Factor VIII or IX Concentrate (60° or 68° for 72-77 Hours)

		No. anti-HIV-positive/total tested		
Blood product	Units/kg/year	1985	1986	1987
Heat-treated	>300	0/5	0/14	0/17
concentrate	<300	0/11	0/15	0/22

IX. Conclusion

In our hemophilia center, it was the practice prior to October 1984 to treat all newly diagnosed hemophilia A patients and all those with mild disease who were hepatitis B surface antibody negative with cryoprecipitate until they developed antibodies to hepatitis B. This procedure eliminated acute infection and the chronic carrier state for hepatitis B. In July 1982, Heptavac became available, and we immunized all of our patients who had not yet developed HBsAb. Meanwhile, we were following the status of HIV infections. In January 1985, we found that four of seven patients heavily treated with cryoprecipitate had seroconverted (22). At this point heat-treated factor VIII and IX concentrates were being produced by all four pharmaceutical companies, and we switched our patients not already on heat-treated concentrate to the Cutter and Hyland products. In two and a half years of use of these products exclusively we have seen no further seroconversions (Table 4). This finding documents the efficacy of these heat-treating methods in eradicating infectious HIV from factor concentrates (78).

The high prevalence of anti-HIV antibodies in hemophiliacs and the known median incubation period of HIV infection of over five to seven years suggest that there will be more cases of AIDS in this group in the next several years. Whether the rate of development of the disease in hemophiliacs will differ from other risk groups remains to be determined. Certainly, if some patients received HIV antigen alone, the incidence of disease will be lower. Moreover, the use of exclusively heat-treated, serotested blood products will protect newly diagnosed patients from becoming infected.

References

1. Pool JG, Shannon AE. Production of high-potency concentrates of antihemophilic globulin in a closed-bag system. Assay in vitro and in vivo. N Engl J Med 1965; 273:1443-7.
2. Abildgaard CF, Simone JV, Corrigan JJ, Seeler RA, Edelstein G, Vanderheiden J, Schulman I. Treatment of hemophilia with glycine-precipitated factor VIII. N Engl J Med 1966; 275:471-5.
3. Dallman PR, Pool JG. Treatment of hemophilia with factor VIII concentrates. N Engl J Med 1968;278:199-202.

4. Hoag MS, Johnson FF, Robinson JA, Aggeler PM. Treatment of hemophilia B with a new clotting-factor concentrate. N Engl J Med 1969; 280:581-6.
5. Hilgartner MW, Giardina P. Liver dysfunction in patients with hemophilia A, B, and von Willebrand's disease. Transfusion 1977; 17:495-9.
6. Biggs R. Jaundice and antibodies directed against factors VIII and IX in patients treated for haemophilia or Christmas disease in the United Kingdom. Br J Haematol 1974; 26:313-29.
7. Biggs R, Spooner R. Haemophilia treatment in the United Kingdom from 1969 to 1974. Br J Haematol 1977; 35:487-504.
8. Morfini M, Rafanelli D, Longo G, Messori A, Rossi Ferrini P. Hepatitis-free interval after clotting factor therapy in first infused haemophiliacs. Thromb Haemost 1986; 56:268-70.
9. Craske J, Dilling N, Stern D. An outbreak of hepatitis associated with intravenous injection of factor-VIII concentrate. Lancet 1975; 2:221-3.
10. Fletcher ML, Trowell JM, Craske J, Pavier K, Rizza CR. Non-A non-B hepatitis after transfusion of factor VIII in infrequently treated patients. Br Med J 1983; 287:1754-7.
11. Hay CRM, Preston FE, Triger DR, Underwood JCE. Progressive liver disease in haemophilia: an understated problem? Lancet 1985; 1:1495-8.
12. Centers for Disease Control. *Pneumocystis carinii* pneumonia among persons with hemophilia A. MMWR 1982; 31:365-7.
13. Centers for Disease Control. Surveillance of hemophilia-associated acquired immunodeficiency syndrome. MMWR 1986; 35:669-71.
14. Levine, P. Personal communication 1986.
15. Centers for Disease Control. Update on acquired immunodeficiency syndrome (AIDS) among patients with hemophilia A. MMWR 1982; 31:644-52.
16. Centers for Disease Control. AIDS weekly surveillance report—United States. January 4, 1987. 1-5.
17. Centers for Disease Control. Update: acquired immunodeficiency syndrome—Europe. MMWR 1986; 35:35-46.
18. Barré-Sinoussi F, Chermann JC, Rey F, Nugeyre MT, Chamaret S, Gruest J, Dauguet C, Axler-Blin C, Vézinet-Brun F, Rouzioux C, Rozenbaum W, Montagnier L. Isolation of a T-lymphotropic retrovirus from a patient at risk for acquired immunodeficiency syndrome (AIDS). Science 1983; 220:868-71.
19. Popovic M, Sarngadharan MG, Read E, Gallo RC. Detection, isolation, and continuous production of cytopathic retroviruses (HTLV-III) from patients with AIDS and pre-AIDS. Science 1984; 224:497-500.
20. Levy JA, Hoffman AD, Kramer SM, Landis JA, Shimabukuro JM, Oshiro LS. Isolation of lymphocytopathic retroviruses from San Francisco patients with AIDS. Science 1984; 225:840-2.
21. Kaminsky LS, McHugh T, Stites D, Volberding P, Henle G, Henle W, Levy JA. High prevalence of antibodies to acquired immune deficiency syndrome (AIDS)-associated retrovirus (ARV) in AIDS and related conditions but not in other disease states. Proc Natl Acad Sci USA 1985; 82:5535-9.
22. Koerper MA, Kaminsky LS, Levy JA. Differential prevalence of antibody to AIDS-associated retrovirus in haemophiliacs treated with factor VIII concentrate versus cryoprecipitate: recovery of infectious virus. Lancet 1985; 1:275.

23. Evatt BL, Gomperts ED, McDougal JS, Ramsey RB. Coincidental appearance of LAV/HTLV-III antibodies in hemophiliacs and the onset of the AIDS epidemic. N Engl J Med 1985; 312:483-6.
24. Eyster ME, Goedert JJ, Sarngadharan MG, Weiss SH, Gallo RC, Blattner WA. Development and early natural history of HTLV-III antibodies in persons with hemophilia. JAMA 1985; 253:2219-23.
25. Ragni MV, Tegtmeier GE, Levy JA, Kaminsky LS, Lewis JH, Spero JA, Bontempo FA, Handwerk-Leber C, Bayer WL, Zimmerman DH, Britz JA. AIDS retrovirus antibodies in hemophiliacs treated with factor VIII or factor IX concentrates, cryoprecipitate or fresh frozen plasma: prevalence, seroconversion rate, and clinical correlations. Blood 1986; 67:592-5.
26. Melbye M, Biggar RJ, Chermann JC, Montagnier L, Stenbjerg S, Ebbesen P. High prevalence of lymphadenopathy virus (LAV) in European haemophiliacs. Lancet 1984; 2:40-1.
27. Gürther LG, Wernicke D, Eberle J, Zoulek G, Deinhardt F, Schramm W. Increase in prevalence of anti-HTLV-III in haemophiliacs. Lancet 1984; 2:1275-6.
28. Rouzioux C, Vézinet-Brun F, Couroucé AM, Gazengel C, Vergoz D, Desmyter J, Vermylen J, Vermylen C, Klatzmann D, Geroldi D, Barreau C, Barré-Sinoussi F, Chermann JC, Christol D, Montagnier L. Immunoglobulin G antibodies to lymphadenopathy-associated virus in differently treated French and Belgian hemophiliacs. Ann Intern Med 1985; 102:476-9.
29. Moffat EH, Bloom AL, Mortimer PP. HTLV-III antibody status and immunological abnormalities in haemophilia patients. Lancet 1985; 1:935.
30. Kitchen L, Leal M, Wichmann I, Lissen E, Ollero M, Allan JS, McLane MF, Essex M. Antibodies to human T-cell leukemia virus type III in hemophiliacs from Spain. Blood 1985; 66:1473-5.
31. Baselga JM, Buti M, Esteban R, Tusell J, Vila M, Guardia J. HTLV-III antibodies and Christmas disease. Lancet 1986; 1:1033.
32. Duncombe AS, Savidge GF, Craske J. HTLV-III related illness and Christmas disease. Lancet 1986; 1:447-8.
33. Melbye M, Froebel KS, Madhok R, Biggar RJ, Sarin PS, Stenbjerg S, Lowe GDO, Forbes CD, Goedert JJ, Gallo RC, Ebbesen P. HTLV-III seropositivity in European haemophiliacs exposed to factor VIII concentrate imported from the USA. Lancet 1984; 2:1444-6.
34. Koerper MA, Levy JA. Prevalence of antibodies to AIDS-associated retrovirus (ARV) and recovery of infectious virus from hemophiliacs in San Francisco. Presented at Second International Conference on AIDS, Paris, June 23-25, 1986.
35. Vilmer E, Barré-Sinoussi F, Rouzioux C, Gazengel C, Vézinet-Brun F, Dauguet C, Fischer A, Manigne P, Chermann JC, Griscelli C, Montagnier L. Isolation of new lymphotropic retrovirus from two siblings with haemophilia B, one with AIDS. Lancet 1984; 1:753-7.
36. Gomperts ED, Feorino P, Evatt BL, Warfield D, Miller R, McDougal JS. LAV/HTLV III presence in peripheral blood lymphocytes of seropositive young hemophiliacs. Blood 1985; 65:1549-52.
37. Eyster ME, Whitehurst DA, Catalano PM, McMillan CW, Goodnight SH, Kasper CK, Gill JC, Aledort LM, Hilgartner MW, Levine PH, Edson JR, Hathaway WE,

Lusher JM, Gill FM, Poole WK, Shapiro SS. Long-term follow-up of hemophiliacs with lymphocytopenia or thrombocytopenia. Blood 1985; 66:1317-20.
38. Goldsmith JC, Moseley PL, Monick M, Brady M, Hunninghake GW. T-lymphocyte subpopulation abnormalities in apparently healthy patients with hemophilia. Ann Intern Med 1983; 98:294-6.
39. Luban NLC, Kelleher JF Jr, Reaman GH. Altered distribution of T-lymphocyte subpopulation in children and adolescents with haemophilia. Lancet 1983; 1:503-5.
40. Goldsmith JM, Kalish SB, Green D, Chmiel JS, Wallemark CB, Phair JP. Sequential clinical and immunologic abnormalities in hemophiliacs. Arch Intern Med 1985; 145:431-4.
41. Lederman MM, Ratnoff OD, Scillian JJ, Jones PK, Schacter B. Impaired cell-mediated immunity in patients with classic hemophilia. N Engl J Med 1983; 308:79-83.
42. Menitove JE, Aster RH, Casper JT, Lauer SJ, Gottschall JL, Williams JE, Gill JC, Wheeler DV, Piaskowski V, Kirchner P, Montgomery RR. T-lymphocyte subpopulations in patients with classic hemophilia treated with cryoprecipitate and lyophilized concentrates. N Engl J Med 1983; 308:83-6.
43. Gill JC, Menitove JE, Wheeler D, Aster RH, Montgomery RR. Generalized lymphadenopathy and T cell abnormalities in hemophilia A. J Pediatr 1983; 103:18-22.
44. Weintrub PS, Koerper MA, Addiego JE Jr, Drew WL, Lennette ET, Miner R, Cowan MJ, Ammann AJ. Immunologic abnormalities in patients with hemophilia A. J Pediatr 1983; 103:692-5.
45. Gjerset GF, Martin PJ, Counts RB, Fast LD, Hansen JA. Immunologic status of hemophilia patients treated with cryoprecipitate or lyophilized concentrate. Blood 1984; 64:715-20.
46. Unzeitig JC, Church JA, Gomperts ED, Nye CA, Pasquale S, Richards W. Abnormal T-cell subsets and mitogen responses in hemophiliacs exposed to factor concentrate. Am J Dis Child 1984; 138:645-8.
47. Saidi P, Kim HC, Raska K Jr. T-cell subsets in hemophilia. N Engl J Med 1983; 308:1291-2.
48. deShazo RD, Andes WA, Nordberg J, Newton J, Daul C, Bozelka B. An immunologic evaluation of hemophiliac patients and their wives: relationships to the acquired immunodeficiency syndrome. Ann Intern Med 1983; 99:159-64.
49. Kessler CM, Schulof RS, Alabaster O, Goldstein AL, Naylor PH, Phillips TM, Luban NLC, Kelleher JF, Reaman GH. Inverse correlation between age related abnormalities of T-cell immunity and circulating thymosin α_1 levels in haemophilia A. Br J Haematol 1984; 58:325-36.
50. Weintrub PS, Koerper MA, Addiego JE Jr, Levy JA, Ammann AJ. Interleukin production and response to interleukin in patients with hemophilia A. Submitted for publication.
51. deShazo RD, Daul CB, Andes WA, Bozelka BE. A longitudinal immunologic evaluation of hemophiliac patients. Blood 1985; 66:993-8.
52. Ludlam CA, Tucker J, Steel CM, Tedder RS, Cheingsong-Popov R, Weiss RA, McClelland DBL, Philip I, Prescott RJ. Human T-lymphotropic virus type III (HTLV-III) infection in seronegative haemophiliacs after transfusion of factor VIII. Lancet 1985; 2:233-6.

53. Pitchenik AE, Shafron RD, Glasser RM, Spira TJ. The acquired immunodeficiency syndrome in the wife of a hemophiliac. Ann Intern Med 1984; 100:62-5.
54. Jason JM, McDougal JS, Dixon G, Lawrence DN, Kennedy MS, Hilgartner M, Aledort L, Evatt BL. HTLV-III/LAV antibody and immune status of household contacts and sexual partners of persons with hemophilia. JAMA 1986; 255:212-5.
55. Ratnoff OD, Lederman MM, Jenkins J. Lymphadenopathy in a hemophiliac patient and his sexual partner. Ann Intern Med 1984; 100:915.
56. Melbye M, Ingerslev J, Biggar RJ, Alexander S, Sarin PS, Goedert JJ, Zachariae E, Ebbesen P, Stenbjerg S. Anal intercourse as a possible factor in heterosexual transmission of HTLV-III to spouses of hemophiliacs. N Engl J Med 1985; 312:857.
57. Kreiss JK, Kitchen LW, Prince HE, Kasper CK, Essex M. Antibody to human T-lymphotropic virus type III in wives of hemophiliacs: evidence for heterosexual transmission. Ann Intern Med 1985; 102:623-6.
58. Ragni MV, Bontempo FA, Lewis JH, Spero JA, Rabin BS. An immunologic study of spouses and siblings of asymptomatic hemophiliacs. Blood 1983; 62:1297-9.
59. Pabinger-Fasching I, Lechner K, Bettelheim P, Niessner H, Köller U, Knapp W. T-cell subsets in female sexual partners of asymptomatic hemophiliacs. Thromb Haemost 1984; 51:135.
60. Kreiss JK, Kasper CK, Fahey JL, Weaver M, Visscher BR, Stewart JA, Lawrence DN. Nontransmission of T-cell subset abnormalities from hemophiliacs to their spouses. JAMA 1984; 251:1450-4.
61. Burger H, Weiser B, Robinson WS, Lifson J, Engleman E, Rouzioux C, Brun-Vézinet F, Barré-Sinoussi F, Montagnier L, Chermann JC. Transient antibody to lymphadenopathy-associated virus/human T-lymphotropic virus type III and T-lymphocyte abnormalities in the wife of a man who developed the acquired immunodeficiency syndrome. Ann Intern Med 1985; 103:545-7.
62. Hilgartner MW. Low risk of HIV infection in children of men with hemophilia. N Engl J Med 1986; 315:969.
63. Ragni MV, Urbach AH, Kiernan S, Stambouli J, Cohen B, Rabin BS, Winkelstein A, Gartner JC, Zitelli BZ, Malatack JJ, Bontempo FA, Spero JA, Lewis JH. Acquired immunodeficiency syndrome in the child of a haemophiliac. Lancet 1985; 1:133-5.
64. Ragni MV, Spero JA, Bontempo FA, Lewis JH. Recurrent infections and lymphadenopathy in the child of a hemophiliac: a survey of children of hemophiliacs positive for human immunodeficiency virus antibody. Ann Intern Med 1986; 105:886-7.
65. Lawrence DN, Jason JM, Bouhasin JD, McDougal JS, Knutsen AP, Evatt BL, Joist JH. HTLV-III/LAV antibody status of spouses and household contacts assisting in home infusion of hemophilia patients. Blood 1985; 66:703-5.
66. Dolana G, Tse D, Thomas W, Kingdon HS. Hepatitis risk reduction in hemophilia; a heated factor VIII preparation. Blood 1982; 60 (Suppl 1):210a.
67. Levy JA, Mitra G, Mozen MM. Recovery and inactivation of infectious retroviruses added to factor VIII concentrates. Lancet 1984; 2:722-3.
68. Levy JA, Mitra GA, Wong MF, Mozen MM. Inactivation by wet and dry heat of AIDS-associated retroviruses during factor VIII purification from plasma. Lancet 1985; 1:1456-7.

69. Spire B, Dormont D, Barré-Sinoussi F, Montagnier L, Chermann JC. Inactivation of lymphadenopathy-associated virus by heat, gamma rays, and ultraviolet light. Lancet 1985; 1:188-9.
70. Martin LS, McDougal JS, Loskoski SL. Disinfection and inactivation of the human T lymphotropic virus type III/lymphadenopathy-associated virus. J Infect Dis 1985; 152:400-3.
71. Petricciani JC, McDougal JS, Evatt BL. Case for concluding that heat-treated, licensed anti-haemophilic factor is free from HTLV-III. Lancet 1985; 2:890-1.
72. McDougal JS, Martin LS, Cort SP, Mozen M, Heldebrant CM, Evatt BL. Thermal inactivation of the acquired immunodeficiency syndrome virus, human T lymphotropic virus-III/lymphadenopathy-associated virus, with special reference to anti-hemophilic factor. J Clin Invest 1985; 76:875-7.
73. White GC, Matthews TJ, Weinhold KJ, Haynes BF, Cromartie HL, McMillan CW, Bolognesi DP. HTLV-III seroconversion associated with heat-treated factor VIII concentrate. Lancet 1986; 1:611-2.
74. van den Berg W, ten Cate JW, Breederveld C, Goudsmit J. Seroconversion to HTLV-III in haemophiliac given heat-treated factor VIII concentrate. Lancet 1986; 1:803-4.
75. Dietrich S. Personal communication. 1987.
76. Centers for Disease Control. Survey of non-U.S. hemophilia treatment centers for HIV seroconversions following therapy with heat-treated factor concentrates. MMWR 1987; 36:121-4.
77. Schimpf K, Mannucci PM, Kreutz W, Brackmann HH, Auerswald G, Ciavarella N, Mösseler J, DeRosa V, Kraus B, Brueckmann C, Mancuso G, Mittler U, Haschke F, Morfini M. Absence of hepatitis after treatment with a pasteurized factor VIII concentrate in patients with hemophilia and no previous transfusions. N Engl J Med 1987; 316:918-22.
78. Koerper MA, Levy JA. Clinical observations on HIV seropositive hemophiliacs after four and a half years of followup and efficacy of heat-treated products. Presented at Third International Conference on AIDS, Washington DC, June 1-5, 1987.
79. Centers for Disease Control. AIDS weekly surveillance report—United States, January 18, 1988:1-5.
80. Nicholson NA, Karabus CD, Beatty DW, Becker WB. Immunological studies in haemophilic children. S Afr Med J 1987; 71:567-9.
81. Andrews CA, Sullivan JL, Brettler DB, Brewster FE, Forsberg AD, Scesney S, Levine PH. Isolation of human immunodeficiency virus from hemophiliacs: correlation with clinical symptoms and immunologic abnormalities. J Pediatr 1987; 111:672-7.
82. Regni MV, Urbach AH, Taylor S, Claassen D, Gupta P, Lewis JH, Ho DD, Shaw GM. Isolation of human immunodeficiency virus and detection of HIV DNA sequences in the brain of an ELISA antibody-negative child with acquired immune deficiency syndrome and progressive encephalopathy. J Pediatr 1987; 110:892-4.
83. Berthier A, Chamaret S, Fauchet R, Fonlupt J, Genetet N, Gueguen M, Pommereuil M, Ruffault A, Montagnier L. Transmissibility of human immunodeficiency virus in haemophilic and non-haemophilic children living in a private school in France. Lancet 1986; 2:598-601.

5

AIDS in Transfusion Recipients

Herbert A. Perkins

Irwin Memorial Blood Bank
of the San Francisco Medical Society
and School of Medicine
University of California
San Francisco, California

I. Evidence That AIDS Is Transmitted by Blood Transfusion

The first report from the Centers of Disease Control indicating the existence of multiple cases of acquired immunodeficiency syndrome (AIDS) with no obvious risk factor other than a history of blood transfusion was published in January 1984 (1). Convincing evidence that a virus was responsible for AIDS became accepted later in 1984 (2-4). Until the publication of these reports, there was still much disagreement as to whether AIDS was an infectious disease and, if so, whether it was caused by a single previously unrecognized virus. The concept that it resulted from intense repetitive stimulation of the immune system had considerable support.

Despite these controversies, the possibility that it was an infectious disease, one in which the responsible agent might be present in blood collected for transfusion, had to be considered from the time that AIDS was first recognized as a clinical entity. The populations at primary risk for AIDS (homosexually active males and drug addicts) also have a high frequency of infection with hepatitis viruses, viruses known to be transmitted by blood transfusion. The report in July 1982 of AIDS in three hemophiliacs (5) provided

Table 1 Evidence That AIDS Is Transmitted by Blood Transfusion

AIDS occurs in populations that have a high incidence of infections known to be transmitted by blood transfusion.
The vast majority of hemophiliacs treated with clotting factor concentrates manufactured from pooled human plasma have antibody as evidence of exposure to the AIDS virus (30). Nearly 1% of AIDS cases have occurred in hemophiliacs.
Over 1200 cases of AIDS reported to the Centers for Diseases Control have acknowledged no risk factors other than blood transfusion.
Blood recipients who develop AIDS have almost always received blood from at least one donor who has developed AIDS, has antibody to AIDS virus in his serum, acknowledges membership in an AIDS risk group, or has an abnormally low ratio of T-lymphocyte helper/suppressor cells (8).
AIDS virus has been cultured from 88% of donors identified as the probable cause of AIDS in a blood recipient (9).

support for the possibility that AIDS could be transmitted by a blood product, but the likelihood that it resulted from the immune stimulation of repeated intravenous infusions of foreign and denatured proteins still remained. The recognition by our group in December 1982 of an apparent case of AIDS in an infant who had received a blood component from a donor who later developed AIDS (6,7), however, led blood banks and governmental agencies to act on the assumption that AIDS was caused by an infectious agent which could be transmitted by blood transfusion.

There is now no reason to doubt that AIDS can be transmitted by blood transfusion (Table 1). The 1121 cases of AIDS reported to the Centers for Disease Control (CDC) as of December 28, 1987 have no acknowledged risk factors other than a history of blood transfusion. Moreover, investigation of the donors who provided the components transfused into the patients who later developed AIDS almost always identifies a high-risk individual (8). In our own studies of the first 25 cases of transfusion-associated AIDS in the San Francisco area, 7 received blood from a donor who later developed AIDS, 11 had an indentifiable high-risk donor, and the other cases have donors whom we were not able to contact. The most convincing evidence for transmission of AIDS by transfusion comes from a CDC study in which 25 suspected donors to transfusion-associated AIDS cases were recalled for study, and the AIDS retrovirus was cultured from the blood of 22 of them (88%) (9).

II. Incidence of Transfusion-Associated AIDS

The reports to the CDC of transfusion-associated AIDS (TAA) as of December 28, 1987 totaled 1121. These cases received their transfusions between

1977 and 1985. Since approximately 3,000,000 patients are transfused in this country every year, that number represents roughly one case of AIDS for every 20,000 transfused. Additional cases of TAA transfused during those years can be expected to be reported in the future, since it is now clear that the incubation period can be at least as long as seven years (10). The risk to recipients obviously varied greatly during this period. The frequency of infection in the involved segments of the community was increasing steadily (11), but blood banks began to take steps in the beginning of 1983 to eliminate donors from high-risk groups.

The Irwin Memorial Blood Bank has its headquarters in San Francisco, which has the highest per capita incidence of AIDS of any major city in the United States. As of November 25, 1987, 75 cases of TAA had been reported in which the blood came from Irwin; an additional 191 recipients were anti-HIV-positive. Two-thirds of these patients had been transfused before 1983, before recognition that AIDS might be transmitted by blood transfusion. One-third, however, was transfused after December 1982 when the first steps to eliminate donors from high-risk groups were initiated. The small number of cases whose transfusions were in recent years may be an effect only of the shorter period of observation. The best estimate of the incubation period from transfusion to the diagnosis of AIDS results in a mean of 4.5 years (12).

III. Reducing Risk of Transfusion-Associated AIDS

A. Self-Exclusion of High-Risk Donors (Table 2)

The first official recommendations for decreasing the risk of TAA were listed in a January 13, 1983 statement issued jointly by the three national blood bank organizations in the United States (13). This statement called upon blood banks to include in their donor screening process specific questions to detect possible AIDS or exposure to patients with AIDS and to avoid recruitment of groups that might have a high incidence of AIDS.

On March 24, 1983 the U.S. Food and Drug Administration (FDA) (14) defined the groups at risk for AIDS who should not donate blood: "persons with symptoms and signs suggestive of AIDS, sexually active homosexual or bisexual men with *multiple* partners (emphasis added), Haitian entrants to the United States, present or past users of intravenous drugs (already excluded) and sexual partners of individuals at increased risk of AIDS." They also recommended that individual donors be educated about AIDS risk as part of the screening procedure. The American Association of Blood Banks (AABB) supplemented this last recommendation with the requirement that every prospective blood donor be provided with the necessary information in writing.

Table 2 Methods Used for Self-Exclusion of High-Risk Donors

Education of risk groups
Information sheet for prospective donors that outlines risk factors for being infected with the AIDS virus
Medical history questions related to AIDS
Certification by donor that he/she is eligible based on the information sheet and a truthful medical history
Opportunities to inform blood banks that the blood donated should not be transfused:
Telephone call back
Confidential questionnaire

On September 3, 1985 the FDA (12) further narrowed the definition of eligible donors by recommending exclusion of all men who had sexual contact with another male since 1977.

The definition of who might donate blood thus became progressively more restrictive as new information was obtained. Exclusion was still up to the donor himself; if he failed to tell the truth, the blood bank would have no way of knowing it. The self-exclusion policies, however, were based on intensive educational activities in the homosexual communities, as well as the information sheet for donors that details explicitly who should not donate. This information sheet is required reading for all blood donors before they can be accepted. Self-exclusion policies have eliminated almost all high-risk donors, but it is now apparent that they are not totally effective. Since the routine testing of donor blood for antibody to the AIDS virus began, most of the antibody-positive donors (66% in our experience) have admitted previous high-risk activities and should not have donated. They often do not considered themselves to be homosexual or even bisexual and did not believe they could be at risk for AIDS.

Changes in the donor medical history questions also began in January 1983 (13,14). The donor history now asks about possible intimate sexual contacts with AIDS cases, as well as signs or symptoms which could be a manifestation of infection with the AIDS virus: e.g., purple spots on the skin, white spots in the mouth, enlarged lymph nodes, unexplained weight loss, chronic diarrhea, chronic cough. The donor then has to certify in writing that he gave a truthful history.

Recognition that these voluntary procedures might not be sufficient came with anecdotes of people who continued to donate because they had always been regular donors and were afraid that cessation of donation might lead to a suspicion that they were homosexual, a fact that they strongly wished to keep secret. Two approaches have been used by blood banks to give such donors a confidential means to notify the blood bank that the blood they donated should not be transfused. One approach is to give every donor a receipt that contains a message with a telephone number to call as soon as he or she leaves the blood bank; the note tells the donor that the blood will be discarded and no questions will be asked. The donor need only give the number assigned to the donation, not a name. The second approach, pioneered by the New York Blood Center (16), provides the donor with a second confidential questionnaire with the donation number but not his name. The questionnaire requires all donors to check one of two statements: (1) "My blood may be used for transfusion." or (2) "My blood should only be used for studies." Some blood banks do this with bar code labels applied to the medical history form by each donor in a privacy booth. These labels can be read only by a light pen attached to a computer. Many blood banks use both the call-back and the confidential questionnaire.

B. Autologous Donation

Another approach to providing safer blood is to allow the patient to donate his own blood prior to an elective procedure. The logic behind this procedure has been recognized for many years. Homologous blood carries the risk of serious side effects varying from the transmission of infectious agents to the reactions caused by mismatched red blood cells, white cells, platelets, and plasma proteins. Autologous blood avoids all of those problems. The arrival of AIDS has called the public's attention to the advantages of autologous donations, but AIDS should not be the major impetus to autologous donation. Its occurrence is rare when compared with the reported 10% incidence of posttransfusion hepatitis (17) and its better than 50% chance of resulting in chronic liver disease (18). Of those with liver disease who are biopsied, 10-20% have evidence of cirrhosis, and deaths from the late sequelae of posttransfusion hepatitis are undoubtedly far more common than from posttransfusion AIDS.

C. Designated Donors

Permitting patients to designate relatives or friends as their blood donors is a far more widely requested but less logical approach (Table 3). The three national blood bank organizations went on record as opposed to designated donations for very good reasons.

First, widespread use of designated donors threatens the adequacy of the national blood supply. Anecdotal evidence indicates that, where designated donors are permitted, some previously regular donors no longer give because they are reserving themselves in case they are needed by a relative or friend. The magnitude of this donor loss and of the extent to which it contributes to the reduced rate of blood donation in this country in the past few years is impossible to estimate.

Table 3 Designated (Directed) Donors

Argument against	Argument for
Threatens the blood supply. Donors may reserve themselves for relatives or friends.	Brings new donors to the blood bank.
Logistic confusion, with increased chance for errors.	Hysterical patients cannot be convinced their family and friends are not safer donors than the average.
Increases legal liability for blood bank, hospital, and physician if designated components are misdirected.	Resisting pleas for designated donors waste time and risks loss of patients to an area where they are accepted.
Occasional designated donors are clearly less safe than the average.	The average designated donor is not different from the usual volunteer donor.

Secondly, extensive use of designated donors creates logistic confusion as large numbers of components are saved for specific patients. Extraordinary care must be taken to be certain that such units are available for the designated recipient where and when needed. The resulting confusion increases the chance for errors, and clerical errors are the primary cause of transfusion reactions resulting from the administration of incompatible blood.

A third argument against the use of designated donors is the fear that such donors could be less safe than the usual altruistic volunteers. It seems reasonable to assume that homosexually active men who wish to keep their sexual orientation a secret will be likely to donate blood for transfusion when urged to give for a relative or friend. Without such difficult-to-resist pressures, they could discreetly stay away from the blood bank. A more dangerous donor than usual would also be likely to respond to the confused patient in our area who put up a notice in a local store offering to pay strangers who would donate blood. Routine blood donors are unpaid volunteers who donate for altruistic reasons.

Despite these examples, designated donors are neither better nor worse than the usual blood bank donor on the average. In our experience with our first 10,000 designated donations, the frequency of abnormal laboratory tests (serological test for syphilis, hepatitis B surface antigen, antibody to hepatitis B core antigen, and antibody to the human immunodeficiency virus (HIV) is not significantly different from that found with our routine blood donors (19).

The arguments presented above against the use of designated donors have no influence on the hysterical patient who cannot be convinced that his family will not provide safer donors than those available through the blood bank. Physician pressures to permit designated donations have been prompted by the hours lost trying to convince patients that such donations were not accepted and were not necessary, and by the patients lost to other physicians working in areas where such donations were permitted. At the time of this writing, the majority of blood banks in this country have bowed to these pressures and accept designated donations. In some states, laws require them to do so.

D. Surrogate Tests

At a meeting called in January 1983 by the Centers for Disease Control (within weeks of the first reported case of possible transfusion-associated AIDS), participants suggested that blood banks in high-risk areas investigate the feasibility of surrogate tests. These were, by definition, not specific for AIDS but were positive in a high proportion of populations at risk for AIDS and, at the same time, positive in an acceptably small proportion of normal blood donors (Table 4). They suggested that the test for antibody to hepatitis B core antigen (anti-HBc) might be suitable because of the high frequency of positive results among healthy homosexually active males. Studies carried out in the next few months in San Francisco and New York showed that 6-7% of blood donors would be lost with the use of this test. This loss was a significant threat to the blood supply but one which seemed within the capacity of the blood banks to replace. However, New York studies compared the frequency of abnormal results in donors who stated that their blood could be used for transfusion with those who said it should be used only for laboratory studies. Their results indicated that none of the tests the CDC had suggested distinguish between those two groups (16). The frequency of abnormal results was minimally higher among those who said their blood should not be transfused, and results were normal in the vast majority of both groups.

Table 4 Surrogate Tests

	Percent abnormal		
Test	Controls	Homo-bisexuals	AIDS
Helper/suppressor ratio	3.1	19.7	77.4
No. lymphocytes/ml	~5.0	12.1	69.6
Anti-HBc	~5.0	79.2	88.2
Anti-HBs	~5.0	79.5	81.9
Immune complexes	1.6	62.5	77.8

Abbreviations: anti-HBc, antibody to hepatitis B core antigen; anti-HBs, antibody to hepatitis B surface antigen.
Source: CDC data presented in January 1983.

Attention was next directed to other surrogate tests such as thymosin α_1 (20), acid-labile α interferon (21), β-microglobulin (22), and neopterin (23). The evidence on these tests was still incomplete when the availability of a specific test for the AIDS virus was announced.

Despite the above indicated inadequacies, surrogate tests for AIDS were introduced into a number of blood banks in the San Francisco Bay area prior to the availability of the test for antibody to the AIDS retrovirus. The Stanford University Blood Bank was the first to introduce such a test—in June 1983. They chose to do a T-lymphocyte helper/suppressor ratio on all of their own blood donors in view of the recognized association of a low ratio with AIDS. They chose this test because they had it in routine operation in their research laboratory. One year later, the Irwin Memorial Blood Bank and other blood banks in the San Francisco area began routine testing of all donors with anti-HBc as a surrogate test for AIDS. Anti-HBc was chosen in preference to the helper/suppressor ratio employed by Stanford because it was abnormal in a much higher proportion of risk group members (Table 4), was available commercially, and was much more likely to produce reproducible and standardized results.

Irwin's decision to do a surrogate test for AIDS virus infection occurred, not because of new evidence that it could discriminate between high-risk and normal donors, but as a response to community pressure to do something, and also because of several incidents that proved that education and information would never make self-exclusion completely successful as a means of eliminating high-risk donors. Several donors were encountered who had answered all donor history questions so as to be accepted, but later admitted that they had had homosexual experiences. These donors had not thought they were lying at the time of their medical history. They had convinced themselves that they could not possibly be at risk for AIDS—a form of psychological denial for self-protection. Such donors have been widely recognized since the test for anti-HIV has become available (24).

Irwin concluded at the time that these donors were first encountered that only an arbitrary objective test would prevent transfusing their blood, and elected to use the anti-HBc test with the full recognition that almost everyone it rejected was not from an AIDS risk group. The loss of 6% of its donors was accepted in hopes of preventing a few more cases of TAA. Shortly after initiation of the anti-HBc test in the San Francisco area, the announcement was made that the cause of AIDS had been found and that a specific test would be available to blood banks within six months. Further expansion of surrogate tests for AIDS did not occur. After the test for anti-HIV became available, it became apparent that the test for anti-HBc excluded 37% of donors with Western blot-confirmed antibody to the AIDS virus (Irwin Memorial Blood Bank data, unpublished).

E. Specific Test for AIDS

With unprecedented speed, a test to detect antibody to HIV was developed, licensed by the U.S. Food and Drug Administration, and made available to blood banks in a few weeks less than one year after the recognition that HIV causes AIDS. The test method, designed for the mass screening needs of blood banks, was an enzyme-linked immunosorbent assay (ELISA) test in which a solid surface is coated with a semipurified extract of the virus grown in tissue culture in a susceptible line of cells. Test serum is incubated with the viral antigens to permit attachment of specific antibody. The amount of antibody found is then quantitated by adding anti-human globulin tagged with an enzyme. Each incubation step is followed by thorough washing to remove unbound antibody. A substrate is then added which turns color in proportion to the amount of antibody-tagged enzyme remaining bound to the solid surface. The color is quantitated by optical density in a spectrophotometer. The end point, or optical density cutoff, that separates positives from negatives is set arbitrarily by the manufacturer (with FDA approval) after inspection of results of large numbers of tests on patients with AIDS, with AIDS related-complex (ARC), and normal controls.

The licensed tests made available to blood banks have a very low cutoff (in the range of twice the optical density of the mean negative control) in a deliberate attempt to make the test as sensitive as possible in the hopes that no AIDS virus carriers will be missed. When applied to known cases of AIDS or ARC, these ELISA tests proved to be highly sensitive and specific (25). It was correctly anticipated, however, that a high degree of nonspecificity would occur when the test was applied to the normal blood donor population. False-positive results could be anticipated among the millions of tests done on blood donors each year and would be prominent in comparison with the expected very low incidence of AIDS carriers remaining in the blood donor population.

As experience accumulated in the blood banks, it became apparent that the vast majority of ELISA-positive blood donor tests were false positives. The majority of initial reactive tests were not reproducible. In most of these instances the optical density was very close to the cutoff, being just over the cutoff the first time and just under it on repetition. This lack of reproducibility led to the recommendation by the FDA that all initial reactives should be retested in duplicate. The sample should be considered positive only if one or both of the repeat tests was reactive (26).

False-positive ELISA tests

The frequency of positive (repeatedly reactive or RR) blood donors initially averaged 3.4 per 1,000 in the United States (27), with remarkably little difference between areas where AIDS is relatively common and those where few or no AIDS cases have been seen. This uniformity in frequency resulted from the fact that the vast majority of ELISA positives were false positives. The cause of these false-positive reactions, at least in part, was antibodies directed against surface antigens of the cells in the line used to grow the virus. The first five tests to be licensed used the H9 cell line and the HTLV-III virus supplied by the National Cancer Institute. That cell line is known to express the HLA antigen DR4, and sera with anti-DR4 (and other related HLA antibodies) usually gave a reactive ELISA test result (28). Other antibodies to cell surface antigens, such as autoantibodies, may explain additional false-positive reactions. Thus, the viral extracts used as targets in the first-generation tests for antibody to the AIDS virus appear to have been contaminated with antigens intrinsic to the cell line in which the virus is grown.

The purification techniques used by the five manufacturers to prepare the targets varied and have subsequently been changed to decrease the occurence of false-positive reactions. One licensed ELISA test uses the lymphadenopathy-associated virus (LAV strain of HIV) grown in the CEM cell line which does not appear to express HLA antigens.

Tests should be available shortly in which there is very little possibility of false positives caused by contaminating cellular antigens, since the viral proteins will be individually produced by genetic engineering techniques. Such preparations, however, still leave the possibility of a positive reaction caused by natural antibodies in some individuals that cross-react with AIDS virus proteins even though these antibodies were not stimulated by the AIDS virus itself. It is hoped that an appropriate pattern of responses to different viral proteins will prove to be specific.

F. Confirmatory Tests

Until tests that are very specific are available, blood banks generally have relied on the results of a separate confirmatory test to distinguish true from false positives. The favored confirmatory test is the Western blot. This procedure differs from the ELISA screening test primarily in the fact that the viral proteins have first been separated by size by electrophoresis on sodium dodecyl sulfate agar gel and then blotted onto nitrocellulose strips. These strips are exposed to test serum, and then to labeled antiglobulin as in the ELISA screening test. The antiglobulin may be tagged with an enzyme or a radioisotope. Antibody to the AIDS virus reacts with a characteristic series of viral proteins (the gp160 envelope protein with its gp120 and gp41 breakdown products; the p55 and the p25 *gag* protein and others). Ninety percent of the time the true-positive reactions clearly demonstrate multiple bands in the expected areas. Unfortunately 5-10% of Western blot results are still equivocal.

The significance of a weak band in the p25 area only is particularly difficult to interpret since it may be the only evidence of AIDS antibody but also could result from non-HIV-related cross-reacting antibody.

Another test useful for confirmation that agrees very closely with the Western blot is the immunofluorescence assay (IFA) (29). Here the test serum is exposed to a slide containing a cell line infected with AIDS virus mixed 1:1 with uninfected cells. After exposure to fluorescein-tagged antiglobulin, the slide is inspected under an ultraviolet microscope. The pattern of fluorescence in the cells and the absence of stain in uninfected cells is highly specific to the experienced eye.

One further confirmatory test, with relatively little published information, is the radioimmune precipitation (RIP) test. Test serum is incubated with tagged viral proteins and then electrophoresed as in the Western blot. The RIP test works best at detecting antibody to the high molecular weight, highly immunogenic envelope proteins gp160 and gp120.

The first evidence confirming the ability of the Western blot to discriminate true-positive from false-positive reactions in a blood donor population was obtained in a study done by the Centers for Disease Control and the Atlanta Red Cross (30). For a period of approximately six months all consenting ELISA-positive blood donors at the Atlanta Red Cross were referred to the CDC for interview and for an attempt to culture AIDS virus from their lymphocytes. The most significant finding was that strongly ELISA positives (with an optical density at least six times mean negative control) were almost always Western blot or culture positive (86.7%), in contrast to moderately and weakly reactive specimens (1.9%). Virus could not be cultured from 50 samples that were ELISA negative nor from 227 samples that were ELISA reactive on an initial test but nonreactive in two further repeats with the same sample. The conclusion was that strongly ELISA positives are likely to be true positives and that the majority of antibody producers are carrying virus.

IV. The Antibody-positive Individual

Based on the above results, many public health clinics have reported antibody results from the ELISA results only, but require a positive/negative optical density ratio of at least seven to consider a test positive. Blood banks, requiring a test as sensitive as possible, abide by the much lower cutoff specified by the manufacturer. Any unit with a repeatedly positive ELISA reaction is discarded (regardless of the result of any further confirmatory tests) and some blood banks even go to the extreme of discarding a donation based on an initial reactive result. Most blood banks have a Western blot test done on all positive ELISAs, and tell the donors they have antibody to the AIDS virus only if the Western blot confirms that fact. Such Western blot-positive donors should be told that they most probably can infect others and should take appropriate precautions (31).

A. Informing Donors with False-Positive Reactions

Initially blood banks focused on the problem of donors whose ELISA-positive tests were confirmed by Western blot. Blood from ELISA-positive donors not confirmed by Western blot was discarded, but those donors were not informed because of uncertainty as to what the results meant. Within months, however, large numbers of ELISA-positive, Western blot-negative donors were returning to give again, and were being accepted with the full knowledge of the blood banks that the units would be discarded. Blood banks are now facing the fact that they may have to tell their ELISA-positive, Western blot-negative donors their test results. It is not fair to let these donors waste their time and undergo the minor discomforts and risks of blood donation on the mistaken assumption that they are doing something useful. It is wrong to let such donors assume all previous tests have been normal, since they have been permitted to return. It must be acknowledged, nonetheless, that this group is a particularly difficult one to inform. The donor has to be told that the result is believed to be a false positive, but that a guarantee that it is false cannot be given. Further studies on such blood donors, especially large-scale viral cultures and subsequent antibody testing, are under way to provide more definitive information for them.

B. The True Positive

When the test was first introduced, the initial frequency of Western blot confirmed antibody to HIV among American blood donors averaged about 1 in 4000, varying from about 1 in 1000 in high-incidence areas to no confirmed positives in many small blood banks in low-incidence areas. An urgent question that immediately arose was "Who are these antibody-positive blood donors?" Do they represent the first clear evidence of widespread extension of the infection into the heterosexual community or a failure of the self-exclusion process? The evidence from all sites is clearly for the latter explanation. The antibody-positive donors are largely from the recognized AIDS risk groups. The vast majority will admit to homosexual contacts; regretably a few of the donors had been transfused in the past seven years.

Why did these antibody-positive donors lie when their medical history was taken? According to them, they did not realize nor believe that they had given false information. They were certain they could not be ar risk for AIDS.

In our experience many were primarily heterosexual in orientation or had been exposed to few partners whom they knew well, but there were others who were exclusively homosexual and admitted to multiple partners. Either these donors had not read the information they were presented before donation or they were unable to accept it. They appear to have set up an unconscious psychological protection that allowed them to deny the risk of AIDS. In any case, the final result indicates that self-exclusion of high-risk donors was not completely effective.

We should not, however, belittle the usefulness of the self-exclusion procedure. Unquestionably these procedures did remove almost all high-risk donors. They unquestionably reduced the chance of transmitting AIDS by blood transfusion to far below what it would have been in the absence of the self-exclusion precedures.

V. The False Negatives

The self-exclusion procedures remain in effect at the present time despite the routine use of the test for antibody to HIV. The need for continuing self-exclusion policies is dictated by the possibility of false-negative ELISA screening tests. When an individual is infected with the AIDS virus, it may take six to eight weeks before antibody appears, and in some cases possibly longer (see Chapter 8). (Overt AIDS, of course, may take years to manifest itself.) The virus is present from the time of exposure, even in the absence of antibody. Evidence that an antibody-negative blood donor may transmit HIV to a recipient before the donor turns antibody positive has been presented (32).

VI. The Current Risk of AIDS from Blood Transfusions

The possibility of false-negative ELISA tests bring us to the ultimate question of how safe is the blood supply now? Currently licensed tests detect over 99% of patients with AIDS (25). It is, therefore, unlikely that more than 1% of healthy blood donors who are chronic carriers of the virus test nonreactive for anti-HIV. Of greater concern is the possibility that persons who have engaged in activities that put them at risk for AIDS may have been recently infected, but have not yet had time to develop detectable antibody (32). A recent publication from the CDC (33) estimates that as many as one in every 40,000 recipients in this country is currently at risk of HIV infection from the transfused blood. Further reduction of the risk will require a more sensitive test for the presence of the virus itself or some method to destroy the virus in a donated unit. The latter approach has been applied with some success to concentrates of blood coagulation factors manufactured to treat hemophilia (34) (see Chapter 4), but no physical or chemical approach to destroy intracellular viruses without harming the cells is available at this time.

VII. Special High-Risk Recipient Groups

A. Prior Recipients of Blood from Donors Who Later Develop AIDS

The first case of suspected transfusion-transmitted AIDS (5) had received blood from 19 different donors, one of whom proved to be on the list of AIDS patients at the San Francisco Health Department. The Irwin Memorial Blood Bank then entered into an agreement with the San Francisco Health Department to compare all reported cases of AIDS with the blood bank donor files in a deliberate attempt to identify all donors since January 1, 1979 who had later developed AIDS. As of June 2, 1986, 96 donors have been identified. Their blood was transfused into 426 recipients (multiple donations, multiple components per donation). When first sought, 230 of these recipients were dead, almost all from the illnesses for which they were transfused. As of the time of this writing, 123 are alive and 73 are of unknown status. Of the 353 whose status is known, nine have developed AIDS. Forty-six additional recipients have been tested for antibody to AIDS virus and 27 (59%) were reactive. Clearly recipients of blood components from donors who later develop AIDS are at very high risk for infection and disease (35).

In this small group of recipients, AIDS infection appears to have been transmitted by red blood cells, by platelet concentrates, and by fresh frozen plasma (confirming previous reports by the CDC) (1). The chance of a recipient becoming infected was lower the longer the interval between transfusion and the onset of AIDS in the donor. If the donor developed AIDS within one year of the transfusion, 90% of the recipients had either AIDS or antibody to the virus. If AIDS occurred in the donor between one and five years after giving the blood, 55% of the recipients were infected. Thus far, no recipient has been recognizably infected if the interval was over five years but the numbers examined are small.

B. Prior Recipients of Blood from Donors Who Now Have Antibody

As indicated above, donors with antibody are highly likely to carry virus. Therefore, their prior recipients appear to be at as high a risk as prior recipients of donors who later develop AIDS. The majority of donors who appear to have transmitted AIDS do not have AIDS themselves. In our series of 34 recipients with AIDS (as of June 28, 1986), only nine had a donor who later developed AIDS. In all other cases in which investigation of the donors has been completed, it has been possible to identify an anti-HIV-positive donor who admits prior risk activities for AIDS.

C. Recipients of Blood Containing Antibody

Recipients of blood containing antibody may be at the highest risk of all, since there is no possibility that their donors had not yet been infected at the time they gave the blood. Such recipients are available for study only in instances where blood was transfused before the test became available but the donor serum had been saved. In one such national study now underway, sera from 200,000 donors at blood banks in areas at high risk for AIDS have been saved, and the recipients of positive units and controls are being followed.

VIII. The Obligation to Inform

Our blood bank began the above studies among potentially exposed blood recipients as a research endeavor with informed consents. As experience accumulated it became apparent to us and others that there is an obligation to inform recipients of potentially infected blood that they may have been exposed. In numerous meeting with ethicists, clinicians, lawyers, and other community leaders, there was unanimous opinion that there is a duty to tell a patient information that could affect the patient's health, and that the information should be transmitted through the patient's personal physician. This is true even when the emotional hysteria associated with AIDS makes the information psychologically traumatic and even though there is no effective therapy for AIDS. Even more important is the fact that knowledge of infection by the AIDS virus can lead recipients to take precautions to protect their sexual contacts.

Any decision that it will do more harm than good to tell a patient of potential exposure to the AIDS virus must be made by the patient's personal physician who knows the patient well, and is willing to accept the additional legal liability of not passing on the information. The national blood bank organizations have taken the position that the blood bank whose donor has been found infected should notify the hospitals to which the donor's prior components were sent.

IX. Final Comments

The rise of AIDS has presented blood banks, hospitals, and physicians with demands for actions to make the blood supply safe prior to the availability of data on which logical decisions could be based. All are agreed that the safety of the blood supply is of foremost concern, but the public must be aware that blood transfusions will be complicated by morbidity and mortality quite apart from AIDS, and that AIDS is far from the most common cause of such complications. Equally important to safety is the adequacy of the blood supply, since patients will surely die if blood is not available. Blood donations decreased substantially in this country after AIDS appeared. This fact reflects in part the large number of previous donors who are no longer eligible and in part the completely mistaken notion that there is a risk of acquiring AIDS by donating blood. Moreover, the vast majority of people whose blood is safe to transfuse are reluctant to take the time to give it or are unwilling to accept the minor transient discomfort of the needle insertion.

Total elimination of transfusion-transmitted AIDS will require a better test for donor blood than is now available—one that will miss no carrier of the AIDS virus. The test for HIV p25 antigen does not meet this goal. An acceptable test must also have a very small proportion of false-positive results (ideally none). False-positive results mean blood donations lost and donors unnecessarily alarmed.

The fate of recipients of blood components containing the AIDS virus is still to be ascertained. The data available to us at the present time on proportions with antibody, with ARC, and with AIDS are minimum figures. There has been no large-scale testing of recipients in general. Those recipients who have been potentially exposed to blood containing AIDS virus (ascertained because a donor developed AIDS or was found to have antibody) have been studied only in small numbers so far and for very brief periods subsequent to the suspect transfusion. How many will ultimately develop AIDS or ARC is still unknown.

The general public needs to put its assumptions about AIDS and blood transfusion into proper prospective. This new disease has always been a very rare complication of blood transfusion, and the risk at the present time under the most pessimistic assumptions is far lower than it was two to three years ago. Finally, the public's concerns, and the problems of transfusion-associated AIDS in general, will be markedly alleviated if successful therapy for AIDS is developed.

References

1. Curran JW, Lawrence DN, Jaffe H, et al. Acquired immunodeficiency syndrome (AIDS) associated with transfusions. N Engl J Med 1984; 310:69-75.

2. Barre-Sinoussi F, Chermann JC, Rey F, et al. Isolation of a T-lymphotropic retrovirus from a patient at risk for acquired immune deficiency syndrome. Science 1983; 220:868-71.
3. Gallo RC, Salahuddin SZ, Popovic M, et al. Frequent detection and isolation of cytopathic retroviruses (HTLV-III) from patients with AIDS and at risk for AIDS. Science 1984; 224:500-3.
4. Levy JA, Hoffman AD, Kramer SM, et al. Isolation of lymphocytopathic retroviruses from San Francisco patients with AIDS. Science 1984; 225:840-2.
5. Centers for Disease Control. *Pneumocystis carinii* pneumonia among persons with hemophilia A. MMWR 1982; 31:365-7.
6. Centers for Disease Control. Possible transfusion-associated acquired immune deficiency syndrome (AIDS)—California. MMWR 1982; 31:652-4.
7. Ammann AJ, Cowan MJ, Wara DW, et al. Acquired immunodeficiency in an infant: possible transmission by means of blood products. Lancet 1983; 253:770-3.
8. Jaffe HW, Sarngadharan MG, DeVico A, et al. Infection with HTLV-III/LAV and transfusion-associated immunodeficiency syndrome. JAMA 1985; 253:770-3.
9. Feorino PM, Jaffe HW, Palmer E, et al. Transfusion-associated acquired immunodeficiency syndrome. Evidence for persistent infection in blood donors. N Engl J Med 1985; 312:1293-5.
10. Information supplied by Centers for Disease Control, 1986.
11. Centers for Disease Control. Update: acquired immunodeficiency syndrome in the San Francisco Cohort Study, 1978-1985. MMWR 1985; 34:573-5.
12. Lur K-J, Lawrence DN, Morgan WM, et al. A model-based approach for estimating the mean incubation period of transfusion-associated acquired immunodeficiency syndrome. Proc Natl Acad Sci 1986; 83:3051-5.
13. American Association of Blood Banks, American Red Cross, Council of Community Blood Centers. Joint statement on acquired immune deficiency syndrome (AIDS) related to transfusion. Arlington, VA: January 13, 1983.
14. Director. Office of Biologics. National Center for Drugs and Biologics, Food and Drug Administration. Recommendations to decrease the risk of transmitting acquired immune deficiency syndrome (AIDS) from blood donors. Letter, March 24, 1983.
15. Director. Office of Biologics Research and Review, Food and Drug Administration: Revised definition of high risk groups with respect to acquired immune deficiency syndrome (AIDS) transmission from blood and plasma donors. Letter, September 3, 1985.
16. Pindyke J, Waldman A, Zang E. Measures to decrease the risk of acquired immunodeficiency syndrome transmission by blood transfusion. Transfusion 1985; 25:3-9.
17. Aach RD, Lander JJ, Sherman LA, et al. Transfusion-transmitted viruses: interim analysis of hepatitis among transfused and nontransfused patients. In: Vyas GN, Cohen SN, Schmid RS, eds. Viral hepatitis. Philadelphia: The Franklin Institute Press, 1978.
18. Alter HJ, Hoffnagle JH. Non-A, Non-B: observations on the first decade. In: Vyas GN, Dienstag JL, Hoofnagle JH, eds. Viral hepatitis and liver disease. Orlando, FL: Grune & Stratton, 1984.

19. Cordell RR, Yalon VA, Cigahn-Haskell C, McDonough BP, Perkins HA. Experience with 11,916 designated donors. Transfusion 1986; 26:484-6.
20. Hersh EM, Reuben JM, Rios A, et al. Elevated serum thymosin alpha-1 levels associated with evidence of immune dysregulation in male homosexuals with a history of infectious diseases or Kaposi's sarcoma. N Engl J Med 1983; 308:45-6.
21. Eyster ME, Goedert JJ, Poon M-C, Preble OT. Acid labile interferon. A possible preclinical marker for the acquired immunodeficiency syndrome in hemophilia. N Engl J Med 1983; 309:583-6.
22. Zolla-Pazner S, William D, El-Sadr W, et al. Quantitation of beta-2 microglobulin and other immune characteristics in a prospective study of men at risk for acquired immune deficiency syndrome. JAMA 1984; 251:2952-5.
23. Wachter H, Fuchs D, Hausen A, et al. Elevated urinary neopterin levels in patients with acquired immunodeficiency syndrome (AIDS). Hoppe-Selyer's Z Physiol Chem 1983; 364:1345-6.
24. Schorr JB, Berkowitz A, Cumming PD, et al. Prevalence of HTLV-III antibody in American blood donors (letter). N Engl J Med 1985; 313:384-5.
25. Barrett JE, Dawson G, Heller J, et al. Performance evaluation of the Abbott HTLV III EIA, a test for antibody to HTLV III in donor blood. AM J Clin Pathol 1986; 86:180-5.
26. Petricciani JC, Director Division of Blood and Blood Products, Food and Drug Administration. Testing for HTLV-III antibody (letter addressed to blood bank associations, received March 18, 1985).
27. Kuritsky JN, Rastogi SC, Faich GA, et al. Results of nationwide screening of blood and plasm for antibodies to human T-cell lymphotrophic III virus, type III. Transfusion 1986; 26:205-7.
28. Hunter JB, Menitove JE. HLA antibodies detected by ELISA HTLV-III antibody kits (letter). Lancet 1985; 2:397.
29. Kaminsky LS, McHugh T, Stites D, et al. High prevalence of antibodies to AIDS-associated retroviruses (ARV) in acquired immune deficiency syndrome and related conditions and not in other disease states. Proc Natl Acad Sci 1985; 82:5535-9.
30. Ward JW, Grindon AJ, Feorino PM, et al. Laboratory and epidemiologic evaluation of an enzyme immunoassay for antibodies to HTLV-III. JAMA 1986; 256:357-61.
31. U.S. Department of Health and Human Services. Public Health Service: Facts about AIDS. August 1985.
32. Centers for Disease Control. Transfusion-associated human T-lymphotropic virus type III/lymphadenopathy-associated virus infection from a seronegative donor—Colorado. MMWR 1986; 35:389-91.
33. Ward JW, Holmberg SD, Allen JR, et al. Transmission of Human Immunodeficiency Virus (HIV) by blood transfusions screened as negative for HIV antibody. N Engl J Med 1988; 318:473-8.
34. Petricciani JC, McDougal JS, Evatt BL. Case for concluding that heat-treated, licensed antihaemophilic factor is free from HTLV-III. Lancet 1985; 2:890-1.
35. Perkins HA, Samson S, Garner J, et al. Risk of AIDS for recipients of blood components from donors who subsequently developed AIDS. Blood 1987; 70:1604-10.

6
Pediatric AIDS

Morton J. Cowan
School of Medicine
University of California
San Francisco, California

Arthur J. Ammann
Genentech, Inc.
South San Francisco, California

I. Definition of Pediatric AIDS

A diagnosis of pediatric AIDS can be established utilizing two criteria: 1) the presence of human immunodeficiency virus (HIV) infection and 2) the presence of B- and T-cell immunodeficiency. Although more complex definitions have been proposed, they have been devised for epidemiological purposes only. Unfortunately, they have been used by medical providers to disallow medical and psychosocial treatment for many severely ill infants and children, who although infected by HIV and immunodeficient fail to fulfill certain criteria established by public health agencies.

II. History of Pediatric AIDS

Pediatric AIDS was independently described in 1983 in three geographically distinct areas associated with three major risk factors: 1) intravenous drug abusing mothers, 2) Haitian ancestry, and 3) blood transfusions (1-5). Subsequently, vertical transmission of an infectious agent was suggested by the discovery of three affected female siblings born to an intravenous drug-abusing, prostitute mother (6). Histocompatibility typing of the siblings and mother indicated that each child had a different father, thereby ruling out a genetic etiology of the immunodeficiency.

Initially, the existence of pediatric AIDS was doubted because of difficulties in proving that patients had a distinct etiology of their immunodeficiency. However, the characteristic immunological phenotype (hypergammaglobulinemia and T-cell immunodeficiency), the presence of risk factors similar to adult AIDS, the occurrence in identical geographic areas, and the rapid increase in numbers of infants and children with unexplained immunodeficiency all strongly suggested that pediatric AIDS was a distinct immunodeficiency disorder in children.

With the discovery of a new retrovirus as the probable cause of AIDS (7-9), retrospective and prospective studies were performed to confirm the original hypothesis that adult and pediatric AIDS had an identical viral association. In addition, antibody testing of sera from a large population of patients with primary immunodeficiency diseases indicated that HIV was not present prior to 1977 in infants and children with immunodeficiency (10). The first serum positive for HIV was obtained in 1978 from a one-year-old child of an intravenous drug-abusing mother from San Francisco. Allowing for a minimum incubation of a year between exposure and symptoms in both mother and infant, it was estimated that HIV must have been present in San Francisco in 1977. This study (10) also provided evidence that HIV was not a cause of immunodeficiency in children in San Francisco prior to 1977.

As the number of adults infected with HIV has increased, there has been a parallel increase in the number of pediatric patients with HIV infection. Today, with the possible exception of protein-calorie malnutrition, HIV infection is the major cause of severe T-cell immunodeficiency in children.

III. Transmission

While the pediatric risk groups differ to some extent from those in adults, the routes of transmission are similar, that is, via blood or sexual contact (Table 1). The most frequent means by which children are infected with HIV is from an infected mother (1-4). Other routes include sexual contact (abuse), infected needles, and infected blood products (5,11,12). It should be pointed out that there are no known cases of paternal transmission of HIV to infants and children other than via sexual abuse. Also, there has been no documented case of transmission of the virus through gammaglobulin preparations or the hepatitis B vaccine (13,14) although two patients with common variable hypogammaglobulinemia receiving intravenous gammaglobulin have been reported from whom retroviruses similar to HIV have been isolated (15).

The most common mode of transmission of HIV in infants is from an infected mother. Perinatal transmission through cervical secretions, and possibly through breast milk, has been suggested (16). In 1981 we noted three half-siblings who developed AIDS (6). Two of the children were delivered vaginally but were separated from their mother at birth, suggesting pre- or perinatal transmission. The third child was delivered by Caesarean section and was not breast-fed, implicating transplacental transmission. Since then there have been cases of children who were symptomatic at birth and reports of HIV in abortion material after as early as 20 weeks' gestation, in-

Table 1 Transmission of HIV in Children

1 Maternal
   a. in utero/transplacental
   b. vaginal secretions
   c. breast milk
2. Blood
   a. transfusions—blood and platelets
   b. clotting factor concentrates
   c. sharing of needles
3. Sexual contact/abuse

dicating infection in utero (17-19). The possibility of infection at birth from vaginal secretions has become quite real since the discovery of HIV in vaginal secretions (18). However, it will be extremely difficult to prove infection through that route unless a method for prenatal detection becomes readily available.

Unequivocal transmission of infection via breast milk has not been proven. However, HIV has beeñ detected in breast milk, and there is at least one reported instance of possible transmission from breast milk (16). In this case, the woman became infected after receiving a postpartum blood transfusion from a subsequently identified infected donor. This was her only known risk factor. The infant received no blood transfusions and its only intimate contact with its infected mother was by nursing for 6 weeks.

In infants and young children, the second most common route of transmission is via transfusion of blood products. In 1983 we reported a child with AIDS who had received a platelet transfusion from a donor who later died of AIDS (5). Subsequently, we located a second child who received a red cell transfusion from this same donation. Three years after the initial transfusion the child developed some signs and symptoms of immunodeficiency and near-fatal varicella infection and now, five years posttransfusion, has evidence for AIDS-related complex (ARC), including thrush and lymphadenopathy.

Of interest has been the observation of a very low incidence of blood-transfusion-acquired HIV infection in infants receiving CMV seronegative blood (62). This is most likely related to the high incidence of CMV seropositivity among HIV-infected adults. In our own unpublished experience with the use of CMV seronegative blood products for neonates, congenitally immunodeficient children, and bone marrow transplant recipients, we have not had a case of HIV infection by blood product exposure.

The other blood product most commonly associated with HIV infections is factor VIII and IX concentrates for patients with hemophilia (20,21) (see Chapter 4). Currently, techniques have been developed for processing concentrates that inactivate HIV (22, 23). These techniques, as well as antibody testing of blood donors, should significantly reduce the incidence of new HIV infection in recipients of these blood products. However, a significant number of individuals have been infected through 1985 (when antibody testing by blood banks began) and are at high risk for developing AIDS over the next three to five years (or longer).

Other potential routes of transmission in infants and children include needles and sexual contact. Increasing intravenous drug abuse in older children and adolescents is a significant problem in transmission of HIV. Transmission from sexual abuse of children has been reported (24).

Although the virus has been detected in saliva, tears, and urine, no documented cases of transmission of infection through casual, nonsexual contact with excretions or secretions have been reported. Several studies have evaluated household contacts and families with infants with AIDS where no special precautions were used, e.g., while changing diapers, kissing, etc. (25, 26) and none has shown any evidence of transmission of HIV. Other studies have looked at health-care workers and found similar results (27).

IV. Groups at Risk

There are five risk groups for HIV infection in infants and children (Table 2). The most common is infants of infected mothers. This group includes drug-abusing mothers, women infected from blood transfusions and through sexual contact, and women of Haitian ancestry (1-4). Currently, it is impossible to predict which infants will become infected from an infected mother. It is estimated that children born to infected mothers have a 50-60% chance of HIV infection (28), but this may be too high. In one limited study of mothers who had had one infected child, 66% of 20 subsequent children were also infected (29). Of importance were the facts that infection of the neonates did not correlate with the clinical status of the mother; some healthy antibody-positive women had infected infants, and some women with AIDS had uninfected offspring. The diagnosis of infection in this study was based on serological or clinical evidence of disease, although not every infected child developed AIDS. Since these findings came from a population of women selected on the basis of a previously infected child, there may be a bias toward overestimating the incidence of transmission for other high-risk populations. In a European study of 13 children (aged 12-20 months) of seropositive mothers, 10 were infected (63). Other case reports indicate that transmission of the virus from an infected mother is not guaranteed even when the mother has been shown to be viremic (30).

Until the results of prospective studies are available, the transmission rate from mother to child will remain unknown. Early results from our prospective study in San Francisco (M. Cowan) of 30 seropositive drug-abusing women indicate a much lower HIV transmission rate (approximately 20%) than previously thought.

Table 2 Groups at Risk for Pediatric AIDS

1. Infants of infected mothers
2. Recipients of blood transfusions 1979-85 (rare cases expected after 1985)
3. Hemophiliacs
4. Sexually abused children
5. IV drug abusers

Other groups at risk are similar to those in adults and include recipients of blood transfusion between 1979 and 1985, hemophiliacs requiring factor VIII/IX transfusion, those with sexual contacts, and intravenous drug abusers. Of particular risk for blood transmission are those children requiring large amounts of blood products, including patients undergoing chemotherapy, open-heart surgery, and bone-marrow transplants, as well as hemophiliacs (31).

V. Pathophysiology

HIV infection in pediatric patients has a clinical course that is similar but not identical to that in adult patients. Estimates of the incubation period for AIDS (exposure to onset of AIDS) have varied from a few years to 15 years. In one analysis in which age at infection was assessed it was found that the mean incubation period for children under 5 years of age was 2 years, compared to 8 years for older children and adults (64). There are many observations that remain unexplained, including the variable progression of the syndrome and the fact that some, but not all, infants born to HIV-positive mothers are infected (28). Some of the variability has been attributed to the presence or absence of other infections (cytomegalovirus, Epstein-Barr virus [EBV]) or possibly to differences in pathogenicity of "strains" of HIV (32) (see Chapter 8).

HIV infects several distinct cell types, including T cells, monocytes, and cells of the central nervous system (33-35). The propensity of HIV isolates to infect different cell types has been shown to vary (35). The presence of the CD4 receptor is probably a prerequisite for infection of certain cell types (36). In vitro, after integration of the virus, replication and dissemination of virus requires antigen stimulation and interleukin-2 (IL-2) (7-9). In vivo, the requirements may be similar with dissemination of the virus occurring following antigen exposure and stimulation of immunity, e.g., by additional infections.

Despite the observation that HIV infects both monocytes and T cells, the earliest immunological abnormality detected in infants is hypergammaglobulinemia (6,65). This polyclonal B-cell activation may result from direct infection of B cells by HIV, viral stimulation of B cells, and/or loss of T-cell regulatory influences. Although unusual, hypogammaglobulinemia is observed more frequently in pediatric AIDS. The etiology of hypogammaglobulinemia is uncertain but may be related to infection of immature B-cells in infants during early embryogensis. The susceptibility to infection is not always correlated with severe immunological abnormalities; observations in individual patients suggest that severe opportunistic infections may occur in infants with minimally impaired T-cell immunity (6).

A major difference between the infections seen in pediatric AIDS compared with adult AIDS is the high frequency of bacterial infections in children (65). This probably results from a lack of acquired immunity in infants to most common pathogens. As the immunodeficiency progresses, there is an increasing susceptibility to opportunistic infections. By the time a diagnosis of classical AIDS is made (immunodeficiency and opportunistic infection), the immune system is severly impaired with deficiency of T-cell antigen and mitogen proloferative responses, monocyte function, monocyte and lymphocyte cytokine production (IL-1, IL-2, interferon-α, interferon-γ, tumor necrosis factor-α and -β), deficient antibody formation, decreased NK-cell activity, and increases circulating immune complexes (37, 38). It has not yet been determined whether all of the immunological abnormalities are a result of HIV infection alone or a result of mulitple infections acting in concert with HIV.

VI. Clinical Manifestations

The incubation period from HIV infection to the development of initial symptoms in children is approximately eight weeks (17). What has been noted in adults but difficult to recognize in infants is a transient influenza-like syndrome characterized by fever and myalgia. However, the time from infection to development of ARC or AIDS varies considerably and may depend on the routes of transmission as well as the dose of virus. In one group of children who were closely followed after a transfusion of contaminated blood, the onset of symptoms ranged from 1 to 29 months (median eight months) (28). In another group of 12 neonates who received blood transfusions from two HIV-infected donors, all developed laboratory and/or clinical evidence of infection within the first year of life (66). Three of the children have remained asymptomatic (with abnormal laboratory studies) for 2½-5 years of followup. In our own experience, seropositive children have remained relatively asymptomatic for as long as four years after a transfusion of blood in the newborn period. The longest reported instance for development of AIDS in a child receiving a blood transfusion was 5.5 years (39). For children infected in utero the median time interval between birth and symptoms is four months.

Many of the clinical manifestations seen in adults infected with HIV are also seen in children, including fevers, weight loss (failure to thrive), malaise, chronic or recurrent diarrhea, lymphadenopathy, hepatosplenomegaly,

Table 3 Pediatric and Adult AIDS Compared

	Pediatric	Adult
Infections		
opportunistic	Frequent	Frequent
bacterial	Frequent	Infrequent
Laboratory		
hypergammaglobulinemia	Frequent	Frequent
lymphopenia	Not always present	Frequent
decreased T4 cells	Not always present	Frequent
abnormal T cell function	Frequent	Frequent
Failure to thrive	Frequent	Frequent weight loss
Malignancy	Rare	Frequenct
Parotitis	Frequent	Rare
Lymphoid interstitial pneumonitis	Frequent	Rare
Central nervous system abnormalities	Frequent	Frequent
Dysmorphic syndrome	Frequent	Not seen

and recurrent or persistent thrush (Table 3). In addition to these systemic manifestations, cardiomyopathy and multiorgan arteriopathy have been reported in children with HIV infection by at least one group (67,68). Susceptibility to bacterial infections in children with HIV infection is often manifested by draining otitis media and/or recurrent episodes of sepsis and meningitis (1-4). These signs and symptoms may last for weeks to months before development of those clinical symptoms indicative of AIDS, that is, opportunistic infection, diffuse interstitial pneumonitis, or malignancy. Children appear susceptible to most, if not all, of the opportunistic infections seen in adults with AIDS. *Pneumocystis carinii* pneumonia (PCP) occurs in 70% of children with AIDS. Other opportunistic infectious organisms that have been seen in children include invasive *Candida* esophagitis, invasive herpes simplex, disseminated varicella, *Cryptosporidium* and atypical mycobacterium.

There are several clinical manifestations of HIV infection in children that may distinguish it from that in adults. One is the incidence of malignancy. While a few cases of Kaposi's sarcoma (KS) have been reported in children (40,69) it appears that aggressive KS is mostly limited to AIDS in adults. Other malignancies, such as lymphoma, are rare. Persistent diffuse parotitis, with only a few exceptions (70) not seen in adults, has been reported in 14-30% of children with AIDS (1-4). The etiology of this clinical manifestation of AIDS in children is unknown. One case that we evaluated with a salivary gland biopsy was consistent with a Sjogren's-like histopathology. Lymphoid interstitial pneumonitis (LIP) is common in children with AIDS (30-60%) and develops anywhere from 3 to 26 months from onset of symptoms of AIDS (41,42). Until recently, LIP was not noted in adults; however, a few recent reports of this AIDS-associated complication in adults have been published (43). It will be interesting to see whether LIP, which is a relatively good prognostic marker in children, will also be the same for adults with HIV infection (42). The etiology of AIDS-related LIP is unknown, although evidence for a direct involvement of the HIV has been reported (71) and the possibility of associated EBV infection has been suggested (72). While there is no definitive treatment for LIP in children with HIV, there has been some apparent successful reduction in severe hypoxemia by using glucocorticoids (73). The long-term consequences of this therapy are unknown.

Two clinical aspects of HIV infection in children warrant comment. The first is the central nervous system (CNS) manifestations (44-46, 74). From 15-50% of children infected with HIV will develop CNS disease characterized by a progressive loss of developmental milestones and acquired microcephaly. Seizures appear to be uncommon but do occur. Pyramidal tract signs may be seen with truncal ataxia. In children infected in utero or perinatally, the median time of onset to symptoms is six months (2-24 months). The computerized tomography scan of the brain either is normal or shows cortical atrophy and/or basal ganglia calcification. In most cases, examination of the cerebrospinal fluid (CSF) is unremarkable. Although it was initially felt that most of the neurological involvement in AIDS was secondary to opportunistic infections, it appears that HIV is a neurotropic virus. The nucleic acid sequences of HIV have been demonstrated in the brains of both children and adults with AIDS encephalopathy (44). HIV has also been isolated in the CSF and neural tissue from AIDS patients (45). Some children (and adults have had neurological disease without clinical manifestations or immunodeficiency (47), while in others HIV infection has occurred in the brain without causing clinical neurological disease (44, 46) (see Chapter 15). The true impact that this potential neurotropic virus has on the developing nervous system in high-risk infants has not yet been studied prospectively. Many infants and children have CNS infection with other infectious agents, e.g., toxoplasmosis, cytomegalovirus, and/or EBV (41, 48).

Recently, a group of children infected via their mothers were noted to have severe dysmorphic features, including microcephaly, a prominent box-like forehead, a flattened nasal bridge, wide palpebral fissures, hypertelorism, blue sclerai, and shortened philtum (49). These features are not specific to all children with HIV infection in utero. Many of these abnormalities are seen in the fetal alcohol and DiGeorge syndromes (50), which presumably occur secondary to an insult (for example, alcohol) during embryogenesis. As the "dysmorphic syndrome" was reported from a center where the affected infants were exclusively born to intravenous drug-abusing mothers it is difficult to determine if drugs and/or HIV infection were the cause of these findings.

A recent study from New York that compared 30 children with perinatally acquired HIV infection to matched uninfected controls found no significant differences with respect to the incidence of craniofacial features and dermatographics (75). Furthermore, there was no difference between those born to drug-abusing women and those born to non-drug-abusing mothers.

VII. Diagnosis: Pediatric AIDS Versus AIDS-Related Conditions (ARC)

Several approaches to the diagnosis of AIDS have been proposed. The earliest recommendation used clinical features indicative of T-cell deficiency (51). More recently, this has been updated to include several categories of disease based on laboratory and clinical signs and symptoms (76). In view of the rapidly expanding clinical features associated with HIV infection, e.g., thrombocytopenia, lymphoid interstitial pneumonia, malignancies, or isolated central nervous system involvement, it would be appropriate to simplify rather than compound diagnostic categories. This fact is especially important now that the etiology of AIDS is known and because previous categorization has resulted in denial of medical and psychosocial care to many severely symptomatic HIV-infected patients.

Consistent with previous methods of classifying immunodeficiency suggested by the World Health Organization, a diagnosis of pediatric AIDS would require only the demonstration of 1)HIV infection and 2)immunodeficiency. Thus, pediatric AIDS could be diagnosed on the basis of laboratory studies alone, just as is true for other immunodeficiency disorders, such as Wiskott-Aldrich syndrome, hypogammaglobulinemia, and chronic granulomatous disease (52).

The laboratory diagnosis of HIV infection can be made by a variety of tests that detect antibody to viral core proteins or membrane glycoproteins (53, 54). Unfortunately, easily detectable IgM antibody to HIV antigens is not found even in infants with intrauterine infection. Therefore, from birth until twelve months of age, antibody to HIV could be from either a maternal or patient source. If it is necessary to prove HIV infection in an infant under twelve months of age, cultures for HIV or detection of HIV antigen should be performed. Once positive, the serum antibody to HIV remains positive indefinitely except in a few terminally ill patients. The ability to culture virus from patients may vary considerably.

A problem that may be of particular importance in pediatrics is that antibody may not be present (or detectable) in some infants infected via maternal transmission (77-79). In a retrospective study we evaluated 16 high-risk infants of HIV-seropositive women for both antibody and the presence of HIV in cultures of peripheral blood mononuclear cells (unpublished).

Table 4 Supportive Treatment of Pediatric AIDS

1. Attempt early diagnosis and aggressive therapy of bacterial and viral infections.
2. Treat *Pneumocystis carinii* prophylactically with trimethoprim-sulfamethoxazole.
3. Admisister gammaglobulin monthly.
4. Do not immunize with live virus.
5. Administer Zoster-immune gammaglobulin for Varicella.
6. Irradiate all blood products.
7. Use CMV-negative blood products.
8. Consider experimental treatment of viral infectin (Ribavirin for RSV; DHPG for CMV).
9. Treat HIV with AZT when approved by FDA.

Two-thirds of these children had clinical and/or laboratory evidence for HIV infection. Of the 10 infected children, one was HIV-culture-positive without detectable antibody by indirect immunofluorescence, enzyme-linked immunoassay, and Western blot. Our results are consistent with several other reports that approximately 10% of children at risk for maternally transmitted HIV infection could be missed by antibody testing alone (80).

Although many immunological abnormalities have been demonstrated in patients with AIDS, the earliest detected in children are polyclonal hypergammaglobulinemia and T-cell immunodeficiency, as evidenced by elevated immunoglobulins and a diminished response of peripheral blood lymphocytes to antigen or mitogen (1-4). Lymphopenia and abnormal helper/suppressor T cell ratios, while frequently present in adult AIDS, may be normal in pediatric AIDS and should not be used to diagnose AIDS in children.

VIII. Treatment

Currently, there is no effective treatment for HIV infection, and therefore supportive care for children with HIV infection is essential and may improve the quality of life as well as prolong survival (Table 4). Opportunistic infections must be diagnosed and treated aggressively with appropriate antibiotics when available. An open-lung biopsy or bronchial lavage must be performed for significant pulmonary symptoms to diagnose treatable infections such as *Pneumocystis carinii*, respiratory syncytial virus, and cytomegalovirus. Trimethoprim-sulfamethoxazole prophylaxis should be given to all high-risk patients with an early symptomatology or evidence for immunodeficiency. Experimental treatment with dihydroxy proxymethyl guanine (DHPG) has been used for adults with cytomegalovirus infection. We have routinely put all of our immunodeficient and/or symptomatic patients on monthly gammaglobulin therapy in spite of their elevated immunoglobulins, since we have found that patients with AIDS are unable to make specific antibodies to polysaccharide or protein antigens (55). Immunizations with live viral vaccines are contraindicated in immunodeficient patients. However, routine live viral immunizations from HIV-infected infants who have not yet developed immunodeficiency are cautiously being recommended by the World Health Organization and the American Academy of Pediatrics (81). Limited experience to date with live polio and measles vaccines has not yet shown any severe complications but should be administered with caution and only after immunological assessment. Finally, all blood products should be irradiated and negative for CMV antibody.

A variety of attempts have been made to irradicate HIV and/or reconstitute immunity in vivo. Although many drugs have been evaluated in a few prospective placebo-controlled trials, none has halted disease progression or restored immune function, including ribavirin and suramin (56, 57). Azidodeoxythymidine (AZT) was of benefit in reducing mortality and HIV antigenemia in limited clinical trials in adults and was approved by the FDA for the treatment of AIDS in adults in 1987. Currently, several cooperative clinical trials are being performed to evaluate the effectiveness of AZT in infants and children. Early results using intravenous AZT in children have been encouraging, and more wide-scale testing of oral AZT in children is planned. Other agents for which trials are under way include additional purine derivatives and foscarnet. Some of these agents interfere with either reverse transcriptase, virus transcription, translation, or assembly. To be effective, an antiviral drug must cross the blood-brain barrier, be relatively non-toxic, and be absorbed orally for chronic use. There have been no detailed studies of any of these antiviral agents in children.

A second approach to treating HIV infection utilizes immunomodulators such as IL-2 and interferon (58, 59). IL-2 has been tested in a controlled study in adults and, while early results were encouraging, the overall assessment indicated no significant and consistent improvement. Interferon-α was effective in about 30% of adults with Kaposi's sarcoma. However, there was no effect in patients with opportunistic infection. Again, there have been no clinical trials of immunomodulators in children with HIV infection.

Immune reconstitution has been attempted in the form of bone-marrow transplantation using adult recipients with syngeneic (twin) donors. Of the approximately eight transplants that have been performed, there is only one preliminary report of improvement posttransplant when used in combination with ribavirin therapy (60). There are no reports of bone-marrow transplantation in the pediatric population with AIDS. Bone-marrow transplantation is unlikely to be successful without an effective antiviral agent.

IX. Prognosis and Incidence

The incidence of AIDS in children ranges from 1.4% in the United States to 2.7% of all cases in Europe. Of the cases in children, the majority (77%) are secondary to maternal risk factors. In the United States the relative percent

Table 5 Clinical Status of Pediatric Patients with HIV Infection Defined by Antibody or Viral Isolation

HIV	Number in group	Died	AIDS	ARC	Failure to thrive	Lymph-adenopathy	Hepatospleno-megaly	Decreased CD4 cells
Antibody-positive, culture-negative	7	1	0	0	0	0	0	0
Antibody-positive, culture-positive	11	2	5	4	3	7	8	8
Antibody-negative, culture-positive	1	1	1	0	1	1	1	1

of pediatric cases has remained stable over the past two years (61). However, recent surveys suggest that the incidence of antibody-positive infants is increasing dramatically in geographic areas with a high incidence of intravenous drug abuse. There is a predominance of cases in males over females (1.6:1) and a greater percent in blacks and Hispanics (54% and 19%, respectively). The majority of cases come from New York, New Jersey, Florida, and California. Nearly 80% of pediatric AIDS cases are under five years of age. Most of the patients in the 5-13-year-old age group are hemophiliacs.

The actual number of children with AIDS, ARC, or HIV infection is unknown but has been estimated to be two to three times what is reported to the CDC. In an attempt to assess the potential magnitude of maternal infection in Massachusetts, the seroprevalence was determined on samples of newborn blood routinely collected for neonatal screening of inborn errors (84). The results of this study suggested that the prevalence of seropositivity among childbearing women was 2.1 per 1000, ranging from 0.9 to 8.0 per 1000 depending on the location of the maternity hospital. Such studies need to be done in other high-risk locations to begin to assess the actual number of potentially infected children. In California, we surveyed major medical centers with pediatric AIDS referral populations and found the number of cases to be three to four times that officially reported for California. Reluctance to report cases may be a consequence of the excessive publicity that surrounds children with AIDS, especially if they are of school age. In terms of HIV infection, there is no reason to believe that the number of infected children is less than that seen in adults, i.e., five to ten times the number with AIDS. With the possible exception of severe protein caloric malnutrition, pediatric AIDS is now the most common severe T-cell immunodeficiency disease of childhood.

The prognosis for children with ARC or AIDS is generally poor. As many as 75% of children who are diagnosed prior to one year of age die. Of those diagnosed after one year of age, 50% die within 18 months of diagnosis. There are some potentially important prognostic features for children with HIV infection. One is central nervous system disease, which implies poor prognosis. Children with LIP may have a better outcome.

Finally, since 1985, we have evaluated children infected with HIV for both antibody to HIV and the presence of HIV in cultures of peripheral blood mononuclear cells (unpublished). We found a group of 11 children (out of 19 with clinical evidence of infection) who had both antibody and virus detected on culture. This group of children was most clinically affected and had the most significant laboratory abnormalities relative to those children who were only antibody-positive without evidence for viremia (Table 5). Whether viremia will prove to be a significant prognostic factor warrants further study.

X. Public Health

Pediatric AIDS is a preventable disease. For this reason, public health measures should be emphasized to prevent the spread of HIV to additional high-risk groups as well as to low-risk individuals. These measures deserve primary emphasis in view of the fact that HIV infection is lifelong and pediatric AIDS, like adult AIDS, is currently 100% fatal. In addition, early diagnosis is essential to institute timely therapy and public health measures.

A. Sexually Transmitted Pediatric AIDS

Sexual transmission of HIV in the pediatric population is relatively rare at the present time but may increase as the number of infected individuals increases. There are several documented cases of sexually abused children who have developed AIDS. For this reason, screening of both the sexually abused child and the sexual offender for evidence of sexually transmitted diseases, including HIV, is necessary. Antibody screening of the sexual offender can be performed at the time of diagnosis but should be performed only after two months following the suspected event in the patient, as antibody to HIV usually does not become positive until four to eight weeks following exposure (60). To be certain that delayed conversion to antibody positivity has not occurred in the patient, a repeat test should be obtained six months following initial evaluation.

Increased numbers of teenaged patients who are either HIV-antibody-positive or who have AIDS are expected to occur. The major risk factors associated with acquistion of HIV in this group are intravenous drug abuse, multiple bisexual or homosexual partners, and prostitution. In the latter case, the search for "safe sex" among younger prostitutes may decrease the risk of HIV infection to prostitutes and, in turn, to their clients.

Approaches directed toward the prevention of AIDS among children should include education measures that directly address the facts that AIDS is fatal, that AIDS is preventable, and that drug abuse and sexual activities are means of acquiring HIV.

B. Maternal Transmission of Pediatric AIDS

The majority of patients with pediatric AIDS have acquired the infection from a maternal source, with intravenous drug abuse as the major maternal risk factor. Currently there are no measures that can prevent transmission of virus from infected mothers to the fetus. Mothers who are antibody-positive should be counseled in relation to the risks of having an infected infant, although precise information regarding risk is currently inadequate. Limited studies suggest that there is a 30 to 50% incidence of HIV antibody positivity in infants born to mothers who have had a previously affected infant, whereas the incidence of HIV infection in an HIV-antibody-positive mother's first pregnancy may be approximately 20%. Additionally, the progression of infection in HIV-antibody-positive infants may be highly variable and, even in the same family, may vary from rapidly fatal disease to long-term survival (greater than five years). Current data do not support a recommendation of routine abortion in HIV-antibody-positive mothers.

Questions have been raised as to whether pregnancy enhances the progression of HIV infection in the mother. Although there are anecdotal cases, no detailed studies have been performed that convincingly answers this question, and recommendations must therefore await further information.

Once an HIV-infected infant is diagnosed, the source of infection should be sought. In most instances this transmission will be due to maternal infection but may be related to a blood transfusion. As some mothers may be asymptomatic and unaware that they have HIV infection, antibody testing of mothers may be necessary to detect the source of HIV infection.

C. Transmission of HIV by Casual Contact

In view of the absence of evidence for casual transmission of HIV, children with AIDS or children who are HIV-antibody-positive should be permitted to attend school without restrictions except as related to their own health. Confidentiality of HIV status should be maintained. Parents should be notified if the child with AIDS is exposed to infections that would be a risk for HIV-infected individuals, e.g., varicella. Appropriate prophylactic therapy should be given (Zoster immune globulin). Detailed public health recommendations are sometimes based on the theoretical possibility that contact with secretions might result in HIV transmission. Many of these recommendations do not take into account the observation that most HIV-infected patients are asymptomatic and that these account for the majority of HIV-antibody-positive individuals. Further, they contradict the evidence that causual transmission of HIV has not occurred.

D. Immunization of Patients with pediatric AIDS

Patients with severe B- and T-cell immunodeficiency do not respond to immunization with antibody formation. Because of lack of efficacy and the risks of immunization with live attenuated vaccines, routine childhood immunization should not be given to infants and children with impaired immunity. Some debate exists as to whether HIV-antibody-positive infants who are otherwise normal should be immunized. Immunization is currently recommended by the WHO and AAP (81). Arguments in favor of immunization include the need to protect these patients from additional infection and to prevent the spread of infectious disease through unimmunized hosts, the lack of reported cases of vaccine-induced disease, and the fact that many HIV-antibody-positive patients may be immunologically normal. However, it would appear that the risk of immunizing HIV-antibody-positive infants—regardless of clinical or immunological status—is greater that the potential benefit. The lack of reported vaccine-related infections in HIV-antibody-positive infants is probably due to the lack of studies directed at attempts to detect virus in pathological tissues, as well as the already low rate of immunization in infants with a potentially fatal illness. Infants can be protected against many infections using killed vaccines (DPT, polio) and against other infections by the administration of prophylactic gammaglobulin or hyperimmune globulin. Since immunodeficiency may appear at any time in HIV-antibody-positive patients, it would appear prudent to utilize only killed vaccines in this group of patients.

Acknowledgments

This work was supported in part by grants from the California State AIDS Task Force, the Pediatric Clinical Research Center (RR-01271), University of California, and NIDA RO1-04331-01.

References

1. Ammann AJ. Is there an acquired immunodeficiency syndrome in infants and children? J Pediatr 1983; 72:430-2
2. Rubinstein A, Sicklick M, Gupta A, Berstein L, Klein N, Rubinstein E, Spigland I, Fructer L, Litman N, Lee H, Hollander M. Acquired immunodeficiency with reversed T4/T8 ratios in infants born to promiscous and drug addicted mothers. JAMA 1983; 249:2350-6.
3. Oleske J Minnefor A, Cooper R, Thomas K, de la Cruz T, Ahdieh H, Guerro I, Joshi VV, Desposito F. Immune deficiency syndrome in children. JAMA 1983; 249:2345-9.
4. Scott GB, Buck BE, Leterman JG, Bloom FL, Parks WP. Acquired immunodeficiency syndrome in infants. N Engl J Med 1984; 310:76-81.

5. Ammann AJ, Cowan MJ, Wara DW, Weintrub P, Dritz S, Goldman H, Perkins HA. Acquired immunodeficiency in an infant: Possible transmission by means of blood product administration. Lancet 1983; 1:956-8.
6. Cowan MJ, Hellmann D, Chudwin D, Wara DW, Chang RS, Ammann AJ. Maternal transmission of acquired immunodeficiency syndrome. Pediatries 1984; 73:382-6.
7. Barre-Sinoussi F, Chermann JC, Rey F, Nugeyre MT, Chamaret S, Gruest J, Dauget C, Alexer-Blin C, Vezinet-Burn F, Rouzioux C, Roxenbaum W, Montagnier L. Isolation of a T lymphotropic retrovirus from a patient at risk for acquired immune deficiency syndrome (AIDS). Science 1983; 220:868-71.
8. Popovic M, Sarngadharan MG, Read E, Gallo RC. Detection, isolation, and continuous production of cytopathic retroviruses (HTLV-III) from patients with AIDS and pre-AIDS. Science 1984; 224:497-500.
9. Levy JA, Hoffman AD, Kramer SM, Landis, JA, Shimabukuro JM. Isolation of lymphacytotropic retrovirus from San Francisco patients with AIDS. Science 1984; 225:840-2.
10. Ammann AJ, Kaminsky L, Cowan M, Levy JA. Anitbodies to AIDS-associated retrovirus distinguish between pediatric primary and acquired immunodeficiency diseases. JAMA 1985; 253:3116-8.
11. Church JA, Isaacs H. Transfusion-associated acquired immune deficiency syndrome in infants. J Pediatr 1984; 105:731-7.
12. Rubinstein A, Bernstein L. The epidemiology of pediatric acquired immunodeficiency syndrome. Clin Immunol Immunopathol 1986; 40:115-21.
13. Zuck TF, Preston MS, Tankersley DL, Wells MA, Wittek AE, Epstein JE, Daniel S, Phelan M, Quinnan GV JR. More on partitioning and inactivation of AIDS virus is immune globulin preparations. N Engl J Med 1986; 314:1454-5.
14. Francis DP, Feorino PM, McDougal S, Warfield D, Getchell J, Cabradilla C, Tong M, Miller WJ, Schultz LD, Baily FJ. The safety of the hepatitis B vaccine. Inactivation of the AIDS virus during routine manufacture. JAMA 1986; 256:869-72.
15. Webster ADB, Malkovsky M, Patterson S, North M, Dalgleish AG, Beattie R, Ashason G, Weiss R. Isolation of retroviruses from two patients with common variable hypogammaglobulinemia. Lancet 1986; 1:581-3.
16. Ziegler JB, Cooper DA, Johnson RD, Gold J. Postnatal transmission of AIDS-associated retrovirus from mother to infant. Lancet 1986; 1:896-9.
17. Thomas PA, Jaffe JW, Spira TJ, Reiss R, Guerrero IC, Auerbach D. Unexplained immunodeficiency in children. JAMA 1984; 252:639-44.
18. Wofsy CB, Cohen JB, Hauer LB, Podian NS, Michaels BA, Evans LA, Levy JA. Isolation of AIDS-associated retrovirus from genital secretions of women with antibody to the virus. Lancet 1986; 1:527-9.
19. Schafer A, Jovaisas E, Stauber M, Lowenthal D, Koch MA. Proof of diaplacental transmission of HTLV III/LAV before the 20th week of pregnancy. Geburtshilfe-Frauenheilkd 1986; 46:88-9.
20. Gill JC, Menitove JE, Anderson PR, Casper JT, Devare SG, Wood C, Adair S, Casey J, Scheffel C, Montgomery RR. HTLV-III serology in hemophilia: relationship with immunologic abnormalities. J Pediatr 1986; 108:511-6.

21. Levine PH. The acquired immunodeficiency syndrome in persons with hemophilia. Ann Intern Med 1985; 103:723-6.
22. Spire B, Dormont D, Barre-Sinoussi F, Montagnier L, Chermann JC. Inactivation of lymphadenopathy assiciated virus by heat, gamma rays, and ultraviolet light. Lancet 1985; 1:188-9.
23. Levy JA, Mitra G, Mozen MM. Recovery and inactivation of infectious retrovirus from factor VIII concentrates. 1984; 2:722-5.
24. Rubinstein A, Bernstein L. The epidemiology of pediatric acquired immunodeficiency syndrome. Clin Immunol Immunopathol 1986; 40:115-21.
25. Friedland GH, Saltzman BR, Rogers MF, Kahl PA, Lessera ML, Maayers MM, Klein RS. Lack of transmission of HTLV III infection to household contacts of patients with AIDS-related complex with oral candidiasis. N Engl J Med 1986; 314:344.
26. Centers for Disease Control. Education and foster care of children infected with human T-lymphotropic virus type III/lymphadenopathy-associated virus. MMWR 1985; 34:517-21.
27. Hirsch MS, Wormser GP, Schooley RT, Ho DD, Felsenstein D, Hopkins CC, Joline C, Duncanson F, Sarngadharan MG, Saxinger C, Gallo RC. Risk of nosocomial infection with human T cell lymphotropic virus III (HTLV-III). N Engl J Med 1985; 312:1-4.
28. Rogers MF. AIDS in children: a review of the clinical epidemiologic and public health aspects. Pediatr Infect Dis 1985; 4:230-6.
29. Scott GB, Fischl M, Klimas N. Mothers of infants with AIDS: Evidence for both symptomatic and asymptomatic carriers. JAMA 1985; 253-63.
30. Minkoff H, Nanda D, Menez R, Fikrig SM. Pregnancies resulting in infants with AIDS and ARC: Clinical course and long term immunologic followup of mothers. Pediatr Res 1986; 20:297A.
31. Curran TW, Lawrence DN, Jaffe H, Kaplan JE, Zyla LD, Chamberlin M, Weinstein R, Lui KJ, Schonberger LB, Spira TJ, Alexander WJ, Swinger G, Ammann AJ, Solomon S, Auerbach D, Mildvan D, Stoneburner R, Jason JM, Haaverkos HW, Evat BL. Acquired immunodeficiency associated with transfusions. N Engl J Med 1984; 310:69-75.
32. Asjo B, Manson-Morfeldt L, Albert J, Biberfeld G, Karlsson A, Lidman K, Fenyo EM. Replicative capacity of human immunodeficiency virus from patients with varying severity of HIV infection. Lancet 1986; 2:660-2.
33. Shannon K, Cowan MJ, Ball E, Abrams D, Volberding P, Ammann AJ. Impaired mononuclear cell proliferation in patients with the acquired immunodeficiency syndrome results from abnormalities of both T lymphocytes and adherent mononuclear cells. J Clin Immunol 1985; 5:239-45.
34. Levy JA, Shimabukuro J, McHugh T, Casavant C, Stites D, Oshiro L. AIDS associated retrovirus (ARV) can productively infect other cells besides human T helper cells. Virology 1985; 147:441-8.
35. Levy JA, Kaminsky LS, Morrow WW, Steiner K, Luciu P, Dina D, Hoxie J, Oshiro L. Infection by the retrovirus associated with the acquired immunodeficienty syndrome. Ann Intern Med 1986; 103:649-9.

36. Dalgleish AG, Beverly PC, Ciapham PR, Crawford DH, Greaves MF, Weiss RA. The CD4(T4) antigen is an essential component of the receptor for the AIDS retrovirus. Nature 1986; 312:763-7.
37. Fauci AS, Macher AM, Lono DL, Lane CL, Rook A, Masus H, Gelmann EP. Acquired immunodeficiency syndrome: epidemiologic, clinical, immunologic, and therapeutic considerations. Ann Intern Med 1984; 100:92-106.
38. Ammann AJ, Abrams D, Conant M, Chudwin D, Cowan MJ, Volberding P, Lewis B, Casavant C. Acquired immune dysfunction in homosexual men: Immunologic profiles. Clin Immun Immunopath 1983; 27:315-25.
39. Maloney M, Cox F, Wray B. AIDS in a child 5½ years after transfusion. N Engl J Med 1985; 312:1256.
40. Buck BE, Scott GB, Valdes-Dapnea M, Parks WP. Kaposi sarcoma in two infants with the acquired immune deficiency syndrome. J Pediatr 1983; 103:911-13.
41. Johsi VV, Oleske JM, Minnefor AB, Singh R, Bokhari T, Rapkin RH. Pathology of suspected acquired immune deficiency in children: A study of eight cases. Pediatr Pathol 1984; 2:71-87.
42. Rubinstein A, Morecki R, Silverman B, Charytan M, Krieger BZ, Andiaman W, Ziprkowski MN, Goldman H. Pulmonary disease in children with acquired immune deficiency and AIDS related complex. J Pediatr 1986; 108:498-503.
43. Grieco MH, Chinoy-Acharya P. Lymphocytic interstitial pneumonia associated with the Acquired Immunodeficiency Syndrome. Am Rev Respir Dis 1985; 131:952-5.
44. Shaw GM, Harper ME, Hahn BE, Epstein LG, Gadjudusek DC, Prince RW, Navia BA, Petito CK, O'Hara CJ, Groopman JE, Cho ES, Oleskek JM, Wong-Stall F, Gallo RC. HTLV-III infection in brains of children and adults with AIDS encephalopathy. Science 1985; 227:177-81.
45. Levy J, Hollander H, Shimbukuro J, Mills J, Kaminsky L. Isolation of AIDS associated retrovirus from cerebrospinal fluid and brains of patients with neurologic symptoms. Lancet 1985; 2:586-8.
46. Barnes DM. Brain function decline in children with AIDS. Science 1986; 232:1196.
47. Carne CA, Tedder RS, Smith A, Sutherland S, Elkington SG, Daly HM, Preston FE, Crask J. Acute encephalopathy coincident with seroconversion for anti-HTLV III. Lancet 1985; 2:1206-8.
48. Andiman WA, Eastman R, Martin K, Katz BZ, Rubinstein A, Pitt J, Pahwa S, Miller G. Opportunistic lymphoproliferations associated with Epstein Barr viral DNA in infants and children with AIDS. Lancet 1985; 2:8469-70.
49. Marion RW, Wiznia AA, Hutcheon G, Rubinstein A. Human T cell lymphotropic virus III (HTLV-III) embryopathy. A new dysmorphic syndrome associated with intrauterine HTLV-III infection. Am J Dis Child 1986; 140:638-40.
50. Ammann AJ, Wara DW, Cowan MJ, Barrett DJ, Stiehm ER. The DiGeorge Syndrome and the fetal alcohol syndrome. Am J Dis Child 1982; 136:906-9.
51. Centers for Disease Control: Provisional case definition for acquired immunodeficiency syndrome in children. MMWR 1983; 32:691.
52. Ammann AJ. The acquired immunodeficiency syndrome in infants and children. Ann Intern Med 1985; 103:734-7.
53. Petricciani JC. Licensed tests for antibody to human T lymphotropic virus III. Ann Intern Med 1985; 103:726-9.

54. Weiss SH, Goedert JJ, Sarngadharan MG, Bodner AJ, Gallo RC, Blattner WA. Screening test for HTLV-III (AIDS agent) antibodies. JAMA 1985; 253:221-5.
55. Ammann AJ, Schiffman G, Abrams VP, Ziegler J, Conant MB. B-cell immunodeficiency in acquired immune deficiency syndrome. JAMA 1984; 251:1447-9.
56. Hirsch MS, Kaplan JC. Prospects of therapy for the infections with human T lymphotropic virus. Ann Intern Med 1985; 103:750-5.
57. Gutpa S, Gottlieb MS. Treatment of the acquired immunodeficiency syndrome. J Clin Immunol 1986; 6:183-93.
58. Ernst M, Kern P, Flad HD, Ulmer AJ. Effects of systemic *in vivo* interleukin 2 (IL-2) reconstitution in patients with acquired immunodeficiency syndrome (AIDS) and AIDS related complex (ARC) on phenotypes of peripheral blood mononuclear cells (PBMC). J Clin Immunol 1986; 6:170-81.
59. Krown SE, Real FX, Cunningham-Rundles S, Myskowski PL, Fein S, Mittelman A, Oettgen HF, Safai B, Koziner B. Preliminary observations on the effect of recombinant leukocyte A interferon in homosexual men with Kaposi's sarcoma. N Engl J Med 1983; 508:1071-5.
60. Lane HC, Fauci AS. Immunologic reconstitution in the acquired immunodeficiency syndrome. Ann Intern Med 1985; 103:714-8.
61. Hardy AM, Allen JR, Morgan M, Curran JW. The incidence rate of acquired immunodeficiency syndrome in selected populations. JAMA 1985; 253:215-20.
62. Brady MT, Ng A. Protection of neonates from transfusion-associated AIDS by the use of CMV-seronegative blood before availability of specific serologic tests for HTLV-III (HIV). Am J Perinatol 1987; 4:305-7.
63. Constantopolous P, Gabaude B, Duforestel T, Fuzibet J, Mourey C, Lefebvre J, Cassuto J, Gillet J. Positive HIV serology in the pregnant woman: current data on its management. Rev Fr Gynecol Obstet 1987; 82:453-62.
64. Medley G, Anderson R, Cox D, Billard L. Incubation period of AIDS in patients infected via blood transfusion. Nature 1987; 328:719-21.
65. Pawha S, Fikrig S, Menex R, Pahwa R. Pediatric acquired immunodeficiency syndrome; demonstration of B lymphocyte defects in vitro. Diagn Immunol 1986; 4:24-30.
66. Saulsbury F, Wykoff R, Boyle R. Transfusion-acquired immunodeficiency virus infection in twelve neonates: epidemiologic, clinical and immunologic features. Pediatr Infect Dis J 1987; 6:544-9.
67. Joshi V, Pawel B, Connor E, Sharer L, Oleske J, Morrison S, Marin-Garcia J. Arteriopathy in children with acquired immune deficiency syndrome. Pediatr Pathol 1987; 7:261-75.
68. Joshi V, Gadol C, Connor E, Oleske J, Mendelson J, Marin-Garcia J. Dilated cardiomyopathy in children with acquired immunodeficiency syndrome: a pathology study of five cases. Hum Pathol 1988; 19:69-73.
69. Malekzadeh M, Church J, Siegel S, Mitchell W, Opas L, Lieberman E. Human immunodeficiency virus-associated Kaposi's sarcoma in a pediatric renal transplant recipient. Nephron 1987; 47:62-5.
70. Colebunders R, Francis H, Mann J, Bila K, Kandi K, Lebughe I, Gigase P, Van Marck E, Macher A, Quinn T. Parotid swelling during human immunodeficiency virus infection. Arch Otolaryngol Head Neck Surg 1988; 114:330-2.

71. Chayt K, Harper M, Marselle L, Lewin E, Rose R, Oleske J, Epstein L, Wong-Staal F, Gallo R. Detection of HTLV-III RNA in lungs of patients with AIDS and pulmonary involvement. JAMA 1986; 256:2356-9.
72. Joshi V, Kauffman S, Oleske J, Fikrig S, Denny T, Gadol C, Lee E. Polyclonal polymorphic B-cell lymphoproliferative disorder with prominent pulmonary involvement in children with acquired immune deficiency syndrome. Cancer 1987; 59:1455-62.
73. Rubinstein A, Bernstein L, Charytan M, Krieger B, Ziprkowski M. Corticosteroid treatment for pulmonary lymphoid hyperplasia in children with the acquired immune deficiency syndrome. Pediatr Pulmonol 1988; 4:13-7.
74. Epstein L, Sharer L, Goudsmit J. Neurological and neuropathological features of human immunodeficiency virus infection in children. Ann Neurol 1988; 23 (suppl):S19-23.
75. Qazi Q, Sheikh T, Fikrig S, Menikoff H. Lack of evidence for craniofacial dysmorphism in perinatal human immunodeficiency virus infection. J Pediatr 1988; 112:7-11.
76. Classification system for human immunodeficiency virus (HIV) infection in children under 13 years of age. MMWR 1987; 36:225-30.
77. Pahwa R, Good R, Pahwa S. Prematurity, hypogammaglobulinemia, and neuropathology with human immunodeficiency virus infection. Proc Natl Acad Sci USA 1987; 84:3826-30.
78. Espanol T, Garcia-Armui R, Bofill A, Sune J, Bertran J. Hypogammaglobulinemia and negative anti-HIV antibodies in AIDS. Arch Dis Child 1987; 62:853-4.
79. Goetz D, Hall S, Harbison R, Reid J. Pediatric acquired immunodeficiency syndrome with negative human immunodeficiency virus antibody response by enzyme-linked immunosorbent assay and Western blot. Pediatrics 1988; 81:356-9.
80. Borkowshy W, Krasinski K, Paul D, Moore T, Bebenroth D, Chandwani S. HIV infections in infants negative for anti-HIV by enzyme-linked immunoassay. Lancet 1987; 1:1168-71.
81. vonReyn C, Clements C, Mann J. Human immunodeficiency virus infection and routine childhood immunisation. Lancet 1987; 2:669-72.
82. Curran J, Jaffe H, Hardy A, Morgan W, Selik R, Dondero T. Epidemiology of HIV infection and AIDS in the United States. Science 1988; 239:610-6.
83. Rogers M, Thomas P, Starcher E, Noa M, Bush T, Jaffe H. Acquired immunodeficiency syndrome in children: report of the CDC National Surveillance, 1982 to 1985. Pediatrics 1987; 79:1008-14.
84. Hoff R, Berardi V, Weiblen B, Mahoney-Trout L, Mitchell M, Grady G. Seroprevalence of human immunodeficiency virus among childbearing women. Estimation by testing samples of blood from newborns. N Engl J Med 1988; 318: 525-30.

7

Heterosexual Transmission of HIV

Judith B. Cohen and Constance B. Wofsy

San Francisco General Hospital
and School of Medicine
University of California
San Francisco, California

I. Introduction

From the earliest days of the epidemic, the acquired immunodeficiency syndrome (AIDS) has primarily been a sexually transmitted disease. The rapid spread of AIDS in U.S. populations of homosexual men led to a variety of explorations into aspects of their lifestyle and environment that might account for transmission within the group. It is now clear that it is the pattern of sexual partners and practices that has facilitated sexual transmission of human immunodeficiency virus (HIV) within this population. However, viruses, including this relatively newly identified retrovirus, do not recognize gender or sexual preference; therefore, the possibility for sexual transmission of the AIDS virus exists among all persons who are sexually active.

The probability of sexual transmission of HIV appears to vary from a high of 60% among homosexual men to less than 10% among hemophiliac mates with considerable variability among population groups and geographic areas (1). Sexual transmission between homosexual and bisexual males is the most efficient. In partner studies among intravenous drug users (IVDUs),

Table 1 Prevalence of HIV Antibody in Sexual Partners of Men in Specific AIDS Risk Groups

Risk group	Number studied	Number of index seropositive or with AIDS	Number (%) of partners seropositive	Reference
Hemophiliac	42	21	2 (9%)	26
Hemophiliac	43	34	2 (6%)	27
Hemophiliac	148	148	10 (7%)	29
IVDU	7	7	6 (86%)	31
IVDU	Unknown	48 men	17 (35%)	57
		9 women	4 (44%)	
IVDU	21	12	1 (8%)	34
Haitian	17 men	17	11 (65%)	18
	82 women	82	50 (61%)	
Bisexual	55 women	51	12 (22%)	38
Household	15	15	6 (40%)	41
Household	Unknown	28 men	15 (54%)	60
		17 women	11 (65%)	

Abbreviation: IVDU, intravenous drug user.

estimates of transmission range from 10% to 40%, although sexual partners who don't share needles appear to be at less risk of virus transmission than their needle-sharing partners. Sexual transmission to female partners of other high-risk men, such as hemophiliacs, appears to be even lower (Table 1).

In the United States, where 93% of AIDS cases are male and there is more opportunity for male-to-female heterosexual transmission, the incidence of heterosexual transmission has remained low. In other parts of the world, particularly central Africa and Haiti, AIDS appears to be heterosexually transmitted, and the ratio of male-to-female transmission approaches 1:1 (see Chapters 2, 3).

The rate of spread of any epidemic of sexually transmitted disease depends on the efficiency of transmission, the prevalence of infection already in the population, and the relative frequency of opportunity for transmission to occur. There is now a growing body of information about the relative efficiency of transmission of this virus as part of heterosexual activity, but the role of the cofactors is less clear. The virus has been identified in blood, semen, and vaginal and cervical secretions; however, concurrent systemic or genital infection, local trauma, or sex during menses are possible cofactors that may facilitate viral transmission or disease expression. The prevalence of HIV infection in most heterosexual populations is now estimated to be less than 1%, but the potential for spread of infection to more of the heterosexual population is great.

The relationship between the number of heterosexual partners and acquisition of the virus is now being explored. Much concern has been expressed about the extent of AIDS virus infection among prostitutes and their role as transmitters of infection. The evidence available is greatly exceeded by the conjectural claims in the media, and since diversity of sexual practices and the use of protection such as condoms are both characteristic of many people with multiple partners, the role of number of partners per se may be obscured by these related factors.

II. System of Classification of AIDS Cases Attributed to Heterosexual Transmission

Attribution of transmission for persons diagnosed with AIDS generally follows standards set by the Centers for Disease Control (CDC) (2). In identifying the source of transmission for any person diagnosed with AIDS, the Centers utilize a descriptive system that is hierarchical and mutually exclusive. A newly diagnosed adult (or next of kin) is asked about homosexuality or bisexuality, drug use, hemophilia or other clotting disorders, blood transfusions, and ethnic/geographic origin (Haiti or central Africa, in particular). If the response to any of these is positive for a point in time that is within a reasonable incubation period for AIDS (since 1978), attribution of transmission is designated to the single circumstance highest on the list. For example, if a man with AIDS admits bisexuality and intravenous (IV) drug use, his AIDS transmission is counted as of bisexual origin; if he has been an IVDU and is also Haitian, his transmission is counted as due to drug abuse. Thus, heterosexual transmission is considered causal only if the person has none of the preceding characteristics of risk exposure.

Centers for Disease Control attribute an AIDS case in a male as due to heterosexual transmission only if a man diagnosed with the disease has never had homosexual or bisexual experiences, never used drugs IV, or never had a transfusion of blood or blood components, but has had sexual contact with at least one woman with AIDS or AIDS-related complex (ARC) or who was in a "risk" group (3). Cases in men with AIDS who meet the above exclusionary criteria but with multiple female sex partners of unknown risk status are not defined as due to heterosexual transmission, but are categorized as "other." As of May 30, 1988, 1132 cases of AIDS in adult men had been classified as due to heterosexual transmission (Table 2) (2). Their small proportion (2%) among total male cases has remained essentially the same over time (4).

Attribution to heterosexual transmission among U.S. women with AIDS is reported by the CDC if the woman has never used IV drugs or never had a transfusion, but has been a sexual partner of a man with AIDS or ARC, or

Table 2 U.S. AIDS Cases Attributed to Heterosexual Transmission: May 30, 1988

Category	
Heterosexual cases, total 2574 (4% of total)	
Male	1132
Female	1142
Heterosexual cases since January 1988	
Male	220
Female	336
Multiple risk factors:	
Heterosexual *and*	
Homosexual/bisexual male	658
Homosexual/bisexual male, IVDU	240
IVDU	1020
Blood transfusion	128

Abbreviation: IVDU, intravenous drug user.
Source: Ref. 2.

at risk for these. As of July 29, 1986, 402 cases, or 27% of all U.S. cases of adult women with AIDS, were attributed to heterosexual contact (2). Specifically, the CDC reported that the risk exposure of such women was due to the following circumstance:

	%
Partner with IV drug use	61
Partner who was bisexual	16
Partner from another country where heterosexual transmission is more frequent	4
Partner with hemophilia or who had a blood transufsion	1
Partner with HIV or AIDS but unknown risk group	7
Partner risk circumstances unknown	11

In terms of geographic distribution, four states have 80% of all heterosexual cases. In rank order, they are New York, New Jersey, Florida, and California (5).

The one location within the United States where heterosexual transmission appears to be a major source of AIDS is in the community of Belle Glade, Florida (6). This is an economically depressed area with a resident population of approximately 20,000 and a seasonal migrant agricultural labor force of 10,000 Caribbean workers. The majority of AIDS cases there do not appear to be due to homosexual transmission, and the ratio of men to women is nearer 2:1 (5). Conditions of environmental sanitation and heterosexual transmission appear to be more similar to those in Haiti and central Africa than to the rest of the United States.

A. Characteristics of U.S. AIDS Cases Classified as Due to Heterosexual Contact

In February 1984, Guinan et al. (1), using the CDC mutually exclusive stratification, compared four AIDS patient groups: homosexual men, IV drug users, Haitians, and those with no identified risks. Haitians and many other males with no identified risk reported multiple sexual partners in Haiti and/or New York. In November 1984, Chamberland et al. (4) characterized the first 201 AIDS cases in the category of no identified risk reported to the CDC between June 1981 and January 1984. (At this time, the CDC had not established risk categories for "heterosexual transmission" or "blood transfusion" cases.) Patients with AIDS in "no known risk" groups were more likely than patients in known risk groups to be female and nonwhite, and to reside outside of the areas with the highest rates of AIDS. They were also much more likely to present with opportunistic infection than with Kaposi's sarcoma (KS). Of the 201 patients, 35 (17%) had received blood transfusions within five years of diagnosis. Another 30 (15%, 28 women, two men) had been sexual partners or spouses of persons known to be at increased risk for developing AIDS. The remaining patients included 89 for whom detailed information was not available. The authors concluded that these 89 were primarily persons "who had either undetected risk factors or were sexual partners of persons in high-risk groups." An early, well-documented case of heterosexual transmission was reported by Groopman et al. (7) who described a 24-year-old Black woman with KS whose only risk exposure was a sexual relationship with an asymptomatic but HIV-positive Haitian partner (7).

B. Implications for Family and Children

In these early reports, the emerging evidence for infection in women and heterosexuals with families raised the issues of transmission to other family members, particularly infants and young children, as well as prenatal AIDS virus transmission. Many studies have reported household members of patients with AIDS and ARC, including families with infants with AIDS, and those in which sleeping and personal hygiene facilities were shared; among all of them, there is not a single documented instance of nonsexual household virus transmission (8,9).

Prenatal and perinatal transmission are also effective means of transmission. Human immunodeficiency virus has been identified in amniotic fluid (10) and fetal tissue (11). A dysmorphic syndrome in congenitally infected infants has been described (12). Most early research identified mothers only after their infants were diagnosed with AIDS or ARC. Scott and coworkers (13) followed 16 mothers of 22 infants with AIDS or ARC. All mothers but one were clinically well at delivery, but five developed AIDS and seven developed ARC during an average followup period of 30 months. Under these circumstances, the probability of a subsequent child also being infected may be as high as 60%. Furthermore, the progression from asymptomatic HIV infection to ARC or to AIDS may be much more rapid in pregnant seropositives than in nonpregnant asymptomatic women. However, it appears that a seropositive father poses no risk to the infant unless the mother has been infected.

Prospective studies are underway of risk of *in utero* AIDS infection in HIV antibody-positive women. One such study from New York presented preliminary findings at the Third International AIDS Conference in Washington, D.C. in June 1987. Selwyn (14,63) reported on 78 pregnancies among IVDU women with known HIV antibody status prior to or during pregnancy. Of 33 seropositive mothers, 14 elected to terminate the pregnancy, three aborted spontaneously, and 16 had live births. Of these 16, at a mean of 34 weeks, six remained seropositive and six became negative. Six of these 12, including one seronegative infant, were symptomatic at follow-up.

C. Case Identification Due to Heterosexual Contact

Heterosexual Contact Cases in Europe

All European countries presently have some AIDS surveillance; most of these now use the CDC case definition and report data quarterly to the World Health Organization collaborating Centre on AIDS in France.

By June 1986, European countries reported over 1500 cases of AIDS. Early in the epidemic a significant proportion of these, especially in Belgium, France, and the Netherlands, were heterosexually transmitted cases from Zaire and the Congo in Africa (15). A more current estimate is that 12% of European AIDS cases are African patients from 21 countries (16).

The prevalence of HIV infection in European populations remains lower than in the United States. Earliest reports were from The Netherlands and France, followed by the Scandinavian countries, then by countries on the Mediterranean, i.e., Greece and Italy (15). As in the United States, the most rapid growth of heterosexually transmitted cases parallels increased HIV seroprevalence among heterosexual IVDUs, especially in such major cities as Paris, London, Amsterdam, and Berlin.

Heterosexual Contact Cases in the Caribbean

Virtually all of the AIDS cases initially reported from the Caribbean were among people residing in Haiti, and among Haitian immigrants to the United States and Canada (17) (see Chapter 3). AIDS was reported from Haiti prior to 1980, and in contrast to the experience in the United States and Europe, the majority of cases have not been due to homosexuality, IV drug use, or blood transfusions. The male to female ratio of AIDS cases in Haiti is approximately 3:1 (17). One study of heterosexual sex partners of Haitian AIDS patients reported that 61% (51/82) of female sex partners of male AIDS patients and 65% (11/17) of male sex partners of female AIDS patients were seropositive (18). In this regard, the prevalence and transmission of HIV in Haiti resembles that of Africa.

Heterosexual AIDS Cases in Africa

Evidence is accumulating that AIDS seroprevalence has reached alarming levels in some urban areas of central Africa, and that the predominant mode of transmission is via heterosexual contact (19,20) (see Chapter 2). Cases of AIDS first appeared in 1980-1981 among affluent African patients treated at Belgian and French hospitals, and since then have followed the same doubling in cumulative frequency pattern observed in the United States and Europe (16). Although diagnostic capabilities within Africa vary considerably, 10-fold epidemic increases in AIDS have been reported from Kigali, Rwanda and from Kinshasa, Zaire since 1980, and from adjacent Zambia and Tanzania since then (16,20,21). A current estimate is that AIDS incidence in Zaire is in the range of 60-100 cases per 100,000, which is 50-100 times greater than in most European countries (16).

Bidirectional heterosexual transmission as the likeliest source of spread is supported by research that demonstrates a strong association between HIV antibody or AIDS/ARC with concurrent sexually transmitted diseases (STDs) and/or increased average numbers of sexual contacts (22). Further, in these countries, where prostitutes do not use barrier protection and untreated STDs are frequent, several studies have reported rates of HIV seropositivity among prostitutes and among their customers ranging from 54% to 88% (22,23,24,25). Other risk factors in this part of the world include the use of unsterilized needles and unsafe blood and blood products (see Chapter 2).

III. Population Groups at Increased Risk for Heterosexual Transmission

A. Heterosexual Transmission to Partners of Hemophiliacs

Four reports have been published on heterosexual transmission of the virus in partners of hemophiliacs. Kreiss and co-workers (26) reported on 42 couples whose relationships had lasted an average of 11 years (range 2-40 years). Of the 42 males, 21 (50%) were antibody-positive, including 10 with AIDS or ARC. Two female partners or 10% were seropositive; both had partners who were seropositive but did not have AIDS or ARC. Neither had engaged in rectal intercourse.

Jason and co-workers (27) studied both sexual and casual/household contacts of 43 hemophiliacs. Among the men, 9 were seronegative and 34 had evidence of HIV infection (17 were antibody-positive only, 5 had ARC, and 12 had AIDS). Of the 33 seropositive males with consistent sexual partners, two spouses (6%) were affected; one had AIDS, and one had ARC. None of the sexual partners were HIV seropositive, although some had indicators of low immune function.

Melbye and co-workers (28) reported briefly on 29 hemophiliac households in Denmark, noting that although 14 of 29 hemophiliac males were antibody-positive, only one female sexual partner among all household members was seropositive (28).

The AIDS-hemophilia French study group reported that among the wives or partners of 148 seropositive patients with hemophilia who responded to a national epidemiologic survey, 10 (6.8%) were confirmed as antibody-positive (29). No information on specific sexual or contraceptive practices was reported.

One additional report about heterosexual transmission from a hemophiliac man to his spouse is of interest because it describes a transient antibody response (30). The husband had antibody to HIV, reduced T-helper lymphocytes, and lymphadenopathy syndrome when his wife was first examined. She showed mildly decreased T-helper cells and had a positive enzyme-linked immunosorbent assay (ELISA) antibody response to the virus confirmed by Western blot. Subsequently, the husband lost his antibody response and was also diagnosed with AIDS (*Pneumocystis carinii* pneumonia [PCP]). The couple continued to have intercourse but used condoms. Three months later, her serum no longer had detectable antibody, and her absolute number of T4$^+$ cells had risen to within normal limits. She has continued to be antibody-negative and was clinically well for six subsequent months of followup. The possibility of exposure only to HIV antigens must also be considered.

B. Heterosexual Transmission from IV Drug Abusers

Although hemophiliac spouses were among the earliest heterosexual transmission cases reported, there is now ample evidence that other cases reported early in the epidemic represented the major risk group for heterosexual transmission of HIV in the United States and Europe, namely heterosexual IVDUs and their sexual partners. The first report of "immunodeficiency" in partners of men with AIDS was in May 1983. Harris and co-workers (31) described seven steady sexual partners of IVDU men with AIDS; none of the seven spouses acknowledged IV drug use or had any other AIDS risk exposure. At the time, no test for antibody to the virus was available, but among the seven women partners, one had a full AIDS syndrome (PCP, oral candidiasis, lymphadenopathy) and another had persistent generalized lymphadenopathy, lymphopenia, cutaneous anergy, and a decreased helper/suppressor ratio. Only one of seven women was free of any AIDS-related signs and symptoms.

Since that time, many reports of heterosexual transmission of HIV have documented that infection is likely and can occur in either direction: male to female or female to male. Current surveillance information from the United States and several countries in Europe indicates that the majority of AIDS cases attributed to heterosexual transmission are from a needle-sharing IV drug abusing person to a sexual partner who does not use drugs. Des Jarlais and co-workers (32) estimate from New York AIDS data that at least 58% of the estimated 11,000 male IVDUs in the city have prolonged, stable heterosexual relationships (32). If female partners involved in short-term relationships and male sexual partners of female IVDUs are included as potential heterosexual risk partners, the total persons at potential risk for heterosexual transmission in New York City alone exceeds 10,000 persons.

Heterosexual AIDS incidence observed in New York City has provided an opportunity to assess the relative efficiency of heterosexual transmission in comparison with homosexual or needle-sharing risk. Des Jarlais et al. (32) estimated early in the New York City epidemic that the relative risk of AIDS transmission to heterosexual partners of IVDUs was approximately 9%, less than one-third the risk from sharing needles in that city. A 1985 estimate by Hardy et al. (33) put the relative risk of contracting the AIDS virus as 1 among heterosexual partners who share sexual relations only and 17 among homosexual men, compared with 20 among those who share both IV drug use and sexual relationship. Similarly, a report from Europe indicated that among 14 couples where only one used drugs, one partner (8%) was seropositive, but among 14 couples where drug abuse was also shared seven partners (50%) were seropositive (34).

It is apparent that among heterosexual IVDUs sharing drug use represents significantly greater transmission risk for AIDS than does sexual activity. However, the extensive numbers of non-drug-using sexual partners of IVDUs represent the largest single at risk heterosexual transmission group.

C. Transmission from Bisexual Partners

In the United States, among HIV seropositive men who define themselves as bisexual or homosexual, many have had at least some sexual contact with heterosexual women partners. For example, one study of the epidemiology of AIDS among men in San Francisco found that among gay and homosexual men, over 10% reported one or more (median = 2.9) female sexual partners during the previous two years (35). Thus, it is reasonable to estimate that thousands of heterosexual women who have had sexual contact with bisexual men may have been exposed to HIV in such areas where seroprevalence is high as in New York, San Francisco, Los Angeles, and Miami.

One example of a transmission chain beginning with a bisexual man has been reported by Calabrese and Gopalakrishna (36). A bisexual man from Ohio traveled frequently to New York City where he engaged in homosexual activity. He developed AIDS and died in 1983. After his death, his heterosexual monogamous spouse of 10 years was examined and advised that she had no signs of impaired immune function. She subsequently established a mutually monogamous sexual relationship with another heterosexual man. Eighteen months later she developed AIDS and died. The serum of her male partner is strongly reactive for HIV antibody; he has a low helper/suppressor ratio, generalized lymphadenopathy, and oral thrush.

No population studies that would permit estimates of infectivity in this risk group have yet been reported, although several studies are underway (37,38). Given the health and behavioral characteristics of the bisexual population, the rate of infectivity is likely to be between those for partners of IVDUs and partners of hemophiliacs.

D. Transmission from Unspecified Sexual Partners

There are studies of sexual partner transmission without regard to the major risk group of the infected partner as classified by the CDC. Redfield and coworkers (39) have studied AIDS and ARC cases in members of the U.S. military and their spouses. In the first report, they documented HIV infection in five of seven wives of men with AIDS or ARC; three of the five seropositive women also had clinical evidence of ARC (39). All relationships had lasted longer than two years. In a subsequent report, two more women and 10 men were described as heterosexual transmission cases (40). However, whereas all five women had a partner with AIDS or an identifiable risk group sexual partner, only 1 of the 10 men identified a specific risk relationship (with a Haitian immigrant). The remaining nine gave histories of multiple sexual partners, including prostitutes in the United States and other countries; therefore, no definitive attribution of their exposure is possible. All 15 denied receptive anal intercourse. Another report of 42 heterosexual partners of AIDS and ARC patients found that 47% were antibody-positive (41).

In these studies, the proportions of sexual partners who were seropositive ranged from 45% to 72%. No association with increased risk was found for specific sexual practices (e.g., anal intercourse) or with duration of the relationship, although the partnerships described were usually of two years or longer.

E. Risk of Transmission from Multiple Partners

Among homosexual men the relative risk for AIDS is associated with increased numbers of sexual partners. However, the role played by multiple partners in heterosexual transmission of the virus is less clear and more controversial. In part, this is because data from the United States and Europe cannot be directly compared to reports from Africa. In part, also, the question is clouded by incomplete information on numbers of partners and sexual behavior patterns from most studies of heterosexually transmitted cases. Finally, the role attributed to prostitutes in heterosexual transmission reflects more controversy and confusion than information.

At the present time, there are no reports from the United States that document the role of multiple partners in heterosexual transmission. However, in populations and areas where virus prevalence is higher, increased numbers of heterosexual partners may represent increased risk potential. For example, one report of 229 AIDS cases and controls in Haiti found that the 93 men and 35 women with AIDS who were not homosexual or IVDUs were significantly more likely than controls to report more heterosexual partners per year (17). Cases were also more likely than controls to have had nonmedical injections (e.g., vitamins), but it was not clear whether these injections were associated with early morbidity from AIDS.

Information from several countries in central Africa is also consistent on this point. Two reports in 1984 from Zaire (23) and Rwanda (24) found a male to female ratio near 1:1 for AIDS, and seropositivity was associated with higher numbers of sexual contacts than negative controls.

A more recent and thoroughly documented study from Zaire compared 58 male cases with controls; AIDS patients reported a mean of 32 sexual partners per year compared with an annual average of three for control males (42). Other factors, such as history of injections, did not differ between the groups.

Among those concerned with heterosexual transmission of AIDS, especially in Africa, the boundaries between "multiple sexual partners," "promiscuity," and "prostitution" are far from clear. Some researchers, for example, define any unmarried sexually active women as a prostitute. Others group together any "sexual contact with multiple partners, including prostitutes" (39). To add to the confusion, some health jurisdictions include such AIDS cases as heterosexual in origin, whereas others classify them as "no identifiable risk." The following studies concerned with the role of prostitution in AIDS transmission are part of this confusion and controversy.

F. Transmission via Prostitutes

There are no reports from the United States at present that permit systematic assessment of the role of multiple partners in heterosexual transmission. The Centers for Disease Control (Jan 17, 1986) reported that among the "other" cases of AIDS completely interviewed, 35% (39/111) reported histories of STD, and 26% (15/57) of males in the group reported contact with one or more prostitutes (41). Since there are no population data for the frequency of these characteristics among people of the same age and residence who do not have AIDS, the relative significance of these reports is not clear. Throughout the course of the epidemic, however, the proportion of these "other" potential multiple-partner cases has been much smaller than the heterosexual transmission cases where a single high-risk partner has been identified. This fact suggests that when general population prevalence of the virus is low, the increased risk conveyed by additional sexual partners is not very significant.

Reserach information on prostitution and AIDS is fragmentary and controversial. Further, it is limited to information about female prostitutes, although male prostitution has undoubtedly contributed to homosexual transmission of the disease in the United States. Although a great deal of concern

Table 3 HIV Antibody in Female Prostitutes in the United States, Europe, and Africa

Site	Source	Number tested	Positive (%)	IVDU (%)	HIV-positive who are IVDU (%)	Reference
Seattle	Jail	92	5	Unk	Unk	3
Miami	AIDS clinic	25	40	Unk	80	3
San Francisco	various	87	4	32	100	52
Germany[a]		NA	1	Unk	Unk	47
Germany[b]		NA	20-50	Unk	Unk	47
Greece[c]		200	6	0	NA	48
Italy	Clinic	24	46	58	100	49
London	STD clinic	50	0	6	NA	45
Paris	Street prostitutes	56	0	0	NA	46
Kenya	STD clinic	50	55	0	0	44
Rwanda	STD clinic	84	80	0	0	24

Abbreviations: IVDU, intravenous drug user; NA, not applicable; STD, sexually transmitted disease; Unk, unknown.

[a]Registered prostitutes.

[b]Unregistered prostitutes near the train station.

[c]Intravenous drug abuse.

has been expressed about prostitution as a mechanism for spread of the AIDS virus into the heterosexual community, the CDC has noted that nearly all heterosexual transmission cases in the United States have been among sexual partners of men and women with the diagnosed disease or in high-risk groups (3).

In the United States and Europe, reports about prostitution and HIV infection have been based on seroprevalence surveys from jails, STD clinics, or other sites where prostitutes congregate (Table 3) (44-49). There is a strong association between personal IV drug use and seropositivity. A multicenter study of U.S. prostitutes in cities was coordinated by the Centers for Disease Control during 1986-1987. Preliminary results were reported in March 1987 (49a). HIV infection rates varied from 57% among prostitutes recruited from intravenous drug use treatment centers in New Jersey to 0% among 34 brothel employees in Nevada. Again, HIV infection was strongly associated with sharing of needles in IV drug use and was also higher among black and Hispanic IV drug-using women than among whites.

Despite evidence that there are indeed some prostitutes in the United States and Europe infected (mostly IV drug users), no case has been confirmed of direct transmission from a female prostitute to a male partner. The strongest inference has come from Redfield who reported high levels of heterosexual activity including use of prostitutes by United States servicemen with AIDS. Nine servicemen who denied any other risk activity indicated extensive heterosexual activity, including use of female prostitutes, primarily in Germany, as the only other possible risk for exposure to the AIDS virus (39). These findings generated considerable debate about their reliability at interview, and about the prevalence of AIDS virus infection in German prostitutes with estimates ranging from 1% to 20-50% (47). However, the CDC still includes men reporting contacts with a female prostitute as the only possible risk in "less probable heterosexual transmission cases" in the "other" category (2). Of the 32 women with AIDS interviewed in the "other" category, none acknowledged payment for sex within the five years prior to diagnosis (50).

Evidence Linking AIDS Virus and Prostitution in Africa

In 1983, clusters of AIDS cases in Kinshasa, Zaire, in central Africa indicated a male to female ratio of 1:1 and first suggested bidirectional spread of the AIDS virus within central Africa (23). African female prostitutes were thought to be at particular risk, because four out of nine women with AIDS diagnosed in Rwanda in 1983 considered themselves prostitutes (24). At the same time, 17 men in Rwanda were diagnosed with AIDS and 11 of these 17 reported contact with prostitutes but denied other risk behaviors (24).

By 1985, Belgian researchers working in Zaire stated that "in central Africa, infection with HTLV-III or lymphadenopathy-associated virus is linked to heterosexual promiscuity and female prostitution" (42). In their study, 24% of 40 African women with AIDS were prostitutes who had no history of addiction to oral or intravenous drugs. Compared with 81% of 58 male AIDS patients, only 34% of 58 control males had visited a prostitute. However, male patients reported a mean of 32 sexual partners per year versus three partners per year by the control males. Unspecified cofactors were suspected to play a role in the acquisition of viral infection and expression of disease. Further studies in central Africa confirm the greater prevalence of HIV antibody in African female prostitutes and male customers of prostitutes than in controls (Table 3) (22,42).

In 1985, Kreiss et al. (44) studied 90 female prostitutes in Nairobi, Kenya, East Africa. Prevalence of the AIDS virus was high and was related to the socioeconomic status of the prostitute. Sixty percent of lower-status prostitutes were infected versus 31% of higher-class prostitutes; in comparison, rates were 8% of all clinic patients and 2% of medical personnel. There was a significant association between seropositivity and contact with males from central Africa, suggesting a pattern of geographical spread of the infection within Africa. Vaginal intercourse without condoms was the reported means of contact in all cases. Sexually transmitted diseases were found in 40% of the lower socioeconomic class prostitutes with a strong correlation between seropositivity and venereal disease. Venereal disease is widespread in Africa (16). The role, however, of venereal disease as a cofactor in virus acquisition or expression of disease remains undetermined. Nevertheless, caution should be used in extrapolating data from Africa to other parts of the world, and making more general suppositions about AIDS in prostitutes.

IV. Disease Expression in Heterosexual Transmission Cases

Information to date on the natural history of HIV infection has come largely from studies of male homosexuals and from AIDS cases in intravenous drug abusers who are also primarily males. Heterosexually transmitted cases, especially seropositive women without disease are less available for study. One striking population difference is the absence of KS among women. Since heterosexuals present with opportunistic infections, they have shorter average survival after definitive AIDS diagnosis. Female AIDS mortality during the year after diagnosis is 59% compared with 49% mortality among males (50).

A. Viral Infectivity in Blood, Semen, Cervical/Vaginal Secretions

The most infectious bodily secretions are blood and semen/seminal fluid, although the virus has been identified in most other bodily secretions. HIV has been isolated in semen but has not been isolated from spermatozoa (51). Recently, researchers in two laboratories have grown HIV from female genital secretions (51,52). Thus, there is potential for viral transmission from female secretions, although the absolute amounts of virus in these secretions were relatively low. The efficiency of transmission from male to female versus from female to male is probably affected by the relative infectivity of these different secretions, as well as sex during menses, specific sexual practices (e.g., vaginal versus anal intercourse), the relative integrity of skin and mucosal surfaces involved, and possibly the presence of other sexually transmitted diseases.

Little is known about the relative importance of these factors in AIDS transmission heterosexually at this time. However, these issues can be addressed indirectly by looking at HIV transmission among heterosexual IVDUs. The proportion of female AIDS cases attributed to contact with a male IVDU is 5.4%, compared with the proportion of male cases from a female IVDU of 3.7%. Comparison of these two rates gives an estimate of approximately 70% efficiency for transmission from female to male compared with from male to female (53). Interestingly, a very similar estimate of 71%, based on much more limited numbers, comes from transmission cases among partners of blood transfusion recipients (54).

B. Relationship of HIV Infection and Pregnancy and Cofactors for Infection

Immune function during the perinatal period is of particular concern both for the mother and for the infant (see Chapter 6). The natural history of HIV infection may be affected by pregnancy in the same ways that pregnancy affects malignant and immune-compromised conditions. Pregnancy is associated with alterations in immune function, and these may accelerate the progression of infection in the mother. An early study followed 15 women who were asymptomatic at delivery but had infants who developed AIDS or ARC in the postnatal period (13). In the 30 months of followup, only three remained asymptomatic; five developed AIDS, and seven developed ARC.

Another study of women with ARC and AIDS observed unusually high maternal morbidity and mortality among pregnant women (55). These reports are consistent with published case reports about women who were diagnosed with opportunistic infections during pregnancy, and whose disease progressed rapidly to death despite treatment (56). The risk of prenatal transmission from an infected mother to a fetus may be as high as 60% (13). Over three-quarters of infants diagnosed with AIDS have contracted the disease prenatally from an infected mother.

Information on heterosexually transmitted cases in Africa suggests another role for coinfection in sexual transmission. In one study, over half of the persons found to be positive for HIV antibody also had evidence of active STD infection, and symptoms included open genital lesions (44). Clearly, populations where such conditions are prevalent offer different opportunities for HIV transmission sexually than ones in which STDs are infrequent, and treatment is readily available.

V. Behavioral Factors Affecting Heterosexual Transmission

Natural history studies of AIDS transmission among homosexual men indicate that the sexual behavior patterns most strongly associated with increased risk of transmission are receptive anal intercourse and large numbers of sexual partners (see Chapter 1). In areas such as New York and San Francisco, the high prevalence of HIV infection in gay and bisexual men as well as IVDAs means that heterosexual transmission risk may also be increased with increased numbers of heterosexual partners. This prediction is supported by reports from countries where heterosexual transmission appears to be the most prevalent form of transmission. One study from Haiti, for example, compared sexual partners for AIDS patients without other risk exposure (homosexuality and/or IV drug use) to controls (17). Among males, 52% (16/31) reported 10 or more partners per year compared with 30% (19/62) among controls. Among female AIDS patients without other risk factors, there was no pronounced difference in numbers of partners, compared with controls. Another study of African AIDS patients in Brussels and Rwanda with matched controls reported that significantly more cases than controls reported "significant heterosexual promiscuity" defined as more than 30 sexual partners per year (22).

However, several reports on prevalence of HIV antibody among sexually active women including prostitutes have not found infection to be associated with increased numbers of sexual partners. Kreiss et al. (44) studied 90 female prostitutes in Nairobi, Kenya, and found that the 50 seropositive women did not differ from the 40 seronegatives on duration of prostitution or number of sex acts per year. A study from the United States of 400 sexually active women including prostitutes, reporting a seroprevalence rate of 4%, found no differences in seropositivity between prostitutes and nonprostitutes, and no increased risk of seropositivity with increased numbers of male sexual partners (52).

Evidence is also incomplete on the role of specific sexual practices in heterosexual transmission of AIDS. However, a partner study of 57 drug users found no statistical association between seroconversion and rectal sex or sex during menses (57). Case reports and limited series studies of sexual partners of hemophiliacs have also demonstrated seroconversion (27) and the development of AIDS (26) when sexual behavior did not include anal sex.

Prevention

Evidence is beginning to accumulate on the effectiveness of barrier methods in preventing AIDS virus transmission. One laboratory study, which simulated the pressures during intercourse on six kinds of condoms, showed that HIV did not pass through either latex or lambskin condoms (58). The spermicide nonoxynol-9, widely used in vaginal creams and jellies, and as a condom lubricant ingredient, has also been demonstrated to be viricidal in vitro (59). A case report has been cited earlier in this chapter of a woman whose antibody to HIV returned to negative following her utilization of condoms for sexual intercourse with her HIV-infected spouse (30). However, seroconversion happened within one month of safe sex practices, and most authorities feel that her serological status was unrelated to implementation of condom use per se. Finally, a study of antibody-negative sexual partners of HIV-infected persons reported that among sexual partners who used barrier protection, one seroconversion occurred among 10 antibody-negative partners during 24 months of followup (60).

Counseling for people at risk primarily involves teaching how HIV is transmitted heterosexually and how to avoid, or minimize exposure. Basic guidelines, reflecting our knowledge of possible HIV spread at this time, are presented in Table 4.

Referral to a drug treatment program is indicated for men and women who use IV drugs and want to stop. Those who continue to use IV drugs should be encouraged not to share needles and should be taught how to appropriately clean needles and works.

Table 4 Sexual Practice Guidelines for Men and Women at Risk of Sexual Exposure to HIV

For persons who do not know whether a sex partner is infected:

- Realize that intimate sexual expression can be achieved without exchanging secretions or having penetration.
- Don't allow partner's blood (including menstrual blood), semen, urine, vaginal secretions, or feces to enter your vagina, anus, or mouth.
- Use condoms for vaginal, rectal, and oral sex.
- Use contraceptive foams, jellies, or creams that contain the spermicide nonoxynol-9 in conjunction with a condom.
- Know your sex partner. Ask questions about past sexual history and drug use.

For persons who think or know that they might be infected:

- Realize that sexual expression can be achieved without exchanging secretions or having penetration.
- NEVER allow your semen, blood, urine, vaginal secretions, or feces to enter another person's body. Always use a condom for sex.

These guidelines also apply to men and women who are themselves infected.

Men and women at risk may want to be tested for antibodies to HIV. They will need counseling to help assess what implications a positive or negative test result would have for their lives. Women at risk who are considering pregnancy should be encouraged to be screened for HIV antibody.

Guidelines for heterosexual people who are seropositive have been published by the CDC (61). These guidelines should be made available to all people known to be infected. The concerns expressed most frequently by seropositive heterosexuals are the fear of becoming ill, the fear of transmitting HIV to their sexual partners and children, the difficulty of communicating with potential sexual partners and of remaining sexually active, and the potential loss of future childbearing possibilities.

The CDC recommends that seropositive women avoid pregnancy until more is known about perinatal transmission of HIV. For a pregnant woman with evidence of HIV infection, the risk of perinatal transmission, although not inevitable and not predictable, is estimated to be 20-50% (62). Infected pregnant women must therefore decide whether to run the risk of delivering an infected baby or to terminate the pregnancy.

With the exception of known IV drug users, heterosexual men and women at risk for AIDs are living throughout the community and cannot be targeted as a circumscribed group. Education and counseling about AIDS should be readily available in all health care settings that serve sexually active women and men. AIDS should be included as an STD in all educational materials about venereal disease, including STD education programs in the public schools. Health care settings most likely to serve those at risk are drug treatment programs, family planning facilities, STD clinics, prenatal clinics, women's health and other primary care clinics, and doctors' offices. Prisons and jails also house many people at high risk. All of these facilities should provide information about AIDS and heterosexual transmission appropriate for their clients. Individual counseling on risk education and antibody testing should be available for persons at risk by staff who are specially trained in order to provide effective AIDS prevention counseling.

Organizations that provide AIDS education and support services must design materials and other programs specifically geared toward heterosexual families. More important, however, are general education campaigns geared toward the public at large. Public service announcements on radio and television should attempt to educate all people about AIDS and publicize available resources. Existing educational efforts directed at people known to be at risk have been effective and desirable, but have also fostered the notion that AIDS is "somebody else's problem." This disease is a major public health problem in our society, and, if current predictions are accurate, it will become an increasingly large problem in the years to come. As the epidemic grows, more heterosexual men and women and their children will be affected by AIDS. Therefore AIDS prevention education must reach all people potentially at risk.

Acknowledgment

This work was performed with the support of funds provided by the State of California allocated on the recommendation of the Universitywide Task Force on AIDS.

References

1. Guinan MF, Thomas PA, Pinsky PF, Goodrich JF, Selik RM, Jaffe HW, Haverkos HW, Noble G, Curran JW. Heterosexual and homosexual patients with the acquired immunodeficiency syndrome: a comparison of surveillance, interview, and laboratory data. Ann Intern Med 1984; 100:213-8.
2. Centers for Disease Control. AIDS Weekly Surveillance Report, July 29, 1986.
3. Centers for Disease Control. Heterosexual transmission of human T-lymphotrophic virus type III/lymphadenopathy-associated virus. MMWR 1985; 34: 351-3.
4. Chamberland ME, Castro KG, Haverkos HW, Miller BI, Thomas PA, Reiss R, Walker J, Spira TJ, Jaffe HW, Curran JW, et al. Acquired immunodeficiency syndrome in the United States: an analysis of cases outside high-incidence groups. Ann Intern Med 1984; 101:617-23.
5. Centers for Disease Control. Unpublished data.
6. Castro KG, Lieb S, Calisher C, Witte J, Jaffe HW. The Field Study Group. AIDS and HIV Infection, Belle Glade, Florida. In: Third International Conference on AIDS, Washington, DC, 1987:106.
7. Groopman JE, Sarngadharan MG, Salahuddin SZ, Buxbaum R, Huberman MS, Kinniburg J, Sliski A, McLane MF, Essex M, Gallo RC. Apparent transmission of human T-cell leukemia virus type III to a heterosexual woman with the acquired immunodeficiency syndrome. Ann Intern Med 1985; 102:63-6.
8. Sande MA. Transmission of AIDS: the case against casual contagion. N Engl J Med 1986; 314:380-2.
9. Peterman TA, Stoneburner RL, Allen JR. Risk of HTLV-III/LAV transmission to household contacts of persons with transfusion-associated HTLV-III/LAV infection. In: Second International Conference on AIDS, Paris, France, 1986:107.
10. Sprecher S, Soumenkoff G, Puissant F, Degueldre M, et al. Vertical transmission of HIV in 15 week fetus. Lancet 1986; 2:288.
11. Jovasias E, Koch MA, Schafer A, Stauber M, Lowenthal D. LAV/HTLV-III in 20 week fetus. Lancet 1985; 2:1129.
12. Marion RW, Wiznia AA, Hutcheon G, Rubenstein A. Human T-cell lymphotropic virus type III (HTLV-III) embryopathy: a new dysmorphic syndrome associated with HTLV-III infection. Am J Dis Child 1986; 140:638-40.

13. Scott CB, Fischl MA, Klimas N, Fletcher MA, Dickinson GM, Levine RS, Parks WP. Mothers of infants with the acquired immunodeficiency syndrome: evidence for both symptomatic and asymptomatic carriers. JAMA 1985; 253: 363-66.
14. Selwyn PA, Schoenbaum EE, Mayers MM, Rogers MF, Klein RS, Friedland GH. HTLV-III/LAV infection and pregnancy outcomes in intravenous drug abusers. In: Second International Conference on AIDS, Paris, France, 1986: 111.
15. Brunet JB, Ancelle RA. The international occurrence of the acquired immunodeficiency syndrome. Ann Intern Med 1985; 103:670-4.
16. Clumeck N. Epidemiological correlations between African AIDS and AIDS in Europe. Infection 1986; 14:97-9.
17. Pape JW, Liautaud B, Thomas F, Mathurin JR, St. Amand MM, Boncy M, Pean V, Pamphile M, LaRoche C, DeHoritz J, Johnson WD. The acquired immunodeficiency syndrome in Haiti. Ann Intern Med 1985; 103:674-8.
18. Johnson WD, Liautaud B, Thomas F, Robert-Guroff M, Dehoritz J, Goncy M, Pamphile M, Deschamps MM, Stanback ME, Verdier RI, Blattner W, Pape J, Gheskio M. Heterosexual transmission of HTLV-III in Haiti. In: Program and Abstracts of the 25th Interscience Conference on Antimicrobial Agents and Chemotherapy, Minneapolis, Minnesota. Washington, DC: American Society for Microbiology, 1985:130, abstract no. 218.
19. Norman C. Politics and science clash on African AIDS. Science 1985; 230: 1140-2.
20. Biggar RJ. The acquired immunodeficiency syndrome in Africa. Lancet 1986; 1:79-82.
21. Serwadda D, Mugwera RD, Sewankambo NK, Lwegaba A, Carswell JW, Kirya GB, Bayley AC, Downing RG, Tedder RS, Claydon SA, Weiss RA, Dalgleish AG. Slim disease. a new disease in Uganda and its association with HTLV-III infection. Lancet 1985; 1:849-52.
22. Clumeck N, Robert-Guroff M, Van dePerre P, Jennings A, Sibomana J, Demol P, Cran S, Gallo RC. Seroepidemiological study of HTLV-III antibody prevalence among selected groups of heterosexual Africans. JAMA 1985; 254:2599-602.
23. Piot P, Quinn TE, Taelman H, Feinsod FM, Minlangv KB, Wobin O, Mbendi N, Mazebo P, Ndangi K, Stevens W, Kalambayi K, Mitchell S, Bridts C, McCormick JB. Acquired immunodeficiency syndrome in a heterosexual population in Zaire. Lancet 1984; 1:65-9.
24. Van de Perre P, Rouvroy D, Lepage P, Boggerts J, Kestelyn P, Kayihigi J, Hekker AC, Butzler JP, Clumeck N. Acquired immunodeficiency syndrome in Rwanda. Lancet 1984; 1:62-5.
25. Kreiss JK, Koech DK, Plummer F, Holmes KK, Piot P, Ronald AR, Ndinya-Achola JO, D'Costa W, Quinn TC, et al. HTLV-III infection in Kenyan prostitutes. In: Program and Abstracts of the 25th Interscience Conference on Antimicrobial Agents and Chemotherapy, Minneapolis, Minnesota. Washington, DC: American Society for Microbiology, 1985:131, abstract no. 227.

26. Kreiss JK, Kitchen LW, Prince HE, Kasper CK, Essex M. Antibody to human T-lymphotropic virus type III in wives of hemophiliacs: evidence for heterosexual transmission. Ann Intern Med 1985; 102:623-6.
27. Jason JM, McDougal JS, Dixon G, Lawrence DN, Kennedy MS, Hilgartner M, Aledort L, Evatt BL. HTLT-III/LAV antibody and immune status of household contacts and sexual partners of persons with hemophilia. JAMA 1986; 255:212-5.
28. Melbye M, Ingersley J, Biggar RJ, Alexander S, Sarin PS, Goedert JJ, Zachariae E, Ebbesen P, Stenbjerg S. Anal intercourse as a possible factor in heterosexual transmission of HTLV-III to spouses of hemophiliacs. N Eng J Med 1986; 312:857.
29. Allain JP. Prevalence of HTLV-III/LAV antibodies in patients with hemophilia and in their sexual partners in France. N Engl J Med 1986; 315:517.
30. Burger H, Weiser B, Robinson WS, Lifson J, Engleman E, Rouzioux C, Brun-Vezinet F, Barre-Sinoussi F, Montagnier L, Chermann J. Transient antibody to lymphadenopathy-associated virus/ human T-lymphotropic virus type III and T-lymphocyte abnormalities in the wife of a man who developed the acquired immunodeficiency syndrome. Ann Intern Med 1985; 103:545-7.
31. Harris C, Small CB, Klein RS, Friedland GH, Moll B, Emeson EE, Spigland I, Steigbigel NH. Immunodeficiency in female sexual partners of men with the acquired immunodeficiency syndrome. N Engl J Med 1983; 308:1181-4.
32. desJerlais, DC, Chamberland ME, Yancovitz SR, Weinberg P, Friedman SR. Heterosexual partners: a large risk group for AIDS. Lancet 1984; 2:1346-7.
33. Hardy AM, Allen JR, Morgan WM, Curran JW. The incidence rate of acquired immunodeficiency syndrome in selected populations. JAMA 1985; 253:215-20.
34. Tirelli T, Vaccher E, Carbone A, et al. Heterosexual contact is not the predominant mode of HTLV-III transmission among intravenous drug abusers. JAMA 1986; 255:2289.
35. Winkelstein W, Wiley JA, Padian N, Levy J. Potential for transmission of AIDS-associated retrovirus from bisexual men in San Francisco to their female sexual contacts. JAMA 1986; 255:901.
36. Calabrese LH, Gopalakrishna KV. Transmission of HTLV-III infection from man to woman to man. N Engl J Med 1986; 314:987.
37. Cohen JB, Hauer LB, Poole LE, Wofsy CB. Sexual and other practices and risk of HIV infection in a cohort of 450 sexually active women in San Francisco. In: Third International Conference on AIDS, Washington, DC, 1987:119.
38. Padian NS, Marquis L, Francis DP, Anderson RE, Rutherford GW, O'Malley PM, Winkelstein W. Male-to-Female Transmission of Human Immunodeficiency Virus. JAMA 1987; 258:788-90.
39. Redfield RR, Markham PD, Salahuddin SZ, Sarngadharan MG, Bodner AJ, Folks TM, Ballou WR, Wright DC, Gallo RC. Frequent transmission of HTLV-III among spouses of patients with AIDS-related complex and AIDS. JAMA 1985; 253:1571-3.
40. Redfield RR, Markham PD, Salahuddin MS, Wright DC, Sarngadharan MG, Gallo RC. Heterosexually acquired HTLV-III/LAV disease (AIDS-related com-

plex and AIDS) epidemiologic evidence for female-to-male transmission. JAMA 1985; 254:2094-6.
41. Harris CA, Cabradilla CD, Robert-Guroff M, Klein RS, Friedland GH, Getchell JP, Saltzman BR, Kalyanaraman VS, Catalano MT, Hewlett JM, Gallo RC, Steigbigel NH. HTLV-III/LAV infection and AIDS in heterosexual partners (hp) of AIDS patients. In: Programs and Abstracts of the 25th Interscience Conference on Antimicrobial Agents and Chemotherapy, Minneapolis, Minnesota. Washington, DC: American Society for Microbiology, 1985:130, abstract no. 219.
42. Clumeck N, Van de Perre, P, Carael M, Rouvroy D, Nzaramba D. Heterosexual promiscuity among African patients with AIDS. N Engl J Med 1985; 313: 182.
43. Centers for Disease Control. Update: Acquired immunodeficiency syndrome—United States. MMWR 1986; 35:17-21.
44. Kreiss JK, Joech D, Plummer FA, Holmes KK, Lightfoote M, Piot P, Ronald AR, Ndinya-Achola JO, D'Costa LJ, Roberts P, Ngugi EN, Quinn TC. AIDS virus infection in Nairobi prostitutes: spread of the epidemic to East Africa. N Engl J Med 1986; 314:414-8.
45. Barton SE, Underhill GS, Gilchrist C, Jeffries DJ, Harris JR. HTLV-III antibody in prostitutes. Lancet 1985; 2:1424.
46. Brenky-Fadeux D, Fribourg-Blanc A. HTLV-III antibody in prostitutes. Lancet 1985; 2:1424.
47. James JJ, Morgenstern MA, Hatten JA. HTLV-III/LAV antibody positive soldiers in Berlin. N Engl J Med 1986; 314:55-6.
48. Papaevangelou G, Roumeliotou-Karayannis A, Kallinikos G, Papoutsakis G. LAV/HTLV-III infectiion in female prostitutes. Lancet 1985; 1:1018.
49. Tirelli U, Vaccher E, Carbone A, DePaoli P, Santini G, Monfardini S. HTLV-III antibody in prostitutes. Lancet 1985; 2:1424.
49a. Cohen JB, Wofsy C, Gill P, et al. Antibody to human immunodeficiency virus in female prostitutes. MMWR 1987; 36:157-60.
50. Centers for Disease Control. Unpublished data.
51. Vogt MW, Craven DE, Crawford DF, Witt DJ, Byington R, Schooley RT, Hirsch MS. Isolation of HTLV-III/LAV from cervical secretions of women at risk for AIDS. Lancet 1986; 1:525-7.
52. Wofsy CW, Cohen JB, Hauer LB, Padian NS, Michaelis BA, Evans LA, Levy JA. Isolation of AIDS-associated retrovirus from genital secretions of women with antibodies to the virus. Lancet 1986; 1:527-9.
53. Centers for Disease Control. Update: acquired immunodeficiency syndrome—United States. MMWR 1986; 35:17-20.
54. Norman C. AIDS trends: projections from limited data. Science 1985; 230: 1081-21.
55. Kapila R, Grigoriu A, Kloser P. Women with AIDS/ARC. In: Second International Conference on AIDS, Paris, France, 1986:154.
56. Minkoff R, deRegt RH, Landesman S, Schwartz RH. Pneumocystis carinii pneumonia associated with acquired immunodeficiency syndrome in pregnancy: a report of three maternal deaths. Obstet Gynecol 1986; 67:284-7.

57. Saltzman BR, Harris CA, Klein RS, Friedland GH, Kahl PA, Steigbigel NH. Risk of HTLV-III/LAV transmission to household contacts of persons with transfusion-associated HTLV-III infection. In: Second International Conference on AIDS, Paris, France, 1986, 210.
58. Conant M, Hardy D, Sernatinger J, Spicer D, Levy JA. Condoms prevent passage of AIDS-associated retrovirus. JAMA 1986; 255:1708.
59. Hicks DR, Martin LS, Getchell JP, Heath JL, Francis JP, McDougal JS, Curran JW, Voeller B. Inactivation of HTLV-III/LAV infected cultures of normal human lymphocytes by nonoxynol-9 in vitro. Lancet 1985; 2:1422-33.
60. Fischl MA, Dickinson GM, Scott GB, Klimas N, Fletcher MA, Parks W. Evaluation of heterosexual partners, children, and household contacts of adults with AIDS. JAMA 1987; 257:640-4.
61. Centers for Disease Control. Additional recommendations to reduce sexual and drug abuse-related transmission of human T-lymphotropic virus type III/lymphadenopathy-associated virus. MMWR 1986; 35:152-5.
62. Centers for Disease Control. Recommendations for assisting in the prevention of perinatal transmission of HTLV-III/LAV and AIDS. MMWR 1985; 34: 721-6, 731-2.
63. Selwyn PA, Schoenbaum EE, Feingold AR, Mayers M, Davenny K, Rogers M, et al. Perinatal Transmission of HIV in Intravenous Drug Abusers (IVDAs). In: Third International Conference on AIDS, Washington, DC, 1987:157.

8

The Human Immunodeficiency Viruses
Detection and Pathogenesis

Jay A. Levy
Cancer Research Institute
School of Medicine
University of California
San Francisco, California

I. Introduction: The Search for the AIDS Agent

The first official reports on the disease now known as acquired immunodeficiency syndrome (AIDS) were made by the Centers for Disease Control (CDC) in 1981. This agency responded to information from California and New York about an unusually high prevalence of *Pneumocystis carinii* pneumonia (PCP) and of Kaposi's sarcoma (KS) in young homosexual men (1-4) (see Chapters 13, 17). In searching for the reason for the sudden increase in these diseases, our laboratory first studied KS. We cultivated over 30 cell lines from KS biopsies in attempts to find the causative agent; cytomegalovirus (CMV) was suspected (5) (see Chapter 19). The cultured cells had endothelial cell characteristics, including Factor VIII antigen production, and histologically they appeared to be derived from KS tissue (Table 1). However, they failed to show characteristics of *malignant* cells; they did not grow in soft agar or induce tumors in nude mice. Whether these results reflected the suspected "benign" nature of KS (6) or an inability to isolate the true malignant

Table 1 Kaposi's Sarcoma-Derived Cell Lines

Source	No.	Factor VIII	UEA	RT	CMV	Agar growth	Nude mouse
Skin	13	7/13	5/12	0/13	0/2	0/2	0/3
Lymph node	18	14/16	ND	0/18	0/6	0/4	0/5

Small pieces (1-3 mm) of Kaposi's sarcoma tissue were washed free of blood and minced into small fragments using forceps. They were then cultured in 30-mm Falcon plastic dishes under a cover slip in the presence of RPMI 1640 medium with 10% fetal calf serum, 2 mM glutamine, and antibiotics (penicillin and streptomycin). The monolayer cells that grew out from these small pieces were maintained in culture for several weeks with frequent passages until enough cells were available for evaluation.

Detection of Factor VIII and *Ulex europaeus* antigens (UEA) performed by Dr. Jay Beckstead (UCSF). Reverse transcriptase assays (RT) conducted by standard procedures on culture supernatants (25). Presence of CMV investigated using virus-specific radioactive probes in the laboratory of Dr. Jay Nelson. Growth in agar conducted using the methyl cellulose procedure. Inoculation of 6-10 million cells under the skin of nude mice conducted in collaboration with Dr. Paul Arnstein (California State Laboratory, Berkeley, California).

cell was not known. Neither CMV nor any other virus was isolated from the cells, and molecular studies did not consistently show a CMV genome in the cell lines or in the KS tissue (J. Nelson and J. Levy, unpublished observations).

By 1982, several immunological studies, particularly the measurement of helper (CD4+) and suppressor (CD8+) T cells (see Chapter 10), indicated that AIDS primarily involved a compromise in immune function (3,4). PCP and KS were epiphenomena. Because the T-helper lymphocyte appeared to be the major cell reduced in the new disease, this cell type was considered the target for the cytopathic events in AIDS. Initially, several hypotheses for the cause of T-cell death were considered, including the use of inhaled nitrates ("poppers"), infection by multiple known infectious agents [e.g., Epstein-Barr virus (EBV), CMV, herpes simplex virus, hepatitis B virus, or adenovirus], and exposure to sperm through multiple sexual encounters (7-9). An infectious agent eventually became accepted as the most likely cause. Because common viruses had already been recognized for many years in homosexual men, the primary group at risk for AIDS, their role in the disease seemed secondary. While some investigators pursued the possibility that a variant of these viruses caused AIDS, our laboratory supported the hypothesis that a new agent was involved and it infected T lymphocytes. At first, a variety of virus families were considered; we concentrated on the parvoviruses and retroviruses. The former were studied because of their known association with immune deficiency in cats, dogs, and mice (10,11), and because of the epidemic of canine parvovirus in the United States in 1977 (12), a year before the believed onset of AIDS. The latter, the retroviruses, were well known as immune-suppressing agents in birds, mice, and cats (10,13). These viruses can be detected in cell culture by reverse transcriptase assays (see below). The isolation of parvoviruses in vitro, however, is difficult. Usually, induction of disease in hamsters and mice is needed for their detection. Thus, to look for these viruses, we initially inoculated peripheral blood mononuclear cells (PMC) from AIDS patients into a variety of small animals by several routes. After 3 years of observation, no evidence of an infectious agent was found (14) (see Section XII).

In April of 1983, two groups of investigators—one at the Pasteur Institute in Paris and the other at the National Cancer Institute in Bethesda, Maryland—reported the isolation of retroviruses from individuals with the persistent generalized lymphadenopathy syndrome (PGL) (15) or with AIDS (16). The French group detected a virus after culturing the lymph node of an individual with PGL. Using a variety of reagents directed against the already known human retrovirus, the human T-cell leukemia virus type I (HTLV-I) (17-18), they determined that a slight but not conclusive cross-reaction with the PGL virus could be observed. Because their human retrovirus was isolated from T cells, they considered it a T-lymphotropic virus, but perhaps of a type different from HTLV-I (15). The group at the National Institutes of Health (NIH) isolated agents that had all the characteristics of HTLV-I, including morphology and antigenic properties (16-18). Moreover, evidence for integration of the HTLV-I genome in infected lymphocytes was presented (19). From these reports it was assumed that HTLV-I had been isolated from these patients and the question remained whether this virus could be the cause of AIDS.

For several reasons, HTLV-I did not appear to be the likely candidate. First, it was an agent that had been recognized in Japan, the Caribbean, and the southeastern United States for several years (13,18,20,21), and no consistent association with immune deficiency was found in the large majority of infected individuals. Second, the virus, HTLV-I, is highly cell-associated and cannot be passed easily in cell-free culture (20-22). Thus, the transmission of this virus and AIDS to hemophiliacs through Factor VIII concentrates (made from plasma) (23) did not seem possible (see Chapter 4). Third, HTLV-I transforms T-helper cells into cells undergoing continuous growth and does not generally kill them (17,18,21); therefore, the loss of T-helper cells in AIDS patients could not be explained. Finally, the antibody data did not indicate a substantial concurrence of antibodies to HTLV-I with the presence of AIDS or the AIDS-related complex (ARC) (16).

Our laboratory, once equipped and certified for biohazard research in October 1983, was able to seek a new virus in the PMC of AIDS patients. We were then aware of more recent information from the Paris group on the characteristics of their retrovirus, which was now called lymphadenopathy-associated virus (LAV) (24). In contrast to HTLV-I, this virus had a different morphology and grew to high titer in culture. Thus, it was not solely cell-associated. Moreover, instead of immortalizing the infected T lymphocytes into an established cell line, a characteristic of HTLV-I, this agent caused cytopathic changes in the T lymphocytes that resulted in cell death (15,24). It therefore had properties consistent with an AIDS-inducing agent.

Within a month, our laboratory isolated from the blood of AIDS patients retroviruses that we called the AIDS-associated retroviruses (ARV). These viruses grew to high titer in culture and gave cytopathic effects in PMC (25), as had been reported by the Pasteur Institute group. Using antiserum provided by Dr. Barré-Sinoussi, we evaluated whether our agents cross-reacted with the first French isolate (LAV_{BRU}). Some of the isolates showed a relationship, as determined by indirect immunofluorescence assays (IFA) (see Section XIII). However, these studies were hindered by the lack of a good cell line for reproducible viral antibody assays. All the procedures were conducted with cultured PMC infected with LAV or ARV. Nevertheless, what was evident from these and other antibody studies was that ARV did not cross-react with HTLV-I (25).

Because ARV could have represented another opportunistic infection in AIDS, we had to determine if the virus was found in all patients with AIDS and in individuals coming from the known risk groups for the disease. In particular, it was important to know whether retroviruses could survive the preparation involved in producing Factor VIII concentrates. Otherwise, AIDS in many hemophiliacs could not be explained. The procedures for obtaining this clotting factor were known to inactivate herpesviruses which, like retroviruses, are enveloped lipid-containing viruses (26).

In collaboration with Drs. Mozen and Mitra at Cutter Laboratories, we spiked serum and plasma with high titers of the mouse xenotropic retrovirus and then assayed the concentrated material for residual infectious virus at each step during the purification of Factor VIII. This virus was used as a prototype of ARV because it was available in high titer and could be easily quantitated in culture (27). These studies (reviewed in Chapter 4) indicated in March 1984 that, in contrast to herpesviruses, retroviruses could survive Factor VIII concentration and remain infectious in a lyophilized form (28). This result provided supportive evidence that a retrovirus could induce AIDS in hemophiliacs and placed greater emphasis on ARV as the causative agent.

In May 1984, Dr. Gallo and his associated at the NIH reported the isolation of a new human retrovirus associated with AIDS (29-31). This AIDS virus did not have the biological or antigenic properties of HTLV-I but was named human T-cell lymphotropic virus type III (HTLV-III) because of its presumed preferential growth in T lymphocytes and suspected relationship to HTLV-I. At that time, no evidence of a relationship of HTLV-III to the already described LAV was provided, although their reported characteristics appeared similar. That same month we announced our findings on ARV at the American Association for Cancer Research (AACR) meeting in Toronto and subsequently published a report on the isolation of over 20 different ARV from individuals from all the known risk groups for AIDS (25). In that paper, we demonstrated for the first time that infectious virus can be found in asymptomatic individuals. This finding suggested the existence of a "carrier" state. We also reported the complete association of serum antibodies to ARV with AIDS and the detection of these antibodies only in individuals from the known risk groups. These latter studies were possible because we found that ARV could infect and replicate in the established HUT-78 human T-cell line (25,32). An infected cell line (E) was grown in continuous culture and used for IFA and immunoblot procedures (see Section XIII). We did not know then whether ARV was similar to HTLV-III, but assumed it was related to LAV as indicated by our initial IFA studies (25).

In time, the biological features of all three prototype AIDS viruses (LAV, HTLV-III, and ARV) became known and they appeared to be similar. The viruses had the same morphology by electron microscopy (Figure 1) and replicated to high titer in T-helper lymphocytes. They caused cytopathology in infected cells characterized by formation of multinucleated cells and balloon degeneration (Figure 2), and they had distinct viral proteins (see below). Electron microscopic examination of these viruses also showed their resemblance to an agent detected by Karpas in 1983 in AIDS tissues (33).

Other observations made with colleagues in Australia documented for the first time the transmission of ARV from one healthy individual to another; the incubation time for development of symptoms was 3 years (34). Furthermore, that study suggested that the individual was most contagious (via seminal fluid) during the asymptomatic period, since sexual contacts of this patient when he had persistent lymphadenopathy syndrome, and subsequently AIDS, did not become infected by the virus. Moreover, in 1984, the role of retroviruses in immune deficiency in macaque monkeys was appreciated (35,36). Finally, further studies indicated that the newly recognized human retrovirus could be recovered from members of all the groups known to be at risk for AIDS and from individuals coming from many different parts of the world, including Africa (37-39). Its association with AIDS became well documented.

Both molecular and immunological studies conducted in 1984-1985 further confirmed that LAV, HTLV-III, and ARV were very similar viruses (40) (see Chapter 9). Their characteristics best placed them in a lentivirus subfamily of human retroviridae (Table 2) (40-42). These included the induction of disease after a long incubation period, the association with encephalopathies,

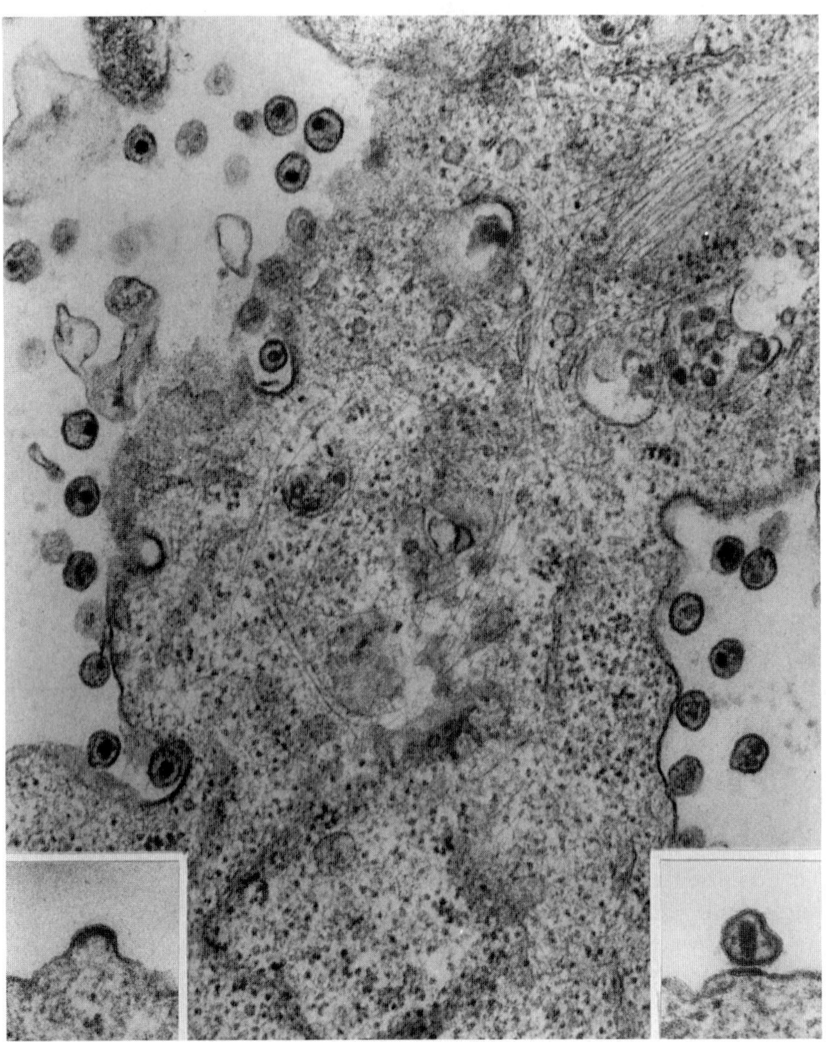

Figure 1 Electron micrograph of HIV_{SF2} (formerly ARV-2) replicating in a human lymphocyte (×32,000). The cylindrical nucleoid shows a small central core on cross-section (left inset, ×54,000) and a bar-shaped nucleoid on tangential section (right inset, ×54,000). (Courtesy of Dr. Lyndon Oshiro, Berkeley, California. From Levy JA. In: Rosenblum M et al., eds. AIDS and the Nervous System. New York: Raven Press, 1988:328.)

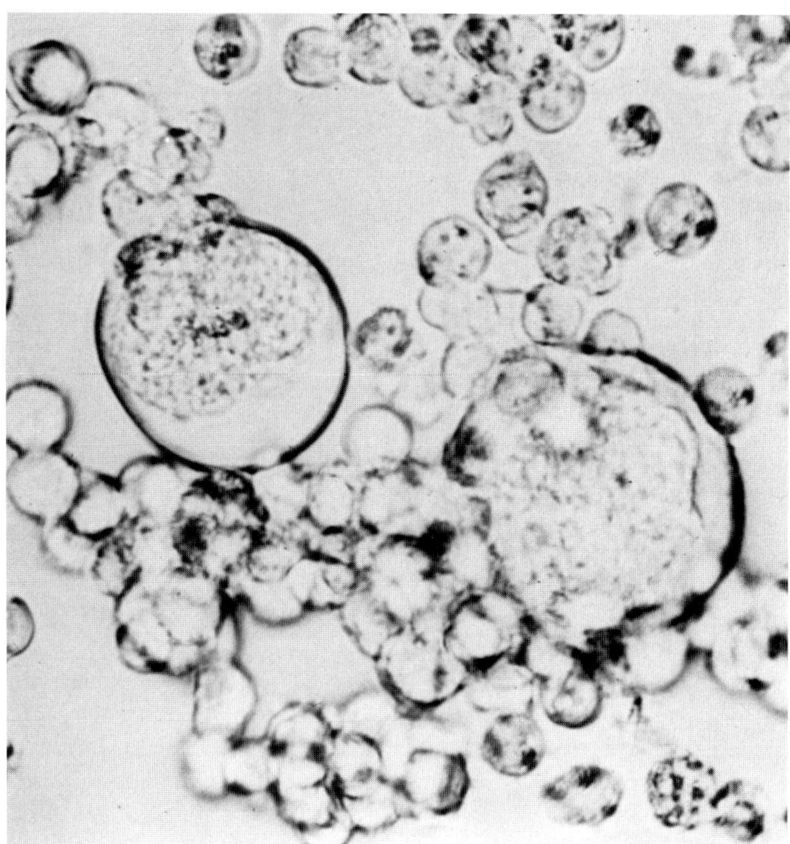

Figure 2 HIV-infected HUT 78 cells showing typical cytopathic effects. Note the large multi-nucleated cells created by syncytial formation (fusion) and the ballooning of infected cells ($\times 50$).

a long viral genome (9.7 kb), and the existence of additional open reading frames between the *pol* and *env* genes. (The molecular properties of HIV are discussed in further detail in Chapter 9.) In this chapter we will review some of the biological, serologic, and molecular features of this AIDS virus, which has now been termed the human immunodeficiency virus (HIV) (43), as suggested by a subcommittee of the International Committee for Taxonomy of Viruses (ICTV). In following that recommendation, ARV has been renamed $HIV_{San\ Francisco}$ or HIV_{SF}.

Table 2 Characteristics Common to HIV and Lentiviruses

Clinical
1. Association with a disease with a long incubation period
2. Involvement of hematopoietic system
3. Involvement of the central nervous system
4. Association with immune suppression

Biological
1. Cytopathic effect in certain infected cells, e.g., T-helper cells (fusion, multinucleated cells)
2. Infection of macrophages
3. Accumulation of unintegrated circular and linear forms of proviral DNA in infected cells
4. Latent infection in some infected cells
5. Morphology of virus particle by electron microscopy: cylindrical nucleoid

Molecular
1. Large provirus size (9.7 kb)
2. Primer binding site, $tRNA^{lys}$
3. Truncated *gag* gene: several processed *gag* proteins
4. Similar genomic base composition
5. Polymorphism, particularly in the envelope region
6. Novel central open reading frame in the viral genome that separates the *pol* and *env* regions

II. The Virion

HIV, as discussed in Chapter 9, has a general structure common to all retroviruses. Its RNA codes for major retroviral structural proteins such as those of the internal core (*gag*), polymerase (*pol*) and envelope (*env*). The viral genome also contains open reading frames for at least five other viral proteins (see Chapter 9). The structural proteins have been located in specific regions of the virion particle by immunoelectron microscopy (44) (Figure 3). The outside envelope consists of small projections (or spikes) containing the 120,000 Mr glycoprotein (gp120) or external region of the envelope gene. Virus neutralization generally involves this surface protein (45-49). As with other retroviruses, this protein is attached to the virion via an *env* transmembrane glycoprotein of 41,000 Mr (gp41). This latter protein also has external and cytoplasmic domains. Because a portion of gp41 is exposed on the outside of the virion, antibodies to it have also been found to neutralize the virus (49,50). As detailed below, infection requires the interaction of these envelope glycoproteins with the cell surface.

Of interest is the presence of the HIV p17 *gag* protein just below the viral membrane but not within the core of the virion (Figure 3). This location

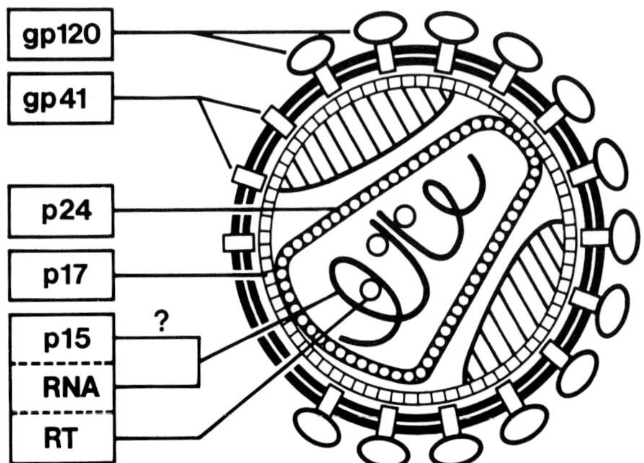

Figure 3 The structure of the human immunodeficiency virus (HIV). This model reflects the basic structure of a retrovirus, although differences among subfamilies can be observed. As a lentivirus, HIV has a cylindrical inner core, in which is found the diploid RNA strands closely associated with reverse transcriptase (RT). A basic nucleoprotein of 15,000 Mr (p15) is also localized in the nucleoid. The core structure itself contains a 25,000 Mr protein (p25 or p24). The *gag* p17 is outside the core and covers the inner surface of the envelope of HIV. The surface of the virion contains about 70-80 slightly convex knobs containing the envelope glycoprotein of 120,000 Mr (gp120). The knobs, about 50 nm in diameter and 9 nm in height, are connected to a transmembrane glycoprotein of 41,000 Mr (gp41) of the viral envelope. This gp41 has both external and cytoplasmic domains. (From Ref. 44.)

of a *gag* protein is unusual for a retrovirus and may be responsible for the observations suggesting that antibodies to p17 can also neutralize HIV (51). The major *gag* protein of 25,000 Mr (p25 or p24) makes up the core shell. Within the core are other *gag* proteins that are primarily phosphorylated (e.g., p15). Associated closely with the viral RNA is the polymerase (*pol*) or RNA-directed DNA polymerase (reverse transcriptase). This viral gene product directs the synthesis of a DNA copy (cDNA) of the viral RNA—essentially the reversal of conventional gene transcription. The coding for this enzyme in viruses gives them the name *retrovirus* (Greek *retro*, "backward") (for review, see Ref. 13). The presence of the other HIV gene products has not yet been demonstrated in the virion; they may be regulatory proteins found only in infected cells (see Chapter 9).

III. Virus Detection

The initial detection of HIV was achieved through procedures that measured particle-associated reverse transcriptase activity in cell culture supernatants

(15,25,29). Once a virus infection was suspected, conventional procedures for recognition of the agent were conducted, including IFA, immunoblot analyses of suspected infected cells, and electron microscopy. All these procedures have since been perfected to be more sensitive and, as noted below, can be modified to detect virus in the blood of nearly all infected individuals. Because in some instances HIV may be present in a latent stage (see Section VI.C), procedures for detecting the integrated viral genome in infected cells need to be perfected. The recent derivation of a DNA-enhancing technique that depends on amplification of the probe detecting the integrated viral copy has been promising (52,52a). Using this procedure, the eventual detection of HIV in all samples of infected blood may be easily achieved, and the process could be used for demonstrating virus in individuals who show no antibodies to the agent (285). It is more sensitive than standard in situ hybridization methods that generally detect virus only when sufficient replication is taking place to permit measurement of viral RNA (53). In the following two sections, HIV recovery from PMC and the antigen assay are described; they are common methods for virus detection and each involves different approaches.

A. Isolation of HIV from Blood

Initially, a variety of methods were developed to demonstrate the presence of infectious HIV in blood even when small numbers of PMC were used. The first recommended procedure for virus culture involved the separation of an individual's PMC on Ficoll-Hypaque gradients followed by stimulation with the mitogen phytohemagglutinin (PHA) for 3 days. Subsequently, the cells were washed and cultivated for up to 30 days in appropriate medium (15,25,29). The mitogen enhances virus release from infected cells (54). After 7-10 days, if the culture did not maintain a sufficient number of viable cells, mitogen-stimulated PMC from seronegative individuals were added. Using this procedure, we and others were able to isolate HIV from many but not all seropositive individuals (25,37,38). Moreover, the state of disease in these individuals appeared to determine the ability to isolate virus. Patients in the early stages of ARC or AIDS yielded virus readily. AIDS patients with advanced disease (e.g., PCP) and asymptomatic individuals yielded virus from their PMC in about 50% of cases (37). The reason for this reduced success in virus isolation is probably twofold. In severe AIDS, an insufficient number of virus-producing CD4+ cells (T-helper lymphocytes and some macrophages) are present in the patient's PMC. In healthy individuals, a strong cellular immune response (CD8+ T-suppressor cells), activated by PHA, appears to suppress HIV release (55) (see Section XIII.B).

To bypass these constraints on virus recovery, modifications in isolation procedures have been developed. For optimal virus recovery, PHA is not added to the patient's PMC; instead, these PMC are initially cocultivated with at least equal amounts of mitogen-stimulated PMC from seronegative individuals. In this way, the activation by PHA of CD8+ cells is minimized and the stimulated CD4+ cells added are immediate fresh targets for transfer of HIV from any number of infected cells. Also, the HLA differences between the two PMC can lead to antigenic stimulation of the cells and better release of virus (56). This new procedure has given a recovery rate from seropositive individuals of over 90% (57). Moreover, by using small culture dishes or wells, even low numbers of infected PMC can give efficient virus recovery, since good cell density is achieved (57).

Finally, for those seropositive individuals who do not yield HIV by either technique, purification of CD4+ cells or elimination of CD8+ cells by the panning technique (58) will almost always yield virus (55,59) (see Section XIII.B). By this latter procedure, mouse monoclonal antibodies to either CD4 or CD8 antigens are attached to the surface of a plastic dish. Separated PMC are added to the dish and selective removal or purification of the cell type is achieved by their attachment to the monoclonal antibody (58). Virus production by purified CD4+ cells can occur unchallenged by antiviral CD8+ cells. Essentially, all PMC or purified lymphocytes are maintained in culture with RPMI-1640 medium containing 10% fetal calf serum, 10% IL-2, and, where needed, antibiotics (100 U/ml of penicillin, 100 μg/ml streptomycin). Currently, our laboratory is able to isolate HIV from all infected individuals by one of these procedures. Moreover, by the initial method using PHA, the cellular immune response of the individual to HIV infection can be assessed. Finally, freezing and thawing PMC has been reported to be a good method for virus recovery (60), although its efficacy with small numbers of infected PMC was not studied. The procedure may kill CD8+ cells as well as release virus present in intracellular vacuoles (e.g., in macrophages) (see Section VIII.A). Details on these optimal procedures for recovery and cultivation of HIV have been described (57,60).

B. HIV Antigen Detection Assays

Recently, enzyme-linked immunosorbent assay (ELISA) procedures have been developed to detect HIV in cell culture fluids and in infected cell extracts and blood. Both a sandwich and competition ELISA have been described (61,62). The first type of procedure involves the detection of HIV by specific attachment of a viral protein to antibodies that are fixed to a solid phase (plastic dish or beads). This reaction is then monitored by a second labeled antiviral protein antibody. In the competition assay (62), a biotin-labeled viral protein (e.g., p25) is used with plates containing small amounts of antiviral antibodies. When virus-containing fluid or unlabeled infected cell extracts are added, the viral antigens compete with the labeled p25 for the antibody binding sites on the plate. Thus, a quenching of the color reaction indicates the presence of HIV.

These assays are helpful in measuring the degree of virus replication or expression in body fluids. As little as 30 pg of viral antigen and 100 infectious particles can be detected. Viral antigen assays on sera have also been used to follow the course of infection (63,64), and to measure the in vivo effect of antiviral drugs (65). The results on blood samples suggest that progression of disease correlates with the presence of high levels of p25 in the serum (63,64). Whether this finding results from the observed loss of anti-p25 antibody in AIDS patients with advanced disease (64; see below), real antigen excess, or both, is still not clear. Moreover, it may be apparent only in certain patients or population groups (65a). The explanation will come when the sensitivity of these procedures for measuring HIV antigens in blood have been optimized to account for immune complexes that can block p25 detection (66).

IV. Presence of HIV in Tissues of Infected Individuals

A. HIV in Hematopoietic Cells

The detection of HIV and its recovery from the blood and bone marrow (25) have been optimized by the procedures described above (Section III.A). Detection of the virus depends on factors affecting its replication and the number of infected lymphocytes, macrophages, and other hematopoietic cells present in the blood (see Section VIII.A). In situ hybridization studies suggest that 0.01-0.001% of the PMC contain the HIV genome (53). This low amount of HIV-infected cells has posed a question as to why progressive CD4+ cell loss is observed during HIV infection. Other factors, including cell fusion (67,68) or autoantibody production (69), may be involved (see Section XIV.B). Moreover, recent studies suggest that only a fraction of the infected cells are detected by in situ hybridization techniques. By titrating PMC from infected individuals onto susceptible target cells, some studies have found that as high as 1% of cells may actually be infected (69a). Furthermore, DNA-enhancing techniques (52a) have suggested that many cells contain HIV (perhaps in a latent state), but conventional detection procedures do not show this infection. These observations and those involving cultivation procedures, sometimes with purified CD4+ cells (59), strongly suggest that the PMC of every seropositive individual carry HIV; however, the number of infected white cells varies.

B. HIV in the Brain

Early in 1984, because some seropositive individuals presented only with neurological findings without an indication of immune deficiency, we considered the possibility that HIV, like other lentiviruses (13,70), could infect the brain and induce neurological disease. For these initial studies, cerebrospinal fluids (CSF) and a brain biopsy from individuals presenting with neurological symptoms were examined for virus. The results indicated conclusively that HIV infection of the brain occurs, and that infectious virus is present, often in high titer, in the CSF and brain tissue (71) (see Chapter 15). These studies supported the observations by Shaw et al. (72) of HIV DNA in brain tissues. Subsequent reports (73,74) demonstrated that infectious HIV can be found in the brains of patients with several neurological diseases, including acute encephalitis. Moreover, studies indicating *de novo* synthesis in the CSF of immunoglobulins directed against HIV further confirmed that the nervous system could be infected (75). In general, the presence of HIV in CSF is associated with neurological findings, although virus has been recovered from the CSF of asymptomatic individuals or those with only fever or headache (74). In some individuals, the virus may be transiently present in the CSF (e.g., coming from the blood) since they never show neurological findings. Alternatively, the individuals may subsequently develop symptoms. Another explanation for the lack of clinical signs could be the biological features of the particular HIV (see Section IX). The cells in the brain infected by HIV (reviewed in Chapter 15) appear to be macrophages, capillary endothelial cells, and glial cells (76-80). The susceptibility of astrocytes and oligodendrocytes (76,79,80) to HIV (see Section VIII.B) demonstrates its neurotropism, its similarity to other lentiviruses, and a mechanism by which HIV can directly cause neurological damage. Astrocytes, the immune cell counterparts in the brain (81), maintain the integrity of the blood-brain barrier (82) (see Chapter 15). Oligodendrocytes produce myelin required for good nerve transmission.

C. HIV in Other Tissues

By electron microscopy, HIV-like particles have been observed in lymph node dendritic cells, salivary glands, the prostate, and the testes (83,84). Other studies have shown that infectious virus can be found in cells of the cornea and retina (85,86) and that HIV can infect blood dendritic cells (286) and Langerhans' cells of the epidermis (87). This latter observation must be confirmed but is not surprising since Langerhans' cells have macrophagelike function in the integument.

Recently, we isolated infectious HIV from two of four rectal mucosa biopsies obtained from individuals presenting with diarrhea (88). And, in collaboration with Drs. Wiley and Nelson in San Diego, California, we have detected, using in situ hybridization techniques, infected epithelial cells in the rectum and duodenum from five of 10 patients who presented with chronic diarrhea (88). The cells infected are located in the bowel crypt, which contains goblet and columnar epithelial cells and enterochromaffin cells. The latter cell type, derived during embryogenesis from the neural crest, appears to be one of the cells susceptible to HIV. Finally, in the lamina propria, infected cells—probably macrophages—were also detected (88).

HIV in bowel epithelium adds further emphasis to the gastrointestinal tract as a site for transmission of the virus through anal/genital contact as well as a source of infection. Its presence in the intestinal epithelial cells of the rectum also supports the observation from epidemiological studies that douching (lavage) of the anal canal before receptive anal intercourse is an independent risk factor for infection of an individual with HIV (89). Moreover, the results implicate HIV in intestinal endocrinological problems that could be responsible for chronic diarrhea, characteristic of "slim disease" in Africa (90); enterochromaffin cells have endocrine functions that play a role in bowel mobility and digestion. Also, the presence of HIV in the duodenum suggests that the virus can be responsible for HIV-associated malabsorption syndromes.

Most recently, the possible presence of HIV in endothelial cells of the cervix has been reported (90a). Finally, whether HIV is involved in adrenal

Table 3 Cells Susceptible to HIV

Hematopoietic
T lymphocytes
B lymphocytes
Macrophages
Promeylocytes
Megakaryocytes
Dendritic cells
Brain
Macrophages (microglia)
Astrocytes
Capillary endothelial cells
Oligodendrocytes
Other
Bowel epithelial cells
Bowel enterochromaffin cells
? Cervical endothelial cells
? Prostate, salivary gland, testes
? Myocardium, Langerhans' cells

Cells listed are those found to be infected in vivo by HIV or sensitive to infection in vitro.

and cardiac cell dysfunction also needs to be investigated, since some infected individuals show adrenal insufficiency (91) and cardiomyopathy (92). Also, HIV has been recovered from the myocardium of a patient with congestive cardiomyopathy (92a). All these studies with human cells and tissues indicate not only that HIV is lymphotropic, but that it can also infect many other cells of the body (Table 3). They emphasize the difficulty in controlling this virus after infection has taken place.

V. HIV Recovery from Body Fluids

As noted above, HIV can be found in substantial titer in the cerebrospinal fluid (71,74). Based on the kinetics of virus replication in culture, we estimate the amount of virus to vary between 100 and 10,000 infectious particles (IP) per milliliter. Thus, HIV appears to replicate efficiently in brain cells.

When other body fluids are examined for the presence of infectious virus, varying results are obtained. For instance, plasma and serum, which are the source of infectious virus for hemophiliacs through Factor VIII concentration, actually contain very small amounts of detectable infectious HIV. Only about 30% of serum or plasma yields virus (93,94), at levels of less than 50 IP/ml. In rare cases, titers as high as 25,000 IP/ml have been found; however, the levels are far below those observed with hepatitis B virus (HBV), in which titers as high as 10^9 IP/ml can be detected (95). This fact supports the extremely low risk of transmission of HIV versus HBV following a needlestick injury (96) (see Section XVI).

Studies of saliva (42,97,98), tears (42,99), milk (100), urine (42), and ear secretions (cerumen) (D. Sooy, L. Evans, and J. Levy, unpublished observations), have also demonstrated only low levels of free virus—about 10-100 times less than in blood and in relatively few samples (see Table 4). No HIV has been isolated from feces (L-Z. Pan and J. Levy, unpublished observations). These studies suggest that the virus in these body fluids is not a source of contagion. The detection of HIV in saliva brought immediate concern to the public. However, results from our laboratory and others have indicated that the amount of infectious virus in this body fluid is extremely low and is present in at most only 10% of saliva from infected individuals (42,98). We estimate that the titer of virus, if present, is much less than 1 IP/ml and thus would not be a risk for infection. Furthermore, incubation of infectious HIV for 30 minutes with saliva reduces its titer by 50% (L. Evans, unpublished observations). Finally, in seminal and vaginal fluid, free infectious virus in low titer can be detected (42,101-105). In some studies, about 30% of semen and 50% of cervical/vaginal specimens are positive (Table 4); in others, no free virus has been found (105). Moreover, when present, the estimated number of infectious particles is again low—fewer than 100 IP/ml (42,104).

Table 4 Isolation of HIV from Body Fluids

	Virus isolation (no. positive/no. samples)	Estimated quantity of HIV[a]
Cell-free fluid		
Plasma	3/9	10-50
Serum	20/78	10-50
Tears	2/5	<1
Ear secretions	1/8	1-10
Saliva	2/39	<1
Urine	1/5	<1
Vaginal/cervical	6/16	<1
Semen	5/15	10-50
Milk	1/5	<1
Infected cells		
Blood (PMC)	87/90	0.01-0.001%
Saliva	3/20	<0.01%
Bronchial	3/24	NK[b]
Vaginal/cervical	7/16	NK[b]
Semen	11/28	0.01-5%

[a]Expressed as infectious particles (IP)/ml or percent of infected cells observed. Amount of free virus estimated by kinetics of virus replication after infection of PMC. Low levels of virus take over 30 days to reach a detectable level, and extremely small amounts (1 IP/ml) may need to be passed one or two times in PMC before identification of virus can be made. Infected cells detected by in situ hybridization (76). Results reflect representative sampling conducted in author's laboratory.
[b]Not known.

Whereas body fluids have small amounts of free virus, they all can contain virus-infected cells, including pulmonary secretions. In most cases, the frequency of fluids with infected cells is low. Lavage specimens from the lung, for instance, have shown only virus-infected cells, and not free virus, in fewer than 10% of cases (106). Thus, coughing poses no evident source of contagion. In genital secretions, however, these infected cells appear to be the major source of HIV transmission (Figure 4) (102-105,107). In our laboratory, up to 5% of the cells in some seminal fluids have been found infected (M. Tateno and J. Levy, unpublished observations), whereas peripheral white cells, by the same method, generally show virus in only 0.01 to 0.001% of cells (53). Obviously, the risk of sexual transmission of HIV will depend on the number of infected cells in genital secretions. Normal seminal fluid contains at least 3×10^6 white cells per milliliter (108). Cervical secretions contain less. However, any condition that increases white cells in these secretions in HIV-infected individuals would enhance transmissibility of the

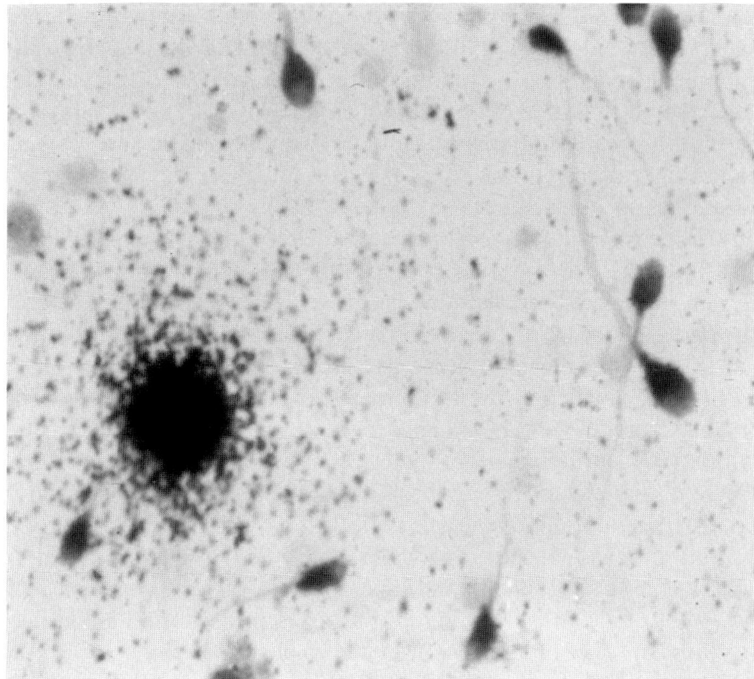

Figure 4 By in situ hybridization, an HIV-infected cell can be detected in seminal fluid (×40).

agent. Sexually transmitted diseases, therefore, are a major cofactor to be considered; the presence of genital ulcers, in particular, correlates with an increased risk of virus spread (109,110) (see Section XVI).

VI. Features of HIV Replication

A. Infection of the Cell

The infectious cycle for HIV is summarized in Chapter 9. As with all retroviruses, the envelope protein(s) serve as an attachment site of the virion to the cell surface. Most data indicate that the CD4 antigen complex (first recognized as a marker for T-helper lymphocytes) is the major cellular receptor for HIV (111-113). Certain specific epitopes on this molecule appear to be involved (114). Monoclonal antibodies to these antigens block viral infection (114), and complexes consisting of viral gp120 and the CD4 antigen are precipitated when antibodies to either protein are used (115,116). Furthermore, a loss (or suspected down-regulation) of the CD4 protein is a major characteristic of HIV infection (111-116). The reason and site for this effect are unclear. Some believe it results from the gp120:CD4 antigen complexes (115, 116); others have implicated the orf-B protein of HIV (117) (see Chapter 9). Nevertheless, this feature of HIV infection may not be a basic one, since recent studies have indicated that some HIV do not affect the expression of the CD4 antigen in infected cells (see Section XV).

The CD4 protein is also present on the surface of macrophages, Langerhans' cells, and B cells, as well as some brain cells and intestinal cells (42, 118-122,162); these cells are also susceptible to HIV infection (see below). Thus, the participation of this cellular protein in HIV infection seems likely. Nevertheless, work in our laboratory has shown that some cultured brain cells that lack any evidence of CD4 antigen production (by both IFA and Northern blot analysis) can be infected by the virus (Table 5) (79). These cells contain glial fibrillary acid protein (GFAP), a characteristic of astrocytes. These results and others (see Section IX) suggest that other receptors or alternative mechanisms for virus entry are involved in HIV infection.

In addition to gp120, the transmembrane protein gp41 has been implicated in HIV entry of cells, since antibodies to this protein also prevent HIV infection (49,50). The gp41 could serve as a fusion protein (123). Sequences similar to those of other fusogenic viruses are found in this region of the HIV envelope (124). Like paramyxoviruses (125), the AIDS virus may interact with the cell at two sites. One protein (gp120) attaches to the cell surface (via CD4) and another protein (gp41) helps the virus enter the cell by fusion (using a different cellular site) (see Figure 5). Thus, antibodies to either portion of the HIV envelope would reduce virus infection; antibodies to both

Table 5 HIV Replication in Cultured Human Brain Cells

	U343MGA	U251MG	SF407	SF612
Surface CD4	–	–	–	–
Cytoplasmic CD4	–	–	–	–
CD4 mRNA	–	–	ND[a]	ND[a]
HIV_{SF2}	–	+	+	+
HIV_{SF117}	+	+	+	–
HIV_{SF128A}	+	+	+	–
HIV_{SF301A}	+	–	–	+

Expression of CD4 antigen determined by standard indirect immunofluorescence assays. Presence of CD4 messenger RNA (mRNA) evaluated using Northern blot procedures by Dr. Dan Littman (UCSF). + indicates replication of HIV in glioma cell lines (U343MGA, U251MG) or in early passaged fetal brain cells (SF407, SF612). Virus production demonstrated by cocultivating infected brain cells with mitogen-stimulated PMC and assaying supernatant for reverse transcriptase activity (See Ref. 79).
[a]Not done.

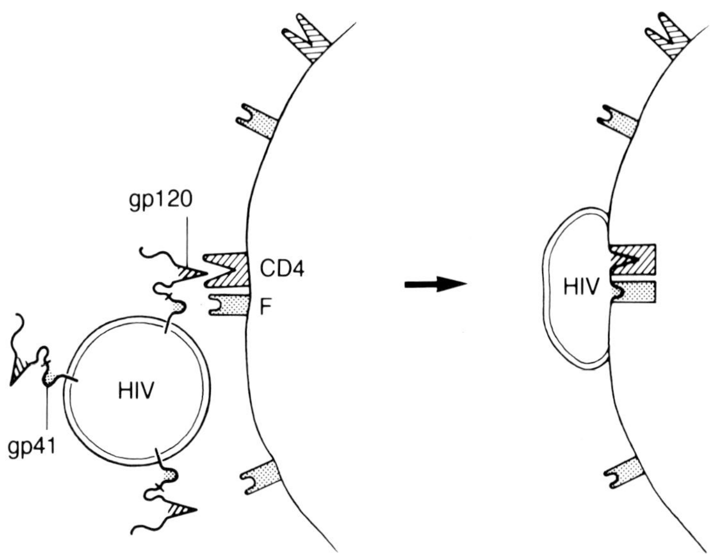

Figure 5 Proposed model for the entry of HIV into a cell. Attachment of the virion to the cell surface takes place via the gp120:CD4 receptor; fusion occurs mediated by the transmembrane gp41 and perhaps a separate cell receptor (F). When both proteins interact with the cell, efficient entry takes place. (From Ref. 227.)

would be most effective. The gp41 may be involved in infection of the CD4-negative cells (Table 5). Cell-to-cell fusion that causes formation of multinucleated cells (syncytia) (67,68,126,127) (Figure 2) may also result from the same virus:cell interaction. Both viral envelope proteins are found on the surface of infected cells (44).

While attachment and fusion by HIV have been studied in some detail, the factors involved in the actual penetration of cells by HIV have not been defined. This step in HIV infection appears distinct from virus attachment. For example, mouse cells transfected with the CD4 gene and expressing this antigen receptor on the cell surface cannot be infected by HIV (120, J. Levy and D. Littman, unpublished observations). Nevertheless, the transformed human HeLa cell lines treated in the same way are infectible (120). Since attachment to both cell types would be possible, it appears that other events (perhaps fusion) necessary for the eventual penetration of the cells by HIV are not feasible with mouse cells. Alternatively, this resistance of mouse cells reflects the nonpermissive nature of the intracellular compartment (see Section VI.B).

Once infection has taken place, the molecular events involved in replication appear similar to those for other retroviruses, particularly lentiviruses

(13,70). These include the release of RNA from the virion core and the production of a single-stranded DNA copy of the viral genome using reverse transcriptase. Subsequently, this single-stranded DNA is duplicated using the same viral enzyme. The cDNA then circularizes, either in the cytoplasm or nucleus, and integrates into the host chromosome. Each of these events requires specific enzymes that could differ among various retroviruses (see Chapter 9). Moreover, as noted below (Section VI.B), cellular factors can influence the events leading to viral reverse transcription, integration, and subsequent virus replication. Once integration takes place, HIV can exist in either a latent state (see below) or enter productive infection in which the integrated proviral DNA produces both messenger and virion RNA genomes and, eventually, infectious viruses (see Chapter 9 for details of the replicative cycle). As with other retroviruses, integration is a random event and does not appear to occur at a specific site for HIV.

One characteristic that has been observed during acute infection of established cell lines with HIV and other lentiviruses is the accumulation of unintegrated proviral copies (both circular and linear forms) in the cytoplasm and nucleus (42,128,129). At the same time, extensive cytopathology and cell death are observed. Eventually, some cells (often clones) survive the cytopathic effects (CPE) and continuously produce substantial amounts of infectious virus (130). These cells contain few, if any, unintegrated proviral forms, and have one to several integrated copies of HIV. The presence of large quantities of unintegrated viral forms appears to correlate with the development of CPE in the infected cells (42) (Figure 2), whereas virus integration is associated with chronic viral infection.

A similar event has been observed with cultured normal T lymphocytes acutely infected with HIV (131). In the first 2 to 3 weeks, most of the cells show CPE and die, but eventually some infected T lymphocytes emerge. They divide readily and can persist in releasing HIV for up to 4 months in culture. These results indicate three important points: 1) cytopathology is not a necessary sequela of HIV infection; 2) HIV infection is not lytic but cytocidal; and 3) integration without the accumulation of proviral forms may lead more readily to the emergence of chronically infected viable cells. Furthermore, the experiments with normal T cells demonstrated the induction of a persistent and perhaps even latent HIV infection; some infected T cells showed very little evidence of HIV infection (e.g., protein expression) until after several cell passages in culture (131) (see Section VI.C on latency).

The association of these unintegrated viral forms with cell death resembles observations reported with the spleen necrosis virus, an avian retrovirus (132). It is conceivable that the unintegrated proviral forms are responsible for the known emergence of variants of HIV (see Sections IX, X). An unintegrated genome would be much more likely to undergo mutations and recombinations than an integrated one. The phenomenon could explain the lack of substantial changes to HIV after long-term passage in cell lines in the laboratory (287). In individuals, the replicating HIV becomes modified through frequent acute infections of host cells.

Finally, work with the animal lentivirus visna (133) has suggested that integration is not necessary for virus replication. Since nondividing macrophages can be infected with HIV (see Section VIII.A), this observation could also be true for HIV but has not been reported.

B. Intracellular Control of Virus Infection

Productive virus infection results not only from the ability of HIV to attach and penetrate the cells but also from events occurring within the intracellular milieu that determine if the cell is *permissive* or *nonpermissive* for virus replication. Thus, the eventual production of virions depends on the particular virus isolate itself, and the specific cell infected.

The ability of HIV to infect different cell types, including lymphocytes from many animal species besides human, has been examined (118,134). These experiments indicated that only primate PMC were susceptible to HIV. Moreover, despite the presence of the CD4 antigen on certain rhesus monkey and baboon PMC, HIV replication in these cells was extremely limited; only a rare HIV isolate replicated to any extent. Some investigators have found efficient growth of HIV in several different primate PMC (134), but these unusual results probably reflect the particular HIV used (see Section IX). Generally, high levels of HIV production are found in only human and chimpanzee PMC. Because virus attachment and penetration seem feasible after the initial interaction with CD4 protein, the observations with rhesus monkey and baboon cells appear to reflect the importance of the intracellular milieu in permitting virus replication in only some primate cells. The same conclusion on intracellular control can be drawn from tissue culture studies with PMC, macrophages, or other cells obtained from different individuals. Variations in virus replication can be noted depending on the cell (coming from a particular individual) and the virus isolate used (see Sections VIII, IX).

In evaluating the nature of this potential intracellular control of HIV infection, we transfected, by standard calcium/phosphate procedures, a biologically active DNA clone of HIV into a variety of animal cells (135). This cDNA (see Chapter 9), upon introduction into treated cells, can become integrated into the cellular genome and subsequently produce infectious HIV. The procedure is commonly used for the transfer of viral genomes into resistant cells. These studies suggested that the relative ability to replicate virus after transfection depends on the taxonomic class of the animal whose cells are used. Primate and human cells showed the best replication of HIV, mink cells showed less, and mouse cells were the least capable of replicating virus (135). The growth of HIV in these rodent cells was detected only when they were mixed with normal human PMC. Thus, once the surface receptor-mediated control of virus infection was bypassed (including penetration), the intracellular compartment appeared to show an effect on HIV production. These latter observations suggested that mouse cells either lacked an important factor needed for HIV replication or made a factor that suppressed HIV replication. These possibilities are currently under study and could lead to some important insights into ways of controlling HIV infectivity. Finally, some recent studies have defined certain cellular factors that directly affect HIV replication (136,137,137a,288). The role of these and other regulatory cellular proteins in influencing HIV pathogenesis merits further attention.

C. Latency and Persistent Infection

One important biological characteristic of retroviruses is their ability to remain "silent," or latent, in a cell (13). In this state, very little, if any, viral RNA or protein is made and the infected cells containing the viral genome replicate without releasing infectious virus; thus, they may not be recognized by the immune system. Latent HIV infection has been demonstrated in vitro with infected peripheral blood lymphocytes (131) and established T-cell lines (79,139). In some cases, methylation of the virus appears to be the mechanism for latency (13,138), but the reason for latency observed in HIV infection is not yet certain. In a latent state, the presence of an *infectious* HIV can be demonstrated by activation of the integrated genome using known inducers of retroviruses such as halogenated pyrimidines (iododeoxyuridine) or 5-azacytidine (13,80,139). Alternatively, some cellular factors might induce virus production (140). Latency has been suspected as one reason for the long incubation period in some individuals, and perhaps a persistent seronegative state (141), but a true latent state in vivo has not been well documented. We have proposed that latency results from a high-level expression of the HIV orf-B protein (p27) (142). Deletions in this region of the viral genome (see Chapter 9) yield HIV mutants that replicate to levels 5-10 times higher than those of the parental virus. The p27, therefore, appears to down-regulate HIV expression.

In some cultures of HIV, a persistent, *low-level* replication of the virus occurs. HIV is not detected unless the cells are cocultivated with an appropriate target cell, such as mitogen-stimulated PMC from seronegative donors. The PMC serve to amplify the replication of HIV. This low-level replication of HIV (which differs from latency, in which no infectious virus is made) has been observed with some infected macrophages (80), perhaps due to virus budding into intracellular vacuoles (see Section VIII.A), cultured brain cells (79), and certain human epithelial and fibroblast cells infected in culture (see Section IX). Once again, this control of virus replication most likely involves an interaction of the particular HIV genome with regulating factors within the cell (see Section II.B). These control mechanisms may be modified by cytokines (140) or any factor that affects the activation or differentiation of the infected cell (see Section VIII.A).

VII. Cytopathology

When the initial isolation of HIV was described (15), an inability to maintain the infected PMC for a long period of time in culture was noted. This observation was later shown to be due to the CPE that HIV induces in cultured PMC (Figure 2) (143). It is characterized by the formation through cell fusion of large multinucleated cells that may extravasate their nuclei, leaving empty cell structures. Ballooning of cells often occurs, most likely from membrane permeability changes with ion influx (159). As noted above, the fusion appears to be mediated by the interaction of viral gp41 and gp120 with cell surface receptor(s), particularly the CD4 antigen complex (67,68). The multinucleated cells can continue to produce infectious virus (42) but eventually they die. The cause of cell death has not yet been determined (see Section VI.A), but cell fusion does not appear to be a necessary requirement (144). Most important, the fact that syncytial cells and infected T cells alone continue to release HIV for extended periods of time after infection (Figure 6) indicates that this virus causes cytocidal, but not cytolytic, infection. The distinction is important, since lytic infection would eliminate much earlier the infected cell that can serve as a reservoir for continual virus spread.

HIV isolates that differ in their production of CPE have been observed. Some have fewer syncytial-inducing properties or they are delayed in CPE induction (145-147,165). The CPE-inducing property of HIV appears to correlate with isolates' ability to replicate quickly in cells, to infect T-cell lines, and to plaque in the MT-4 cell line (146,148). This latter assay, first developed by Harada et al. (149), uses an established HTLV-I-infected human T-cell line, which is plated as a monolayer on poly-L-lysine-treated culture dishes. Only viruses that replicate rapidly and to high titer in these cells induce plaques in the monolayer that represent concentrated areas of syncytial formation (Figure 7). This ability of some isolates to produce CPE appears to correlate with their virulence in the host (146) (see Section XIV). Nevertheless, some isolates that replicate well in MT-4 cells (but with a slightly delayed cycle) and induce some CPE in PMC do not plaque. Obviously, several genes must govern the biological properties observed with HIV. Moreover, certain pathogenic HIV, particularly those recovered from the brain, may not plaque because they replicate well only in macrophages, not in T cells

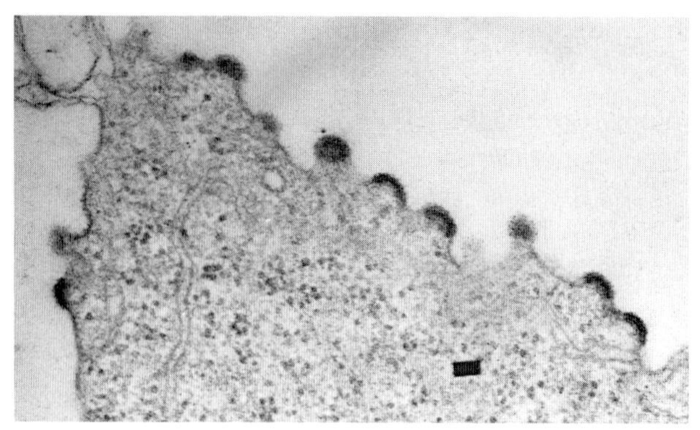

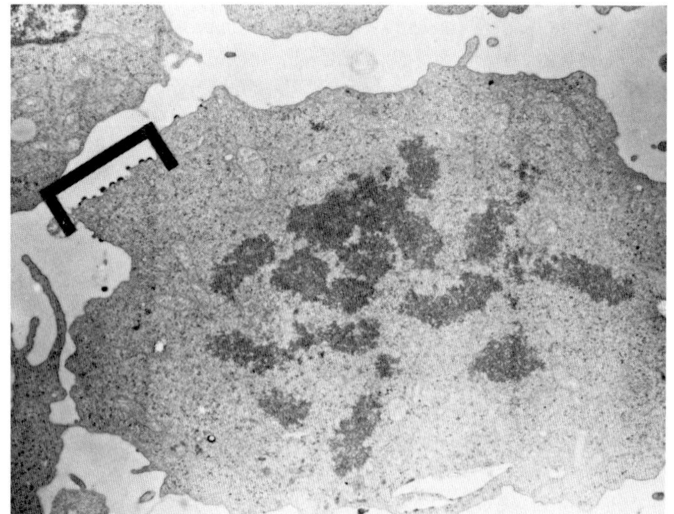

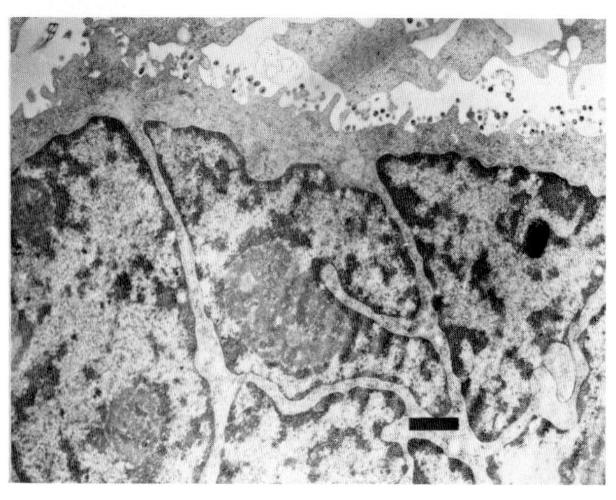

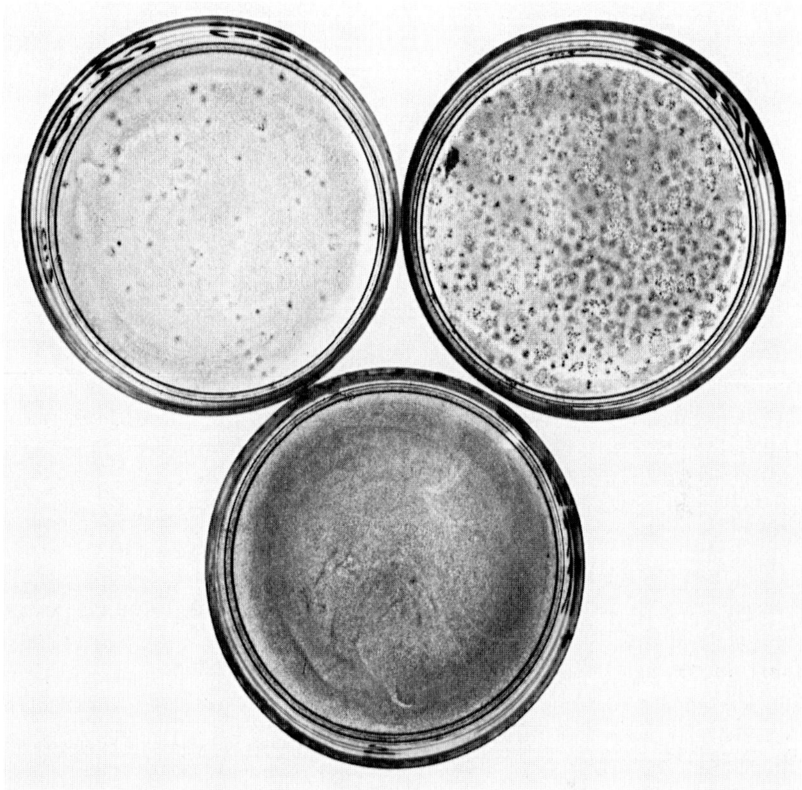

Figure 7 Plaque formation in the MT-4 cell line. Note the small numbers of plaques in the left plate, the multiple plaques in the top right plate, and the absence of plaques in the bottom plate. The last culture was infected with a non-plaque-forming HIV. Studies conducted by M. Tateno (148).

Figure 6 Cultured peripheral mononuclear cells infected with HIV_{SF2} (lead citrate and uranyl acetate stain). (Top) Particles on the surface of a multinucleated cell (original magnification, ×6400; scale = 1000 nm). (Middle) Cell undergoing mitosis with budding HIV particles on plasma membrane (original magnification, ×7300; scale = 1000 nm). (Bottom) Higher magnification of budding viral particles shown bracketed in the middle panel (original magnification, ×27,000; scale = 100 nm). (From Ref. 42.)

(147,150). In studying the genes responsible for this CPE, a "noncytopathic" HIV has been derived by molecular techniques (151). It was modified in the gp41 region and appears to cause fusion without immediate cell death. These observations need further evaluation.

VIII. Susceptibility of Cultured Human Cells to HIV Infection

A. Hematopoietic Cells

The initial attempts to recover a virus from individuals with AIDS focused on the PMC because of the immunologic abnormalities observed in the peripheral white cells. These studies indicated that CD4+ (helper) and not CD8+ (suppressor) T lymphocytes were responsible for production of high titers of the AIDS retrovirus (111) and emphasized the CD4 antigen complex as a potential receptor for HIV. Cultured PMC, presumably CD4+ lymphocytes, were then used to grow HIV, and variations in the sensitivity of these cells from different individuals to virus infection were observed (see Section IX). HIV was subsequently found in peripheral blood macrophages (42,152), but coculturing of the macrophages with normal PMC was often necessary to demonstrate the low level of virus production (42). The established U-937 human macrophage cell line (which also expresses the CD4 antigen) was then found susceptible to some HIV (118), and antibodies to the CD4 molecule were shown to block that infection (118). A loss of CD4 antigen expression on the surface of U-937 cells following infection has also been noted recently (118a). Several groups subsequently demonstrated that normal blood macrophages can be directly infected by HIV (80,150,153,154), and these cells, cultured from different individuals, also varied in their sensitivity to infection by an HIV (154; C. Cheng-Mayer, unpublished observations). Because most isolates do not kill macrophages, this infection can establish a reservoir for HIV spread in the host. Further studies have shown that some HIV grow only in macrophages (155) and may represent a specific subtype; other HIV, particularly those isolated from the brain, preferentially grow in these hematopoietic cells (147,150) (see Section IX). Also, those HIV that replicate to high titer in macrophages can cause CPE consisting of multinucleated cells and sometimes vacuole formation (154,156; B. Castro and J. Levy, unpublished observations). Many of the cells contain virus particles budding into intracellular vacuoles (156). This latter observation could explain why freezing and thawing infected PMC can be an efficient method for recovering HIV (60). Finally, recent studies have indicated that some infected macrophages may release substantial quantities of virus *only* when treated with cytokines (140) or when cocultivated with PMC (80). These results suggest that cell-to-cell contact or communication is required for some HIV to be released and transferred by macrophages to other cells.

Tissue culture and electron microscopic studies have also indicated that HIV can infect B lymphocytes (42,118,157), the promyelocyte line, HL60 (118), and probably megakaryocytes (J. Levy and D. Morgan, unpublished observations) (158); therefore, many different cells of the hematopoietic system are susceptible to the virus. B cells carrying EBV appeared to be most susceptible to infection; they express the CD4 antigen.

B. HIV Infection of Cultured Brain Cells

As noted in Section IV.B, one glial cell that appears susceptible to HIV is the astrocyte. Both established glioma cell lines and cultured fetal brain cells expressing the GFAP astrocyte marker were found susceptible to various trains of HIV (79) (Table 5). The ability to infect these cells did not appear to correlate with recovery of the viruses from the brain, since HIV obtained from both PMC and CSF could replicate in these cells. Instead, the same kind of heterogeneity of virus replication noted with established hematopoietic cell lines was found (see below). Other studies using different brain-derived cell lines have confirmed this neurotropism of HIV (160).

C. HIV Infection of Human Epithelial and Fibroblast Cells

Recently, some HIV isolates, particularly those that are highly cytopathic, and plaque in MT-4 cells, have been grown in the human osteosarcoma (HOS) line, in the human rhabdomyosarcoma (RD) line, and in human foreskin fibroblast cells (161). Replication is limited and virus detection usually requires cocultivation of uninfected human PMC with the infected monolayer cells. Nevertheless, the observations do suggest that epithelial and fibroblast cells could be infected in vivo by HIV. Our detection of HIV in bowel epithelium (88) and the infection of cultured human bowel carcinoma cell lines with HIV (162) support this conclusion. In addition, these studies have indicated that virus infection can take place in cells lacking CD4 antigen expression.

IX. Biological Heterogeneity of HIV

The above sections describe the ability to isolate virus from individuals infected with HIV and to infect a wide variety of human cells with the AIDS virus. They have referred to the relative capacity of different HIV isolates to grow in a variety of cultured human cells. The extent of virus replication in PMC or other cells cultured from an individual depends on both the intra-

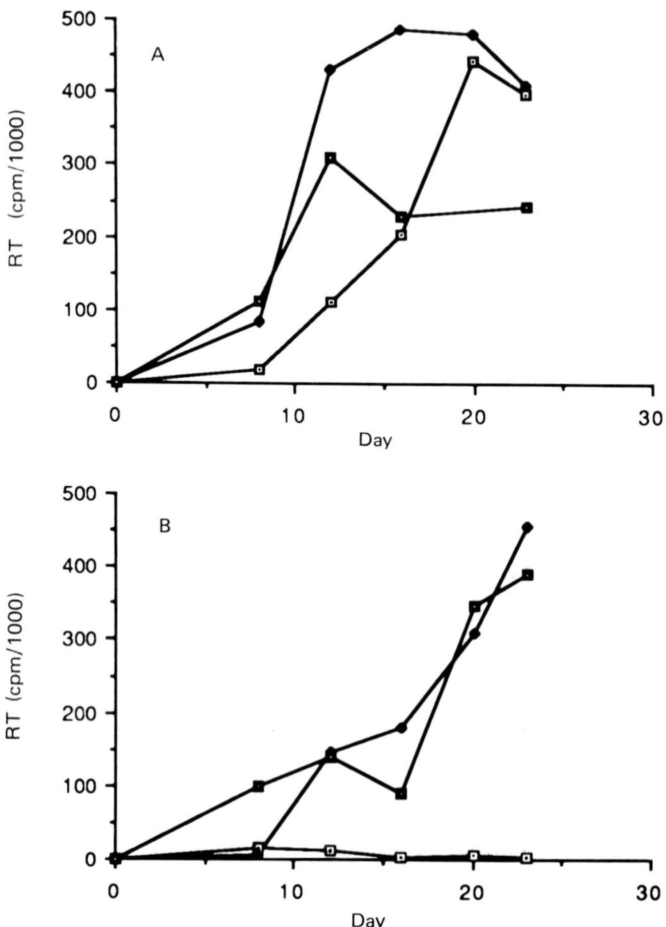

Figure 8 Three different HIV isolates were inoculated onto two EBV-transformed B-cell cultures (A,B) established from donor lymphocytes. A similar quantity of virus was used for inoculation, as determined by the amount of reverse transcriptase (RT) activity per milliliter of virus-containing fluid. (◘) HIV_{SF2}, (□) HIV_{SF3}, (◙) HIV_{SF66}. Viral replication was measured by particle-associated RT activity in the B-cell culture supernatants (25). Note that HIV_{SF2} only replicated in the A cell line. (From Levy et al., *Vaccines* 1987; 5:168.)

cellular milieu and the genetic nature of the particular HIV. Clearly, differences observed in HIV infection reflect specific genetic properties of the virus as well as the host cell involved. Generally, a virus that grows in one established T-cell line will replicate to varying degrees in other T-cell lines (163) but not necessarily in macrophages or B cells (146,147). Moreover, the same B- or T-cell line may be infectable by some HIV and not by others (80,163) (Figure 8). In addition, the replicating ability of the virus in a cell, as reflected in time of initial virus production and extent of progeny release, may vary (118,163,165). These differences in virus infection do not necessarily correlate with expression of CD4 antigen on the cell surface; even cell lines with a high-density expression selectively replicate only certain HIV (163,166). As noted above, intracellular factors and the particular HIV used influence the extent of infection. A similar heterogeneity of HIV replication has been observed with brain-derived cells (79) (Table 5), primary macrophages (154) (see Section VIII.A), and PMC from different seronegative individuals (163). Not only was the time for peak virus replication found to vary depending on the virus isolate and PMC employed, but also the extent of virus replication differed (163). Thus, even with target cells very sensitive for HIV, distinct properties of various isolates, defined by kinetics and extent of replication, can be noted by their interaction with cells from a particular individual (see also Section VI.B).

In additon, the differential ability of individual HIV to infect and replicate in certain hematopoietic types, as noted above, has been reported. While some viruses may preferentially grow in T cells, others, particularly those from the brain, grow best in primary macrophages (80,147,150). Finally, we have found that only certain HIV (e.g., HIV_{SF33}) will replicate in baboon or gorilla PMC or, as noted above (Section VIII.C), in colonic carcinoma cells or human fibroblast cells. These observations suggest that the CD4 receptor need not govern virus infection and that HIV may enter all human cells, but the subsequent steps leading to virus replication vary for each subtype. These differences observed in HIV infection obviously involve specific virus:host cell interactions.

Using these biological features of HIV, we have attempted to classify the virus into biological subtypes. When isolates from the blood were compared with HIV recovered from the brain, distinct differences were appreciated (147) (Table 6). Most HIV from blood replicate in established T-cell lines but not in primary macrophages. In contrast, brain-derived isolates, as noted above, replicate best in primary macrophages and not in established human T-cell lines. Moreover, the blood isolates are often very cytopathic in PMC and induce plaques in the MT-4 cell line (see below), whereas the brain isolates are not (145,147). Serologic properties also appear to distinguish the

Table 6 Potential Characteristics of a Neurotropic HIV

	HIV isolate	
	Blood	Brain
Sensitivity to serum neutralization	+ + +	+
Growth in T-cell lines	+ + +	−
Growth in macrophages[a]	+	+ + +
Plaque in MT-4 cells	+ +	−

[a]From peripheral blood.

Number of plus signs indicates relative ability of isolates from the blood or the brain to have the characteristics listed (see Ref. 147).

brain-derived HIV (147) (see Section XIII.A); they are less sensitive to serum neutralization than is virus recovered from PMC. Finally, these biological differences can identify virus with varying pathogenic properties (146) (see Section XIV).

X. Molecular Heterogeneity of HIV

One of the first observations made when the three prototype AIDS viruses (LAV, HTLV-III, and ARV-2) were identified was that ARV differed by restriction enzyme mapping from LAV/HTLV-III (40,128,129,167,167a). Moreover, two other isolates from San Francisco, ARV-3 and ARV-4 (HIV_{SF3}, HIV_{SF4}), showed restriction maps that were different from ARV-2 as well as LAV/HTLV-III (128). In contrast, LAV and HTLV-III had very similar restriction enzyme maps—an observation that still represents an exception to the findings with other HIV. This heterogeneity in molecular structure has been noted with all isolates from different individuals (see Chapter 9). However, studies in which multiple isolates have been recovered over time from the same individual have shown only limited changes in restriction enzyme sensitivity patterns (146,168). Generally, the constant pattern observed in several regions strongly suggests that the isolates recovered from one patient are variants of the initial HIV transmitted. Furthermore, in cases in which an isolate from one individual has been transmitted to another individual (e.g., from mother to child), a similarity in restriction enzyme patterns has also been noted, but differences were observed (168). The data suggest that viruses introduced into a new host undergo more molecular changes than those maintained in the same host. They also suggest that an individual can be infected by only one isolate and this virus either enters initially with different related variants or evolves into these variants over time within the host. Conceivably, multiple distinct HIV infect an individual but they would become evident only by selective growth in a cell type different from that of the initial isolate (see Section IX). Moreover, studies with chimpanzees have indicated that superinfection with a different HIV can take place (169).

With the few isolates that have been fully sequenced, the heterogeneity in the molecular structure of HIV has been confirmed (40,170-173). Although HTLV-III and LAV are highly similar (differing by only 1%), ARV-2 (HIV_{SF2}) and all other HIV isolates identified show a divergence of 6-10%. For many isolates, only the envelope region has been sequenced (174), because this portion of the virus has shown the greatest degree of divergence (40). In general, variations in the amino acids deduced from the changes among HIV in the envelope region can be as high as 26%. These findings place further emphasis on the need to determine the different envelope serotypes of HIV for the eventual development of a vaccine (see Section XIII.A).

XI. Cofactors in HIV Infection

As has been observed with other viral infections, not all individuals infected with HIV develop disease. While they may in time show symptoms, the reason for a long incubation period is not apparent. One cause may be the existence of a latent infection or the action of T-suppressor lymphocytes (Section XIII.B). Another possible explanation is the role of certain cofactors in determining the progression of disease. We have hypothesized that HIV is itself an opportunistic infection (9). Individuals with an intact immune system will resist the virus-induced disease, as do "survivors" in other virus infections. Others will develop symptoms if their immune system is already affected by immune-compromising factors. These could include the individual's basic genetic background governing the intensity of immune response, the use of drugs that are immunosuppressive or immunoenhancing, and infection by other pathogenic agents. In the last case, the immune system may be so compromised by invading organisms that it cannot resist HIV. These possibilities are being considered by epidemiological programs (see Chapter 1).

Recent work has focused as well on the possible direct interaction of other viruses with HIV that could lead to enhanced virus replication and spread. These studies have employed the HIV long terminal repeat (LTR) (promoter) region linked to the chloramphenicol acetyl transferase (CAT) enzyme (see Chapter 9). They have demonstrated that this construct, transfected into cultured cells, is activated when the cells are superinfected with herpes and papova viruses (175-177). The results suggest that these DNA viruses produce a factor that transactivates the HIV LTR (but at a region different from that for *tat*) (see Chapter 9). These experimental studies need further investigation, but are the first to suggest a potential role of other viruses in HIV infection and spread.

Finally, in cell culture studies, it has been shown that infection of B cells with EBV increases their sensitivity to HIV (see Section VIII.A). In addition, some cells infected with HTLV-I show enhanced replication or become susceptible to HIV. Superinfection of the HTLV-I-infected MT-2 and MT-4 cell lines by HIV are examples of increased virus production by co-infected cells (178). Infection of T-suppressor cells with HTLV-I demonstrates how this infection can make cells sensitive to HIV even though they lack the CD4 antigen complex (179; C. Walker and J. Levy, unpublished observations). Thus, as shown by the experiments with other cultured human cells (Table 5), HIV can infect cells lacking the CD4 antigen. In some HTLV-I-infected individuals, the spread of HIV may be greatly enhanced by this mechanism. This possibility is now being evaluated in patients coming from HTLV-I-endemic areas of the world who are infected by both retroviruses (180).

XII. Animal Studies

In the initial attempts to identify the causative agent of AIDS, we inoculated PMC and whole blood from AIDS patients into a variety of small animals (mice, rats, hamsters, and guinea pigs) as well as primates. We included the small tree shrew (*Suncus suncus*), which is related to primates. These

Table 7 Susceptibility of Animals to HIV

	Number studied	Result
Small animals		
Mouse	328	–
Rat	30	–
Hamster	16	–
Guinea pig	14	–
Rabbit	18	–
Musk shrew	9	–
Primates		
Rhesus monkey	4	–
Baboon	8	–
Chimpanzee	6	6[a]

[a]Seroconversion within 1-6 months; infectious HIV recovered from all animals within 3 months after virus inoculation. HIV has been isolated intermittently from these animals. None of the infected chimpanzees has developed any clinical symptoms or laboratory abnormalities during 3 years of observation.

Except for chimpanzees, both newborn and adult animals were used. Animals were inoculated with HIV or materials containing HIV (14,181). A minus sign indicates that no antibodies to HIV or virus itself were recovered from the animals.

studies (Table 7) indicated that only chimpanzees were susceptible to infection and replication of HIV (14,181). The PMC from other primates may show sensitivity to the virus (118), but successful infection has not been achieved. The chimpanzees can be infected within 1 month and seroconvert within 1 to 3 months after infection (181-186). Nevertheless, after 3-5 years of study, none of the HIV-infected animals in the world have developed signs of AIDS despite attempts at suppressing their immune system (181). The results have indicated that chimpanzees can carry and release HIV from their PMC and yet resist the progression to AIDS. The reason for this resistance to viral pathogenesis is not yet known, but it may be related to the presence of antibody-mediated, complement-dependent cytotoxicity (ACC) in this animal system (186). Humans do not appear to have this immune response. Other possible explanations include the absence of autoantibodies or a very strong control of HIV replication by CD8+ lymphocytes (55,181).

Several research groups have used macaques and chimpanzees in which to study immune responses to HIV. In all these studies, both neutralizing and cell-mediated immune responses have been elicited against the virus or its envelope proteins (169,187,188), but protection to challenge of HIV has never been achieved (188). Moreover, a chimpanzee infected by one HIV has been superinfected by another HIV despite the presence of neutralizing antibodies (169). In many cases, the immune response was selective for the type of HIV used in the study. In some situations, however, infection by one HIV has given rise to low titers of neutralizing antibodies against other HIV (181,186). Nevertheless, these animal models do not give encouragement for the use of classic vaccine approaches for HIV prevention. Perhaps studies with simian immunodeficiency virus (SIV), the primate counterpart to HIV (189), will provide helpful information for antiviral therapies for the human lentivirus infection.

XIII. Immune Reactions to HIV

The outcome of any viral infection depends not only on the virulence of the pathogen but also on the strength of the antiviral response by the infected host. Both the humoral and cellular arms of the immune system are involved in this antiviral reaction (see Chapter 10). When measuring the humoral (antibody) response to HIV, a variety of tests have been developed that detect reaction with viral antigens themselves, or, in the case of infectivity, assess the ability to neutralize the virus. The cellular immune responses are generally the most important in controlling a virus after infection has taken place. With HIV, this fact appears especially true, since HIV-infected cells are the primary source of infection and transmission (107).

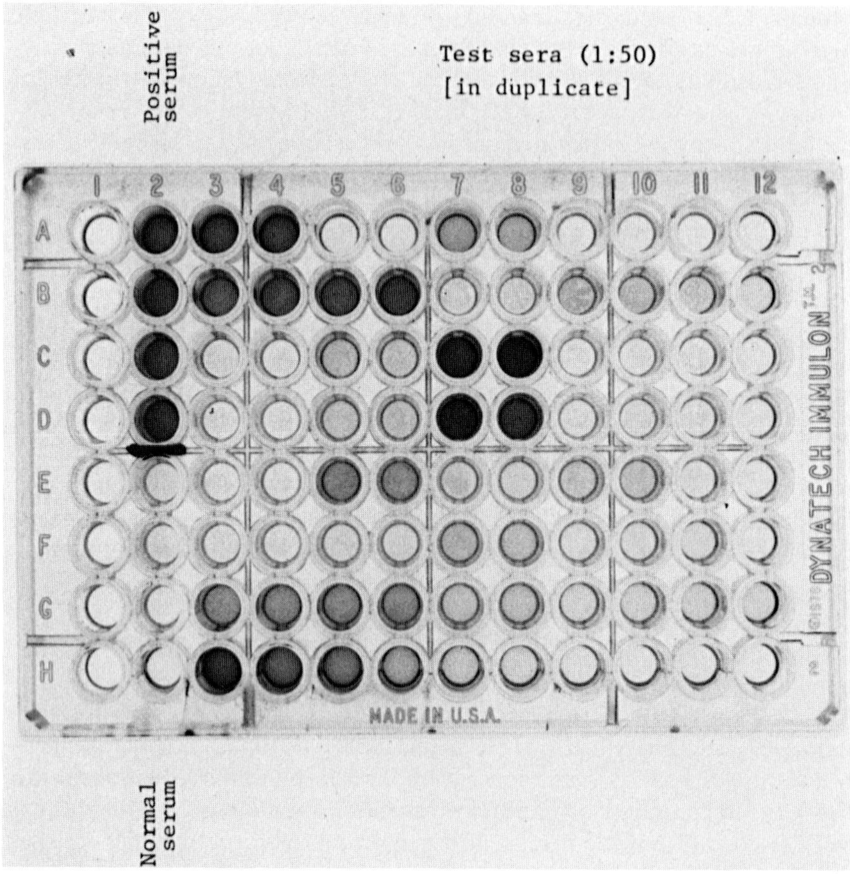

Figure 9 The ELISA test adapted to measure antibodies to HIV. The dark immunoperoxidase stain denotes human antibodies that are reactive with the viral proteins fixed to the bottom of the wells.

A. Humoral Immune Responses

Enzyme-Linked Immunosorbent Assay

One of the first procedures adapted for the detection of antibodies to HIV was the ELISA, which can be used as an automated method for screening sera (190). For this assay, virus is purified from cell culture and disrupted with detergent. The viral proteins are fixed to a 96-well plate or to beads and reacted with the test serum. The binding of the antiviral antibodies to the viral proteins is then measured by an enzyme-linked antihuman antibody.

The reaction is read by a colorimetric procedure (Figure 9). For this procedure, HIV grown in established human T-cell lines (e.g., H9, HUT-78, CEM) has been most useful. The CEM cell line offers some advantages over the others because it lacks HLA antigen expression on the cell surface. Nevertheless, all the ELISA tests using virus from infected human cell lines exhibit a certain degree of false-positive reactions due to antibodies to normal cellular proteins present in some human sera. Since the virus buds from the cell surface (Figure 1), it can incorporate some cellular proteins in its viral coat. Moreover, even purified viral components can be contaminated by cellular proteins carried along by the budding process. At this time, a positive ELISA is repeated, and then confirmed by other antibody tests (see below). In the future, ELISA tests with recombinant viral antigens will be available; because they are free of cellular proteins, they should offer better specificity.

Immunofluorescence Assay

A conventional method for detecting viral antigens or antibodies is to react serum with infected cells fixed on slides or plates. The binding of the antibody is subsequently measured using a fluorescein-labeled antihuman antibody. Our laboratory developed an IFA for the AIDS virus using HIV_{SF2}-infected HUT-78 cells (130). This assay offers the advantage that a specific pattern of attachment of the antibodies to HIV antigens can be read and thus nonspecific reactions can be detected. Moreover, by mixing infected with uninfected cells (1:1), a staining of normal T cells can be noted if more than 50% of the cells are positive. In this situation, absorption with uninfected T cells is performed before repeating the IFA. The IFA is rapid (it can be done in 30 minutes) and specific (130,191,192). Nevertheless, it is not automated and does require some experience in reading. However, IFA is often the best method for detecting early antibody responses after acute HIV infection (193). Moreover, in many developing countries, only fluorescent microscopes are available and thus this assay might be the only screening test available.

Western Blot (Immunoblot)

A relatively new procedure for measuring antiviral antibody responses involves the use of specific viral antigens. For these studies, virus is purified from culture fluid and disrupted with detergent, as described above. The proteins are then placed on a polyacrylamide gel and under electrophoresis migrate according to size. These proteins are transferred to a nitrocellulose filter by a blotting technique and subsequently reacted with serum from the individual. The attachment of the antibodies to specific viral proteins can then be detected using antihuman antibody reagents. The specificity of the antibodies can be distinguished from antibodies to cellular proteins by their

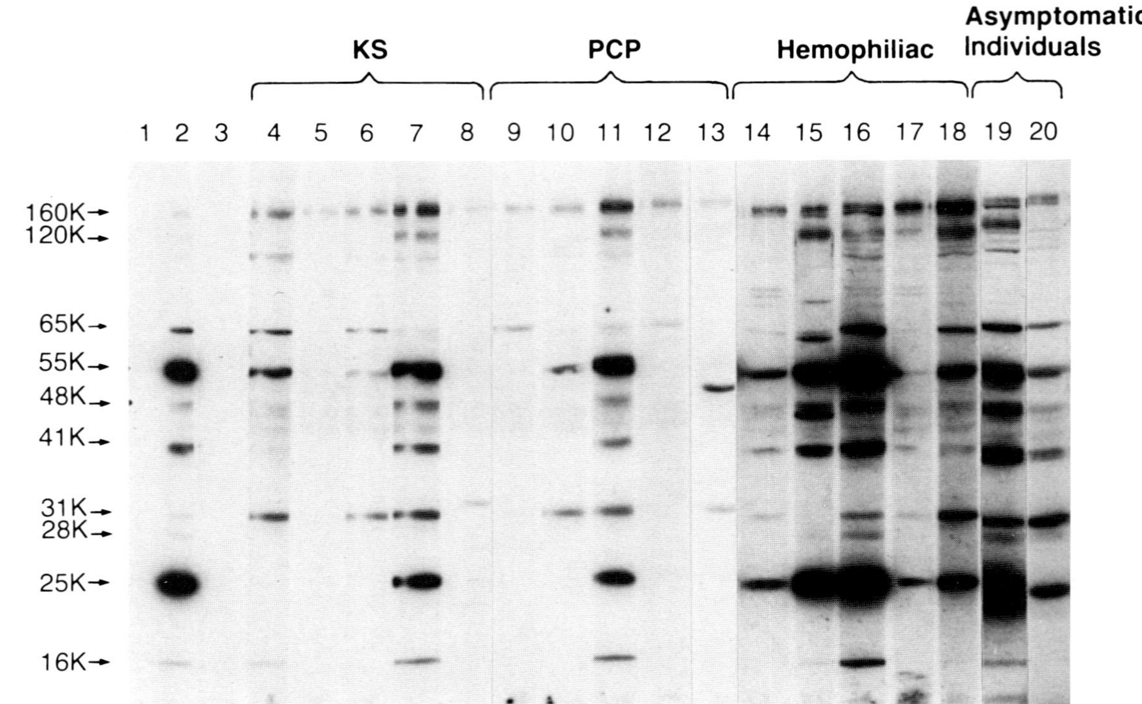

Figure 10 A profile of the antibody reaction to HIV proteins as demonstrated by immunoblot procedures. The figures at the left denote the major viral proteins: envelope (gp160, gp120, gp41), reverse transcriptase (p65, p53, p31), and the core proteins (p55, p40, p25). (From Ref. 194.)

position on the filter and by the use of positive control sera. A positive reaction is detected either through a colorimetric procedure or through radioactively labeled antihuman antibodies (e.g., iodinated staph A).

As noted above, the immunoblot procedure (Figure 10) is very helpful in distinguishing antibody responses to specific viral proteins (194). One potentially important result obtained from these studies supports the observations from others that antibodies to the *gag* p25 protein appear to decrease as the clinical state worsens (64,194-197). One other noteworthy observation is the continual presence of antibodies to the envelope protein throughout the clinical course. In particular, we have found the consistent presence of antibodies to gp160 (the nonprocessed envelope precursor protein) in all patients even in the terminal stages of AIDS (194) (Figure 10). This result suggests that the antigen expressed at the cleavage site of the gp120 and gp41 proteins may be highly immunogenic in infected individuals. The presence of these antienvelope antibodies mirrors observations of neutralizing antibodies present even in sera of severely ill patients (see below). The immunoblot procedure has also recently been used as well to detect IgM antibodies (198), but this method needs further evaluation.

Radioimmune Precipitation and Radioimmune Assay

The radioimmune precipitation assay (RIPA) involves the solubilization of cells or pelleted virus by detergents and reacting them with antibodies either pooled or produced against a particular viral protein (45,199). For this assay, the proteins of infected cells are labeled in culture and the cells are subsequently extracted. The reaction of these lysates with antibodies to viral proteins can then lead to the precipitation of even small amounts of labeled proteins that might not be detected by the immunoblot procedure. The RIPA has indicated the high prevalence of antibodies to the HIV envelope protein (199a). The assay has also been used effectively in distinguishing HIV-1 and HIV-2 proteins (200), and in examining long precursor viral polypeptides (199). It gives results comparable to those of immunoblot but differs in utilizing native rather than denatured proteins.

Radioactive reagents can also be used in a competition assay in which the extent of prevention of the interaction of labeled antigen or labeled antibodies is measured. This radioimmune assay (RIA) reflects the reduction in a labeled reactant (complex) when unlabeled (cell lysate or antibody) is added (201). The competition curves can be extrapolated to give the amount of antigen or antibody present.

Neutralization Assays

The ability of the host to produce neutralizing antibodies to HIV can be assessed by a variety of procedures. These include the measurement of reduced p25 production in infected cells (67), reverse transcriptase (RT) activity in cell culture (202,203), or plaque formation (204,205). In general, serum at an appropriate dilution is mixed with virus for 30-60 minutes at room temperature. The mixture is diluted 5-10-fold and added to target cells. Control cultures receive the virus incubated with serum from uninfected individuals. A reduction of at least 66% in RT activity or plaques is used as a measure of neutralization. Fifty-percent reduction in p25 antigen production is regarded as indicating neutralization by that procedure. While initially the presence of neutralizing antibodies to HIV was not easily detected (202, 204), recent evidence using well-defined systems has often shown high titers of serum neutralization, even in severely ill patients (203,206). In particular, some strains of HIV, for example, HIV_{SF2} (ARV-2), appear to be very sensitive to neutralization; antiviral levels in serum can approach titers of 1:20,000 (203).

The site or sites on the virion sensitive to neutralizing antibodies has not yet been defined. As noted above, regions of the gp120, gp41, and perhaps the core protein, p17, may mediate virus infection of cells. Antibodies to any of these proteins could affect infection. Recent evidence has indicated that neutralization can involve a portion of the gp120 not responsible for virus attachment (205a,205b). Mutations in the second conserved region of gp120 or antibodies to this region prevent virus infection without blocking virus binding to cells.

Serologic Differences Among HIV

The above-described neutralization tests have led to the evaluation of potential HIV serotypes where identification would be important for vaccine development. Preliminary studies using three different sera have indicated that certain viruses can be grouped according to their sensitivity to neutralization (203) (Table 8). Subgroup A includes all virus isolates that were easily neutralizable, subgroup B viruses are susceptible to only two of the sera, and subgroup C to only one. Finally, an African isolate (HIV_{SF170}) was not found susceptible to neutralization by any of the three sera tested (subgroup D). This latter virus is sensitive to neutralization only by some African sera. These studies begin to unravel the question of serotyping and suggest that a finite number of antigenically distinct HIV will be found.

Using these serologic properties for distinguishing HIV, we evaluated (as noted above) some of our blood- and brain-derived isolates. These studies indicated that isolates from PMC were much more sensitive to serum neutralization than those from the brain (Table 6). Whether these serologic features can further differentiate specific biological or molecular subtypes needs evaluation.

Table 8 Neutralization of HIV Infectivity by Anti-HIV-1 Sera

Proposed serotype	HIV_{SF}	Source	Serum 1	Serum 2	Serum 3
A	2	PMC (SF, 1983)	>1000	100	10
	33	PMC (Ph, 1984)	>1000	100	10
	66	PMC (SF, 1984)	>1000	100	10
	117	PMC (SF, 1985)	>1000	100	10
	301A	CNS (SF, 1986)	>1000	100	100
B	97	PMC (SF, 1985)	80	20	–
	171	PMC (Af, 1985)	20	10	–
C	98	CNS (SF, 1985)	20	–	–
	128A	CNS (SF, 1985)	20	–	–
	162	CNS (SF, 1985)	100	–	–
	153	PMC (Af, 1985)	20	–	–
	247	PMC (DR, 1985)	100	–	–
D	170	PMC (Af, 1985)	–	–	–

HIV isolates tested for sensitivity to neutralization by standard procedures (see Ref. 203). Sera came from three seropositive individuals. Number represents reciprocal of end-dilution of serum that reduced by more than 67% particle-associated reverse transcriptase activity in inoculated cultures when compared to control cultures receiving virus incubated with normal serum. In general, 10-fold dilutions were used for initial screening and then twofold dilutions defined end-titers for some of the isolates. Ph, Philadelphia; Af, Africa; DR, Dominican Republic.

B. Cellular Immune Response: Control of HIV Infection

The cellular immune system, consisting of T lymphocytes, macrophages, and NK cells, is concerned with cell-mediated immune reactions (Chapter 10). One of its responses is linked to antibody production: antibody-dependent cellular cytotoxicity (ADCC). This reaction during HIV infection involves a cytotoxic response of host effector cells against anti-*env* antibody-coated infected cells (207-210). While the level of antibodies involved in ADCC does not appear to reflect a clinical state (208,210), a decrease in effector cells in the infected individual may correlate with development of AIDS. This possibility needs to be evaluated.

Certain laboratories have demonstrated the presence of cytotoxic cellular responses to infected cells, presumably by CD8+ lymphocytes (211,212). Some of these studies were performed with target cells that had been manipulated in the laboratory to express viral antigens (e.g., infection of cells using a vaccinia virus vector). It is not yet clear whether these in vitro observations mirror events occurring in the host.

Our emphasis has been on the possible role of lymphocytes in suppressing HIV replication. In an early evaluation of seropositive, asymptomatic individuals, we noted that about 50% did not readily release HIV from their cultured PMC (37). In the search for an explanation of this observation, the T-suppressor (CD8+) cell, which limits infection by many viruses (including EBV) (213), appeared to be a good candidate.

In a limited group of subjects from whose PMC HIV could not recovered, CD8+ cells were removed by panning (58). These studies indicated that, whereas unseparated PMC did not yield virus, the CD8-depleted cells released substantial amounts of HIV (55). As expected, the purified CD8+ cells did not produce virus. Conclusive proof that the CD8+ cells were indeed controlling the retrovirus infection was obtained by adding back purified CD8+ cells to virus-releasing cultures. HIV replication was suppressed by a dose-response effect; only substantial numbers of CD8+ cells reduced virus production. Moreover, CD8+ cells cultured for 3 weeks in flasks could suppress HIV when added back to CD4+ cells releasing virus (55). This observation suggested that, as in lymphokine-activated killer (LAK) cell therapy in cancer (214), adoptive transfer might be helpful, at least for experimental purposes, in controlling HIV infection in some individuals lacking this immune response. Finally, in some individuals, removal of CD8+ cells did not lead to recovery of HIV from the depleted PMC. Subsequent studies indicated that there were 10-15% CD8+ cells still remaining in their PMC after panning. Only after selection for the CD4+ cells by panning could virus be recovered (59). These studies emphasized the fact that a small number of the CD8+ cells in certain individuals may be able to control HIV replication.

Using Marbrook chambers, our group has shown that one mechanism for the suppression of virus release is a diffusible factor made by CD8+ cells. The CD8+ lymphocytes were placed in the bottom chamber and CD4+ cells in the top. A filter prevented contact between the two populations. In the presence of the filter, CD8+ cells still substantially reduced HIV replication (215). While the nature of the diffusible factor is under study, the possibility that cell-to-cell contact is a more effective means of inhibiting virus replication needs to be evaluated.

Suppression of virus replication in the host appears to reduce progression of disease, and prolong the asymptomatic course (64). In one individual we have been studying since October 1984, virus release has been under suppression by CD8+ lymphocytes since February of 1985. After 3 years, he remains asymptomatic, and his CD4+ cells have gone from 300 to a normal count of more than 1000 cells per cubic millimeter (80). How long this control of HIV production will last is being followed closely. Understanding the mechanism of this control may be helpful in the care of other infected individuals.

Table 9 Heterogeneity of HIV

1. Cell tropism
2. Replication efficiency
3. CD4 antigen modulation
4. Cytopathic properties
5. Latency
6. Antigenic properties
7. Restriction enzyme sensitivity
8. Sequence variation

Characteristics can differ for specific HIV and form the basis for classification of individual isolates.

Table 10 Factors Influencing Pathogenesis

Virus characteristics
1. Replication: host range
2. Cytopathology
3. Latency
Host response
1. Autoantibody production
2. Hyperresponse: lymphoma, KS
3. Hyporesponse: carcinomas, infections
4. Humoral immunity against virus: neutralizing antibodies, ADCC
5. Cellular immunity against virus: cytotoxic and suppressive responses

Factors define characteristics of HIV that can influence its virulence and features of host response that may affect the pathogenic properties of the virus. Essentially, immune responses can enhance pathogenesis (e.g., autoantibody production, immune complex formation) or reduce it (e.g., neutralizing antibodies, antibody-dependent cellular cytotoxicity [ADCC], cellular immune responses).

XIV. Features of HIV Pathogenesis

The preceding sections have dealt with the heterogeneous characteristics of HIV (Table 9), the variations in sensitivity of different cells to infection, and how the host responds to the virus. Obviously, these two components (virus and host) determine the outcome of infection. In evaluating the major aspects of HIV-induced disease, we need to appreciate the factors associated with the virulence of the pathogen and the strength of the antiviral response by the host (Table 10).

A. Biological Changes in HIV over Time

Molecular changes in HIV have been detected through restriction enzyme mapping of virus isolates recovered from the same individual over a defined

Table 11 Change in HIV Over Time in an Infected Individual

Virus	Clinical state	Host range	Cytopathology	Plaque formation	Neutralization
HIV_{SF2}	Oral Candida	HUT 78 U937	+	–	+ +
HIV_{SF13}	KS PCP	same[a]	+ +	+	+ +

[a]Also grows in B cells and peripheral blood macrophages.

Initial isolate (HIV_{SF2}) obtained from infected individual who presented with yeast infection of the mouth (oral candidiasis). This virus had a wide host range, was not cytopathic in cell culture, did not form plaques in the MT-4 cell line, and was easily neutralized by serum antibodies (see Table 8). The sequential isolate (HIV_{SF13}) recovered 5 months later from the same individual when he had KS and PCP had an even wider host range with ability to grow in B cells and peripheral blood macrophages. This virus grew rapidly to high titer in infectious cells and was highly cytopathic in PMC. It formed plaques in MT-4 cells but had the same neutralization pattern as initial HIV_{SF2} isolate (see Ref. 146).

period of time (168). In our laboratory we have also evaluated, first by biological and serologic and then by molecular procedures, viruses isolated from the same individual on at least two occasions. In three patients in whom severe disease developed, the sequential virus isolate differed in its biological properties but did not show major differences in its molecular or serologic features (146). For example, in one case, HIV_{SF2} isolated from an individual with oral candidiasis replicated less efficiently and was less cytopathic than HIV_{SF13} isolated 5 months later when the same patient had developed KS and PCP. The second isolate has a greatly enlarged host range with replication in B cells and primary macrophages. It grows rapidly to high titer in infected cells and it produces plaques in MT-4 cells (Table 11). These biological characteristics would be expected for a more virulent virus. Molecular studies indicate that HIV_{SF13} and HIV_{SF2} are related and not distinct HIV. The two other cases gave similar results with disease progression correlating with a highly replicating, cytopathic virus. In contrast, an individual who remained asymptomatic has had an HIV with low cytopathic properties for over a year (146). Thus, it appears likely that the biological properties of HIV can play a major role in the pathogenic process.

B. Autoantibodies

When a virus infects an individual, both immune-suppressing and immune-enhancing consequences can develop. In HIV infection, both features of virus interaction with the immune system can be observed. With immune suppression, opportunistic infections and, in some cases, cancers occur. In immune

Table 12 Autoantibodies in HIV Infection

Target	Clinical sign[a]
Red blood cells	Anemia
Neutrophils	Neutropenia
Lymphocyte	Immune deficiency
Platelet	Immune thrombocytopenic purpura
Peripheral nerve	Neuropathy
Lupus anticoagulant (phospholipid)	Thrombosis ? Neurological disease
Nucleus (ANA)	Autoimmunity

[a]Autoimmune syndromes that have been recognized in individuals infected with HIV.

Table 13 HIV and Autoantibody Production

Shared region	Location[a]
IL-2	LTR, *env*
γ-Interferon	LTR
HLA antigens	*env*
α-1 Thymosin	*gag*
Neuroleukin (Phosphohexose	*env*
isomerase)	*env*
Peptide T[b]	isomerase
HLA antigens	virion surface[c]

[a]Region of HIV that has potential cross-reaction with normal cellular protein as deduced from sequence analyses.
[b]May be homolog of vasoactive intestinal polypeptide (219a).
[c]Incorporated into viral envelope from cell surface.

enhancement, proliferation of certain cells of the immune system takes place, leading to malignancies such as Kaposi's sarcoma (endothelial cells of lymph channels) and B-cell lymphomas (see Chapters 13, 14). This hyperimmune response is also mirrored by increased production of cytokines such as thymosin and alpha interferon as well as immunoglobulins (9). In newborn children, for instance, hypergammaglobulinemia is a frequent first sign of HIV infection (216) (see Chapter 6). In adults, this hypergammaglobulinemia can be reflected by high titers of antibodies to known viruses such as EBV and CMV. It can also be revealed by the presence of autoimmunity.

A number of autoimmune syndromes associated with HIV infection have been recognized (see Chapter 10) (Table 12). Moreover, HIV itself shares several regions of its genome with that of normal cellular proteins (51,217-221,289,290) (Chapter 10) (Table 13). Thus, immunization with purified HIV might lead to autoimmune syndromes. For this reason, the recent trials of vaccination with recombinant viral gp160 produced in insect cells (222) are important; they can evaluate the potential production of autoantibodies in the vaccinated individuals.

Among the autoantibodies observed during HIV infection are those directed against lymphocytes (223-225). Initially, they appear to react primarily with T-helper cells, but, with more progressive disease, antibodies to all T cells have been detected (223; D. Kiprov, personal communication). Recently, antilymphocyte antibodies were found to react with an 18,000 Mr protein (p18) on the surface of activated CD4+ cells (69). Unstimulated (e.g., mitogen-treated) CD4+ cells, B lymphocytes, and macrophages do not express this antigen. Neither stimulated nor unstimulated CD8+ cells make p18. Activated macrophages, however, can express p18 on their cell surface (R. Stricker, unpublished observations). This selective expression of the p18 protein on activated CD4+ cells has also been observed when unstimulated CD4+ cells are infected with virus, either HIV or a mouse retrovirus (69). Thus, an interrelationship among virus infection, CD4+ cell activation, and autoantibodies has been observed. Subsequent studies have indicated that this anti-p18 antibody selectively kills CD4+ cells and not CD8+ cells in the presence of complement. Finally, the presence of the anti-p18 antibody correlates with disease in the HIV-infected patient. Asymptomatic seropositive individuals lack evidence of the autoantibody (69).

We have hypothesized that HIV infection of CD4+ cells serves, via a "carrier-hapten" mechanism (226), to induce antibodies to the p18 protein that is normally made on activated CD4+ cells (227). When the immune system responds to the viral antigens on the surface of the infected cell, it also recognizes p18, which has now been made immunogenic (Figure 11). The resulting anti-p18 autoantibodies then kill not only virus-infected cells but also CD4+ cells activated by other factors such as concomitant infections. The production of these autoantibodies is important since they can hasten the progression of disease by further destruction of the CD4+ cells. Their existence offers one explanation for the small number of CD4+ cells found in AIDS.

C. Immune Complexes

Besides autoantibodies, hypergammaglobulinemia can lead to the formation of antibody:antigen complexes that circulate in blood. These appear to be more commonly found in HIV-infected individuals whether asymptomatic or with disease (228,229). These complexes can contain viral antigens (229,230) and, in some cases, appear to carry infectious virions (229). The complexes can inhibit the detection of viral proteins in an antigen assay (see Section III.B) and can compromise the immune system by blocking the reticuloendothelial

HIV AND AUTOIMMUNITY

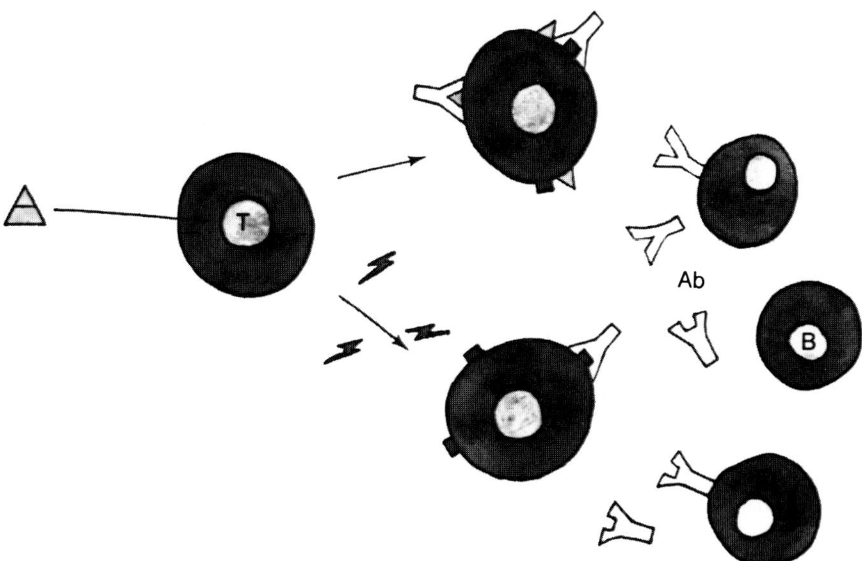

Figure 11 Carrier-hapten mechanism for autoantibody production. The virus (◬) after infection of the T helper lymphocyte induces not only viral antigens (Δ) on the cell surface but also the expression of a normal cellular protein (■) (e.g., p18) (69). This same antigen is produced when T-helper cells are activated by mitogens or other factors. The immunogenicity of this normal cellular protein is enhanced by its expression on virus-infected cells. Antibodies are made against the viral protein and the normal cellular protein. Thus, when this cellular protein is expressed following activation of T lymphocytes, the autoantibodies react with these cells as well as with the virus-infected cells.

system, as occurs in other immune-complex diseases. Formation of antibody: p25 complexes may explain the decrease in antibodies to p25 observed in individuals with progressive disease (Section XIII.A). The assumption is that viral p25 made in large quantities attaches to the anti-p25 antibody. Which factor comes first in the pathogenesis of the disease, however, has not been elucidated.

D. Summary

All these observations on the biological, serologic, and molecular heterogeneity of HIV (Table 9) and the variety of host responses to the virus are important features of HIV pathogenesis (Table 10). From the initial virus infection of the cell via a surface receptor to the various intracellular controls of virus replication, different HIV subtypes can be identified and the infection in a particular cell becomes established or aborted. Efficient spread of the virus with death of infected cells enhances progression of disease. Finally, the immune responses to the host can be detrimental (autoantibodies, immune complexes) or helpful (cytotoxic or suppressor CD8+ cells). These factors indicate the complexity of HIV infection and should be considered in developing appropriate antiviral therapy.

XV. The HIV-2 Subtype

In 1986, after HIV had been identified in the United States, the Caribbean, and Central Africa, a new type of retrovirus associated with AIDS was reported in regions of western Africa. The existence of a different human AIDS virus was first suggested by reports of antibodies to SIV in prostitutes in Senegal (231). Antibodies to the prototype HIV (now called HIV-1) did not cross-react substantially with SIV. Subsequent evaluation by Montagnier and his associates of AIDS patients in Portugal who had originally come from Guinea Bissau or Cape Verde suggested the existence of a new type of HIV (200). These individuals had very little or no antibody reactivity to HIV-1. Suspecting that the patients had a poor antibody response to HIV, the investigators isolated an infectious retrovirus from one patient's PMC and evaluated the viral antigenic properties by immunoblot assay. These studies indicated that this AIDS patient had high titered antibodies to his own viral proteins but not to HIV-1. In particular, the envelope proteins of the west Africa isolate (called LAV-2) were distinct antigenically as well as by size. They were gp140 and gp36 rather than the conventional gp120 and gp41 of HIV-1. The *gag* protein also had a molecular weight of about p27 rather than the p25 (p24) of HIV-1, but, like the *pol* gene products, the *gag* proteins cross-reacted with antibodies to HIV-1. Furthermore, when antiserum from the west African patient was reacted with purified proteins from SIV, a reaction with several of these proteins, including the envelope, was noted (200). And, antibodies to SIV recognized some of the proteins of this virus isolate (200). That same year, Kanki and associates (232), having suspected another HIV-related virus in prostitutes in Senegal (231), isolated a new type of retrovirus from one asymptomatic woman. They named it HTLV-IV, because of its lymphotropism and similarity to HTLV-III; it cross-reacted best with anti-

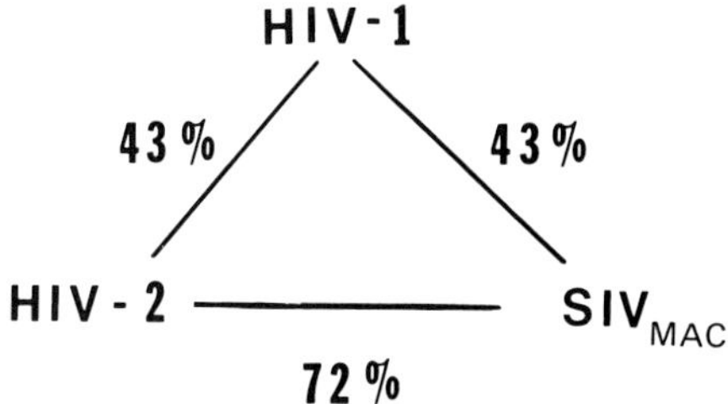

Figure 12 Diagram of the amino acid differences among the human and simian immunodeficiency viruses (HIV, SIV).

bodies to SIV. Finally, a third isolate, SBL-6669, was recently recovered from a west African patient; it showed a similar relationship to SIV and HIV-1 as did LAV-2 (233).

The cloning and sequencing of both the French isolate (LAV-2) (234) and HTLV-IV (235,236) have provided the following information: By amino acid analysis, LAV-2 shows 73% similarity to SIV and 43% similarity to HIV-1; HIV-1 and SIV also differ by about 57% (Figure 12). HTLV-IV, however, shows more than 99% sequence homology to SIV. Recently, as was suspected (236), HTLV-IV has been identified as a primate virus contaminant of the cell cultures used for the isolation of the Senegalese virus (237). Based on a 55% difference in sequences between LAV-2 (and SBL-6669) and HIV-1 (234), a new subtype of the human AIDS virus has been recognized and designated HIV-2. Because SIV most closely resembles HIV-2, some investigators are now searching among the primate populations in Africa for an HIV-1-type of simian agent.

The transmission and pathogenesis of HIV-2 appears similar to those of HIV-1 (238). Certain isolates may not be as cytopathic as others and, according to some investigators, this AIDS virus subtype may not produce disease in many infected individuals (239). Nonetheless, the time period of following patients infected with HIV-2 has been short and may be insufficient to permit the incubation time already known to be necessary for HIV-1-induced disease (now estimated at a mean of 5 years; see Chapter 1). HIV-2 appears to productively infect monkey cells and may be transmitted to primates other than chimpanzees (240). This feature probably reflects its SIV-like properties. In our laboratory we have identified HIV-2-like viruses from AIDS and ARC patients in the Ivory Coast; as expected, their antibodies and their viral proteins cross-react best with those of SIV and not HIV-1 (241). Most interestingly, some individuals in the Ivory Coast seem to be infected by both AIDS viruses since they have antibodies reacting with HIV-1 and HIV-2 isolates (241,242). One of our Ivory Coast isolates (HIV-2_{UC1}) is not cytopathic and does not substantially reduce CD4+ antigen expression in infected cells (241). In this regard, it is different from the HIV-1 and the other HIV-2 isolates described; it may be an unusual subtype of HIV-2. Recently, however, some HIV-1 isolates, particularly those recovered from the brain, also have been found not to affect CD4 antigen expression in infected CD4+ peripheral blood cells (L. Evans and C. Cheng-Mayer, unpublished observations). Thus, modulation of CD4 antigen expression may be another feature that distinguishes different HIV-1 and HIV-2 isolates. The possibility that HIV-2_{UC1} is a less pathogenic or a neurotropic strain is under study; the individual from whom we isolated the virus died with neurological symptoms.

Recently, using synthetic peptides made from a specific region of the gp41 of each AIDS virus subtype, investigators have distinguished immune reactions to HIV-1 and HIV-2 (243). This ELISA will be very helpful in screening sera for both viruses; it confirms serologic studies we have performed using immunoblots. Because some individuals who make antibodies to HIV-2 may show responses only to the envelope protein, an ELISA using just HIV-1 antigens would not be sufficient to detect these infected individuals. Thus, blood banks throughout the world will soon need to add an HIV-2 antigen (presumably the envelope) to the ELISA test to detect blood from HIV-2-infected individuals. At the time of this writing, serologic evidence of HIV-2 infection has been found primarily in west Africa, particularly Senegal, Guinea Bissau, and the Ivory Coast (238,239). Its presence in parts of Europe and Brazil has also been reported, and just recently in a west African patient living in the United States (244).

XVI. HIV Transmission

As discussed in Chapter 1, HIV infection has been linked to exposure only to blood or genital secretions; there is no evidence at all for HIV transmission by saliva, tears, urine, or other body fluids (245). Moreover, heat treatment of clotting factors (Chapter 4) (28,246) and the usual procedures for preparation of immunoglobulins for therapy eliminate infectious virus (247).

During sexual activity, the highest risk for infection of homosexual men is incurred by the receptive partner in anal/genital contact (89); the insertive partner rarely shows infection by HIV. Anal lavage appears to be an independent variable in this transmission rate (89). These observations support the detection of HIV in bowel epithelial cells (88). This tissue, being both friable and sensitive to virus, can be an important site for infection. And, as noted in Section V, the infected cell in genital secretions appears to be the primary source for this virus transmission (107).

When heterosexual activity has been evaluated (see Chapter 7), anal contact for a woman has been shown to carry the same risk that it does for men. However, vaginal intercourse carries less risk for both men and women. A frequency at least 10 times lower by this route than by anal contact has been estimated (248). For women, infection can occur if an infected cell in the seminal fluid finds entrance into the cervical os to meet resident macrophages and lymphocytes in the endometrium. This event could occur in sexual activity, particularly during or shortly after menses when the mucosal plug of the cervical canal is not present. Recent studies also suggest that endothelial cells of the cervix might be infected directly by HIV (90a). The virus could be transmitted to men through contact with infected women if the men have abrasions or lesions on their penile epithelium or along the urethral canal; white blood cells once infected by contact with the vaginal secretions could then recirculate in the host. This route of infection is not common and the risk is low, as it is for insertive partners in anal/genital contact. Some epidemiologists believe that the foreskin, with its mucosal lining, may be a site of entry for the AIDS virus (249). In fact, recent data from Africa link a higher risk of HIV transmission to uncircumcised men (110).

Several studies have looked specifically at casual contact as a source of contagion, and none has provided any evidence. Thus, health-care workers in hospitals having close contact with HIV-infected patients rarely have shown seroconversion—and only when a needle stick was involved (96,245). These investigations suggest that the risk for seroconversion after needle sticks is 1/1000 (96). In 1987, three nurses became infected after having prolonged exposure to large amounts of blood from HIV-infected individuals (250). These three women, however, had eczema or open wounds on their hands that could have been a site for infection.

Insects, while considered by some to be possible vectors of HIV (251), are highly unlikely transmitters because of the extremely small amount of blood potentially present on their mouth parts (252). Moreover, if insects were a source of infection, one would expect cases of AIDS in African children who spend most of their time outside and are continually exposed to insect bites. However, those without the known risk factors of maternal transfer or transfusion are not infected by the virus (245,252).

Finally, it should be appreciated that HIV is very sensitive to heat, lipid solvents, and common antiseptics (253). Thus, eliminating virus from medical instruments, hospital supplies, and areas exposed to contaminated materials is not a difficult task.

XVII. Acute HIV Infection

Cooper et al., studying individuals who had recently been exposed to HIV, described the clinical characteristics of acute HIV infection (254,291) (Table 14). They include atypical lymphocytosis, lymphadenopathy, fever, malaise, myalgias, and other features commonly seen in a viral disease. The

Table 14 Characteristics of Acute HIV Infection

1. Mononucleosislike illness
2. Fever, sweats, lethargy, malaise, arthralgias, myalgias, headache, and sore throat—followed by generalized lymphadenopathy
3. Macular, erythematous eruption
4. Increased T suppressor cells → decreased H/S ratio
5. Possible occurrence within 1 week after infection, duration of 1-2 weeks
6. Possible recurrence in 3 weeks to 3 months

syndrome often presents with a macular erythematous rash, usually on the trunk, but sometimes on the extremities. This rash may be caused by the deposition in the skin of immune complexes. These symptoms of acute HIV infection generally last 1 to 2 weeks and can recur 3 weeks to 3 months later. Prospective studies of individuals presenting with this syndrome showed that seroconversion to HIV occurred within 6 days to 2 months after infection (193,255). The antibody test used influenced the detection time; IFA and IgM antibody assays generally showed seroconversion earlier than did ELISA and immunoblot procedures (193,198). For a period of time after HIV infection, the presence of viral antigens (e.g., p25) or infectious HIV in the blood in the absence of antibodies can be observed (42,255-257). Probably about 30% of individuals acutely infected with HIV show symptoms. Recent HIV infection can also be reflected by an acute encephalitis with marked pleocytosis in the CSF (258). Subsequent resolution of this syndrome can result in long-term periods in which the invididual shows no further signs of brain involvement.

XVIII. Treatment

Because of the known severity of AIDS, many pharmaceutical companies have attempted to develop an effective antiviral drug. The steps in HIV infection that could be affected are described in Chapter 9. Whereas tissue culture studies have shown the efficacy of many products (259-269), only 3-azidothymidine (AZT) (Zidovidine) has shown promise in clinical trials (270). This drug appears to be much more active against virus reverse transcriptase than cellular polymerases, but unfortunately it can be toxic (271). In the first 6 months of treatment severe bone-marrow depression requiring blood transfusions can frequently occur, particularly in severely ill patients. Moreover, in cell culture it does not show long-lasting effects and thus may not give prolonged clinical help (272). In addition, it is less effective in reducing HIV infection of macrophages, since these cells lack the enzymes needed to activate AZT (273). AZT has shown efficacy in prolonging life in some individuals with PCP and late-stage KS (269); thus, it is now prescribed widely for individuals showing signs of severe disease. Most recently, this drug is being evaluated in trials of individuals who are asymptomatic to determine if it will delay the course of a disease and show less toxicity.

Interferons alpha and beta can reduce HIV replication in cell culture (268,269), but this effect is often short-lived; after 10 days virus production can re-emerge (269). Thus, prolonged use may not show any substantial antiviral effect. In fact, the results of clinical trials with interferon, aside from antitumor effects in KS (274), have not been promising. Suramin, which showed activity against HIV in cell culture (261), was not effective in vivo and proved very toxic; it caused death in some treated individuals (275). Recently, ribavirin has given transient clinical improvement to some patients, and is under further study (276). As is desirable for an anti-HIV drug, ribavirin does cross the blood-brain barrier. Finally, some investigators have recently suggested the use of solubilized CD4 antigens as antiviral therapy (277). This immunological recognition site, however, is important in immune response, and flooding the blood with the CD4 protein might further compromise normal immune function. Thus, all these new approaches suggested by cell culture studies require careful monitoring in animals and then human subjects. Further work on new antiviral therapy is needed, but in the rush to try a new drug its potential adverse side effects should not be overlooked. In general, many investigators believe that treatment using both immunomodulating agents and antiviral drugs will be the best approach for arresting and controlling HIV infection.

XIX. Prospects for Antiviral Therapy

This chapter has reviewed the discovery and characterization of the AIDS virus as a lentivirus. It has described the presence of HIV in several cells and tissues of the body, not just T lymphocytes, and its heterogeneity, as demonstrated by biological, serologic, and molecular features. The recent identification of a second variant of HIV, HIV-2, is noteworthy. Whether it presages still other HIVs remains to be determined. (For other recent reviews on HIV, see 278, 279.) The effect of HIV on the immune system as both an immune-depressing and an immune-stimulating agent must be appreciated. Moreover, the importance of the host's response to HIV in determining the course of the disease must be understood. A strong cellular antiviral response is vital for survival (292).

Because of the wide host range of this agent and its ability to infect and integrate into the genome of the cell, HIV poses a major problem for both antiviral therapy and a vaccine. For both approaches, the infected cell must be recognized and killed. If, however, the virus establishes a latent infection,

Table 15 Approaches to HIV Vaccines

1. Natural nonpathogenic variants
2. Laboratory-produced nonpathogenic mutants
3. Inactivated virus (natural or engineered)
4. Subunit vaccine—natural product
   a. Envelope glycoprotein gp120
   b. Envelope/transmembrane antigen complex
   c. *gag* protein
5. Genetically engineered viral proteins (yeast, bacteria, mammalian cells)
6. Viral proteins in infectious recombinant virus (e.g., *Vaccinia*)
7. Sequence-derived peptides of neutralizing epitopes
8. Anti-idiotypes of neutralizing monoclonal antibodies

viral proteins would not be made in sufficient amounts to be detected by the immune system. HIV could then remain unnoticed and passed to daughter cells for long periods of time. In this state, the individual could experience a long incubation period. However, some activating event could bring about virus production, leading eventually to the spread of HIV and induction of disease. Antiviral approaches could be helpful in maintaining this "latent" state or suppressing the virus sufficiently so that its spread is checked. The constant use of antiviral drugs will probably be needed for this effect. Alternatively, immunomodulating drugs may provide a means for enhancing T-suppressor-cell activity to limit virus replication.

In consideration of a vaccine against HIV, several different procedures are being evaluated (280,281) (Table 15; see also Chapter 21). Both beneficial and adverse responses to these procedures must be appreciated. Most investigators agree that the use of killed virus (effective in the past to control other human diseases) would not be appropriate because of the potential for an infectious virus surviving the inactivation process. Moreover, with some viruses, this approach can lead to more severe disease when infections occur, because of a selective immune response of the host (281,282). Yet the presentation of HIV in its intact three-dimensional form may be the best mechanism for inducing a strong antiviral response—both humoral and cellular. Some have considered the possibility of deleting certain genes from the HIV genome through molecular procedures to obtain replicating virions that are not infectious. Once again, immunization with these particles may pose the danger of viruses that can integrate into the host genome, where they might recover their infectivity and pathogenesis through interaction with resident cellular genes. To avoid viral genetic information, the purification of viral proteins, the induction of these proteins by recombinant engineering techniques in other cells, and their synthesis as peptides from cloned genetic fragments are other approaches being considered. Moreover, genetic engineering can make use of other viruses as vectors for HIV protein expression, such as vaçcinia, adenovirus, varicella-zoster, and, recently, the baculovirus system (222). They can introduce HIV genes into a cell for their expression in large amounts. The most successful production of viral proteins mirroring that found on the virion is through the use of mammalian cells, where the proper glycosylation takes place. Nevertheless, even these purified proteins may not take on the three-dimensional form required for an effective antiviral response in the host.

Finally, a recent approach for producing antiviral responses is an anti-idiotype vaccine (283). By this procedure, antibodies that neutralize HIV could be used as immunogens in animal hosts to induce an antibody that binds to the initial antibody region that attaches to the virus. This antibody would then, by definition, be very similar to the virus binding site itself. Immunizing with this purified anti-idiotype could then produce antibodies to the virus. This vaccination procedure would avoid the potential danger of being exposed to any portion of the actual HIV virion. This anti-idiotype approach has been used effectively in producing neutralizing antibodies to hepatitis B virus (284). It is highly speculative but is being considered for a vaccine against HIV (see Chapter 21).

Clearly, in the 7 years since AIDS was recognized and in the 5 years since the virus was isolated, a great deal of information has been amassed on this newly recognized human retrovirus. Results from studies of similar viruses in other animal systems have been helpful, particularly those dealing with lentiviruses (e.g., in sheep, goats, cows, cats, monkeys, and horses) (13). With the emphasis by scientists all over the world on this major threat to public health, one should expect great advances in the near future. Studies of HIV and other animal retroviruses have already led to very important observations in the fields of virology, cell biology, cancer, and immunological disease. They have encouraged new technological advancements for virus detection and protein expression in vitro. Certainly, work in this field should benefit the fight not only against AIDS but also against other human diseases.

XX. Recent Developments

In rare situations, previously seropositive healthy individuals have lost antibodies to HIV over time (285). In some, virus was still detected in their PMC by the polymerase chain reaction (PCR). In others, HIV could not be detected by either in situ hybridization or PCR. This latter encouraging observation suggests that the individual has eliminated HIV from the body; however, most likely the virus is present in some other tissue site. These findings suggest that HIV can go into a latent state and, over time, fail to elicit an immunological reaction. Whether this situation can produce an asymptomatic course for the lifetime of the infected individual and the mechanisms involved merit attention. Recently, the observations on CD8 + cells suppressing HIV have been confirmed in SIV-infected monkeys (293). Also, studies have shown that in HIV-immunized animals, infected chimpanzees, and HIV-infected individuals, antibodies can be found that enhance HIV infection of T cells and macrophages. The mechanism seems most likely via the Fc and complement receptors (294,295). These observations are important since the epitope on the viral envelope mediating this means of infection must be removed from candidate vaccines. Zagury et al., in the first experiments on immunization of humans against HIV-1, have shown that additional immunizations with paraformaldyhyde-fixed autologous cells infected in vitro produced neutralizing antibodies to divergent HIV-1 strains, as well as group-specific cell-mediated immune reactions (296).

Acknowledgments

The research cited in this chapter conducted by the author and his associates was supported by grants from the National Institutes of Health (RO1-AI-24499, PO1-AI-24286, and NO1-AI-62541), the California Universitywide Task Force on AIDS, and the American Foundation for AIDS Research. The author would like to thank Dr. Cecilia Cheng-Mayer for her comments, and Ms. Christine Beglinger and Mr. James Harris for their help in the preparation of the manuscript.

References

1. CDC. Pneumocystis pneumonia. MMWR 1981; 30:250-2.
2. CDC. Kaposi's sarcoma and Pneumocystis pneumonia among homosexual men. MMWR 1981; 30:305-8.
3. Gottlieb MS, Schroff R, Schanker H, et al. Pneumocystis carinii pneumonia and mucosal candidiasis in previously healthy homosexual men. N Engl J Med 1981; 305:1425-30.
4. Masur H, Michelis MA, Greene JB, et al. An outbreak of community-acquired Pneumocystis carinii pneumonia. N Engl J Med 1981; 305:1431-8.
5. Giraldo G, Beth E, Kyalwazi SK. Etiological implications of Kaposi's sarcoma. Antibiotic Chemother 1981; 29:12-29.
6. Costa J, Rabson AS. Generalised Kaposi's sarcoma is not a neoplasm. Lancet 1983; 1:58-9.
7. Jorgensen KA. Amyl nitrate and Kaposi's sarcoma in homosexual men. N Engl J Med 1982; 307:893-4.
8. Hurtenback U, Shearer GM. Germ cell-induced immune suppression in mice: effect of inoculation of syngeneic spermatozoa on cell-mediated immune responses. J Exp Med 1982; 155:1719-29.
9. Levy JA, Ziegler JL. Acquired immune deficiency syndrome (AIDS) is an opportunistic infection and Kaposi's sarcoma results from secondary immune stimulation. Lancet 1983; 2:78-81.
10. Notkins A, Mergenhagen S, Howard R. Effect of virus infections on the function of the immune system. Ann Rev Microbiol 1970; 24:525-37.

11. McMaster G, Beard P, Englers H, Hirt B. Characterization of an immunosuppressive parvovirus related to the minute virus of mice. J Virol 1981; 38:317-26.
12. Kramer JM, Meunier PC, Pollock RV. Canine parvovirus: update. Vet Med Small Anim Clin 1980; 75:1541-55.
13. Levy JA. The multifaceted retrovirus. Cancer Res 1986; 46:5457-68.
14. Morrow WJW, Wharton M, Lau D, Levy JA. Small animal species are not susceptible to HIV infection. J Gen Virol 1987; 68:2253-7.
15. Barre-Sinoussi F, Mugeyre M, Dauguet C et al. Isolation of a T-lymphotropic retrovirus from a patient at risk for acquired immune deficiency syndrome. Science 1983; 220:868-71.
16. Gallo R, Sarin P, Gelmann E, et al. Isolation of human T-cell leukemia virus in acquired immune deficiency syndrome (AIDS). Science 1983; 220:865-7.
17. Poiesz BJ, Ruscetti FW, Gazdar AF, et al. Detection and isolation of type C retrovirus particles from fresh and cultured lymphocytes of a patient with cutaneous T-cell lymphoma. Proc Natl Acad Sci USA 1980; 77:7415-9.
18. Hinuma Y, Nagata K, Hanaoka M, et al. Adult T cell leukemia: antigen in an ATL cell line and detection of antibodies to the antigen in human sera. Proc Natl Acad Sci USA 1981; 78:6476-80.
19. Gelmann EP, Popovic M, Blayney D, et al. Proviral DNA of a retrovirus, human T-cell leukemia virus, in two patients with AIDS. Science 1983; 220:862-5.
20. Tajima K, Tominaga S, Suchi T, et al. Epidemiological analysis of the distribution of antibody to adult T cell leukemia-virus-associated antigen: possible horizontal transmission of adult T-cell leukemia virus. Gann 1982; 73:893-901.
21. Gallo RC, Kalyanaraman VS, Sarngadharan MG, et al. Association of the human type C retrovirus with a subset of adult T-cell cancers. Cancer Res 1983; 43:3892-9.
22. Yamanouchi K, Kinoshita K, Moriuchi R, et al. Oral transmission of human T-cell leukemia virus type-I into a common marmoset (Callithrix jacchus) as an experimental model for milk-borne transmission. Jpn J Cancer Res 1985; 76: 481-7.
23. Evatt BL, Ramsey RB, Laurence DN, et al. The acquired immunodeficiency syndrome in patients with hemophilia. Ann Intern Med 1984; 100:499-504.
24. Montagnier L, Chermann J, Barre-Sinoussi F, et al. A new human T-lymphotropic retrovirus: characterization and possible role in lymphadenopathy and acquired immune deficiency syndromes. In: Gallo RC, Essex ME, Gross L, eds. Human T-cell leukemia/lymphoma virus. New York: Cold Spring Harbor, 1984: 363-79.
25. Levy JA, Hoffman AD, Kramer SM, et al. Isolation of lymphocytopathic retroviruses from San Francisco patients with AIDS. Science 1984; 225:840-2.
26. Weintrub PS, Koerper MA, Addiego JE, Jr, et al. Immunologic abnormalities in patients with hemophilia A. J Pediatr 1983; 103:692-5.
27. Levy JA, Xenotropic type C viruses. Curr Top Microbiol Immunol 1978; 79: 111-213.
28. Levy JA, Mitra G, Mozen MM. Recovery and inactivation of infectious retroviruses added to factor VIII concentrates. Lancet 1984; 2:722-3.
29. Popovic M, Sarngadharan MG, Read E, Gallo RC. Detection, isolation and continuous production of cytopathic retroviruses (HTLV-III) from patients with AIDS and pre-AIDS. Science 1984; 224:497-500.

30. Gallo RC, Salahuddin S, Popovic M, et al. Frequent detection and isolation of cytopathic retroviruses (HTLV-III) from patients with AIDS and at risk for AIDS. Science 1984; 224:500-2.
31. Sarngadharan MG, Popovic M, Bruch L, et al. Antibodies reactive with human T-lymphotropic retroviruses (HTLV-III) in the serum of patients with AIDS. Science 1984; 224:506-8.
32. Gazdar AF, Carney DN, Bunn PA, et al. Mitogen requirements for the in vitro propagation of cutaneous T-cell lymphomas. Blood 1980; 55:409-17.
33. Karpas A. Unusual virus produced by cultured cells from a patient with AIDS. Mol Biol Med 1983; 1:457-9.
34. Cooper DA, Gold J, May W, et al. Contact tracing in the acquired immune deficiency syndrome: Evidence for transmission of virus and disease by an asymptomatic carrier. Med J Aust 1984; 141:579-82.
35. Daniel MD, King NW, Letvin RD, et al. A new type D retrovirus isolated from macaques with an immunodeficiency syndrome. Science 1984; 223:602-5.
36. Marx PA, Maul DH, Osborn KG, et al. Simian AIDS: isolation of a type D retrovirus and transmission of the disease. Science 1984; 223:1083-6.
37. Levy JA, Shimabukuro J. Recovery of AIDS-associated retroviruses from patients with AIDS, related conditions, and clinically healthy individuals. J Infect Dis 1985; 152:734-8.
38. Salahuddin SZ, Markham PD, Popovic M, et al. Isolation of infectious human T-cell leukemia/lymphotropic virus type III (HTLV-III) from patients with acquired immunodeficiency syndrome (AIDS) or AIDS-related complex (ARC) and from healthy carriers: A study of risk groups and tissue sources. Proc Natl Acad Sci USA 1985; 82:5530-4.
39. Benn S, Rutledge R, Folks T, et al. Genomic heterogeneity of AIDS retroviruses isolated from North America and Zaire. Science 1985; 230:949-51.
40. Rabson A, Martin M. Molecular organization of the AIDS retrovirus. Cell 1985; 40:477-80.
41. Gonda M, Wong-Staal F, Gallo R, et al. Sequence homology and morphologic similarity of HTLV-III and visna virus, a pathogenic lentivirus. Science 1985; 173-7.
41a. Sonigo P, Alizon M, Staskus K, et al. Nucleotide sequence of the visna lentivirus: Relationship to the AIDS virus. Cell 1985; 42:369-82.
42. Levy JA, Kaminsky LS, Morrow WJW, et al. Infection by the retrovirus associated with the acquired immunodeficiency syndrome. Ann Intern Med 1985; 103:694-9.
43. Coffin J, Haase A, Levy JA, et al. Human immunodeficiency viruses. Science 1986; 232:697.
44. Gelderblom HR, Hausmann EHS, Ozel M, et al. Fine structure of human immunodeficiency virus (HIV) and immunolocalization of structural proteins. Virology 1987; 156:171-6.
45. Lasky LA, Groopman JE, Fennie CW, et al. Neutralization of the AIDS retrovirus by antibodies to a recombinant envelope glycoprotein. Science 1986; 233: 209-12.
46. Matthews TJ, Langlois AJ, Robey WG, et al. Restricted neutralization of divergent human T-lymphotropic virus type III isolates by antibodies to the major envelope glycoprotein. Proc Natl Acad Sci USA 1986; 83:9709-13.

47. Putney SD, Matthews TJ, Robey WG, et al. HTLV-III/LAV-neutralizing antibodies to an *E. coli*-produced fragment of the virus envelope. Science 1986; 234:1392-5.
48. Krohn K, Robey WG, Putney S, et al. Specific cellular immune response and neutralizing antibodies in goats immunized with native or recombinant envelope proteins derived from human T-lymphotropic virus type IIIB and in human immunodeficiency virus-infected men. Proc Natl Acad Sci USA 1987; 84:4994-8.
49. Ho DD, Sarngadharan MG, Hirsch MS, et al. Human immunodeficiency virus neutralizing antibodies recognize several conserved domains on the envelope glycoproteins. J Virol 1987; 61:2024-8.
50. Chanh TC, Dreesman GR, Kanda P, et al. Induction of anti-HIV neutralizing antibodies by synthetic peptides. EMBO J 1986; 5:3065-71.
51. Sarin PS, Sun DK, Thornton AH, et al. Neutralization of HTLV-III/LAV replication by antiserum to thymosin alpha-1. Science 1986; 232:1135-7.
52. Kwok S, Mack DH, Mullis KB, et al. Identification of human immunodeficiency virus sequences by using in vitro enzymatic amplification and oligomer cleavage detection. J Virol 1987; 61:1690-4.
52a. Ou C-Y, Kwok S, Mitchell SW, et al. DNA amplification for direct detection of HIV-1 in DNA of peripheral blood mononuclear cells. Science 1988; 239: 295-7.
53. Harper ME, Marselle LM, Gallo RC, et al. Detection of lymphocytes expressing human T-lymphotropic virus type III in lymph nodes and peripheral blood from infected individuals by in situ hybridization. Proc Natl Acad Sci USA 1986; 83:772-6.
54. Zagury D, Bernard J, Leonard R, et al. Long-term cultures of HTLV-III infected T cells: a model of cytopathology of T-cell depletion in AIDS. Science 1986; 231:850-3.
55. Walker CM, Moody DJ, Stites DP, Levy JA. CD8+ lymphocytes can control HIV infection in vitro by suppressing virus replication. Science 1986; 234:1563-6.
56. Margolick JB, Volkman DJ, Folks TM, Fauci AS. Amplification of HTLV-III/LAV infection by antigen-induced activation of T cells and direct suppression by virus of lymphocyte blastogenic responses. J Immunol 1987; 138:1719-23.
57. Castro B, Weiss C, Wiviott L, Levy JA. Optimal conditions for recovery of the human immunodeficiency virus from peripheral blood mononuclear cells. J Clin Microbiol (in press).
58. Wysocki LJ, Sato VL. Panning for lymphocytes: a method for cell selection. Proc Natl Acad Sci USA 1978; 75:2844-8.
59. Walker CM, Moody DJ, Stites DP, Levy JA. Low number of CD8+ cells can inhibit HIV replication in cultured autologous CD4+ cells. Submitted.
60. Gallo D, Kimpton JS, Dailey PJ. Comparative studies on use of fresh and frozen peripheral blood lymphocyte specimens for isolation of human immunodeficiency virus and effects of cell lysis on isolation efficiency. J Clin Microbiol 1987; 25:1291-4.
61. Allain J-P, Laurian Y, Paul DA, et al. Long-term evaluation of HIV antigen and antibodies to p24 and gp41 in patients with hemophilia. N Engl J Med 1987; 317:1114-21.

62. Homsy J, Thomson-Honnebier GA, Cheng-Mayer C, Levy JA. Detection of human immunodeficiency virus (HIV) in serum and body fluids by sequential competition ELISA. J Virol Methods 1988; 19:34-65.
63. Goudsmit J, Lange JMA, Paul DA, Dawson GJ. Antigenemia and antibody titers to core and envelope antigens in AIDS, AIDS-related complex and subclinical human immunodeficiency virus infection. J Infect Dis 1987; 155:558-60.
64. Lange JMA, Paul DA, Huisman HG, et al. Persistent HIV antigenaemia and decline of HIV core antibodies associated with transition to AIDS. Br Med J 1986; 293:1459-62.
65. Chaisson RE, Allain J-P, Leuther M, Volberding PA. Significant changes in HIV antigen level in the serum of patients treated with azidothymidine. N Engl J Med 1986; 315:1610-2.
65a. Baillou A, Barin F, Allain J-P, et al. Human immunodeficiency virus antigenemia in patients with AIDS and AIDS-related disorders: A comparison between European and Central African populations. J Infect Dis 1987; 156:830-3.
66. Lange JMA, Paul DA, de Wolf F, et al. Expression, antibody production and immune complex formation in human immunodeficiency virus infection. AIDS 1987; 1:15-20.
67. Lifson JD, Feinberg MB, Reyes GR, et al. Induction of CD4-dependent cell fusion by the HTLV-III/LAV envelope glycoprotein. Nature 1986; 323:725-8.
68. Sodroski J, Goh WC, Rosen C, et al. Role of the HTLV-III/LAV envelope in syncytium formation and cytopathicity. Nature 1986; 322:470-4.
69. Stricker RB, McHugh TM, Moody DJ, et al. An AIDS-related cytotoxic autoantibody reacts with a specific antigen on stimulated CD4+ T cells. Nature 1987; 327:710-3.
69a. Ulrich PP, Busch MP, El-Beik T, et al. Assessment of human immunodeficiency virus expression in cocultures of peripheral blood mononuclear cells from healthy seropositive subjects. J Med Virol 1988; 25:1-10.
70. Haase A. The slow infection caused by visna virus. Curr Top Microbiol Immunol 1975; 72:101-56.
71. Levy JA, Hollander H, Shimabukuro J, et al. Isolation of AIDS-associated retrovirus from cerebrospinal fluid and brain of patients with neurological symptoms. Lancet 1985; 2:586-8.
72. Shaw G, Harper M, Hahn B, et al. HTLV-III infection in brains of children and adults with AIDS encephalopathy. Science 1985; 227:177-82.
73. Ho D, Rota T, Schooley R, et al. Isolation of HTLV-III from cerebrospinal fluid and neural tissues of patients with neurologic syndromes related to the acquired immunodeficiency syndrome. N Engl J Med 1985; 313:1493-7.
74. Hollander H, Levy JA. Neurologic abnormalities and human immunodeficiency virus recovery from cerebrospinal fluid. Ann Intern Med 1987; 106:692-5.
75. Resnick L, diMarzo-Veronese F, Schupbach J, et al. Intra-blood-brain-barrier synthesis of HTLV-III specific IgG in patients with neurologic symptoms associated with AIDS or AIDS-related complex. N Engl J Med 1985; 313:1498-504.
76. Wiley CA, Schrier RD, Nelson JA, et al. Cellular localization of the AIDS retrovirus infection within the brains of acquired immune deficiency syndrome patients. Proc Natl Acad Sci USA 1986; 83:7089-93.

77. Gyorkey F, Melnick JL, Gyorkey P. Human immunodeficiency virus in brain biopsies of patients with AIDS and progressive encephalopathy. J Infect Dis 1987; 155:870-6.
78. Koenig S, Gendelman HE, Orenstein JM, et al. Detection of AIDS virus in macrophages in brain tissue from AIDS patients with encephalopathy. Science 1986; 233:1089-93.
79. Cheng-Mayer C, Rutka JT, Rosenblum ML, et al. The human immunodeficiency virus (HIV) can productively infect cultured glial cells. Proc Natl Acad Sci USA 1987; 84:3526-30.
80. Levy JA, Evans L, Cheng-Mayer C, et al. The biologic and molecular properties of the AIDS-associated retrovirus that affect antiviral therapy. Ann Inst Pasteur 1987; 138:101-11.
81. Massa PT, Dorries T, ter Meulen V. Viral particles induce Ia antigen expression in astrocytes. Nature 1986; 320:543-6.
82. Fontana A, Fiierz W, Wekerie H. Astrocytes present myelin basic protein to encephalitogenic T-cell lines. Nature 1984; 307:273-6.
83. Armstrong JA, Horne R. Follicular dendritic cells and virus-like particles in AIDS related lymphadenopathy. Lancet 1984; 2:370-2.
84. Lecatsas G, Houff S, Macher A, et al. Retrovirus-like particles in salivary glands, prostate and testes of AIDS patients. Proc Soc Exp Biol Med 1985; 178:653-5.
85. Salahuddin SZ, Palestine AG, Heck E, et al. Isolation of the human T-cell leukemia/lymphotropic virus type III from the cornea. Am J Ophthalmol 1986; 101:149-52.
86. Pomerantz RJ, Kuritzkes DR, de la Monte SM, et al. Infection of the retina by human immunodeficiency virus type I. N Engl J Med 1987; 317:1643-7.
87. Taschachler E, Groh V, Popovic M, et al. Epidermal Langerhans cells: A target for HTLV-III/LAV infection. J Invest Dermatol 1987; 88:233-7.
88. Nelson JA, Wiley CA, Reynolds-Kohler C, et al. Human immunodeficiency virus detected in bowel epithelium of patients with gastrointestinal symptoms. Lancet 1988; 1:259-62.
89. Winkelstein W Jr, Lyman DM, Padian N, et al. Sexual practices and risk of infection by the human immunodeficiency virus: The San Francisco men's health study. JAMA 1987; 257:321-5.
90. Serwadda D, Mugerwa RD, Sewandambo NK, et al. Slim disease: A new disease in Uganda and its association with HTLV-III infection. Lancet 1985; 2: 849-52.
90a. Pomerantz RJ, de la Monte SM, Donegan SP, et al. Human immunodeficiency virus (HIV) infection of the uterine cervix. Ann Intern Med 1988; 108:321-7.
91. Greene LW, Cole W, Greene JB, et al. Adrenal insufficiency as a complication of the acquired immunodeficiency syndrome. Ann Intern Med 1984; 101:149-52.
92. Cohen IS, Anderson DW, Virmani R, et al. Congestive cardiomyopathy in association with the acquired immunodeficiency syndrome. N Engl J Med 1986; 315:628-30.
92a. Calabrese LH, Proffitt MR, Yen-Lieberman B, et al. Congestive cardiomyopathy and illness related to the Acquired Immunodeficiency Syndrome (AIDS) associated with isolation of retrovirus from myocardium. Ann Intern Med 1987; 107:691-2.

93. Michaelis B, Levy JA. Reocvery of human immunodeficiency virus from serum. J Am Med Assoc 1987; 257:1327.
94. Falk LM Jr, Paul DA, Landay A, Kessler H. HIV isolation from plasma of HIV-infected persons. N Engl J Med 1987; 316:1547.
95. Alter HJ, Seeff LB, Kaplan PM, et al. Type B hepatitis: the infectivity of blood positive for e antigen and DNA polymerase after accidental needlestick exposure. N Engl J Med 1976; 295:909-13.
96. Gerberding JL, Bryant-LeBlanc CE, Nelson K, et al. Risk of human immunodeficiency virus, cytomegalovirus, and hepatitis B virus transmission to health care workers exposed to patients with acquired immunodeficiency syndrome (AIDS) and AIDS-related conditions. J Infect Dis 1987; 156:1-8.
97. Groopman JE, Salahuddin SZ, Sarngadharan MG, et al. HTLV-III in saliva of people with AIDS-related complex and healthy homosexual men at risk for AIDS. Science 1984; 226:447-9.
98. Ho DD, Byington RE, Schooley RT, et al. Infrequency of isolation of HTLV-III virus from saliva in AIDS. N Engl J Med 1985; 313:1606.
99. Fujikawa LS, Palestine AG, Nussenblatt RB, et al. Isolation of human T-lymphotropic virus type III from the tears of a patient with acquired immunodeficiency syndrome. Lancet 1985; 2:529-30.
100. Thiry L, Sprecher-Goldberger S, Jonckheer T, et al. Isolation of AIDS virus from cell-free breast milk of three healthy virus carriers. Lancet 1985; 2:891-2.
101. Ho DD, Schooley RT, Rota TR. HTLV-III in the semen and blood of a healthy homosexual man. Science 1985; 226:451-3.
102. Zagury D, Bernard J, Leibowitch J, et al. HTLV-III in cells cultured from semen of two patients with AIDS. Science 1984; 226:449-51.
103. Vogt M, Craven D, Crawford D, et al. Isolation of HTLV-III/LAV from cervical secretions of women at risk for AIDS. Lancet 1986; 1:525-7.
104. Wofsy CB, Cohen JB, Hauer LB, et al. Isolation of the AIDS-associated retrovirus from vaginal and cervical secretions from women with antibodies to the virus. Lancet 1986; 1:527-9.
105. Vogt MW, Witt DJ, Craven DE, et al. Isolation patterns of the human immunodeficiency virus from cervical secretions during the menstrual cycle of women at risk for the acquired immunodeficiency syndrome. Ann Intern Med 1987; 106:380-2.
106. Dean NC, Golden JA, Evans L, et al. Human immunodeficiency virus recovery from bronchoalveolar lavage fluid in patients with AIDS. Chest 1988, in press.
107. Levy JA. The transmission of AIDS: The case of the infected cell. JAMA 1988; 259:3037-8.
108. Olsen GP, Shields JW. Seminal lymphocytes, plasma and AIDS. Nature 1984; 309:116.
109. Quinn TC, Mann JM, Curran JW, et al. AIDS in Africa: An epidemiologic paradigm. Science 1986; 234:955-63.
110. Cameron DW, Plummer FA, Simonsen JN, et al. Female to male heterosexual transmission of HIV infection in Nairobi (abstrct). III International Conference on AIDS, June 1-5, 1987, Washington, DC, p 25.

111. Klatzmann D, Barre-Sinoussi F, Mugyre M, et al. Selective tropism of lymphadenopathy-associated virus (LAV) for helper-inducer T-lymphocytes. Science 1984; 225:59-62.
112. Dalgleish A, Beverley P, Clapham P, et al. The CD4 (T4) antigen is an essential component of the receptor for the AIDS retrovirus. Nature 1984; 312:763-6.
113. Klatzmann D, Champagne E, Chamaret S, et al. T-lymphocyte T4 molecule behaves as receptor for human retrovirus LAV. Nature 1984; 312:767-71.
114. Sattentau QJ, Dalgleish AG, Weiss RA, Beverley P. Epitopes of the CD4 antigen and HIV infection. Science 1986; 234:1120-3.
115. McDougal JS, Kennedy M, Sligh J, et al. The binding of HTLV-III/LAV to T4+ T cells by a complex of the 110 kD viral protein (gp110) and the T4 molecule. Science 1986; 231:382-5.
116. Hoxie J, James D, Alpers J, et al. Alterations in T4 (CD4) protein synthesis and mRNA synthesis in cells infected with HIV. Science 1986; 234:1123-7.
117. Guy B, Kieny MP, Riviere Y, et al. HIV F/3′ *orf* encodes a phosphorylated GTP-binding protein resembling an oncogene product. Nature 1987; 330:266-9.
118. Levy JA, Shimabukuro J, McHugh T, et al. AIDS-associated retroviruses (ARV) can productively infect other cells besides human T helper cells. Virology 1985; 147:441-8.
118a. Clapham PR, Weiss RA, Dalgleish AG, et al. Human immunodeficiency virus infection of monocytic and T-lymphocytic cells: Receptor modulation and differentiation induced by phorbol ester. Virology 1987; 158:44-51.
119. Wood GS, Warner NL, Warnke RA. Anti-leu-3/T4 antibodies react with cells of monocyte/macrophage and Langerhans lineage. J Immunol 1983; 131:212-6.
120. Maddon PJ, Dalgleish AG, McDougal JS, et al. The T4 gene encodes the AIDS virus receptor and is expressed in the immune system and the brain. Cell 1986; 47:333-48.
121. Dewhurst S, Stevenson M, Volsky DJ. Expression of the T4 molecule (AIDS virus receptor) by human brain-derived cells. FEBS Lett 1987; 213:133-7.
122. Funke I, Hahn A, Rieber EP, et al. The cellular receptor (CD4) of the human immunodeficiency virus is expressed on neurons and glial cells in human brain. J Exp Med 1987; 165:1230-5.
123. Kowalski M, Potz J, Basiripour L, Dorfman T, et al. Functional regions of the envelope glycoprotein of human immunodeficiency virus type I. Science 1987; 237:1351-5.
124. Gonzalez-Scarano F, Waxham MN, Ross AM, Hoxie JA. Sequence similarities between human immunodeficiency virus gp41 and paramyxovirus fusion proteins. AIDS Res Human Retroviruses 1987; 3:245-52.
125. Portner A, Scroggs RA, Naeve CW. The fusion glycoprotein of Sendai virus: Sequence analysis of an epitope involved in fusion and virus neutralization. Virology 1987; 157:556-9.
126. Lifson J, Coutre S, Huang E, Engleman E. Role of envelope glycoprotein carbohydrate in human immunodeficiency virus (HIV) infectivity and virus-induced cell fusion. J Exp Med 1986; 164:2101-6.

127. Yoffe B, Lewis DE, Petrie BL, et al. Fusion as a mediator of cytolysis in mixtures of uninfected CD4+ lymphocytes and cells infected with the human immunodeficiency virus. Proc Natl Acad Sci USA 1987; 84:1429-33.
128. Luciw PA, Potter SJ, Steimer K, et al. Molecular cloning of AIDS-associated retrovirus. Nature 1984; 312:760-3.
129. Shaw GM, Hahn BH, Arya S, et al. Molecular characterization of human T-cell leukemia (lymphotropic) virus type III in the acquired immune deficiency syndrome. Science 1984; 226:1165-71.
130. Kaminsky LS, McHugh T, Stites D, et al. High prevalence of antibodies to AIDS-associated retroviruses (ARV) in acquired immune deficiency syndrome and related conditions and not in other disease states. Proc Natl Acad Sci USA 1985; 82:5535-9.
131. Hoxie JA, Haggarty BS, Rackowski JL, et al. Persistent noncytopathic infection of human lymphocytes with AIDS-associated retrovirus (ARV). Science 1985; 229:1400-2.
132. Keshet E, Temin HM. Cell killing by spleen necrosis virus is correlated with a transient accumulation of spleen necrosis virus DNA. J Virol 1979; 31:376-88.
133. Harris JD, Blum H, Scott J, et al. The slow virus visna: reproduction in vitro of virus from extrachromosomal DNA. Proc Natl Acad Sci USA 1984; 81: 7212-5.
134. McClure MO, Sattentau QJ, Beverley PCL, et al. HIV infection of primate lymphocytes and conservation of the CD4 receptor. Nature 1987; 330:487-9.
135. Levy JA, Cheng-Mayer C, Dina D, Luciw PA. Replication of AIDS-associated retrovirus (ARV-2) in human and animal fibroblast cells transfected with a molecular clone of the virus. Science 1986; 232:998-1001.
136. Jones KA, Kadonaga J, Luciw PA, Tjian R. Activation of the AIDS retrovirus promoter by the cellular transcription factor, Sp1. Science 1986; 232: 755-9.
137. Nabel G, Baltimore D. An inducible transcription factor activates expression of human immunodeficiency virus in T cells. Nature 1987; 326:711-3.
137a. Garcia JA, Wu FK, Mitsuyasu R, Gaynor RB. Interactions of cellular proteins involved in the transcriptional regulation of the human immunodeficiency virus. EMBO J 1987; 6:3716-7.
138. Bednarik DP, Mosca JD, Raj BK. Methylation as a modulator of expression of human immunodeficiency virus. J Virol 1986; 61:1253-7.
139. Folks T, Powell DM, Lightfoote MM, et al. Induction of HTLV-III/LAV from a non virus-producing T-cell line: implications for latency. Science 1986; 231:600-2.
140. Folks TM, Justement J, Kinter A, et la. Cytokine-induced expression of HIV-1 in a chronically infected promonocyte cell line. Science 1987; 238:800-2.
141. Ranki A, Krohn M, Allain JP, et al. Long latency precedes overt serroconversion in sexually transmitted human-immunodeficiency-virus infection. Lancet 2:589-93.
142. Luciw PA, Cheng-Mayer C, Levy JA. Mutational analysis of the human immunodeficiency virus (HIV): the orf-B region down-regulates virus replication. Proc Natl Acad Sci USA 1987; 84:1434-8.
143. Lifson JD, Reyes GR, McGrath MS, et al. AIDS retrovirus induced cytopath-

ology: giant cell formation and involvement of CD4 antigen. Science 1986; 232:1123-7.

144. Somasundaran M, Robinson HL. A major mechanism of human immunodeficiency virus-induced cell killing does not involve cell fusion. J Virol 1987; 61: 3114-9.
145. Anand R, Reed DC, Forlenza S, et al. Non-cytocidal natural variants of human immunodeficiency virus isolated from AIDS patients with neurological disorders. Lancet 1987; 2:234-6.
146. Cheng-Mayer C, Seto D, Tateno M, Levy JA. Biologic features of HIV-1 that correlate with virulence in the host. Science 1988; 240:80-82.
147. Cheng-Mayer C, Levy JA. Distinct biologic and serologic properties of HIV isolates from the brain. Ann Neurol 1988; 23:s58-61.
148. Tateno M, Levy JA. MT4 plaque formation distinguishes HIV subtypes. Virology (in press).
149. Harada S, Koyanagi Y, Yamamoto N. Infection of HTLV-III/LAV in HTLV-I-carrying cells MT-2 and MT-4 and application in a plaque assay. Science 1986; 229:563-6.
150. Gartner S, Markovits P, Markovitz DM, et al. The role of mononuclear phagocytes in HTLV-III/LAV infection. Science 1986; 233:215-9.
151. Fisher AG, Ratner L, Mitsuya H, et al. Infectious mutants of HTLV-III with changes in the 3′ region and markedly reduced cytopathic effects. Science 1986; 233:655-9.
152. Gyorkey F, Melnick JL, Sinkovics JG, Gyorkey PA. Retrovirus resembling HTLV in macrophages of patients with AIDS. Lancet 1985; 1:106.
153. Ho DD, Rota RT, Hirsch MS. Infection of monocyte/macrophages by human T-lymphotropic virus type III. J Clin Invest 1986; 77:1712-5.
154. Crowe S, Mills J, McGrath MS, et al. Quantitative immunocytolfuorographic analysis of CD4 surface antigen expression and HIV infection of human peripheral blood monocyte/macrophages. AIDS Res Human Retroviruses 1987; 3:135-45.
155. Popovic M, Gartner S. Isolation of HIV-1 from monocytes but not T lymphocytes. Lancet 1987; 2:916-7.
156. Gendelmann HE, Orenstein JM, Martin MA, et al. Efficient isolation and propagation of human immunodeficiency virus on recombinant colony-stimulating factor 1-treated monocytes. J Exp Med 1988; 167:1428-41.
157. Montagnier L, Gruest J, Chamaret S, et al. Adaption of lymphadenopathy associated virus (LAV) to replication in EBV-transformed B lymphoblastoid cell lines. Science 1984; 225:63-6.
158. Gyorkey F, Melnick JL. AIDS retrovirus and other viruses in brain and hematopoietic cells of patients in early and late stages of the acquired immune deficiency syndrome. In: Kurstak E, Kipowski ZJ, Morozov PV, eds. Viruses, Immunity, and Mental Disorders. New York: Plenum, 1987:109-21.
159. Garry RF, Ulug ET, Bose HR, Jr. Membrane-mediated alterations of intracellular NA^+ and K^+ in lytic virus-infected and retrovirus-transformed cells. Bioscience Rep 1982; 2:617-23.
160. Dewhurst S, Sakai K, Bresser J, et al. Persistent productive infection of human glial cells by human immunodeficiency virus (HIV) and by infectious molecular clones of HIV. J Virol 1987; 61:3774-82.

161. Tateno M, Levy JA. The susceptibility of non-hematopoietic cell lines to HIV infection. IV International Conference on AIDS, June 1988 (abstract).
162. Adachi A, Koenig S, Gendelman HE, et al. Productive, persistent infection of human colorectal cell lines with human immunodeficiency virus. J Virol 1987; 61:209-13.
163. Evans LA, McHugh TM, Stites DP, Levy JA. Differential ability of human immunodeficiency virus isolates to productively infect human cells. J Immunol 1987; 138:3415-8.
164. Dahl K, Martin K, Miller G. Differences among human immunodeficiency virus strains in their capacities to induce cytolysis or persistent infection of a lymphoblastoid cell line immortalized by Epstein-Barr virus. J Virol 1987; 61: 1602-8.
165. Asjo B, Albert J, Karlsson A, et al. Replicative capacity of human immunodeficiency virus from patients with varying severity of HIV infection. Lancet 1986; 2:660-2.
166. Kikikawa R, Koyanagi Y, Harada S, et al. Differential susceptibility to the acquired immunodeficiency syndrome retrovirus in cloned cells of human leukemic T-cell line Molt-4. J Virol 1986; 57:1157-62.
167. Alizon M, Sonigo P, Barre-Sinoussi F, et al. Molecular cloning of lymphadenopathy-associated virus. Nature 1984; 312:757-60.
167a. Hahn B, Shaw G, Ayra S, et al. Molecular cloning and characterization of the HTLV-III virus associated with AIDS. Nature 1984; 312:166-9.
168. Hahn BH, Shaw GM, Taylor ME, et al. Genetic variation in HTLV-III/LAV over time in patients with AIDS or at risk for AIDS. Science 1986; 232:1548-53.
169. Fultz PN, Srinivasan A, Greene CR, et al. Superinfection of a chimpanzee with a second strain of human immunodeficiency virus. J Virol 1987; 61: 4026-9.
170. Sanchez-Pescador R, Power MD, Barr PJ, et al. Nucleotide sequence and expression of an AIDS-associated retrovirus (ARV-2). Science 1985; 227:484-92.
171. Ratner L, Haseltine W, Patarca R, et al. Complete nucleotide sequence of the AIDS virus, HTLV-III. Nature 1985; 313:277-84.
172. Wain-Hobson S, Sonigo P, Danos O, et al. Nucleotide sequence of the AIDS virus, LAV. Cell 1985; 40:9-17.
173. Muesing MA, Smith DH, Cabradilla CD, et al. Nucleic acid structure and expression of the human AIDS/lymphadenopathy retrovirus. Nature 1985; 313: 450-8.
174. Starcich BR, Hahn BH, Shaw GM, et al. Identification and characterization of conserved and variable regions in the envelope gene of HTLV-III/LAV, the retrovirus of AIDS. Cell 1986; 45:637-48.
175. Gendelman HE, Phelps W, Feigenbaum L, et al. Trans-activation of the human immunodeficiency virus long terminal repeat sequence by DNA viruses. Proc Natl Acad Sci USA 1986; 83:9759-63.
176. Mosca JD, Bednarik DP, Raj NBK, et al. Herpes simplex virus type-1 can reactivate transcription of latent human immunodeficiency virus. Nature 1987; 325:677-80.

177. Ostrove JM, Leonard J, Weck KE, et al. Activation of the human immunodeficiency virus by herpes simplex virus type 1. J Virol 1987; 61:3726-32.
178. Harada S, Koyanagi Y, Yamamoto N. Infection of human T-lymphotropic virus type-1 (HTLV-I)-bearing MT-4 cells with HTLV-III (AIDS virus): chronological studies of early events. Virology 1985; 146:272-81.
179. de Rossi A, Franchini G, Alsovini A, et al. Differential response to the cytopathic effects of human T cell lymphotropic virus type III (HTLV-III) superinfection in T4+ (helper) and T8+ (suppressor) T-cell clones transformed by HTLV-1. Proc Natl Acad Sci USA 1986; 83:4297-301.
180. Kanner SB, Parks ES, Scott GB, Parks WP. Simultaneous infections with human T cell leukemia virus type I and the human immunodeficiency virus. J Infect Dis 1987; 155:617-25.
181. Morrow WJW, Homsy J, Eichberg JW, et al. Immunosuppressive therapy did not induce disease in baboons, rhesus monkeys, and chimpanzees inoculated with the human immunodeficiency virus (HIV). Submitted.
182. Alter JH, Eichberg JW, Masur H, et al. Transmission of HTLV-III infection from human plasma to chimpanzees: an animal model for AIDS. Science 1984; 226:549-52.
183. Francis DP, Feorino PM, Broderson JR, et al. Infection of chimpanzees with lymphadenopathy-associated virus: a potential model for acquired immunodeficiency syndrome. Lancet 1984; 2:1276-7.
184. Gadjusek DC, Gibbs CJ, Rodgers-Johnson P, et al. Infection of chimpanzees by human T-lymphotropic retroviruses in brain and other tissues from AIDS patients. Lancet 1985; 2:55-6.
185. Fultz PN, McClure HM, Swenson RB, et al. Persistent infection of chimpanzees with human T-lymphotropic virus type III lymphadenopathy-associated virus: a potential model for acquired immunodeficiency syndrome. J Virol 1986; 58:116-24.
186. Nara PL, Robey WG, Arthur LO, et al. Persistent infection of chimpanzees with human immunodeficiency virus: serological responses and properties of reisolated viruses. J Virol 1987; 61:3173-80.
187. Arthur LO, Pyle SW, Nara PL, et al. Serological responses in chimpanzees inoculated with human immunodeficiency virus glycoprotein (gp120) subunit vaccine. Proc Natl Acad Sci USA 1987; 84:8583-7.
188. Hu S-L, Fultz PN, McClure HM, et al. Effect of immunization with a vaccinia-HIV *env* recombinant on HIV infection in chimpanzees. Nature 1987; 328: 721-3.
189. Kanki PJ, McLane MF, King NW Jr, et al. Serologic identification and characterization of a macaque T-lymphotropic retrovirus closely related to HTLV-III. Science 1985; 228:1199-1201.
190. Weiss S, Goedert J, Sarngadharan M, et al. Screening test for HTLV-III (AIDS agent) antibodies. JAMA 1985; 253:221-5.
191. Lennette ET, Karpatkin S, Levy JA. Indirect immunofluorescence assay for antibodies to the human immunodeficiency virus (HIV). J Clin Microbiol 1987; 25:199-202.
192. McHugh TM, Stites DP, Casavant CH, et al. Evaluation of the indirect immunofluorescent assay as a confirmatory test for detecting antibodies to the AIDS-associated retrovirus. Diag Immunol 1986; 4:233-40.

193. Cooper D, Imrie AA, Penny R. Antibody response to human immunodeficiency virus after primary infection. J Infect Dis 1987; 155:1113-8.
194. Pan L-Z, Cheng-Mayer C, Levy JA. Patterns of antibody response in individuals infected with the human immunodeficiency virus. J Infect Dis 1987; 155:626-32.
195. Kalyanaraman VS, Cabradilla CSD, Getchell JP, et al. Antibodies to the core protein of lymphadenopathy-associated virus (LAV) in patients with AIDS. Science 1984; 225:321-3.
196. Schupbach J, Haller O, Vogt M, et al. Antibodies to HTLV-III in Swiss patients with AIDS and pre-AIDS and in groups at risk for AIDS. N Engl J Med 1985; 312:265-70.
197. Steimer KS, Puma JP, Power MD, et al. Differential antibody responses of individuals infected with AIDS-associated retroviruses surveyed using the viral core antigen p25 gag expressed in bacteria. Virology 1986; 150:283-90.
198. Joller-Jemelka HI, Joller PW, Muller F, et al. Anti-HIV IgM antibody analysis during early manifestations of HIV infections. AIDS 1987; 1:45-7.
199. Allan JS, Coligan JE, Barin F, et al. Major glycoprotein antigens that induce antibodies in AIDS patients are encoded by HTLV-III. Science 1985; 228: 1091-4.
199a. Barin F, McLane MF, Allan JS, et al. Virus envelope protein of HTLV-III represents major target antigen for antibodies in AIDS patients. Science 1985; 228:1094-7.
200. Clavel F, Guetard D, Brun-Vezinet F, et al. Isolation of a new human retrovirus from West African patients with AIDS. Science 1986; 233:343-6.
201. Kanner SB, Cheng-Mayer C, Geggin RB, et al. Human retroviral env and gag polypeptides: serologic assays to measure infection. J Immunol 1986; 137: 674-8.
202. Robert-Guroff M, Giardina PJ, Robey WG, et al. HTLV-III neutralizing antibody development in transfusion-dependent seropositive patients with B-thalassemia. J Immunol 1987; 138:3731-6.
203. Cheng-Mayer C, Homsy J, Evans LA, Levy JA. Identification of HIV subtypes with distinct patterns of sensitivity to serum neutralization. Proc Natl Acad Sci USA 1988; 85:2815-9.
204. Weiss RA, Clapham PR, Cheingson-Popov R, et al. Neutralization of human T-lymphotropic virus type III by sera of AIDS and AIDS-risk patients. Nature 1985; 316:69-72.
205. Harada S, Purtilo DT, Koyanagi Y, et al. Sensitive assay for neutralizing antibodies against AIDS-related viruses (HTLV-III/LAV). J Immunol Methods 1986; 92:177-81.
205a. Ho DD, Kaplan JC, Rackauskas IE, Gurney ME. Second conserved domain of gp120 is important for HIV infectivity and antibody neutralization. Science 1988; 239:1021-3.
205b. Willey RL, Smith DH, Lasky LA, et al. In vitro mutagenesis identifies a region within the envelope gene of the human immunodeficiency virus that is critical for infectivity. J Virol 1988; 62:139-47.
206. Weiss RA, Clapham PR, Weber JN, et al. Variable and conserved neutralization antigens of human immunodeficiency virus. Nature 1986; 324:572-5.

207. Rook AH, Clifford HL, Folks T, et al. Sera from HTLV-III/LAV antibody-positive individuals mediate antibody-dependent cellular cytotoxicity against HTLV-III/LAV infected T cells. J Immunol 1987; 138:1064-7.
208. Ljunggren KB, Bottinger, Biberfeld G, et al. Antibody-dependent cellular cytotoxicity (ADCC)-inducing antibodies against human immunodeficiency virus (HIV): presence at different clinical stages. J Immunol 1987; 139:2263-7.
209. Ojo-Amaize EA, Nishanian P, Keith DE, Jr., et al. Antibodies to human immunodeficiency virus in human sera induce cell-mediated lysis of human immunodeficiency virus-infected cells. J Immunol 1987; 139:2458-63.
210. Evans LA, Thomson-Honnebier G, Steimer K, et al. Antibody-dependent cellular toxicity (ADCC) is directed against envelope proteins of the human immunodeficiency virus. Submitted.
211. Walker B, Chakrabarti S, Moss B, et al. HIV-specific cytotoxic T lymphocytes in lung disorders. Nature 1987; 328:345-8.
212. Plata F, Autran B, Martins LP, et al. AIDS virus-specific cytotoxic T lymphocytes in lung disorders. Nature 1987; 328:348-51.
213. Rickinson AB, Yao QY, Wallace LE. The Epstein-Barr virus as a model of virus-host interactions. Br Med Bull 1985; 41:75-9.
214. Rosenberg SA, Lotze MT, Muul LM, et al. Observations on the systemic administration of autologous lymphokine-activated killer cells and recombinant interleukin-2 to patients with metastatic cancer. N Engl J Med 1985; 313:1485-92.
215. Walker CW, Moody DJ, Stites DP, Levy JA. Low numbers of cytotoxic/suppressor CD8+ lymphocytes prevent HIV replication in autologous purified CD4+ lymphocytes. III International Conference on AIDS, June 1-5, 1987, Washington, DC, p 214.
216. Ammann A, Levy JA. Laboratory investigation of pediatric acquired immunodeficiency syndrome. Clin Immunol Immunopathol 1986; 40:122-7.
217. Reiher WE, Blalock JE, Brunck TK. Sequence homology between acquired immunodeficiency syndrome virus envelope protein and interleukin 2. Proc Natl Acad Sci USA 1986; 83:9188-92.
218. Lee MR, Ho DD, Gurney ME. Functional interaction and partial homology between human immunodeficiency virus and neuroleukin. Science 1987; 237:1047-51.
219. Pert CB, Hill JM, Ruff MR, et al. Octapeptides deduced from the neuropeptide receptor-like pattern of antigen T4 in brain patently inhibit human immunodeficiency virus receptor binding and T-cell infectivity. Proc Natl Acad Sci USA 1986; 83:9254-8.
219a. Ruff MR, Martin BM, Ginns EI, et al. CD4 receptor-binding peptides that block HIV infectivity cause human monocyte chemotaxis. Relationship to vasoactive intestinal polypeptides. FEBS Letters 1987; 211:17-22.
220. Hoxie JA, Fitzharris TP, Youngbar PR, et al. Nonrandom association of cellular antigens with HTLV-III virions. Hum Immunol 1987; 18:39-52.
220a. Naylor PH, Maylor CW, Badamchian M, et al. Human immunodeficiency virus contains an epitope immunoreactive with thymosin alpha 1 and the 30-amino acid synthetic p17 group-specific antigen peptide HGP-30. Proc Natl Acad Sci USA 1987; 84:2951-5.

221. Starcich B, Ratner L, Josephs SF, et al. Characterization of long terminal repeat sequences of HTLV-III. Science 1985; 227:538-40.
222. Rusche JR, Lynn DL, Robert-Guroff M, et al. Humoral immune response to the entire human immunodeficiency virus envelope glycoprotein made in insect cells. Proc Natl Acad Sci USA 1987; 84:6924-8.
223. Kloster BE, Tomar RH, Spira TJ. Lymphocytotoxic antibodies in the acquired immune deficiency syndrome (AIDS). Clin Immunol Immunopathol 1984; 30: 330-5.
224. Dorsett B, Cronin WE, Chuma V, Ioachim HL. Anti-lymphocyte antibodies in patients with the acquired immune deficiency syndrome. Am J Med 1985; 78: 621-6.
225. Kiprov DD, Anderson RE, Morand PR, et al. Antilymphocyte antibodies and seropositivity for retroviruses in groups at high risk for AIDS. N Engl J Med 1985; 312:1517.
226. Lindenmann J. Viruses as immunological adjuvants in cancer. Biochem Biophys Acta 1974; 49:355-75.
227. Levy JA. The human immunodeficiency virus and its pathogenesis. Infect Dis Clin North Am 1988; 2:285-97.
228. McDougal JS, Hubbard M, Nicholson JK, et al. Immune complexes in the acquired immunodeficiency syndrome (AIDS): relationship to disease manifestation, risk group, and immunological defect. J Clin Immunol 1985; 5:130-8.
229. Morrow WJW, Wharton M, Stricker RB, Levy JA. Circulating immune complexes in patients with acquired immune deficiency syndrome contain the AIDS-associated retrovirus. Clin Immunol Immunopathol 1986; 40:515-24.
230. Ujhelyi E, Buki B, Salavecz V, et al. A simple method for detecting HIV antibodies hidden in circulating immune complexes. AIDS 1987; 1:161-5.
231. Barin F, M'Boup S, Denis F, et al. Serological evidence for virus related to simian T-lymphotropic virus type III in residents of West Africa. Lancet 1985; 2: 1387-9.
232. Kanki PJ, Barin F, M'Boup S, et al. New human T-lymphotropic retrovirus related to simian T-lymphotropic virus type III (STLV-III AGM). Science 1986; 232:238-43.
233. Albert J, Bredberg U, Chiodi F, et al. A new human retrovirus isolate of West African origin (SBL-6669) and its relationship to HTLV-IV, LAV-II, and HTLV-IIIB. AIDS Res Retroviruses 1987; 3:3-8.
234. Guyader M, Emerman M, Sonigo P, et al. Genome organization and transactivation of the human immunodeficiency virus type 2. Nature 1987; 326:662-9.
235. Kornfeld H, Riedel N, Viglianti GA, et al. Cloning of HTLV-4 and its relation to simian and human immunodeficiency viruses. Nature 1987; 326:610-3.
236. Hahn BH, Kong LI, Lee S-W, et al. Relation of HTLV-4 to simian and human immunodeficiency-associated viruses. Nature 1987; 330:184-6.
237. Kestler HW, III, Li Y, Naidu YM, et al. Comparison of simian immunodeficiency virus isolates. Nature 1988; 331:619-21.
238. Clavel F, Maninho K, Chamaret S, et al. Human immunodeficiency virus type 2 infection associated with AIDS in West Africa. N Engl J Med 1987; 316:1180-5.
239. Kanki PJ, M'Boup S, Ricard D, et al. Human T lymphotropic virus type 4 and the human immunodeficiency virus in West Africa. Science 1987; 236:827-31.

240. Letvin NL, Daniel MD, Sehgal PK, et al. Infection of baboons with human immunodeficiency virus 2 (HIV-2). J Infect Dis 1987; 156:406-7.
241. Evans LA, Moreau J, Odehouri K, et al. Characterization of a non-cytopathic HIV-2 strain with unusual effects on CD4 antigen expression. Science 1988; 240:1522-5.
242. Denis D, Barin F, Gershy-Damet G, et al. Prevalence of human T lymphotropic retroviruses type III (HIV) and type IV in Ivory Coast. Lancet 1987; 1:408-11.
243. Gnann JW, Jr, McCormick JB, Mitchell S, et al. Synthetic peptide immunoassay distinguishes HIV type 1 and HIV type 2 infections. Science 1987; 237: 1346-9.
244. CDC. AIDS due to HIV-2 infection—New Jersey. MMWR 1987; 37:969-72.
245. Friedland GH, Klein RS. Transmission of the human immunodeficiency virus. N Engl J Med 1987; 317:1125-35.
246. Levy JA, Mitra GA, Wong MF, Mozen MM. Survival of AIDS-associated retrovirus (ARV) during factor VIII purification from plasma: Inactivation by wet and dry heat procedures. Lancet 1985; 1:1456-7.
247. Mitra G, Wong MF, Mozen MM, et al. Elimination of infectious retroviruses during preparation of immunoglobulins. Transfusion 1986; 26:394-7.
248. Padian NS. Heterosexual transmission of acquired immunodeficiency syndrome: international perspectives and national projections. Rev Infect Dis 1987; 9:947-60.
249. Fink AJ. A possible explanation for heterosexual male infection with AIDS. N Engl J Med 1986; 315:1167.
250. CDC. Update: human immunodeficiency virus infections in health-care workers exposed to blood of infected patients. MMWR 1987; 36:295-9.
251. Lyons SF, Jupp PG, Schoub BD. Survival of HIV in the common bedbug. Lancet 1986; 2:45.
252. Zuckerman AJ. AIDS and insects. Br Med J 1986; 292:1094-5.
253. Resnick L, Veren K, Salahuddin Z, et al. Stability and inactivation of HTLV-III/LAV under clinical and laboratory environments. JAMA 1986; 255:1887-91.
254. Cooper DA, Gold J, Maclean P, et al. Acute AIDS retrovirus infection: Definition of a clinical illness associated with seroconversion. Lancet 1985; 1:537-40.
255. Gaines H, Sonneerborg A, Czajkowski J, et al. Antibody response in primary human immunodeficiency virus infection. Lancet 1987; 1:1249-53.
256. Gaines H, Albert J, von Sydow M. HIV antigenaemia and virus isolation from plasma during primary HIV infection. Lancet 1987; 1:1317-8.
257. Salahuddin SZ, Groopman JE, Markham PD, et al. HTLV-III in symptom-free seronegative persons. Lancet 1984; 2:1418-20.
258. Carne C, Smith A, Elkington S, et al. Acute encephalopathy coincident with seroconversion for anti-HTLV-III. Lancet 1985; 2:1206-8.
259. Yarchoan R, Broder S. Development of antiretroviral therapy for the acquired immunodeficiency syndrome and related disorders. N Engl J Med 1987; 316: 557-64.
260. Mitsuya H, Weinhold KJ, Furman PA, et al. 3′-Azido-3′-deoxythymidine (BW A509U): an antiviral agent that inhibits the infectivity and cytopathic effect of human T-lymphotropic virus type III/lymphadenopathy-associated virus in vitro. Proc Natl Acad Sci USA 1985; 82:7096-100.

261. Mitsuya H, Popovic M, Yarchoan R, et al. Suramin protection of T-cells in vitro against infectivity and cytopathic effect of HTLV-III. Science 1984; 226: 172-4.
262. McCormick JB, Getchell JP, Mitchell SW, Hicks DR. Ribavirin suppresses replication of lymphadenopathy-associated virus in cultures of human adult T lymphocytes. Lancet 1984; 2:1367-9.
263. Sansstrom EG, Kaplan JC, Byington RE, Hirsch MS. Inhibition of human T-cell lymphotropic virus type III in vitro by phosphonoformate. Lancet 1985; 2:1480-2.
264. Sarin PS, Gallo RC, Scheer DI, et al. Effects of a novel compound (AL 721) on HTLV-III infectivity in vitro. N Engl J Med 1985; 313:1289-90.
265. Ito M, Baba M, Sato A, et al. Inhibitory effect of dextran sulfate and heparin on the replication of human immunodeficiency virus (HIV) in vitro. Antiviral Res 7:361-7.
266. Walker BD, Kowalski M, Goh WC, et al. Inhibition of human immunodeficiency virus syncytium formation and virus replication by castanospermine. Proc Natl Acad Sci USA 1987; 84:8120-4.
267. Montefiori DC, Mitchell WM. Antiviral activity of mismatched double-stranded RNA against human immunodeficiency virus *in vitro*. Proc Natl Acad Sci USA 1987; 84:2985-9.
268. Ho DD, Rota TR, Kaplan JC, et al. Recombinant human interferon Alfa-A suppresses HTLV-III replication *in vitro*. Lancet 1985; 1:602-3.
269. Michaelis B, Levy JA. Recombinant human interferon beta reduces human immunodeficiency virus replication in peripheral blood mononuclear cells. Proc Am Assoc Cancer Res 1987:460 (abstract).
270. Fischl MA, Richman DD, Grieco MH, et al. The efficacy of 3′-azido-3′-deoxythymidine (azidothymidine) in the treatment of patients with AIDS and AIDS-related complex: a double-blind placebo-controlled trial. N Engl J Med 1987; 317:185-91.
271. Richman DD, Fischl MA, Grieco MH, et al. The toxicity of azidothymidine (AZT) in the treatment of patients with AIDS and AIDS-related complex. N Engl J Med 1987; 317:192-7.
272. Smith MS, Brian EL, Pagano JS. Resumption of virus production after human immunodeficiency virus infection of T lymphocytes in the presence of azidothymidine. J Virol 1987; 61:3769-73.
273. Richman DD, Kornbluth RS, Carson DA. Failure of dideoxynucleosides to inhibit human immunodeficiency virus replication in cultured human macrophages. J Exp Med 1987; 166:1144-9.
274. Abrams DI, Volberding PA. Alpha interferon therapy of AIDS-associated Kaposi's sarcoma. Semin Oncol 1986; 13:43-7.
275. Kaplan LD, Wolfe PR, Volberding PA, et al. Lack of response to suramin in patients with AIDS and AIDS-related complex. Am J Med 1987; 82:615-20.
276. Crumpacker C, Heagy W, Bubley G, et al. Ribavirin treatment of the Acquired Immunodeficiency Syndrome (AIDS) and the Acquired-Immunodeficiency-Syndrome-Related Complex (ARC). Ann Intern Med 1987; 107:664-74.
277. Weiss RA. Receptor molecule blocks HIV. Nature 1988; 331:15.

278. Ho DD, Pomerantz R, Kaplan JC. Pathogenesis of infection with human immunodeficiency virus. N Engl J Med 1987; 317:278-86.
279. Fauci AS. The human immunodeficiency virus: Infectivity and mechanisms of pathogenesis. Science 1988; 239:617-22.
280. Fischinger PJ, Robey WG, Koprowski H, et al. Current status and strategies for vaccines against diseases induced by human T-cell lymphotropic retroviruses (HTLV-I, -II, -III). Cancer Res 1985; 45:4694s-9s.
281. Levy JA. Can an AIDS vaccine be developed? In: Vyas G, ed. Transfusion Medicine Reviews. 1988; in press.
282. Merz DC, Scheid A, Choppin PW. Importance of antibodies to the fusion glycoprotein of paramyxoviruses in the prevention of spread of infection. J Exp Med 1980; 151:275-88.
283. Dreesman GR, Kennedy RC. Anti-idiotypic antibodies: implications of internal image-based vaccines for infectious diseases. J Infect Dis 1985; 151:761-5.
284. Kennedy RC, Eichberg JW, Lanford RE, Dreesman GR. Anti-idiotypic antibody vaccine for type B viral hepatitis in chimpanzees. Science 1986; 232:220-3.
285. Farzadegan H, Polis MA, Wolinsky SM, et al. Loss of human immunodeficiency virus type 1 (HIV-1) antibodies with evidence of viral infection in asymptomatic homosexual men. Ann Intern Med 1988; 108:785-90.
286. Patterson S, Knight SC. Susceptibility of human peripheral blood dendritic cells to infection by human immunodeficiency virus. Virology 1987; 68:1177-81.
287. Robert-Guroff M, Reitz MS, Jr, Robey WG, Gallo RC. In vitro generation of an HTLV-III variant by neutralizing antibody. J Immunol 1986; 137:3306-9.
288. Wu F, Garcia J, Mitsuyasu R, Gaynor R. Alterations in binding characteristics of the human immunodeficiency virus enhancer factor. J Virol 1988; 62:218-25.
289. Golding H, Robey FA, Gates FT, et al. Identification of homologous regions in human immunodeficiency virus I gp41 and human MHC class II beta 1 domain. J Exp Med 1988; 167:914-23.
290. Chaput M, Claes V, Portetelle D, et al. The neurotrophic factor neuroleukin is 90% homologous with phosphohexose isomerase. Nature 1988; 332:454-5.
291. Tindall B, Barker S, Donovan B, et al. Characterization of the acute clinical illness associated with human immunodeficiency virus infection. Arch Intern Med 1988; 148:945-9.
292. Levy JA. The mysteries of HIV: Challenges for therapy and prevention. Nature 1988; 333:519-22.
293. Kannagi M, Chalifoux LV, Lord CI, Letvin NL. Suppression of simian immunodeficiency virus replication in vitro by CD8+ lymphocytes. J Immunol 1988; 140:2237-40.
294. Robinson WE, Montefiori DC, Mitchell WM. Antibody-dependent enhancement of human immunodeficiency virus type 1 infection. Lancet 1988; 1:790-5.
295. Homsy J, Tateno M, Levy JA. Antibody-dependent enhancement of HIV infection. Lancet 1988; 1:1285-6.
296. Zagury D, Bernard J, Cheynier R, et al. A group specific anamnestic immune reaction against HIV-1 induced by a candidate vaccine against AIDS. Nature 1988; 332:728-31.

9

The Molecular Biology of HIV Infection: Clues for Possible Therapy

Arnold B. Rabson

Laboratory of Molecular Microbiology
National Institute of Allergy and Infectious Diseases
National Institutes of Health
Bethesda, Maryland

I. Introduction

In the seven years that have elapsed since the initial clinical description of the acquired immunodeficiency syndrome (AIDS) and the AIDS-related complex (ARC), an extraordinary amount of information has been obtained concerning the epidemiology, clinical course, etiology, and pathogenesis of these disorders. With the identification of the human immunodeficiency virus (HIV) (1) as the etiological agent of AIDS and ARC (2-4), therapeutic approaches directed against this virus could be logically initiated and, more importantly, have already begun to show evidence of efficacy. This chapter will summarize some of the important features of the molecular biology of HIV infection and discuss various therapeutic approaches to HIV infection based on its molecular characteristics.

Any successful therapeutic approach to the treatment of AIDS will, of necessity, involve strategies that address both the clinical immunodeficiency and the replication and persistence of HIV (5). Because HIV is a retrovirus, it retains the potential to persist for years as integrated proviral DNA within the cells of an infected individual; thus, even the possible correction of the immune deficit in AIDS would not constitute sufficient treatment. Direct antiviral therapy will be required and, in the case of reverse transcriptase inhibitors (6), has already been shown to be of value.

Potential antiviral strategies for HIV infection may take many forms. Some of them, such as the development of reverse transcriptase inhibitors, are based upon years of study of the properties of retroviruses. Other experimental approaches, such as the use of synthetic peptides, anti-sense oligonucleotides, or anti-idiotypic antibodies, have developed from recent advances in molecular biology and immunology. Finally, several potential targets for intervention in HIV infection exist for which no therapeutic agents are currently known. These would include viral enzymatic activities such as protease and endonuclease. Whether inhibitors of these unique properties of HIV can be identified, either through rational scientific study or serendipity, may be of great importance in the successful treatment of HIV infection.

II. HIV Replication

The human immunodeficiency virus (HIV) shares many of the basic features of its life cycle and genomic organization with other retroviruses. In particular, many aspects of HIV biology show similarities to other members of the lentivirus family of retroviruses. These viruses, which include visna virus of sheep, equine infectious anemia virus, and a newly described feline immunodeficiency virus, FTLV (7), have similar morphological, biological, and molecular characteristics. Morphologically, the lentiviral particles contain a dense, central cylindrical core. Biologically, these viruses cause slowly progressive, fatal disease in their animal hosts. In vitro, lentiviruses cause marked cytopathic effects, including syncytia formation and cytotoxicity. Similarities in genomic organization include the presence of several novel open reading frames not present in other classes of retroviruses (8) as will be discussed below. Since the initial isolation of HIV as lymphadenopathy-associated virus (LAV, 2), human T-lymphotropic virus type III (HTLV-III, 3), and AIDS-associated retrovirus (ARV, 4), other more distantly related primate and human lentiviruses have been identified. These include the simian immunodeficiency virus (SIV, 9-11) from wild African Green monkeys and laboratory macaques, the closely related HTLV-IV (12) isolated primarily from healthy individuals in West Africa [recently recognized as an SIV contaminant (Nature 1988; 331:621)], and LAV-2 or HIV-2 isolated from patients with AIDS and ARC in West Africa (13) (see also Chapter 8). Molecular characteristics of these viruses have recently been described (14,15) and exhibit many similarities to HIV-1. In the remainder of this chapter, the discussion shall be limited to the initially isolated HIV family (LAV, HTLV-III, ARV, and related viruses), by far the most important cause of human AIDS and related diseases and the viruses about which most is known.

Although HIV exhibits certain special morphological features, the HIV virion has a structure similar to that of other retroviruses. The virion RNA genome is packaged within a core particle whose structural elements are derived from the viral *gag* gene. This core particle is surrounded by a lipid envelope acquired as the virion buds from an infected cell. The viral envelope proteins, gp120 and gp41 (16,17), are found on the surface of the virion particle with the transmembrane protein, gp41, anchored in the viral envelope (18).

The essential features of the HIV life cycle are illustrated in Figure 1. As will be discussed later, each major point in the process of viral replication represents a potential target for therapeutic intervention. The initial step in HIV infection is the binding of the virion particle to the target CD4+ cell, generally a lymphocyte or macrophage. This binding involves the inter-

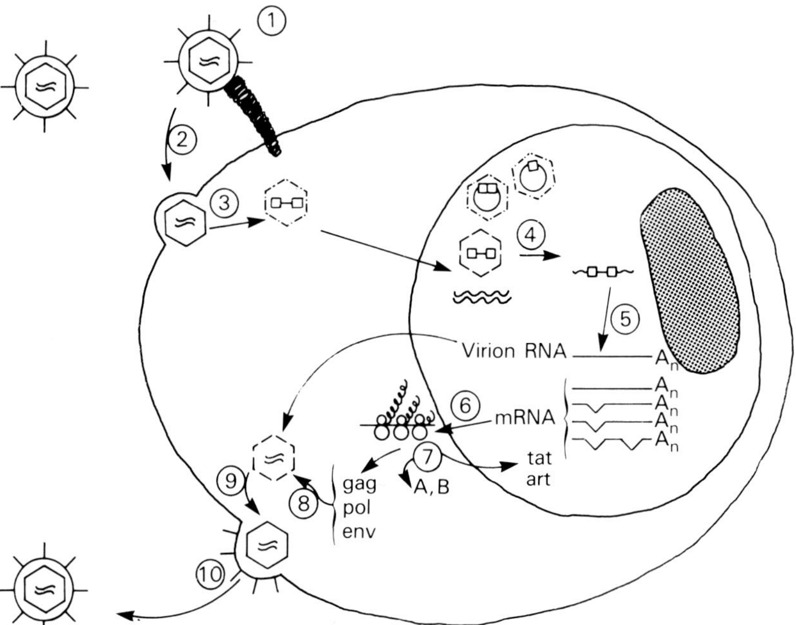

Figure 1 The HIV life cycle. The steps of HIV infection and replication are shown schematically and discussed in the text.

action of the external envelope protein of HIV, gp120, with the CD4 molecule on the surface of the target cell (19-21). That the CD4 molecule is a component of the viral receptor has been clearly demonstrated; however, the failure of mouse cells expressing human CD4 to be productively infected despite binding to the virus (22) raises the possibility that other human proteins may be required for virus internalization. Moreover, some cells lacking CD4 antigen expresion appear to be infected by HIV (Chapter 8); thus, other receptors may also be involved. As depicted in Figure 1, viral binding involves the interaction of a free viral particle with the surface of a target cell; however, direct cell-to-cell spread of HIV from an infected to an uninfected cell is also likely to occur, presumably in part mediated by the binding of gp120 to the CD4 molecule.

After binding of HIV to the target cell surface, the infecting virus must be internalized (step 2). While the details of this process are not understood, it probably requires the interaction of the viral gp41 sequences with the cell membrane and possibly with other cellular proteins. The result of this interaction is the fusion of the viral envelope with the cell membrane in a pH-independent process (23).

Once internalized, the viral RNA genome undergoes reverse transcription (step 3) and integration into the host genome (step 4). Recent data derived from the study of murine leukemia viruses (24) suggest that these enzymatic processes occur in the context of a subviral particle consisting of a nucleoprotein complex that can be found both in the cytoplasm and nucleus. Reverse transcription, catalyzed by the virally encoded reverse transcriptase, involves the synthesis of first-strand DNA primed by a transfer RNA (tRNA) molecule which is bound to the provirus adjacent to the 5′ long terminal repeat (LTR). An intrinsic RNAse H activity degrades the RNA portion of the RNa-DNA hybrid and the second strand of DNA is synthesized after priming from a polypurine tract adjacent to the 3′ LTR. This process results in the generation of three forms of double-stranded DNA genomes: 1) a linear form containing two copies of the viral LTR, present at each end of the DNA provirus, 2) a circular form containing two copies of the LTR, and 3) a circular form containing a single LTR. One of the unusual features of HIV infection, as compared with that of most other retroviruses, is the accumulation of large amounts of unintegrated viral DNA within infected cells. Such an accumulation of unintegrated DNA has been found in only a few other retroviral systems, particularly those causing marked cytopathic effect (CPE), and has been hypothesized to contribute to the cytopathicity of HIV (25).

The integration of retroviral DNA into the host chromosomal DNA is dependent on a virally encoded endonuclease which seems, in vitro, to utilize the linear double-stranded DNA provirus as its substrate (24). The retroviral integration process exhibits features characteristic of transposition such as the generation of a duplication of host DNA sequences at the site of integration (26).

After integration, the DNA provirus undergoes transcription to generate progeny virion RNAs and spliced subgenomic messenger RNAs (mRNAs). The regulation of HIV transcription is complex and involves the interaction of cellular factors and the virally encoded *tat* gene, as will be discussed below. The processing of HIV mRNAs (step 6), which includes RNA splicing, stability, transport, and translatability, also appears to be carefully regulated, in part, by the HIV *art* protein (see below).

Translation of HIV mRNA results in the production of the various HIV proteins (step 7). Some of these proteins, such as *tat* and *art*, have regulatory functions. Others, such as the products of the *gag*, *pol*, and *env* genes, end up in the viral particles (see Figure 2). The functions of the A and B proteins are still unknown. Assembly of progeny virions (step 8) occurs in the cytoplasm and is followed by the budding of newly formed particles from the cell surface (step 9) and the release of these from the cell (step 10).

Thus, in most respects, HIV infection resembles that of other retroviruses; however, a very important feature of HIV infection exhibited by relatively few retroviruses is that productive infection of the target $CD4^+$ cells results in dramatic cytopathic effects including syncytia formation and cell death. Although much of the pathogenesis of AIDS remains to be explained, the cytotoxicity of HIV for $CD4^+$ lymphocytes seems to contribute to the development of the clinical syndrome.

III. HIV Genomic Organization

The organization of the HIV genome was originally deduced on the basis of the DNA sequence of several molecularly cloned HIV proviruses (27-30). Further studies of HIV protein structures and functions and of HIV transcription have resulted in refinements of our understanding of the molecular characteristics of HIV as shown in Figure 2. The HIV genome contains characteristics of all retroviral genomes, including the presence of LTRs, regulatory sequences present at either end of the DNA provirus, and genes encoding viral structural proteins and enzymatic activities, the *gag*, *pol*, and *env* genes. In addition to these regions, the HIV genome contains a number of unique reading frames, including those for the regulatory proteins *tat* and *art* and for the viral proteins referred to as *A* and *B* in Figure 2. Recently, evidence has been presented for an additional gene called R_1 (30a). Some individuals infected with HIV have serum antibodies to an R gene product synthesized in bacteria. In this section, the structural and functional characteristics of each of these segments of the HIV genome and their corresponding proteins will be discussed.

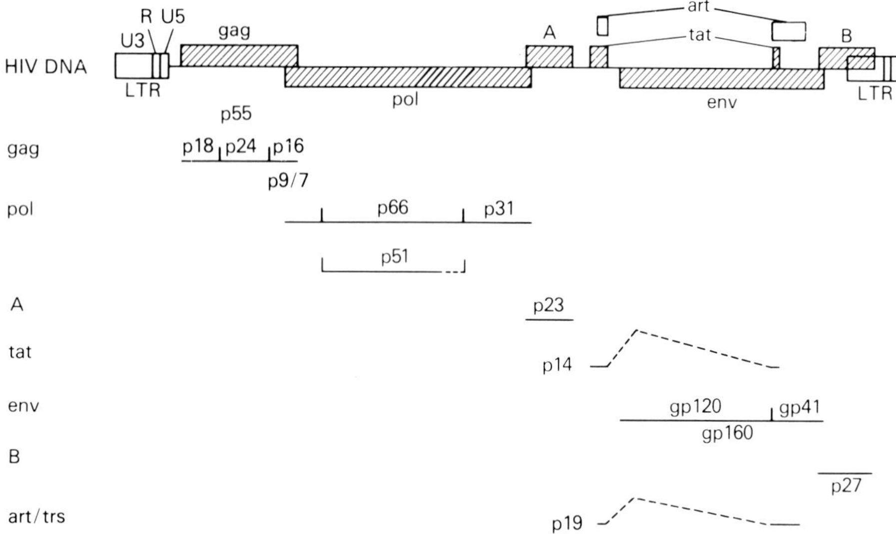

Figure 2 HIV genomic organization. The locations of the viral LTRs and coding sequences are shown. The entire HIV proviral genome is 9.7 kb in length. The identified viral proteins encoded by each gene are shown below.

A. Long Terminal Repeats

The HIV LTRs contain important regulatory segments for viral replication. Each LTR is approximately 630 base pairs (bp) in length and has the same tripartite structure found in other retroviral LTRs. The positions of these segments, and the sites of some of the viral regulatory sequences present in them, are shown in Figure 3. The U3 region is derived from unique sequences present at the 3′ end of the virion RNA molecule and contains a number of

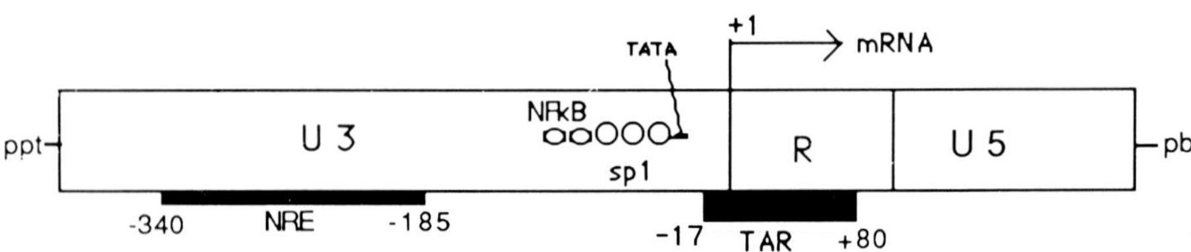

Figure 3 HIV LTR. The structure of the HIV LTRs and the positions of important regulatory sequences are shown. The initiation site for RNA synthesis is numbered as +1; *ppt* refers to the polypurine tract; and *pbs* designates the tRNA primer binding site.

sequences important in the regulation of viral gene transcription. These include a negative regulatory element (NRE) (31), which is present 185-350 bp 5′ to the start of RNA transcription. The deletion of this element seems to result in increased transcription of RNA initiated from the LTR as monitored in transient expression assays (31). The role of this element in viral infection is unclear. Two regulatory regions that have been found to have positive effects on viral RNA transcription are more proximal to the RNA start site. One contains two tandem copies of an 11-bp sequence previously identified as a regulatory sequence in the enhancer of the kappa immunoglobulin gene (32), a portion of which is homologous to the SV40 core enhancer (33). This sequence has been shown by Nabel and Baltimore (34) to bind a nuclear factor called NF-κB. The binding of this factor to the HIV LTR correlates with the activation of the LTR by mitogens and phorbol esters in the Jurkat T cell line (34); thus, it has been suggested that this sequence may play a role in the activation of latent HIV proviruses. Immediately 3′ to the NF-κB binding sites are three copies of a DNA sequence to which the transcription factor, SP1, binds (35). The HIV SP1 binding sites have been shown to be important in both in vitro transcription systems and for LTR-directed RNA synthesis in transient transfection assays (35). Mutations in these sequences significantly decrease LTR activity. In addition to these signals, the U3 region contains a DNA sequence responsible for setting the site of initiation of RNA transcription for most eukaryotic genes. This so called TATA box is present 25 bp 5′ to the RNA start site.

The R region, derived from RNA sequences repeated at the 5′ and 3′ ends of the virion RNA, contains at its 5′ end the site of initiation of RNA transcription (designated as +1). The HIV LTR R region contains an important and unique regulatory sequence, the transactivation response (TAR) region. These sequences, which have been mapped by deletion analysis to lie between −17 in U3 and +54 in R (31,36), constitute the portion of the LTR required for the activation of HIV gene expression by the HIV *tat* gene (see below). A signal for the addition of poly A residues at the 3′ end of the viral RNAs is also present in the R region. The border between R and U5 sequences marks the site of polyadenylation.

The HIV U5 region is 83 bp in length and is derived from sequences present at the 5′ end of the virion RNA. The functions of U5 are unknown. During HIV replication the major transcriptional regulatory sequences are derived from the 3′ LPR.

In addition to these internal LTR signals, important sequences for HIV replication are present immediately adjacent to the LTRs. The site of tRNA primer binding (Figure 3, *pbs*) for the synthesis of the first strand of DNA is present at the 3′ side of the 5′ LTR. A polypurine tract (Figure 3, *ppt*) that serves as the initiation site for the synthesis of the second strand of DNA is present just 5′ to the 3′ LTR. Sequences important for the encapsidation of viral genomic RNA are likely to be present between the 5′ LTR and the *gag* gene, as has been shown for other retroviruses (37,38).

B. *gag* Gene

The most 5′ viral coding sequences constitute the *gag* gene region (Figure 2). This gene encodes the "group-specific antigens" of retroviruses that comprise structural proteins forming the virion core. The *gag* gene transcript is part of a 9.2-kilobase (kb) viral mRNA (39) and is translated as a polyprotein precursor molecule, p55. The p55 undergoes a series of proteolytic cleavages catalyzed by the viral protease (part of the *pol* gene). The complex details of this processing pathway are still being elucidated; however, the major products of the *gag* gene have been identified as p18, p24 (or p25), and p12 (or p16) further processed to p9 and p7 (S. Venkatesan, personal communication).

The p18, p24, and p55 *gag* proteins have been shown to be phosphorylated when expressed in yeast (40). The carboxy-terminal *gag* protein shares a cysteine-rich sequence characteristic of retroviral nucleic acid-binding proteins (41) consistent with a potential role in packaging of the viral RNA genome. Retroviral *gag* proteins often undergo myristylation (42), which may play a role in attachment of the viral core to the lipid envelope.

C. *pol* Gene

The *pol* gene encodes three viral enzymatic functions: a protease, reverse transcriptase (with its associated RNAse H activity), and an endonuclease. The *pol* gene is transcribed as part of the 9.2-kb viral mRNA. Since the *pol* gene is in a different reading frame than the more 5′ *gag* sequences in the 9.2-kb RNA, the virus must adopt a strategy to allow *pol* gene translation. The most likely explanation seems to be the use of a ribosomal frameshift out of the *gag* reading frame into the *pol* frame. Such a mechanism has been shown to occur in the translation of the *pol* gene of the Rous sarcoma virus in vitro (43). Thus, a large *gag-pol* fusion protein is made which is processed both into *gag* polypeptides (as described above) and *pol* gene products.

Based on homologies to other retroviruses and the results of deletion experiments involving HIV *pol* gene constructs (40), the HIV protease appears to be encoded by the 5′ *pol* sequences. The putative protein has a size of 10 kD (E. Lillehoj and S. Venkatesan, manuscript in preparation). The protease is responsible for processing of the *gag* and *gag-pol* precursor molecules. Although the protease cleaves the precursor molecules at several positions, the precise substrate amino acid signals involved in the recognition and cleavage appear to be complex; however, a unique cleavage between Tyr-Pro or Phe-Pro residues seems to be characteristic of retroviral proteases and is utilized in the cleavage of HIV *gag* and *pol* precursors.

The reverse transcriptase (RT) and associated RNAse H activities are encoded by the central portion of the *pol* gene. Two forms of HIV RT have been described (44,45), a p51 and a p66. These share amino-terminal sequences and appear to differ at their carboxy termini. The functional differences between these two RT molecules are currently not known. Recently published site-specific mutagenesis experiments involving the RT sequences have allowed the identification of domains of the RT protein required for reverse transcriptase activity and sensitivity to the inhibitory effects of 3′-azido-3′-deoxythymidine (AZT) and phosphonoacetic acid (46).

A 31-kD protein has been shown to be encoded by the 3′ portion of the *pol* gene (45,47). This region in other retroviral systems is responsible for the endonuclease activity and integration of proviral DNA into the host chromosome. In the context of subviral nuclear particles, the endonuclease of retroviruses is responsible for the staggered nicking of host chromosomal DNA and the ligation of proviral DNA into the host DNA. This process results in the loss of 2 bp from the ends of each LTR and the creation of a duplication of cellular sequences flanking the newly inserted provirus.

D. A/*sor* Gene

The A (48), *sor* (28), or Q (27) gene is transcribed as a 5.0-kb mRNA (39) which is translated into a 23-kD protein (49,50). The A gene product is a basic protein of unknown function. The deletion of portions of the A gene from an infectious HIV DNA clone results in a marked diminution of the ability of virus particles to infect $T4^+$ lymphocytes (51); however, cell-to-cell spread of virus can still occur (52,53). These observations suggest that the A gene product has a role in the structure of infectious virion particles.

E. *tat* Gene

The *tat* gene encodes a 14-kD protein (54,55) that functions as a potent activator of HIV gene expression in *trans* (56,57). The *tat* protein is encoded by a 1.8-kb spliced mRNA containing two coding exons (Figure 2), one located between A and *env*, and the second within the *env* gene in an alternate reading frame (56). The transactivating effect of *tat* was initially observed in transient assays of HIV LTR function as outlined in Figure 4. In these assays, the HIV LTR is ligated to a marker gene such as the bacterial enzyme chloramphenicol acetyl transferase (CAT). The CAT enzyme is not found in mammalian cells, but can be introduced into these cells by the process of calcium phosphate-mediated DNA transfection (Figure 4*A*). After transfection, cells are harvested, lysed, and tested for the activity of the transfected CAT enzyme by assaying the conversion of C-14 chloramphenicol from an unacetylated to an acetylated form on thin-layer chromatography (58). The amount of acetylation of chloramphenicol reflects the degree of expression of the CAT gene in the transfected cells. In Figure 4*B* are shown examples of the

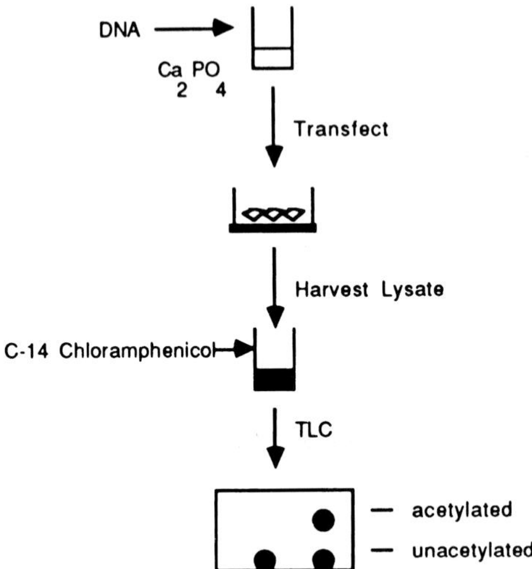

Figure 4 Transactivation of the HIV LTR. (*A*) The CAT assay used to study the activity of the HIV LTR is shown schematically. (*B*) Plasmids used in the CAT assays shown in *C*. pBCAT was constructed by ligating the CAT gene to the +81 position of the HIV LTR at a HindIII site. pSVtat was constructed by ligating a 630-bp HIV genomic fragment containing the first coding exon of *tat* to the SV40 early region promoter. (*C*) Thin-layer chromatograms illustrating transactivation of the HIV LTR by *tat*. The DNAs used for transfection were: lane *1*, salmon sperm DNA; lane *2*, pBCAT DNA; lane *3*, pBCAT and pSVtat DNA.

recombinant plasmids used to assay the activating effect of the *tat* gene on the expression of the HIV LTR in the CAT assay shown in Figure 4*C*. The U3 and most of the R region of the HIV LTR was ligated to the CAT gene to produce pBCAT (59). This plasmid was introduced into a human colon carcinoma cell line, SW480, in the presence or absence of a plasmid capable of expressing functional HIV *tat* protein under the control of the SV40 early promoter. The results of this transfection and CAT assay are shown in Figure 4*C*. In lane *1*, as a negative control, salmon sperm DNA was transfected into SW480 cells, resulting in no CAT activity. In lane *2*, the basal level of CAT activity seen after transfection of the HIV LTR-CAT plasmid is shown. Lane *3* shows the marked (between 40- and 150-fold) increase in CAT gene expression under the control of the HIV LTR when the *tat* gene is simultaneously transfected into these cells. Thus, the *tat* gene product is able to markedly

B

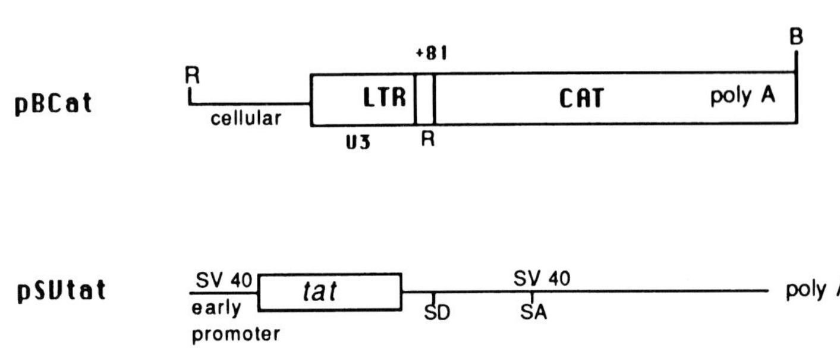

C

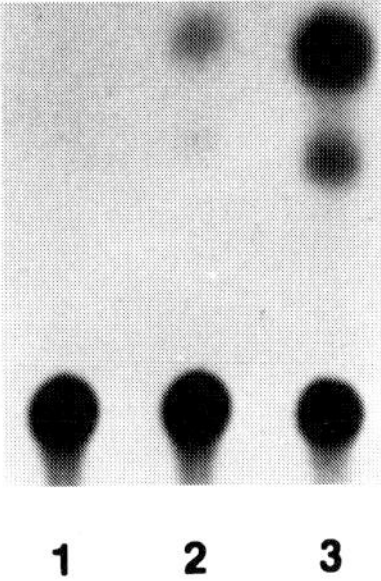

stimulate the expression of genes promoted by the HIV LTR when supplied in *trans*. The precise mechanisms by which the *tat* gene product functions are not known, but may involve a bimodal effect on both RNA synthesis and RNA stability or translatability (60). Significant increases in steady-state levels of RNAs containing HIV LTR sequences can be observed after *tat* co-transfection (55,59,61,62). These increases may reflect increased RNA transcription or stability. Recent studies by Peterlin et al. (63) have suggested that *tat* functions as an antiterminator, overcoming termination of HIV transcription within the R region of the LTR. The presence of stable RNA secondary structure within the TAR sequences forming the 5′ end of viral RNAs is consistent with a model of *tat* activity resulting in increased RNA stability (62). In contrast, increases in LTR-derived RNA in the presence of *tat* may reflect direct transcriptional activation, as suggested by the ability of nuclear extracts prepared from infected cells to enhance transcription of the HIV LTR in vitro (64). Of note in this regard is the fact that the *tat* protein contains a region rich in cysteine residues. These cysteines are arranged in a manner similar to that observed in the metal-binding domain characteristic of certain classes of nucleic acid-binding proteins such as TF IIIA of *Xenopus laevis* (65). Interestingly, the targets of both TF IIIA and *tat* effect lie, at least in part, 3′ to the site of transcription initiation. In addition to its effect on RNA levels, the *tat* gene product may lead to an actual increase in the translation of LTR-containing mRNAs (60,66,67). The unusual RNA secondary structure of the TAR region may be responsible for any effects that *tat* has on translation. Studies of the role of *tat* in HIV replication employing mutated *tat* genes, have shown that the *tat* gene is critical for the high levels of viral replication characteristic of HIV infection of lymphocytes (68,69).

F. *art/trs* Gene

A second transactivating viral regulatory function, referred to as *art* (70) or *trs* (67), was initially detected after deletion mutation analysis of the *tat* gene. These studies revealed the presence of an additional open reading frame overlapping the 3′ end of the first coding exon of *tat* and spliced to sequences overlapping the second *tat* coding exon, but extending further toward the 3′ end of the virus, in a different reading frame. The *art/trs* protein appears to be translated from a 1.8-kb mRNA like that from which *tat* is expressed. When expressed in bacterial (71) or eukaryotic expression systems (72), the *art/trs* reading frame codes for a 19-20-kD protein. The functions of *art/trs* are not clearly delineated, but the *art/trs* protein is required for the processing and translation of *gag* and *env* RNAs. Deletion of *art/trs* has been found to result in reduced (67) levels of *gag* and *env* mRNAs, and markedly decreased *gag* and *env* protein expression (67,70). In transient expression assays, the presence of *art/trs* supplied in *trans* was absolutely required for *env* protein expression (72). This result suggest that *art/trs* has a role in overcoming an inhibition of translation intrinsic to the HIV LTR-*env* mRNA.

G. *env* Gene

The HIV *env* gene is transcribed as a spliced 4.2-kb mRNA (39) that is translated into a precursor protein, gp160, which is processed, probably by a cellular protease, to form the two viral envelope glycoproteins gp120 and gp41 (Figure 5) (16,17). The major external viral glycoprotein, gp120, is present at the surface of the viral particle and is attached to the particle through disulfide bonding to gp41, a transmembrane protein (18). The gp120 contains several domains critical for viral infectivity including a region involved in binding to the CD4 molecule during the attachment of virus to target cells (21). The positions of the CD4 binding domains have been mapped by muta-

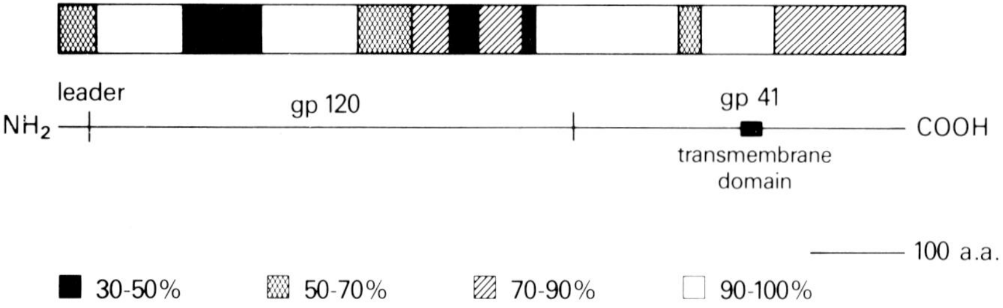

Figure 5 HIV *env* gene variability. The deduced amino acid sequence of the *env* gene of four HIV isolates was compared over consecutive 50 amino acid stretches and the percentage of amino acid conservation was calculated. The degrees of amino acid homologies are shown schematically, as are the positions of the *env* proteins.

tional analysis (73,74) and will be of great importance in defining potential targets for interference with viral replication. It appears that other domains in the gp120 are also important for viral infectivity. For example, alteration of a single amino acid resulting in the elimination of a highly conserved glycosylation site (present in the second conserved region of gp120 shown in Figure 5) leads to a loss of viral infectivity, although gp120-CD4 binding is retained (106). Thus, regions of the gp120 may be important for processes such as viral internalization as well as CD4 binding.

In addition to anchoring the gp120 to the viral particle, the gp41 plays a role in the fusion of attached viral particles with the target cell. In a manner analogous to that of other enveloped viruses such as the paramyxoviruses (75), the amino terminus of the HIV transmembrane protein, gp41, contains a hydrophobic amino acid stretch which may become available to interact with the target cell membrane after cleavage of the gp160 to gp120 and gp41 and binding of the gp120 to the cell. Insertion of this hydrophobic stretch of gp41 into the target cell membrane is likely to be important in allowing the fusion of viral and cellular membranes and internalization of the virus. This process may also be involved in the syncytia formation characteristic of HIV infection of $CD4^+$ lymphocytes. Syncytia can form following the interaction of uninfected $CD4^+$ cells with infected cells expressing the HIV *env* proteins on their surface (76,77). This process of syncytia formation may play an important role in the cytopathicity of HIV (76). The long intracellular carboxy terminus of gp41 has also been implicated in the cytopathicity of HIV as mutants of the virus in which these sequences are deleted demonstrate somewhat reduced cytopathic effect (78).

An important characteristic of the HIV envelope gene is the striking degree of variability in amino acid sequences between different viral isolates

(79-82). Figure 5 shows a schematic representation of a comparison of amino sequence conservation deduced from the DNA sequence of four different HIV isolates (81): the French isolate LAV, a San Francisco isolate (ARV-2), a New York isolate, and a Zairian isolate. As can be seen, the *env* gene contains both highly conserved and highly divergent regions. Divergent regions can share as little as 30-50% homology over 100-200 amino acid stretches. Variability within these divergent regions can readily be identified, even in multiple isolates of HIV obtained from a single patient (83). The presence of such a high degree of *env* variability may have profound clinical implications. If these variable regions play any role in the development of an effective immune response to HIV infection, the appearance of new variant viruses within a patient may preclude the development of effective neutralizing antibodies and cellular immunity and rule out the usefulness of passive immune therapy. The presence of large numbers of HIV strains with extremely variable *env* genes may also create serious difficulties for vaccine development unless constant epitopes capable of inducing an effective immune response can be identified.

As can be seen in Figure 5, a number of highly conserved regions of the *env* gene also exist. It is likely that these contain sequences important for the properties of the *env* gene shared by all HIV isolates. Such properties would include CD4 binding, viral internalization, and syncytia formation as well as the association of gp120 and gp41. Two such domains exist within the 5′ half of gp120. A third includes the 3′ end of gp120, a region that frequently elicits an antibody response in patients (84,85), and is capable of inducing T cell immunity (86). This same conserved domain includes a region of gp120 involved in CD4 binding (73) and spans the gp120/gp41 cleavage site and the 5′ portion of gp41, a region important in membrane fusion. Other conserved regions of the gp41 include the transmembrane region and sequences encompassing the overlap of the *env*, *tat*, and *art/trs* reading frames.

H. B Gene

The B gene (48), also known as F (27) or 3′ *orf* (28), lies 3′ to the end of the *env* and extends into the U3 region of the 3′ LTR. The B gene is transcribed from 1.8-2.0-kb mRNAs (39) and is expressed as a 27-kD protein (87) that has been identified in the cytoplasm of infected cells (88). The function of the B gene has not been clearly established. In one series of experiments, deletions of B sequences did not have major effects on viral replication (89); however, a second set of studies presented data suggesting that the B gene product acted as a negative regulator of viral replication (90). In these latter studies, deletion of segments of the B gene resulted in an approximately fivefold increase in viral replication and in viral DNA synthesis.

Expression of the B gene product by recombinant vaccinia virus vectors has shown that it is myristilated and phosphorylated (91). Furthermore, the B gene product produced in *Escherichia coli* exhibits GTPase, autophosphorylation, and GTP-binding properties similar to those of the *ras* gene family (91). Thus, the B gene may affect the metabolism of HIV-infected cells.

IV. Molecular Approaches to Therapy of HIV Infection

The pathogenesis of AIDS is the result of complex interactions between HIV and the host immune system. Thus, the therapy of AIDS must involve both direct antiviral treatment and therapy aimed at the reconstitution of immune function. The goals of antiviral therapy are the inhibition of intracellular replication of HIV with its associated cytopathicity (in $CD4^+$ lymphocytes) as well as the inhibition of the intercellular spread of the virus within an infected individual. From a conceptual point of view, each of the steps of the viral life cycle outlined in Figure 1 represents a potential target for antiviral therapy as is listed in Table 1. Of particular interest would be those steps,

Table 1 Strategies for Antiviral Therapy of HIV Infection

Potential targets of intervention	Therapeutic approaches
1. Viral binding to target cells	1. Inhibition of gp120-CD4 binding by antibodies or synthetic peptides
2. Fusion of viral and host cell membranes and viral internalization	2. a) Inhibition of gp41 mediated by antibodies, synthetic peptides from "fusigenic sequences" b) Identification and inhibition of interactions between gp120 and other cell surface proteins
3. Synthesis of viral DNA by reverse transcriptase	3. RT inhibitors, especially dideoxynucleosides, antibodies
4. Integration of proviral DNA	4. Identification of endonuclease inhibitors
5-7. Viral RNA transcription, processing, and translation	5-7. a) Search for inhibitors for *tat* and *art/trs* b) Translation arrest by anti-sense RNA molecules c) Modulation of viral gene expression by lymphokines
8, 9. Virion assembly, maturation, and release	8, 9. Identification of inhibitors of viral protease

Abbreviation: RT, reverse transcriptase. Numbers refer to steps of the viral life cycle outlined in Figure 1.

such as reverse transcription or integration, that are dependent on virus-specific enzymes. These processes, unique to the virus, might be inhibited by agents that will not affect normal cellular functions. At this time, the most likely targets for successful antiviral therapy appear to be reverse transcription and viral binding and entry into cells; however, reasons exist for the consideration of potential inhibitors of each step of the viral life cycle, as will be discussed below.

As shown in Figure 1, the first step in the infection of a cell by HIV is the interaction of the virion particle with the CD4 molecule. Blockade of this interaction, either by immunological means or by the use of synthetic peptides, represents an approach to inhibit viral replication. In vitro, monoclonal antibodies directed against certain epitopes of the CD4 molecule, such as OKT4A, have been demonstrated to interfere with gp120-CD4 interactions (19,92,93) and to block viral infectivity. Theoretically, antibodies to the region of the *env* gene involved in binding to CD4 should have the same inhibitory effects. To date, however, high titers of antibody capable of neutralizing viral infectivity have been difficult to demonstrate in patient sera (94). Antibodies produced in animals after immunization with gp160 or gp120 preparations tend to neutralize only the specific HIV isolates from with the immunogen was derived (95,96), consistent with the marked *env* variability discussed above. As the regions of the *env* specifically involved in CD4 binding are clearly delineated, it may be possible to produce immunogens that will elicit higher titers of cross-reactive antibodies capable of neutralizing different HIV strains. Such immunogens might be useful in producing a protective response within already infected individuals or in generating antibodies that could be used in passive therapy of infected patients. Conversely, synthetic peptides corresponding to the binding domains of either gp120 or CD4 may themselves inhibit viral binding and replication. An alternative approach being pursued in several laboratories is the production of anti-idiotypic antibodies. If anti-CD4 antibodies such as OKT4A inhibit gp120-CD4 binding, anti-idiotypic antibodies produced against OKT4A may also inhibit viral adherence to cells by binding to viral particles.

Several important theoretical problems exist with all approaches that focus on blocking the virus-receptor interaction. Most of these approaches might well efficiently block the binding and entry of virus into $CD4^+$ cells; however, it is likely that, in vivo, virus also spreads directly from cell to cell. This may proceed, in part, through gp120-CD4 interactions, but the efficiency by which cell-to-cell spread might be inhibitable is unknown. A second critical consideration relating to the practicality of inhibiting gp120-CD4 interaction as a therapeutic modality relates to the function of the CD4 molecule itself. If the epitopes of CD4 involved in binding to gp120 are the same as, or are sterically related to, the domains of CD4 responsible for its normal role in the immune response, any intervention directed at these sites may interfere with normal CD4 function. In a similar fashion, if the domains of gp120 that bind to CD4 sterically resemble the normal target of CD4 binding in the immune response, inhibition of T4 lymphocyte function might result, mimicking the disease of AIDS itself. For this reason, the use of purified CD4 protein to block HIV infection (107) may not be feasible.

Inhibition of fusion of the viral envelope with the cell membrane represents a potentially more specific means of therapeutic intervention. By analogy with other enveloped viruses, the amino terminus of the transmembrane protein, gp41, is likely to be crucial for this process. In paramyxovirus systems, antibodies against both the amino terminus of the transmembrane protein and peptides corresponding to this domain can inhibit viral infectivity and virally induced syncytia formation (75). The use of such a peptide derived from gp41 offers the intriguing possibility of inhibiting both viral spread and a major component of HIV cytotoxicity: syncytia formation. The recent demonstration that HIV fusion occurs via a pH-independent mechanism suggests that agents such as monensin (97) that block the endocytic uptake of some enveloped viruses (such as vesicular stomatitis virus) will not be effective against HIV. The observation that regions of the gp120 not directly involved in CD4 binding are still required for viral infectivity (R. Willey et al., in press) suggests that additional interactions between the *env* gene products and the cell membrane are required for viral internalization. The identification of any host cell proteins involved in these interactions would represent yet another potential target for the inhibition of viral uptake.

The most successful antiviral agents in HIV infection have been inhibitors of viral reverse transcription (step 3). Of particular value have been a class of nucleoside analogues known as dideoxynucleosides (6). The 2,3-dideoxynucleosides appear to be taken up by T lymphocytes and to undergo phosphorylation to generate 2,3-dideoxynucleoside 5′ triphosphates. These analogues can be utilized by reverse transcriptase and incorporated into an elongating DNA chain; however, the absence of a 3′ OH group on the sugar moiety prevents the formation of the subsequent 5′-3′ phosphodiester bond, resulting in premature chain termination. Retroviral reverse transcriptases appear to be more sensitive to dideoxynucleoside-induced chain termination than do host cell DNA polymerases, thus resulting in the therapeutic usefulness of these compounds. Two particular dideoxynucleosides that have shown clinical promise are 3′-azido, 3′-deoxythymidine (AZT) and 2,3-dideoxycytidine. These compounds can induce long-term inhibition of HIV replication in vitro (98). Of the two, AZT is now widely used in AIDS patients after the clear demonstration of its efficacy in prolonging lifespan in certain groups of AIDS and ARC patients (6). Detailed considerations of the properties of different dideoxynucleoside analogues have recently been reviewed

(6). With the success of these antiviral agents, it can be anticipated that many new inhibitors of reverse transcriptase will soon be evaluated for their therapeutic usefulness in AIDS. Interestingly, the presence of antibodies that inhibit RT catalytic activity has been correlated with improved clinical status, raising the possibility that induction of an anti-RT immune response may provide yet another therapeutic approach (99).

An intriguing target for intervention in HIV infection is the process of integration of proviral DNA (step 4). This process requires a virally specified enzyme, the endonuclease, and appears to be specific for retroviral infection. Thus, inhibition of the viral endonuclease would not be anticipated to interfere with cellular enzymatic activities resulting in a specific antiviral effect. No inhibitors of retroviral endonucleases are known, but the recent description of an in vitro model for the study of retroviral integration (24) provides a system for the assessment of potential inhibitors. However, the potential for replication of HIV without integration also exists.

The expression of HIV genes is dependent on RNA transcription (step 5), RNA processing (step 6), and translation into proteins (step 7). At each step, both cellular and viral factors appear to be involved. Antagonists of the viral gene products required for HIV gene expression could produce a highly specific antiviral effect; however, since the mechanisms of action of *tat* and *art/trs* are, at this time, very poorly understood, it is unlikely that specific inhibitors of these gene products will be readily identified. One known antiviral drug, ribavirin, appears to act through the inhibition of RNA processing. Ribavirin does inhibit HIV replication in vitro (100); however, its clinical efficacy has not yet been proved.

An alternative, specific approach to blocking HIV gene expression is the introduction into infected cells of anti-sense RNA molecules. Such anti-sense RNAs would be the complements of HIV RNAs and are proposed to hybridize to viral RNAs in infected cells, resulting in the inhibition of translation. Anti-sense nucleotides have been shown to have some inhibitory effects on HIV expression in vitro (101); however, it is highly questionable whether it would be clinically feasible to achieve the vast excesses of intracellular anti-sense RNA necessary to significantly inhibit translation.

Expression of HIV can be modulated in vitro by a number of lymphokines. Lymphocyte activation results in increased viral gene expression (102), and lymphokines can stimulate the expression of integrated HIV proviruses (103). Furthermore, treatment of the U937 promonocyte cell line with the lymphokines GM-CSF and γ interferon inhibits HIV replication in these cells (104). Thus, particular lymphokines or combinations of lymphokines may inhibit or enhance the expression of integrated HIV proviruses. Intracellular gene regulatory events can also "turn off" HIV expression. For example, DNA methylation has been shown to be associated with the spontaneous loss of activity of an HIV LTR in tissue culture cells (105).

Virion assembly (step 9) and release (step 10) involve the packaging of virion RNA molecules and processing of viral proteins. A particularly attractive target for antiviral therapy would be the virion-encoded protease responsible for the processing of *gag* and *pol* precursor proteins. The specificity of retroviral proteases suggests that their inhibition might be accomplished with little effect on normal cellular metabolism. Furthermore, much is known of the biochemistry of other proteases and their inhibitors, raising the possibility that this enzyme might be an excellent target for a program of rational drug design.

In summary, while each step in the HIV life cycle offers a potential target for antiviral therapy, certain points appear to be more amenable to intervention. Particularly encouraging is the already demonstrated success of reverse transcriptase inhibitors. In vitro studies suggest that disruption of virus-receptor binding may lead to effective antiviral therapy. Whether any of the other unique and less understood viral enzymes and regulatory molecules prove to be useful targets for inhibitors of HIV replication remains to be seen and will doubtless await further studies of their basic functional characteristics.

Acknowledgments

The author would like to thank Karen Weck for performing the CAT assays in Figure 4; A. S. Rabson, R. L. Kirschstein, and M. A. Martin for critical reading of the manuscript, and Brenda Marshall for editorial assistance.

References

1. Human Retrovirus Subcommittee, International Committee on the Taxonomy of Viruses. Human immunodeficiency viruses. Science 1986; 232:697.
2. Barré-Sinoussi F, Cherman JC, Rey R, Nugeryre MT, Chamaret S, Gruest J, Dauguet C, Axler-Blin C, Brun-Vézinet F, Rouzioux C, Rosenbaum W, Montagnier L. Isolation of a T-lymphotropic retrovirus from a patient at risk for acquired immune deficiency syndrome (AIDS). Science 1983; 220:868-71.
3. Popovic M, Sarngadharan MG, Read E, Gallo RC. Detection, isolation, and continuous production of cytopathic retroviruses (HTLV-III) from patients with AIDS and pre-AIDS. Science 1984; 224:497-500.
4. Levy JA, Hoffman AD, Kramer SM, Lanois JA, Shimabukuro JM, Oskiro LS. Isolation of lymphocytopathic retroviruses from San Francisco patients with AIDS. Science 1984; 225:840-2.
5. Fauci AS. Current issues in developing a strategy for dealing with the acquired immunodeficiency syndrome. Proc Natl Acad Sci USA 1986; 83:9278-83.
6. Mitsuya H, Broder S. Strategies for antiviral therapy in AIDS. Nature 1987; 325:773-8.

7. Pederson NC, Ho EW, Brown ML, Yamamoto JK. Isolation of a T-lymphotropic virus from domestic cats with an immunodeficiency-like syndrome. Science 1987; 235:790-3.
8. Sonigo P, Alizon M, Staskus K, Klatzmann D, Cole S, Danos O, Retzel E, Tiollais P, Haase A, Wain-Hobson S. Nucleotide sequence of the visna lentivirus: relationship to the AIDS virus. Cell 1985; 42:369-82.
9. Kanki PJ, McLane MF, King NW Jr, Letvin NL, Hunt RD, Sehgel P, Daniel MD, Desrosiers RC, Essex M. Serologic identification and characterization of a macaque T-lymphotropic retrovirus closely related to HTLV-III. Science 1985; 228:1199-201.
10. Daniel MD, Letvin NL, King NW, Kannagi M, Sehgal PK, Hunt RD, Kanki PJ, Essex M, Desrosiers RC. Isolation of T-cell tropic HTLV-III-like retrovirus from macaques. Science 1985; 228:1201-4.
11. Kanki PJ, Alroy J, Essex M. Isolation of T-lymphotropic retrovirus related to HTLV-III/LAV from wild-caught African green monkeys. Science 1985; 230: 951-4.
12. Kanki PJ, Barin F, M'Boup S, Allan JS, Romet-Lemoune JL, Marlink R, McLane MF, Lee T-H, Arbeille B, Denis F, Essex M. New human T-lymphotropic retrovirus related to simian T-lymphotropic virus type III (STLV-III AGM). Science 1986; 232:238-43.
13. Clavel F, Guétard D, Brun-Vézinet F, Chamaret S, Rey MA, Santos-Ferreira NO, Laurent AG, Dauget C, Katlama C, Rouzioux C, Klatzman D, Champalimaud JL, Montagnier L. Isolation of a new human retrovirus from West African patients with AIDS. Science 1986; 233:343-6.
14. Guyader M, Emerman M, Sonigo P, Clavel F, Montagnier L, Alizon M. Genome organization and transactivation of the human immunodeficiency virus type 2. Nature 1987; 326:662-9.
15. Hirsch V, Riedel N, Mullins JI. The genome organization of STLV-3 is similar to that of the AIDS virus except for a truncated transmembrane protein. Cell 1987; 49:307-19.
16. Robey WG, Safai B, Oroszlan S, Arthur LO, Gonda MA, Gallo RC, Fischinger PJ. Characterization of envelope and core structural gene products of HTLV-III with sera from AIDS patients. Science 1985; 228:593-5.
17. Allan JS, Coligan JE, Barin F, McLane MF, Sodroski JG, Rosen CA, Haseltine WA, Lee TH, Essex M. Major glycoprotein antigens that induce antibodies in AIDS patients are encoded by HTLV-III. Science 1985; 228:1091-4.
18. DiMarzo-Veronese F, DiVico AL, Copeland TD, Oroszlan S, Gallo RC, Sarngadharan MG. Characterization of gp41 as the transmembrane protein coded by the HTLV-III/LAV envelope gene. Science 1985; 229:1402-4.
19. Dalgleish AG, Beverley PCL, Clapham PR, Crawford DH, Greaves MF, Weiss RA. The CD4 (T4) antigen is an essential component of the receptor for the AIDS retrovirus. Nature 1984; 312:763-7.
20. Klatzman D, Champagne E, Chamaret S, Gruest J, Guétard D, Hercend T, Gluckman J-C, Montagnier L. T-lymphocyte T4 molecule behaves as the receptor for human retrovirus LAV. Nature 1984; 312:767-8.

21. McDougal JS, Kennedy MS, Sligh JM, Cort SP, Mawle A, Nicholson JKA. Binding of HTLV-III/LAV to T4$^+$ T cells by a complex of the 110K viral protein and the T4 molecule. Science 1986; 231:382-5.
22. Maddon PJ, Dalgleish AG, McDougal JS, Clapham PR, Weiss RA, Axel R. The T4 gene encodes the AIDS virus receptor and is expressed in the immune system and the brain. Cell 1986; 47:333-48.
23. Stein BS, Gowda SD, Lifson JD, Penhallow RC, Bensch KG, Engleman EG. pH-Independent HIV entry into CD4-positive T cells via virus envelope fusion to the plasma membrane. Cell 1987; 49:659-68.
24. Brown PO, Bowerman B, Varmus HE, Bishop JM. Correct integration of retroviral DNA in vitro. Cell 1987; 49:347-56.
25. Levy JA, Kaminsky LS, Morrow WJW, Steimer K, Luciw P, Dina D, Hoxie J, Oshiro L. Infection by the retrovirus associated with the acquired immunodeficiency syndrome. Ann Intern Med 1985; 103:694-9.
26. Panganiban AT. Retroviral DNA integration. Cell 1985; 42:5-6.
27. Wain-Hobson S, Sonigo P, Danos O, Cole S, Alizon M. Nucleotide sequence of the AIDS virus, LAV. Cell 1985; 40:9-17.
28. Ratner L, Haseltine W, Patarca R, Livak KJ, Starcich B, Jacobs SF, Doran ER, Rafalski JA, Whitehorn EA, Baumeister K, Ivanoff L, Petteway SR, Pearson ML. Lautenberger JA, Papas TS, Ghrayeb J, Chang NT, Gallo RC, Wong-Staal F. Complete nucleotide sequence of the AIDS virus HTLV-III. Nature 1985; 313:277-84.
29. Sanchez-Pescador R, Power MD, Barr PJ, Steimer KS, Stempien MM, Brown-Shimer SL, Gee WW, Ranard A, Randolph A, Levy JA, Dina D, Luciw PA. Nucleotide sequence and expression of the AIDS-associated retrovirus (ARV-2). Science 1985; 227:484-92.
30. Muesing MA, Smith DH, Cabradilla CD, Benton CV, Lasky LA, Capon DJ. Nucleic acid structure and expression of the human AIDS/lymphadenopathy retrovirus. Nature 1985; 313:430-58.
30a. Wong-Staal F, Chanda PK, Ghrayeb J. Human immunodeficiency virus: the eighth gene. AIDS Research and Human Retroviruses 1987; 3:33-9.
31. Rosen CA, Sodroski JG, Haseltine WA. The location of *cis*-acting regulatory sequences in the human T cell lymphotropic virus type III (HTLV-III/LAV) long terminal repeat. Cell 1985; 41:813-23.
32. Sen R, Baltimore D. Inducibility of κ immunoglobulin enhancer-binding protein NF-κB by a posttranslational mechanism. Cell 1986; 47:921-8.
33. Weiher H, Konig M, Gruss P. Multiple point mutations affecting the SV40 enhancer. Science 1983; 219:626-31.
34. Nabel G, Baltimore D. An inducible factor activates expression of human immunodeficiency virus in T cells. Nature 1987; 326:711-3.
35. Jones KA, Kadonaga JT, Luciw PA, Tjian R. Activation of the AIDS retrovirus promoter by the cellular transcription factor, SP1. Science 1986; 232: 755-9.
36. Muesing MA, Smith DH, Capon DJ. Regulation of mRNA accumulation by a human immunodeficiency virus *trans*-activator protein. Cell 1987; 48:691-701.

37. Watanabe S, Temin HM. Encapsidation sequences for spleen necrosis virus, an avian retrovirus, are between the 5′ long terminal repeat and the start of the *gag* gene. Proc Natl Acad Sci USA 1982; 79:5986-90.
38. Mann R, Mulligan RC, Baltimore D. Construction of a retrovirus packaging mutant and its use to produce helper-free defective retrovirus. Cell 1983; 33: 153-9.
39. Rabson AB, Daugherty DF, Venkatesan S, Boulukos KE, Benn SI, Folks TM, Feorino P, Martin MA. Transcription of novel open reading frames of AIDS retrovirus during infection of lymphocytes. Science 1985; 229:1388-90.
40. Kramer RA, Schaber MD, Skalka AM, Ganguly K, Wong-Staal F, Reddy EP. HTLV-III *gag* protein is processed in yeast cells by the virus *pol*-protease. Science 1986; 231:1580-4.
41. Oroszlan S, Copeland TD, Kalyanaraman VS, Sarngadharan MG, Schultz AM, Gallo RC. Chemical analysis of human T-cell leukemia virus structural proteins. In: Gallo RC, Essex ME, Gross L, eds. Human T-cell leukemia/lymphoma virus. Cold Spring Harbor, New York: Cold Spring Harbor Laboratory, 1984:101-10.
42. Schultz AM, Oroszlan S. In vivo modification of retroviral *gag* gene-encoded polyproteins by myristic acid. J Virol 1983; 46:355-61.
43. Jacks T, Varmus HE. Expression of the Rous sarcoma virus *pol* gene by ribosomal frameshifting. Science 1985; 230:1237-42.
44. DiMarzo-Veronese F, Copeland TD, DeVico AL, Rahman R, Oroszlan S, Gallo RC, Sarngadharan MG. Characterization of highly immunogenic p66/p51 as the reverse transcriptase of HTLV-III/LAV. Science 1986; 231:1289-91.
45. Lightfoote MM, Coligan JE, Folks TM, Fauci AS, Martin MA, Venkatesan S. Structural characterization of reverse transcriptase and endonuclease polypeptides of the acquired immunodeficiency syndrome retrovirus. J Virol 1986; 60: 771-5.
46. Larder BA, Purifoy DJM, Powell KL, Darby G. Site-specific mutagenesis of AIDS virus reverse transcriptase. Nature 1987; 327:716-7.
47. Steimer KS, Higgins KW, Powers MA, Stephens JC, Gyenes A, George-Nascimento C, Luciw PA, Barr PJ, Hallewell RA, Sanchez-Pescador R. Recombinant polypeptide from the endonuclease region of acquired immune deficiency syndrome retrovirus polymerase (*pol*) gene detects serum antibodies in most infected individuals. J Virol 1986; 58:9-16.
48. Rabson AB, Martin MA. Molecular organization of the AIDS retrovirus. Cell 1985; 40:477-80.
49. Lee T-H, Coligan JE, Allan JS, McLane MF, Groopman JE, Essex M. A new HTLV III/LAV protein encoded by a gene found in cytopathic retroviruses. Science 1986; 231:1546-9.
50. Kan NC, Franchini G, Wong-Staal F, DuBois GC, Robey WG, Lautenberger JA, Papas TS. Identification of the HTLV III/LAV *sor* gene product and detection of antibodies in human sera. Science 1986; 231:1553-5.
51. Sodroski J, Goh WC, Rosen C, Tartar A, Portetelle D, Burny A, Haseltine W. Replicative and cytopathic potential of HTLV III/LAV with *sor* gene deletions. Science 1986; 231:1549-53.

52. Strebel K, Daugherty D, Clouse K, Cohen D, Folks T, Martin MA. The HIV "A" (*sor*) gene product is essential for viral infectivity. Nature 1987; 328: 728-30.
53. Fisher AG, Ensoli B, Ivanoff L, Chamberlain M, Petteway S, Ratner L, Gallo RC, Wong-Staal F. The *sor* gene of HIV-1 is required for efficient virus transmission in vitro. Science 1987; 238:888-93.
54. Goh WC, Rosen C, Sodroski J, Ho DD, Haseltine WA. Identification of a protein encoded by the *trans*-activator gene tat III of human T-Cell lymphotropic retrovirus type III. J Virol 1986; 59:181-4.
55. Wright CM, Felber BK, Paskalis H, Pavlakis GN. Expression and characterization of the *trans*-activator of HTLV-III/LAV virus. Science 1986; 234:998-92.
56. Arya SK, Guo C, Josephs SF, Wong-Staal F. *Trans*-activator gene of human T-lymphotropic virus type III (HTLV-III). Science 1985; 229:69-73.
57. Sodroski J, Patarca R, Rosen C, Wong-Staal F, Haseltine W. Location of the *trans*-activating region on the genome of human T-cell lymphotropic virus type III. Science 1985; 229:74-7.
58. Gorman C, Moffat L, Howard B. Recombinant genomes which express chloramphenicol acetyltransferase in mammalian cells. Mol Cell Biol 1982; 2:1044-51.
59. Gendelman HE, Phelps W, Feigenbaum L, Ostrove JM, Adachi A, Howley PM, Khoury G, Ginsberg HS, Martin MA. *Trans*-activation of the human immunodeficiency virus long terminal repeat sequence by DNA viruses. Proc Natl Acad Sci USA 1986; 83:9759-63.
60. Cullen BR. *Trans*-activation of human immunodeficiency virus occurs via a bimodal mechanism. Cell 1986; 46:973-82.
61. Peterlin BM, Luciw PA, Barr PJ, Walka MD. Elevated levels of mRNA can account for the *trans*-activation of human immunodeficiency virus. Proc Natl Acad Sci USA 1986; 83:9734-8.
62. Muesing MA, Smith DH, Capon DJ. Regulation of mRNA accumulation by a human immunodeficiency virus *trans*-activator protein. Cell 1987; 48:691-701.
63. Kao S-Y, Calman A, Luciw PA, Peterlin BM. Anti-termination of transcription within the long terminal repeat of HIV-1 by *tat* gene product. Nature 1987; 330: 489-93.
64. Okamoto T, Wong-Staal F. Demonstration of virus-specific transcriptional activator(s) in cells infected with HTLV-III by an in vitro cell-free system. Cell 1986; 47:29-35.
65. Berg J. Potential metal binding domains in nucleic acid binding proteins. Science 1986; 232:485-7.
66. Rosen CA, Sodroski JG, Goh WC, Dayton AI, Lippke J, Haseltine WA. Post-transcriptional regulation accounts for the *trans*-activation of the human T-lymphotropic virus type III. Nature 1986; 319:555-9.
67. Feinberg MB, Jarrett RF, Aldovini A, Gallo RC, Wong-Staal F. HTLV-III expression and production involve complex regulation at the levels of splicing and translation of viral RNA. Cell 1986; 46:807-17.
68. Fisher AG, Feinberg MB, Josephs SF, Harper ME, Marselle LM, Reyes G, Gonda MA, Aldovini A, Debouk C, Gallo RC, Wong-Staal F. The *trans*-activator gene of HTLV-III is essential for virus replication. Nature 1986; 320:367-71.

69. Dayton AI, Sodroski JG, Rosen CA, Goh WC, Haseltine WA. The *trans*-activator gene of the human T cell lymphotropic virus type III is required for replication. Cell 1986; 44:941-7.
70. Sodroski JG, Goh WC, Rosen C, Dayton A, Terwilliger E, Haseltine W. A second post-transcriptional *trans*-activator gene required for HTLV-III replication. Nature 1986: 321:412-7.
71. Goh WC, Sodroski JG, Rosen CA, Haseltine WA. Expression of the *art* gene protein of human lymphotropic virus type III (HTLV-III) in bacteria. J Virol 1987; 61:633-7.
72. Knight DM, Flomerfelt FA, Ghrayeb J. Expression of the art/trs protein of HIV and study of its role in viral envelope synthesis. Science 1987; 236:837-40.
73. Lasky LA, Nakamura G, Smith DH, Fennie C, Shimaski C, Patzer E, Berman P, Gregory T, Capon DJ. Delineation of a region of the human immunodeficiency virus type 1 gp120 glycoprotein critical for interaction with the CD4 receptor. Cell 1987; 50:975-85.
74. Kowalski M, Potz J, Basiripour L, Dorfman T, Goh WC, Terwilliger E, Dayton A, Rosen C, Haseltine W, Sodroski J. Functional regions of the envelope glycoprotein of human immunodeficiency virus type 1. Science 1987; 237:1351-5.
75. Choppin PW, Scheid A. The role of viral glycoproteins in adsorption, penetration, and pathogenicity of viruses. Rev Infect Dis 1980; 2:40-61.
76. Sodroski J, Goh WC, Rosen C, Campbell K, Haseltine WA. Role of the HTLV-III/LAV envelope in syncytium formation and cytopathicity. Nature 1986; 322: 470-4.
77. Lifson JD, Feinberg MB, Reyes GR, Rabin L, Banapour B, Chakrabarti S, Moss B, Wong-Staal F, Steimer KS, Engleman E. Induction of CD4-dependent cell fusion by the HTLV-III/LAV envelope glycoprotein. Nature 1986; 323: 725-8.
78. Fisher AG, Ratner L, Mitsuya H, Marselle LM, Harper ME, Broder S, Gallo RC, Wong-Staal F. Infectious mutants of HTLV-III with changes in the 3′ region and markedly reduced cytopathic effects. Science 1986; 233:655-9.
79. Alizon M, Wain-Hobson S, Montagnier L, Sonigo P. Genetic variability of the AIDS virus: nucleotide sequence analysis of two isolates from African patients. Cell 1986; 46:63-74.
80. Starcich BR, Hahn BH, Shaw GM, McNeely PD, Modrow S, Wolf H, Parks ES, Parks WP, Josephs SF, Gallo RC, Wong-Staal F. Identification and characterization of conserved and variable regions in the envelope gene of HTLV-III/LAV, the retrovirus of AIDS. Cell 1986; 45:637-48.
81. Willey RL, Rutledge RA, Dias S, Folks T, Theodore T, Buckler CE, Martin MA. Identification of conserved and divergent domains within the envelope genes of the acquired immunodeficiency syndrome retrovirus. Proc Natl Acad Sci USA 1986; 83:5038-42.
82. Desai SM, Kalyanaraman VS, Casey JM, Srinivasan A, Anderson PR, Devare SG. Molecular cloning and primary nucleotide sequence analysis of a distinct human immunodeficiency virus isolate reveal significant divergence in its genomic sequences. Proc Natl Acad Sci USA 1986; 83:8380-4.
83. Hahn BH, Shaw GM, Taylor ME, Redfield RR, Markham PD, Saluhuddin SZ, Wong-Staal F, Gallo RC, Parks ES, Parks WP. Genetic variation in HTLV-III/

LAV over time in patients with AIDS or at risk for AIDS. Science 1986; 232: 1548-53.

84. Crowl R, Ganguly K, Gordon M, Conroy R, Schaber M, Kramer R, Shaw G, Wong-Staal F, Reddy EP. HTLV-III *env* gene products synthesized in *E. coli* are recognized by antibodies present in AIDS patients. Cell 1986; 41:979-86.
85. Putney SD, Matthews TJ, Robey WG, Lynn DL, Robert-Guroff M, Mueller WT, Langlois AJ, Ghrayeb J, Petteway SR Jr, Weinkuld KJ, Fishinger PJ, Wong-Staal F, Gallo RC, Bolognesi DP. HTLV-III/LAV-neutralizing antibodies to an *E. coli*-produced fragment of the virus envelope. Science 1986; 234: 1392-5.
86. Cease KB, Margalit H, Cornette JL, Putney SD, Robey WG, Ouyang C, Streicher HZ, Fischinger PJ, Gallo RC, DeLisi C, Berzofsky JA. Helper T-cell antigenic site identification in the acquired immunodeficiency syndrome virus gp120 envelope protein and induction of immunity in mice to the native protein using a 16-residue synthetic peptide. Proc Natl Acad Sci USA 1987; 84:4249-53.
87. Allan JS, Coligan JE, Lee TH, McLane MF, Kanki PJ, Groopman JE, Essex M. A new HTLV-III/LAV encoded antigen detected by antibodies from AIDS patients. Science 1985; 230:810-3.
88. Franchini G, Robert-Guroff M, Ghrayeb J, Chang NT, Wong-Staal F. Cytoplasmic localization of the HTLV-III *3′ orf* protein in cultured T cells. Virology 1986; 155:593-9.
89. Terwilliger E, Sodroski JG, Rosen CA, Haseltine WA. Effects of mutation within the 3′ *orf* open reading frame of human T-cell lymphotropic virus type III (HTLV-III/LAV) on replication and cytopathogenicity. J Virol 1986; 60:754-60.
90. Luciw PA, Cheng-Mayer C, Levy JA. Mutational analysis of the human immunodeficiency virus: the *orf*-B region down regulates virus replication. Proc Natl Acad Sci USA 1987; 84:1434-8.
91. Guy B, Kieny MP, Riviere Y, Le Peuch C, Dott K, Girard M, Montagnier L, Lecocq J-P. HIV F/3′ *orf* encodes a phosphorylated GTP-binding protein resembling an oncogene product. Nature 1987; 330:266-9.
92. McDougal JS, Nicholson JKA, Cross DG, Cort SP, Kennedy SM, Mawle AC. Binding of the human retrovirus HTLV-III/LAV/ARV/HIV to the CD4 (T4) molecule: conformation dependence, epitope mapping, antibody inhibition, and potential for idiotypic mimicry. J Immunol 1986; 137:2937-44.
93. Sattentau QJ, Dalgleish AG, Weiss RA, Beverly PCL. Epitopes of the CD4 antigen and HIV infection. Science 1986; 234:1120-3.
94. Weiss RA, Clapham PR, Cheingsong-Popov R, Dalgleish AG, Carne CA, Weller IVD, Tedder RS. Neutralization of human T-lymphotropic virus type III by sera of AIDS and AIDS-risk patients. Nature 1985; 316:69-73.
95. Matthews TJ, Langlois AJ, Robey WG, Chang NT, Gallo RC, Fischinger PJ, Bolognesi DP. Restricted neutralization of divergent human T-lymphotropic virus type III isolates by antibodies to the major envelope glycoprotein. Proc Natl Acad Sci USA 1986; 83:9709-13.
96. Weiss RA, Clapham PR, Weber JN, Dalgleish AG, Lasky LA, Berman PW. Variable and conserved neutralization antigens of human immunodeficiency virus. Nature 1986; 324:572-5.

97. Schlegal R, Willingham MC, Pastan I. Monesin blocks endocytosis of vesicular stomatisis virus. Biochem Biophys Res Commun 1981; 102:992-8.
98. Mitsuya H, Jarret RF, Matsukura M, DiMarzo Veronese F, DeVico AL, Sarngadharan MG, Johns DG, Reitz MS, Broder S. Long-term inhibition of human T-lymphotropic virus type III/lymphadenopathy-associated virus (human immunodeficiency virus) DNA synthesis and RNA expression in T cells protected by 2′3′-dideoxynucleosides *in vitro*. Proc Natl Acad Sci USA 1987; 84: 2033-7.
99. Laurence J, Saunders A, Kulkosky J. Characterization and clinical association of antibody inhibitory to HIV reverse transcriptase activity. Science 1987; 235: 1501-4.
100. McCormick JB, Getchell JP, Mitchell SW, Hicks DR. Ribavirin suppresses replication of lymphadenopathy associated virus in cultures of human adult T-lymphocytes. Lancet 1984; 2:1367-9.
101. Zamecnik PC, Goodchild J, Taguchi Y, Sarin PS. Inhibition of replication and expression of human T-cell lymphotropic virus type III in cultured cells by exogenous synthetic oligonucleotide complementary to viral RNA. Proc Natl Acad Sci USA 1986; 83:4143-6.
102. Zagury D, Bernard J, Leonard R, Cheynier R, Feldman M, Sarin P, Gallo RC. Long term cultures of HTLV-III-infected T cells: a model of cytopathology of T cell depletion in AIDS. Science 1986; 231:850-3.
103. Folks TM, Justement J, Kinter A, Dinarello CA, Fauci AS. Cytokine-induced expression of HIV in a chronically infected promonocyte cell line. Science 1987; 238:800-2.
104. Hammer SM, Gillis JM, Groopman JE, Rose RM. In vitro modification of human immunodeficiency virus infection by granulocyte-macrophage colony-stimulating factor and γ interferon. Proc Natl Acad Sci USA 1986; 83:8734-8.
105. Bednarik DP, Mosca JD, Raj NBK. Methylation as a modulator of expression of human immunodeficiency virus. J Virol 1987; 61:1253-7.
106. Willey RL, Smith DH, Lasky LA, et al. In vitro mutagenesis identifies a region within the envelope gene of the human immunodeficiency virus that is critical for infectivity. J Virol 1988; 62:139-47.
107. Weiss RA. Receptor molecule blocks HIV. Nature 1988; 331:15.

10

Immunological Effects of HIV Infection

John F. Krowka, Dewey J. Moody,* and Daniel P. Stites

School of Medicine
University of California
San Francisco, California

I. Introduction

The human immunodeficiency virus (HIV) affects the immune system at many different levels. Its direct inhibitory effects on cells of the immune system, particularly its cytopathic effects on helper T lymphocytes and macrophages expressing the CD4[†] differentiation antigen, play a central role in the pathogenesis of acquired immunodeficiency syndrome (AIDS) and AIDS-related conditions (ARC) (1,2). The plethora of immunological abnormalities observed in HIV-infected individuals are, however, difficult, if not impossible, to reconcile exclusively with direct effects of HIV on CD4-bearing cells. The relationships between many of the immunological abnormalities in HIV-infected individuals and disease are not known.

In contrast to the inhibitory effects of HIV, its ability to stimulate some types of antibody, cytokine, or cytotoxic lymphocyte responses may be beneficial to the infected individual. The existence of some HIV-infected individuals

---

**Current affiliation*: Applied ImmuneSciences, Menlo Park, California.
†CD, cluster of differentiation antigens expressed on leukocyte subpopulations (see Refs. 5 and 6).

who remain asymptomatic for relatively long periods of time suggests that immune responses may control the pathogenic effects of HIV to some degree. Appropriate immune responses to HIV constitute crucial host factors that influence the outcome of infection, but the nature of these antiviral responses are unclear. Effective strategies to prevent or treat HIV infection will require consideration of inhibitory and stimulatory effects of HIV, both direct and indirect, on the many phenotypically and functionally distinct cell types of the immune system.

In the following review we discuss the effects of HIV infection on the immune system. Initially, an outline of the elements and function of the immune system is presented. Then, separate consideration is given to alterations in both *numbers* and *functions* of T lymphocytes, B lymphocytes, macrophages, natural killer (NK) cells, and lymphokines. We also address the hypothesis that autoimmunity directed at the immune system can influence pathogenesis of AIDS and related conditions. Clearly, our knowledge of AIDS is at this point incomplete. New information in this area will hopefully facilitate development of both effective therapeutic and prophylactic strategies.

II. Overview of the Immune System

Immunological responses to infection by HIV might be expected to follow reasonably well-established patterns of antigen processing, T cell-macrophage, T cell-B cell, and T cell-T cell interactions that result in the induction of regulatory and effector T cells and the production of antibodies and lymphokines (3,4). The AIDS virus (HIV) itself, however, perturbs cells of the immune system, particularly those bearing the CD4 marker with subsequent disruption of normal immunoregulatory mechanisms at many levels. A summary of the phenotypes and functions of the major cellular elements of the immune system is presented in Table 1.

III. HIV and T Lymphocytes

A. Effects of HIV on Helper ($CD4^+$) T Lymphocytes

Phenotypical Changes

Soon after the initial report of AIDS (8), a striking association was observed between defects in cellular immunity, subnormal T-lymphocyte helper-to-suppressor ratios ($CD4^+/CD8^+$), and subnormal absolute numbers or percentages of $CD4^+$ lymphocytes in patients with persistent generalized lymphadenopathy (PGL) or AIDS (9-12). Highly significant reductions in the percentages of peripheral blood $CD4^+$ lymphocytes and in the $CD4^+/CD8^+$

Table 1 Laboratory Detection of Immunocytes by Phenotypical and Functional Analysis[a]

Immune cell population	Phenotyping assays	Functional assays
T cells	$CD2^+$ (T11, Leu 5) $CD3^+$ (T3, Leu 4)	Responses to mitogens such as Con A or PHA (see specific subtype)
T helper/inducer cells	$CD4^+$ (T4, Leu 3)	Induction of cell-mediated or antibody responses
T helper	$CD4^+$ $CD45R^-$ (2H4, Leu 8, TQ1) $CDw29^+$ (4B4)	Augmentation of Ig synthesis, IL-2 production
T suppressor/inducer	$CD4^+$ $CD45R^+$ $CDw29^-$	Induction of CD8 cells to suppress Ig synthesis
T suppressor/cytotoxic cells	$CD8^+$ (T8, Leu 2)	Suppression of immune responses or lysis of target cells
T suppressor	$CD3^+$ $CD11b^+$ $OKM1^+$ 9.3^-	Suppression of Ig synthesis
T cytotoxic	$CD8^+$ $CD11b^-$ $OKM1^-$ 9.3^+	Cytotoxicity restricted by MHC antigens
B cells	$B1^+$ $B4^+$ Leu 12^+ Surface Ig^+	Differentiation into plasma cells which produce antibodies
Monocyte-macrophages	Leu $M3^+$ $Mo1^+$ Nonspecific $esterase^+$	Phagocytosis of particles production of IL-1
NK cells	$CD16^+$ (Leu 11) $NKH1^+$ Some HNK $(Leu\ 7)^+$	Killing of tumor cells (particularly K562) in MHC nonrestricted fashion

[a]The phenotypical characteristics of cells were identified by immunofluorescence with monoclonal antibodies (5,6). Functional assays are described in Ref. 7.

Table 2 Comparison of T Lymphocytes and Helper T Lymphocytes in Study Subjects[a]

Lymphocyte subset	Percentage of lymphocytes				
	HIV[-b] heterosexual asymptomatic $n^d = 54$	HIV[-] homosexual asymptomatic n = 63	HIV[+c] homosexual asymptomatic n = 24	HIV[+] homosexual LAS n = 20	HIV[+] homosexual AIDS n = 43
T lymphocytes	64.2	58.9	58.8	65.3	61.0
$CD4^+$[e]	44.3	38.6	26.6[g]	24.1	18.4
$CD4^+$ HLA-DR^+	5.1	4.3	4.6	3.7	4.2
$CD4^+ \kappa\lambda^+$[f]	3.8	3.9	4.5	4.2	3.7
$CD4^+/CD8^+$ ratio	1.8	1.7	0.8[g]	0.6	0.4

[a]See Refs. 13 and 14.
[b]HIV antibody-negative.
[c]HIV antibody-positive.
[d]Number of study subjects.
[e]Cluster of differentiation antigen (see Refs. 5 and 6).
[f]$CD4^+$ cells bearing kappa and lambda chains of immunoglobulin.
[g]The value in this column and in those to its right are significantly different ($p < 0.005$) from the column to the left.

ratios are also observed in asymptomatic HIV antibody-positive individuals in comparison to HIV antibody-negative homosexual or heterosexual males (Table 2 and Refs. 8-17). Subnormal numbers of leukocytes, total lymphocytes, or T cells are frequently observed in AIDS, although reductions in these parameters are not characteristic of less severe manifestations of HIV infections (Table 2 and Refs. 8-17). Reductions in the percentages of $CD4^+$ lymphocytes in the interfollicular and mantle areas of lymph nodes from LAS and AIDS patients have also been reported (18-21). Finally, analysis of lymphocyte subsets in intestinal mucosa also reveal a decrease in the percentage of $CD4^+$ lymphocytes in HIV-infected individuals (22). These studies and others demonstrating subnormal absolute numbers of $CD4^+$ blood lymphocytes in asymptomatic HIV-infected individuals and patients with PGL, ARC, or AIDS (15-17,23-25) clearly illustrate the systemic destructive effects of HIV infection on $CD4^+$ cells in vivo.

During acute HIV infection, however, absolute numbers of $CD4^+$ lymphocytes are not characteristically decreased although the $CD4^+/CD8^+$ ratio may be reduced due to elevation in $CD8^+$ cells (26,27). This pattern is similar to that seen after experimental infection of chimpanzees with lymphadenopathy-associated virus (LAV) (28). Infection with viruses other than HIV such as cytomegalovirus (CMV), hepatitis B virus (HBV), Herpes simplex virus (HSV), or Epstein-Barr Virus (EBV) may also result in transient increases in $CD8^+$ cells with relative decreases in $CD4^+$ cells or $CD4^+/CD8^+$

ratios (29-34). Direct or indirect cytopathic effects of these viruses on CD4$^+$ lymphocytes as well as adaptive responses of CD8$^+$ cytotoxic cells may contribute to these phenotypical abnormalities which are also characteristic of HIV infection.

All subsets of CD4$^+$ lymphocytes are not reduced to the same degree in all HIV-infected individuals. The percentages of activated or immature (HLA DR$^+$) and immunoglobulin-bearing ($\kappa\lambda^+$) CD4$^+$ lymphocytes do not differ substantially from HIV antibody-negative homosexual or heterosexual males and asymptomatic HIV-infected males, and LAS or AIDS patients (Table 2). It is unclear whether the suppressor-inducer subset of CD4$^+$ lymphocytes, defined by the coexpression of CD45R (TQ1, Leu 8, or 2H4; see Table 1 and Refs. 35, 36), is selectively reduced in the peripheral blood of LAS patients (25,37). In AIDS patients, both this suppressor-inducer (CD4$^+$ CD45R$^+$) and the helper-inducer subsets (CD4$^+$ CDw29$^+$) of peripheral blood T cells are decreased (25). Decreases in CD4$^+$ CD45R$^+$ cells in the paracortical areas of lymph nodes from AIDS patients have also been reported (21). It is presently unclear if defects in suppressor-inducer CD4$^+$ cells may contribute to the hypergammaglobulinemia which is associated with HIV infections (12, 15). (See Section IV.) Finally, reductions in the percentages of CD4$^+$ cells that coexpress HB10 have also been reported in AIDS patients (38). The CD4$^+$ HB10$^+$ subset appears to represent resting helper cells but not activated or memory T cells (38). The relationships between these abnormalities of CD4$^+$ lymphocyte subsets and disease progression is not clear. In AIDS all subsets of CD4$^+$ cells are eliminated or functionally incapacitated in an apparently indiscriminate manner by HIV.

It is clear that reductions in CD4$^+$ lymphocytes are strongly associated with HIV infection (12-17). On an individual patient basis, however, an association of phenotypical abnormalities and disease cannot be assumed since considerable heterogeneity with regard to CD4$^+$ cell numbers and CD4$^+$/CD8$^+$ ratios exist in HIV-infected individuals at all stages of the clinical spectrum including AIDS (8-17,39-42). For example, some asymptomatic HIV-infected individuals have very low numbers of CD4$^+$ cells and patients with AIDS may have only slightly subnormal CD4$^+$/CD8$^+$ ratios. These parameters are especially variable among pediatric and hemophiliac patients (39-42).

The etiologic association of HIV with AIDS and the identification of its effects on CD4$^+$ cells provided a framework for understanding both the pathogenetic mechanisms and relationship of HIV to the reductions in CD4$^+$ cells in infected individuals (43-50). In vitro culture systems for HIV demonstrated the replication and direct cytopathic effects of these retroviruses in CD4$^+$ but *not* in CD8$^+$ cells (45,49,50). Further studies indicated that the CD4 molecule is a major receptor for HIV (51,52). Interactions between the envelope glycoprotein (gp120) of HIV and CD4 are involved in the binding of HIV to helper T cells, the formation of multinucleated giant cells, and eventual cell death (53-60). In addition to lysis of $CD4^+$ cells, HIV contributes to the observed phenotypical abnormalities in HIV-infected patients (Table 2) by its ability to drastically reduce CD4 expression in infected cells (59,60).

Functional Changes

Many functional responses associated with helper T lymphocytes are inhibited in HIV infections. These abnormalities may reflect the destruction of $CD4^+$ cells, reduction in interleukin 2 (IL-2) production (see Section VII), or other effects of HIV. Proliferation of lymphocytes in response to concanavalin A (Con A), phytohemagglutinin (PHA), or pokeweed mitogen (PWM) are subnormal in many HIV-infected individuals, particularly in AIDS patients (12,15,17,39,61-66). These mitogens affect both $CD4^+$ and $CD8^+$ cells (67). In comparison to healthy control subjects, substantial reductions in proliferative responses to mitogens by lymphocytes from HIV-infected asymptomatic individuals or patients with LAS have been observed in some studies but not in others (12,15,17,66). No correlation is observed between PHA responses and lymphocyte subset distribution (65). Mitogen responses of separated $CD4^+$ lymphocytes exhibit variability among HIV-seropositive or -seronegative individuals (64,67). Proliferative responses in mixed lymphocyte cultures are also variable among these two groups of individuals although reductions in these responses are frequently observed in AIDS (61,64). The reasons for hyporesponsiveness in some individuals is not known. In general, responses to mitogens or alloantigens are not reliable indices of HIV infection or disease.

In contrast to the variability of responses to mitogens or alloantigens, lymphocytes from AIDS patients consistently show severely reduced ability to proliferate in response to soluble antigens such as keyhole limpet hemacyanin (KLH), tetanus toxoid, or CMV (17,22,64,68). Figure 1 compares the proliferative responses to CMV of HIV antibody-positive and antibody-negative individuals classified with respect to their exposure to CMV and their clinical status. The lymphocytes from healthy individuals who have never been sensitized to either virus fail to proliferate in response to CMV as expected. All healthy HIV-seronegative, CMV-seropositive individuals, in contrast, exhibit significant ($p < 0.001$) proliferation of their lymphocytes in response to CMV. Other studies also demonstrate that most or all healthy CMV-seropositive individuals exhibit T-cell proliferative responses to CMV (69). Lymphocytes from many HIV-infected individuals who have been exposed to CMV as determined by serological analysis, fail to proliferate in response to CMV. All AIDS patients tested demonstrate complete anergy in this antigen-driven test system. Some healthy HIV-seropositive individuals

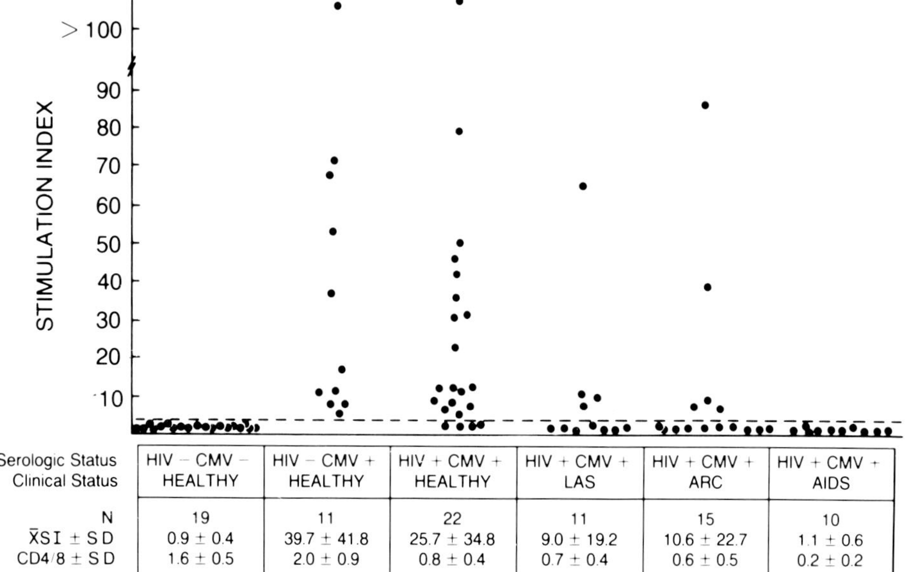

Serologic Status / Clinical Status	HIV − CMV − HEALTHY	HIV − CMV + HEALTHY	HIV + CMV + HEALTHY	HIV + CMV + LAS	HIV + CMV + ARC	HIV + CMV + AIDS
N	19	11	22	11	15	10
$\bar{X}$SI ± SD	0.9 ± 0.4	39.7 ± 41.8	25.7 ± 34.8	9.0 ± 19.2	10.6 ± 22.7	1.1 ± 0.6
CD4/8 ± SD	1.6 ± 0.5	2.0 ± 0.9	0.8 ± 0.4	0.7 ± 0.4	0.6 ± 0.5	0.2 ± 0.2

Figure 1 Lymphocyte proliferation responses to cytomegalovirus. Peripheral blood mononuclear cells (1×10^5) were cultured for 7 days with optimal concentration of UV-inactivated AD169 CMV, generously provided by Dr. John Mills (San Francisco General Hospital). Stimulation indexes (SI) were calculated by dividing the mean ($\bar{X}$) counts per minute of [^{3}H]thymidine incorporated by PBMC cultured with CMV by the $\bar{X}$ counts per minute incorporated by PBMC cultured without antigen. Antibodies to HIV were determined by a commercial ELISA (Abbott Laboratories, N. Chicago, Ill.). Antibodies to CMV were detected by a latex agglutination method (71). The CD4/8 ratios (% Leu 3^+/% Leu 2^+) were determined as described previously (13,14).

and many patients with PGL or ARC also are anergic in their proliferative responses to CMV. These studies indicate that defects in antigen-driven proliferative responses are characteristic of AIDS but may also be observed in other HIV-infected individuals. The ability to induce or augment proliferative responses to CMV in most HIV-infected individuals by the addition of IL-2 suggests that defects related to IL-2 production may play a fundamental role in these deficiencies of lymphocyte proliferative responses (70). Statistical analysis revealed that neither the percentage of $CD4^+$ cells nor the $CD4^+/CD8^+$ ratio or HIV antigen levels correlated highly with proliferative responses to CMV (70).

Studies by Lane and his colleagues (64) demonstrated that both unfractionated peripheral blood mononuclear cells (PBMC) and positively selected $CD4^+$ cells from AIDS patients were unable to proliferate significantly in response to tetanus toxoid. Whether this defect is due to HIV infection of the $CD4^+$ cells or results from other effects of HIV is unclear. A variety of other functional defects related to helper T lymphocytes has been reported in HIV-seropositive individuals, particularly AIDS patients. Deficiencies in the ability of T cells to help antibody responses both in vivo and in vitro have been reported (10,64). These helper defects appear somewhat paradoxical in conjunction with polyclonally elevated levels of immunoglobulins associated with HIV infections (12,15,62). The direct polyclonal activation of B lymphocytes by HIV or EBV may explain this phenomenon at least in part (72-74). Abnormalities in helper T cells that are required for the induction of cytotoxic T lymphocytes (CTL) are also likely to exist although not yet demonstrated.

Not all $CD4^+$ cells are classic "helpers" and some $CD4^+$ CTL have been demonstrated (75). The direct or indirect effects of HIV on $CD4^+$ CTL remain to be defined although it is likely that $CD4^+$ CTL can be infected by HIV. Defects in delayed-type hypersensitivity (DTH) responses that also require the participation of helper T cells (76) are characteristic of AIDS but also occur in other groups of HIV-infected individuals (17). Moreover, impairments in the ability of HIV-infected individuals to produce or respond to lymphokines associated with $CD4^+$ cells have been demonstrated (76-81) (see Section VII). Finally, defects in the potential for clonal expansion of both $CD4^+$ and $CD8^+$ cells from LAS or AIDS patients have also been reported (82,83). These studies demonstrate a wide variety of functional defects in helper T lymphocytes in HIV-infected individuals at all stages of the clinical spectrum.

In addition to infection and lysis of $CD4^+$ cells, direct functional impairment of these $CD4^+$ cells by HIV may occur by a variety of mechanisms. Crude supernatants from HIV-infected H9 cells and semipurified preparations of HIV can inhibit proliferative responses to mitogens, soluble antigens, or alloantigens in vitro (72,84,85). Recently it has been demonstrated that recombinant HIV envelope protein (gp120) and gp120 purified from disrupted HIV are immunosuppressive in vitro (70,86,87). Preliminary studies indicate that gp120 must be glycosylated to exert these immunosuppressive effects (unpublished observations). The binding of gp120 to CD4 may sterically inhibit molecular interactions involved in cellular activation in a manner analogous to inhibition by anti-CD4 antibodies (88,89). It has been suggested that CD4 may function as a negative signal receptor (90), and binding of gp120, which is shed from infected cells (91,92) to CD4, may inhibit some immune responses in this manner. Epitopes of HIV envelope glycoprotein gp41, which are homologous to functionally important regions of IL-2, may compete with IL-2 for its receptor or induce antibodies that inactivate IL-2 (93,94). Although the in vivo effects of gp120 are not known, the results of in vitro studies (70,86,87) indicate that at least HIV proteins gp120 can interfere with immune functions in the absence of cellular infection by HIV. These findings raise important considerations for the development of vaccines and therapy.

In addition to direct inhibitory effects of HIV on $CD4^+$ cells, HIV may indirectly affect their function through its effects on other cell types such as macrophages (95,96) that present nominal antigens in an HLA-restricted context to helper T cells (*vide infra*—Section V). It is not known if blocking antibodies, suppressor cells, or suppressor factors may also contribute to these immunologic deficits (97). As will be discussed in Section VIII, the role of autoimmune phenomena in these abnormalities also merits further consideration.

Because helper T lymphocytes are required for the induction and regulation of both antibody and cell-mediated responses (3,4,76,98,99), the tropism and cytopathic effects of HIV on $CD4^+$ lymphocytes in vitro could lead to the severe defects in specific immune responsiveness observed in AIDS and related diseases. The absence of disease symptoms despite viral replication after experimental infections of chimpanzees (28), however, suggests that infection of $CD4^+$ lymphocytes is necessary but not sufficient to cause disease. Nevertheless, the inhibitory effects of HIV on helper T lymphocytes must play a central role in the disruption of normal immunoregulation and development of immunodeficiency.

Cellular Immune Responses

Besides inhibiting $CD4^+$ cell responses, HIV infection may lead to stimulation of $CD4^+$ and other cells. As activated helper T lymphocytes are required for the generation of most antibody responses (3,4,98), the production of antibodies recognizing HIV in the sera of infected humans and chimpanzees (28,46-48) indicates that HIV can induce specific helper T-cell responses.

In order to determine if helper T cells can be activated by HIV, PBMC were cultured with inactivated $HIV_{SF2^{45}}$ and tested for their ability to incorporate [^{3}H]thymidine as an index of proliferation. Table 3 presents data typical of HIV-seropositive individuals and illustrates the lack of lymphocyte proliferation in vitro in response to HIV antigens. Even in asymptomatic individuals (with > 600 $CD4^+$ cells/mm^3) whose lymphocytes proliferate in response to PHA or *Candida*, negligible responses to HIV antigens were detected (Table 3). Similar results were obtained using PBMC from HIV-seronegative donors (not shown). This proliferative anergy in response to HIV antigens has also been reported by Wahren and his colleagues (101).

Table 3 Lack of Proliferation by Lymphocytes from an Asymptomatic HIV-Seropositive Individual in Response to Sucrose-Gradient-Purified HIV_{SF2}

Antigen or mitogen	[^{3}H]thymidine incorporated (cpm)	Stimulation index
None	1,559	1.0
PHA (1%)	18,472	11.8
Candida extract (50 μg/ml)	17,125	11.0
HIV_{SF2} 0.1 μg/ml	1,343	0.9
1.0 μg/ml	1,997	1.3
10 μg/ml	1.795	1.1
50 μg/ml	2,840	1.8
Control HUT 78 SN (10 μg/ml)	1,956	1.3

Culture and assay conditions were as described in the legend to Figure 1. An extract of *C. albicans* was generously provided by Dr. R. Morelli (San Francisco State University). The HIV_{SF2} isolate (ARV-2)[45] was produced in HUT 78 cells and purified by Dr. Janet Yamamoto (University of California, Davis) on sucrose gradients as described (100). The HIV_{SF2} preparations contained core (p25) and envelope (gp120) antigens as determined by Western blot analysis (100). This experiment is typical of 20 HIV-seropositive individuals tested.

In contrast, nonglycosylated recombinant HIV envelope (ENV2-gp120) (102, 103) or core (*gag*-p25) (104) proteins (provided by the Chiron Corporation, Emeryville, Calif.) were able to stimulate proliferation from some HIV-seropositive individuals (Figure 2). Lymphocytes from HIV-seronegative individuals and AIDS patients did not proliferate in response to these recombinant HIV proteins. Only 4 of 19 (21.0%) HIV-seropositive asymptomatic homosexual males and 5 of 23 (21.7%) PGL or ARC patients exhibited significant ($p < 0.001$) stimulation indices of PBMC proliferation, in response to nonglycosylated recombinant ENV2 (gp120). The PBMC from only 2 of 12 HIV-seropositive asymptomatic individuals and none of the PGL, ARC, or ITP patients proliferated significantly in response to p25 (*gag*). These proliferative responses to recombinant HIV proteins were generally much weaker than responses to recall antigens such as *C. albicans* but nevertheless were significantly different from those of HIV-seronegative individuals. Subsequent studies have demonstrated that $CD4^+$ lymphocytes are required for the generation of proliferative responses to these HIV proteins (not shown). Finally, PBMC from HIV-infected but *not* from any uninfected chimpanzees proliferated in response to both gag (p25) and ENV2 (gp120) proteins of HIV (Figure 3). These studies indicate that proliferative responses to HIV antigens can occur but are not detectable in most infected humans.

Deficiencies in cell-mediated immune responses to HIV are also reflected in the lack of detectable levels of IL-2 released by PBMC from most HIV-seropositive individuals (Figure 4; see also Section VII). The PBMC from all

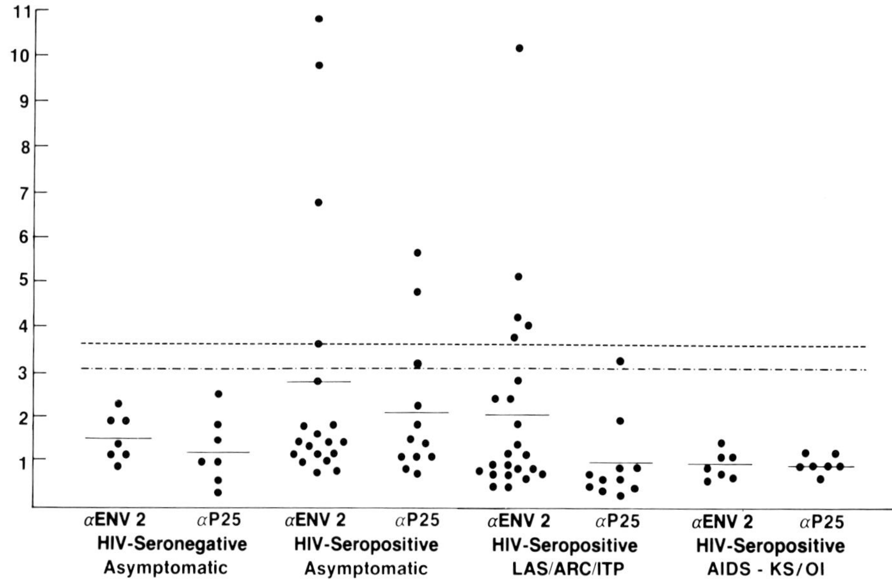

Figure 2 Lymphocyte proliferative responses to recombinant core (p25) and envelope (gp120) proteins of HIV. Culture and assay conditions were performed as described in the legend to Figure 1; 1×10^5 PBMC from HIV-seronegative homosexuals or HIV-seropositive asymptomatic men, LAS, ARC, or AIDS patients were cultured with an optimal concentration (10 μg/ml) of highly purified recombinant p25 (*gag*) (104) or ENV-2 (gp120) (102,103) provided by the Chiron Corporation. Stimulation indexes were calculated as described in the legend to Figure 1. The stimulation indices > 3 SD of the mean proliferative responses of HIV-seronegative individuals to ENV-2 (—•—) and p25 (---) are highly significant ($p < 0.001$) positive responses.

HIV-seronegative or HIV-seropositive asymptomatic individuals and Kaposi's sarcoma (KS) patients did not release detectable levels of IL-2 after stimulation with a nonglycosylated form of the gp120 envelope (ENV2) or with the gag (p25) proteins of HIV. In contrast, 5 of 12 PGL or ARC patients' PBMC released IL-2 in response to an optimal concentration (10 μg/ml) of ENV 2 but not to the p25 core protein. Other defects in antigen- or mitogen-induced IL-2 release in HIV-seropositive individuals have been reported (77-81). Approximately 75% of $CD4^+$ cells and 15% of cytotoxic or suppressor ($CD8^+$) T cells from normal donors are capable of being stimulated to produce IL-2 (106). The phenotypes of the IL-2-producing cells in our studies were not determined.

Zarling and her colleagues have provided evidence of cell-mediated immune responses against HIV in macaques immunized with recombinant vaccinia virus expressing HIV envelope glycoproteins (ENVgp) (107). Moreover,

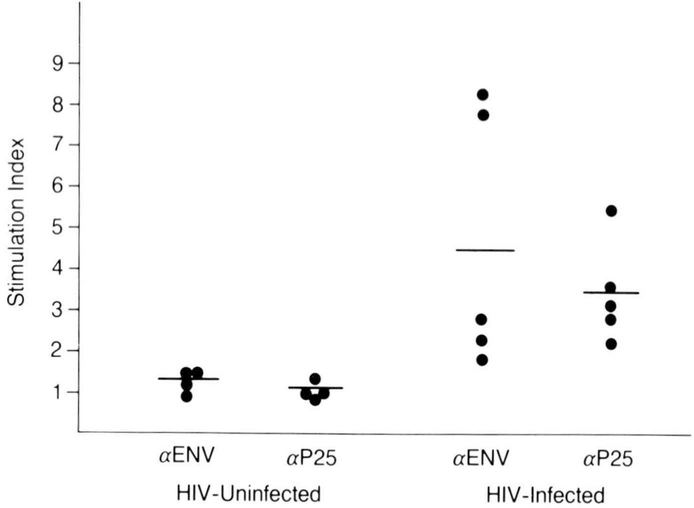

Figure 3 Lymphocyte proliferative responses of chimpanzees to recombinant core (p25) and envelope (gp120) proteins of HIV. One × 10^5 PBMC from HIV-uninfected or experimentally HIV-infected chimpanzees were cultured with an optimal concentration (10 μg/ml) of recombinant ENV-2 (gp120) (102,103) and p25 (*gag*) (104) proteins (Chiron Corporation) for 7 days in medium containing 10% autologous plasma. Assay conditions and calculation of stimulation indexes were performed as described in the legend to Figure 1.

in these studies the proliferative and IL-2 responses to the recombinant virus were much greater than those responses to purified HIV. This finding may reflect a weak ability of ENVgp epitopes on intact virus to stimulate cell-mediated immune responses or may indicate differences in concentrations of the relevant ENVgp epitopes in the two antigen preparations. However, the inability to detect specific proliferation to HIV antigens of PBMC from the majority of HIV-exposed individuals (Table 3, Figure 2) in a test system capable of detecting proliferative responses to CMV and other antigens (Figure 1, Table 3) suggests that HIV-infections do not characteristically induce vigorous helper cell responses in humans. The decreased cell-mediated immune responses to HIV appears similar to the low responses to hepatitis B virus (HBV) (108) but contrasts sharply with the strong proliferative responses induced by CMV or HSV infections (31,69). The mechanisms responsible for these differences and their relevance to pathogenesis or protection against disease are unclear. It is tempting to speculate, however, that the cell-mediated immune responses to HIV of experimentally infected primates may determine the inability to induce serious disease in these animals.

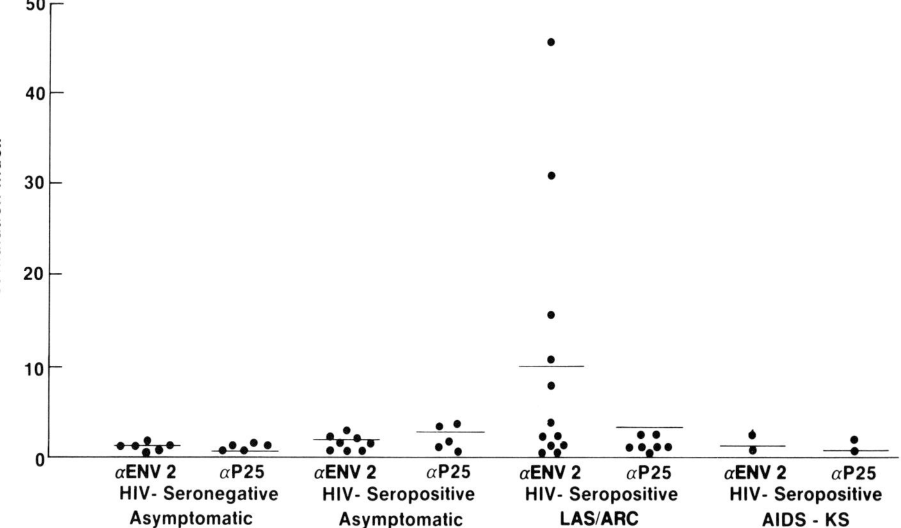

Figure 4 Production of interleukin 2 by lymphocytes in response to recombinant core (p25) and envelope (gp120) proteins of HIV. One × 10^5 PBMC were incubated for 48 hr in the presence or absence of optimal concentrations (10 μg/ml) of recombinant p25 (99) or ENV-2 (gp120) (98) provided by the Chiron Corporation. Supernatants were then collected and assayed for their ability to support the proliferation of 10^4 cells of the IL-2-dependent CTLL line (105). After an additional 48 hr incubation cultures were pulsed with [^{3}H]thymidine and harvested. Stimulation indexes of IL-2 production were calculated by dividing the mean ($\overline{X}$) counts per minute of [^{3}H]thymidine incorporated by CTLL cells cultured with supernatants from ENV2- or p25-stimulated PBMC by the $\overline{X}$ counts per minute incorporated by CTLL cells cultured with supernatants from unstimulated PBMC.

It is clear that both phenotypical and/or functional abnormalities involving CD4$^+$ helper T cells are commonly observed in HIV-infected individuals. The majority of the direct or indirect effects of HIV on CD4$^+$ cells appear to be inhibitory and ultimately may result in the severe immunodeficiency of AIDS and related diseases. Nevertheless, under conditions that remain to be defined, adaptive and specific responses of CD4$^+$ cytotoxic or helper cells might be induced to control the destructive effects of HIV. It may be important for an infected individual to rapidly initiate vigorous immune responses by CD4$^+$ and other cells before the relatively slow-growing HIV can replicate sufficiently to overcome these potentially protective immune responses. Autoimmune reactivity stimulated by HIV may interfere with the induction and/or effector functions of these cells (see Section VIII).

Antigenic stimulation of HIV-infected cells dramatically increases HIV replication and may also impair the ability of CD4$^+$ or other cells to control HIV (85).

B. Effects of HIV on Cytotoxic and Suppressor (CD8$^+$) Lymphocytes

Phenotypical Changes

Lymphocytes expressing the CD8 antigen constitute a functionally and phenotypically heterogeneous group of cells which include CTL, suppressor T lymphocytes, and some NK cells (5,6). Increases in the percentages and absolute numbers of CD8$^+$ lymphocytes are strongly associated with exposure to HIV (10-17,23-27). Table 4 demonstrates that the percentages of CD8$^+$ cells in peripheral blood are significantly elevated in HIV-seropositive asymptomatic homosexual males and HIV-seropositive homosexuals with LAS or AIDS in comparison with HIV antibody-negative individuals. The percentages of CD8$^+$ PBMC do not differ significantly between HIV-seronegative heterosexual or homosexual males. Increases in the percentages of CD8$^+$ cells also occur in the paracortical areas of lymph nodes and in intestinal mucosa of PGL or AIDS patients (18-22). Increases in the percentages and absolute numbers of CD8$^+$ cells and subnormal CD4$^+$/CD8$^+$ ratios also occur after exposure to other viruses such as CMV, HBV, or HSV (32-34).

The percentages of CD8$^+$ lymphocytes that coexpress Leu 7 are significantly elevated in all groups of HIV-seropositive individuals but do not differ

Table 4 Comparison of CD8$^+$ and Leu7$^+$ Lymphocytes in Study Subjects[a]

	Percentage of lymphocytes				
Lymphocyte subset	HIV$^-$ heterosexual asymptomatic n[d] = 54	HIV$^-$ homosexual asymptomatic n = 63	HIV$^+$ homosexual asymptomatic n = 24	HIV$^+$ homosexual PGL n = 20	HIV$^+$ homosexual AIDS n = 43
CD8$^+$	26.8	24.8	38.0[b]	44.2	48.6
CD8$^+$ Leu7$^+$	6.5	8.3	14.6[b]	14.3	20.5
CD8$^+$ CD11b$^-$	32.7	30.4	43.1[b]	50.3	57.0
CD8$^+$ CD11b$^+$	3.0	3.0	3.8	2.3	4.0
CD8$^+$ HLA-DR$^+$	2.7	2.9	7.5[b]	10.9	13.7
CD8$^+$ $\kappa\lambda^-$	26.5	24.4	33.8[b]	41.9	45.0
CD8$^+$ $\kappa\lambda^+$	2.7	2.6	5.1	3.2	5.4
Leu7$^+$	21.5	27.3[b]	34.3	30.2	40.0[b]

[a]See legend to Table 2.
[b]The value in this column and in those to its right are significantly different ($p < 0.005$) from all column to the left.

between HIV-seronegative hterosexual or homosexual males (Table 4 and Refs. 13,14,109). The percentage of Leu7$^+$ cells are increased in HIV-infected asymptomatic homosexual males and patients with LAS or AIDS although there are no significant differences in the percentages of Leu 7$^+$ cells among these three groups. The functional capacities of CD8$^+$ Leu 7$^+$ or Leu 7$^+$ cells in HIV-seronegative and HIV-seropositive individuals remain to be defined. Increases in both of these lymphocyte subsets are also observed after exposure to CMV in HIV-seronegative individuals (34). By clonal analysis we have determined that CD8$^+$ Leu 7$^+$ lymphocytes differentiate into CD3$^+$ CD8$^+$ Leu 7$^-$ cytotoxic lymphocytes in the presence of appropriate "helper" signals (unpublished observations). Based on these and other observations, we suggest that the CD8$^+$ Leu 7$^+$ subset which is significantly elevated in HIV-infected individuals constitutes a CTL precursor population whose differentiation has been prevented by deficiencies in "helper signals." Direct and indirect effects of HIV on CD4$^+$ cells result in these deficiencies.

The CD11b marker, defined by the monoclonal antibody Leu 15, is expressed on CD8$^+$ suppressor T lymphocytes and some NK cells (5,6,110,111). The percentage of CD8$^+$ CD11b$^+$ cells is not significantly elevated in HIV-infected individuals (Refs. 13, 14 and Table 4). In contrast, cytotoxic T lymphocytes (CD8$^+$ 11b$^-$) constitute the major subsets of CD8 cells which is significantly elevated ($p < 0.001$) in HIV-seropositive individuals (Table 4).

The percentage of CD8$^+$ cells that coexpress HLA-DR do not differ between HIV-seronegative heterosexual or homosexual males but are significantly elevated in all groups of HIV-seropositive individuals (Table 4). Since enhancement in HLA-DR expression is associated with T-cell activation, these increases in CD8$^+$ HLA-DR$^+$ lymphocytes may represent an adaptive response against HIV or other pathogens (30). Reduced T-cell ecto-5′ nucleotidase activity and increased OKT10 and HLA-DR expression in association with absence of IL-2 receptors or transferrin receptors on CD8$^+$ PBMC of HIV$^+$ individuals suggests that HLA$^-$ DR$^+$ CD8$^+$ cells may represent a population of "immature" lymphocytes (112). Defects in CD4$^+$ T cells may thus have indirect effects on the maturation of CD8$^+$ cells and other cell types. Similar increases of CD8$^+$ HLA-DR$^+$ lymphocytes are observed after recent exposure to CMV or EBV but are not generally observed in CMV-seropositive, HIV-seronegative individuals (30,34).

Significant increases in CD8$^+$ cells lacking surface-immunoglobulins ($\kappa\lambda^-$) are observed in all groups of HIV-infected individuals (Table 4). Decreases in cells expressing NK-associated markers such as CD16 (Leu 11) have also been observed in AIDS (109). It is not known, however, if differences exist between HIV-seronegative individuals and any groups of HIV-seropositive individuals in their CD8$^+$ cells which coexpress CD16, NKH1, or both of these markers. In summary, infection by HIV stimulates dramatic and persistent increases in lymphocytes expressing cytotoxic phenotypes. The ability of these cells to inhibit HIV requires further characterization.

Functional Changes

Functional abnormalities associated with $CD8^+$ cytotoxic cells have been reported in HIV-infected individuals (68,77,111,113-116). Defects in the ability to generate alloreactive CTL in vitro have been observed in PBMC from patients with AIDS or ARC (111,114-116). The ability to restore CTL responses by the addition of IL-2 or T-cell supernatants to PBMC from all ARC patients, but only in a subset of AIDS patients, indicates that these defects may result from an impaired ability to produce lymphokines, to respond to lymphokines, or both (77,81,111,116). Defects in the ability of lymphocytes from AIDS patients to generate HLA-restricted CTL responses to influenza or CMV have also been reported (68,77,114,115). It is not known if HIV can exert direct inhibitory effects on CTL. Such HIV-specific CTL presumably express HIV antigen receptors on their cell membranes, but it is not known if these cells are susceptible to HIV infection. Direct inhibitory effects of HIV proteins or of non-HIV proteins produced in HIV-infected cells on CTL have also not been analyzed. Infection of helper T cells or macrophages by HIV may impair their ability to collaborate in the generation of CTL. Other indirect effects of HIV such as the induction of suppressor cells or factors or blocking antibodies may also suppress CTL function.

The dramatic increases in $CD8^+$ $CD11b^-$ lymphocytes afer exposure to HIV suggests that CTL may respond adaptively to HIV infection. It is not known, however, if CTL responses to HIV are beneficial or harmful to the HIV-infected individual. Because ENVgp are expressed on the surfaces of HIV-infected cells (91,92,117), these antigens in association with HLA may form target structures for recognition and lysis of HIV-infected cells by CTL or other cytotoxic cells. Reports from a number of laboratories have demonstrated in HIV-infected individuals the existence of HLA-restricted CTL which recognize envelope or core proteins of HIV (118-120). It is not known if other HIV-encoded antigens can stimulate CTL responses. Both *gag*- and ENV-specific CTL are generated in mice in response to infection with the Friend leukemia retrovirus (121). Lysis of HIV-infected cells and production of γ-interferon (γIFN) by CTL or other cytotoxic cells may constitute mechanisms by which the immune system attempts to control HIV infection (122-124). Lysis of HIV-uninfected $CD4^+$ cells which have passively bound ENVgp or other molecules may contribute further to abnormalities of immune regulation and immunodeficiency. In an analogous system it has been demonstrated that cytotoxic lymphocytes can lyse uninfected lymphocytes which have passively bound proteins or peptides of influenza virus (125,126).

Suppressor cell activity in PBMC from patients with AIDS has also been reported (10,97,127). Studies by Hofmann and colleagues (128), however, conclude that suppressor T-cell activity alone cannot account for impaired blastogenic responses of PBMC in AIDS. Recently Walker and his colleagues (129) have demonstrated that $CD8^+$ cells can suppress HIV replication although it is not clear if these "suppressor" cells express CD11 or if they can exert cytotoxic activity against HIV-infected cells. The role of macrophages in this suppression of HIV replication by $CD8^+$ cells is also unclear. The combination of recombinant γ interferon produced by $CD8^+$ cells and macrophage-derived tumor necrosis factor has been demonstrated to effectively inhibit HIV in vitro (212).

The reduced potential for clonal expansion of $CD8^+$ PBMC from PGL or AIDS patients provides further evidence that HIV can inhibit this lymphocyte subset (82,83). Decreases in proliferative responses to mitogens or alloantigens in some HIV^+ individuals may also be related at least in part to direct or indirect inhibitory effects of HIV on $CD8^+$ cells (see Section IIIA).

C. Relationships Between T Cell Abnormalities and Disease Progression in HIV-Infected Individuals

As inhibitory effects of HIV on $CD4^+$ cells play a central role in the development of immunodeficiency, immunological parameters related to numerical and/or functional deficiencies of helper T lymphocytes have received particular attention as prognostic indicators. Individuals with less than 400 $CD4^+$ cells/μl appear to be at greatest risk of developing AIDS (2,130,131). Many HIV-infected individuals fall into this category. In the San Francisco Men's Health Study, 29% of HIV-seropositive men had fewer than 400 $CD4^+$ cells/μl (132). On an individual patient basis, however, this threshhold of 400 $CD4^+$ cells/μl may not necessarily be a point of no return. Studies in San Francisco demonstrate that 13% (4/32) HIV-seropositive men without AIDS but with < 500 helpers/μl had significant increases (> 200 cells/μl) in their absolute $CD4^+$ cell numbers over 2 years. Decreasing levels of $CD4^+$ T cells and progression to ARC or AIDS are, however, seen in most HIV-infected individuals (213).

Immunological parameters including increased numbers of $CD8^+$ cells, low levels of antibody to HIV, high levels of antibody to CMV, or deficiencies in antigen-driven lymphocyte proliferation have also been associated with progression to AIDS (132,133). Among HIV-seropositive asymptomatic men no significant correlation exists between $CD4^+/CD8^+$ ratios and the ability to culture HIV from PBMC (134). In AIDS patients with KS the absolute $CD4^+$ cell numbers and $CD4^+/CD8^+$ ratios are correlated closely with prognosis (135,136). More than 85% of KS patients with > 300 $CD4^{2/3}$ cells/μl and $CD4^+/CD8^+$ ratios > 0.5 survived at least 12 months (136).

Therapeutic strategies that minimize the inhibitory effects of HIV on CD4$^+$ lymphocytes and other cell types as well as those that stimulate protective cell-mediated or antibody responses against HIV may prove useful in slowing down, halting, or reversing progressive immunodeficiency.

IV. HIV and B Lymphocytes

B cells have not been spared from the effects of HIV. Early clinical descriptions of AIDS indicated that many infected individuals had elevated serum immunoglobulins (12,16). It is estimated that 80-90% of the AIDS patients have at least one elevated serum immunoglobulin (Ig) isotype (12). Lane et al. (62), however, report that B cells from AIDS patients fail to produce immunoglobulin in response to in vitro activation with pokeweed mitogen. These two observations highlight the apparently paradoxical effects of HIV on B cells. Data exist that clearly indicate a state of activation in the immune system at the same time when overt immunodeficiency is present. Resolution of this apparent conflict can best be accomplished by separating the direct effects of HIV on B cells (HIV binding or infecting B cells) from the indirect effects (HIV alterations of T-cell control of B-cell function).

In addition to the effects of HIV that interfere with the normal functions of B lymphocytes, infection by HIV results in the induction of antibodies recognizing many different HIV proteins (44,46,48). Some of these antibodies, particularly those recognizing some epitopes of gp120 (102,137, 138), are able to inactivate infectious HIV. Antibodies to most HIV proteins persist throughout the course of infection although antibodies to the p25 (*gag*) protein appear to decrease in association with disease progression (104).

A. Indirect Effects of HIV on B Cells

The profound disruptive effects that HIV has on T-cell regulation almost certainly result in some degree of abnormal control of B-cell function. Immunoglobulin production by B-cells is dependent on the capacity of T cells to provide adequate help or suppression under the appropriate circumstances (34,139). Various phenotypically defined CD4 T-lymphocyte subsets (see Table 1) function as direct helper (CD4$^+$ HB10$^-$), helper-inducer (CD4$^+$ 4B4$^+$), or suppressor-inducer (CD4$^+$ 2H4$^+$) cells for B-cell regulation (38, 140,141). Differential susceptibility of any of these subsets of CD4 cells to HIV infection and inactivation could theoretically produce very different effects on immunoglobulin levels.

A selective decrease in the suppressor-inducer (CD4$^+$ CD45R$^+$) subset of CD4$^+$ cells as may occur in PGL (25) might be expected to result in increased serum immunoglobulin levels. Decreased induction of suppressor T cells combined with the resulting increases in the proportion of helper-inducer

($CD4^+$ Leu 8^-) cells would presumably lead to a state of ''hyper-help'' and concomitant hyperimmunoglobulinemia observed in many HIV-infected individuals. It is also possible that T cell-independent cofactors are also involved in this process.

B. Association with Epstein-Barr Virus

Serological evidence for recurrent infection with EBV has been documented in HIV-infected individuals (142). Birx and colleagues observed that the mean frequency of circulating EBV-infected B cells was 6-10-fold higher in AIDS or ARC patients as compared with healthy controls (143). Direct activation of B cells by EBV can result in the T-independent production of immunoglobulin (74,144). The response to EBV infection in a healthy host would include the development of reactive $CD8^+$ T cells capable of killing virus-infected cells. These cytotoxic cells are dependent, however, on $CD4^+$ cells for maturation and clonal expansion (145). Thus, the loss of the $CD4^+$ subset due to the effects of HIV could influence activation of B cells by EBV with a concomitant reduction in the ability to maintain function of CD8 effector cells. The end result of this process would very likely be polyclonal Ig production.

The connection between EBV, HIV, and B cells was suspected when it became apparent that the incidence of B-cell lymphomas in AIDS patients was much higher than in the general population (146). Analysis of a B-cell lymphoma from a patient with AIDS detected sequences of DNA from the lymphoma which hybridized with EBV-specific probes and showed rearrangement of the c-*myc* oncogene (147). No HIV-specific sequences, however, were detected. This evidence suggests that EBV but not HIV may have a direct role in lymphomagenesis in AIDS.

It would be a mistake to attribute all the Ig production during HIV infection to ''nonspecific activation.'' The vast majority of HIV-infected persons develop readily detectable serum and secretory antibody responses to HIV viral components (16,46-48,102,148). These responses often are detectable, although substantially decreased, in the late stages of the disease (149). This finding is supported by the work of Ammann et al. (150) who demonstrated that 51% of the AIDS patients immunized with a polysaccharide were still capable of recognizing the antigen and developing specific antibodies, albeit at lower titers than healthy controls. These facts highlight the point that even under the influence of abnormal regulation, the B cells present in some HIV-infected people are still capable of mounting specific antibody responses.

C. Direct Effects of HIV on B Cells

There is evidence to indicate that B cells are susceptible to HIV infection. Human B cells, transformed with EBV, express CD4 (the major receptor for HIV—see Section IIIA) and can be infected with HIV (51,151,152).

Examination of lymph nodes from ARC, PGL, and AIDS patients reveals the expected reduction of T-cell zone architecture (153). There is also significant disturbance of the B-cell areas. A small but significant number of patients with PGL were observed to have atrophic or absent germinal centers (153). This finding was also observed in the lymph nodes of AIDS patients. This evidence suggests that the early disease process can result in major losses of B-cell regions of the lymph node. This evidence when considered by itself, would predict that HIV-infected subjects should be Ig deficient rather than Ig overproducers.

Interestingly, the predominant cell type surviving in the lymph nodes of late stage patients is the plasma cell (153). It is possible that susceptible B cells differentiate into a state of HIV resistance but more probably these surviving plasma cells were derived from B cells that were never infected by HIV. Survival of plasma cells even into the very late stages of this disease suggests that the full spectrum of B-cell differentiation may not be open to assault by HIV. Alterations of B-cell populations can occur in the peripheral blood as well as the lymph nodes. Expression of the CD5 antigen (detected by anti-Leu 1) on B cells occurs in higher proportions in the peripheral blood of infected individuals, especially those with AIDS (Table 5). The murine equivalents of these B cells reportedly secrete autoantibodies spontaneously (154). In humans, however, these CD5-bearing B cells are known to exist during fetal development, a period of relative B-cell quiescence (155). It is intriguing to speculate that HIV has the capacity to activate these B cells directly so as to produce spontaneous secretion of autoreactive antibodies, the existence of which has been documented (154). As yet, however, no studies have reported the expression of the CD5 antigen on purified B cells exposed to HIV in vitro.

Table 5 Imbalance of B-Cell Subsets Associated with Elevated Serum Immunoglobulins in HIV-Infected Patients

			Cell populations bearing		Levels of serum		
Group	n	Mean CD4: CD8[a]	CD19	CD5 and CD19	IgG	IgA	IgM
Healthy	10	1.8	11 ± 2[b]	11 ± 2	1,003 ± 55[c]	154 ± 19	173 ± 27
AIDS	8	0.3	10 ± 3	28 ± 5[d]	2,217 ± 429[d]	381 ± 65[d]	263 ± 39

[a]Cluster of differentiation (CD): CD4, Leu3, "helper" T cells; CD8, Leu2, "suppressor/cytotoxic" cells; CD19, Leu12, mature B cells; CD5, Leu1, pan-T cells (see Refs. 5 and 6).
[b]Data expressed as mean percentage of lymphocytes ± SE.
[c]Date expressed as mean mg/dl of serum.
[d]Significantly different, $p < 0.05$.

The ability of HIV to directly affect B cells has been tested with both whole and disrupted (noninfectious) virus preparations. Pahwa et al. (72) reported that disrupted preparations of HIV are capable of activating B cell preparations. At the same time, however, these same preparations are capable of preventing the activation of B cells with other T-independent or T-dependent mitogens. This finding could explain the paradox of poor T-cell help in HIV-infected subjects and a concomitant increase in circulating immunoglobulins. Furthermore, the ability of these preparations to block B-cell activation by other stimulants may explain in part why such a poor *de novo* antibody response is elicited from HIV-infected people (150).

More recently, Schnittman et al. (73) were able to activate B lymphocytes from healthy control subjects using infectious HIV. These B lymphocytes were stimulated to divide as well as to produce and secrete immunoglobulin. There was no indication that these activation effects were related to EBV and they were independent of either T cells or monocytes. Although this data strongly support the hypothesis that B cells are altered as a result of direct viral infection, other studies using noninfectious components of HIV suggest that the virus can also interfere with B-cell function without infecting these cells (72,87). Perhaps the most likely scenario that would encompass HIV effects on B cells would be to accept the existence of both direct and indirect influences. The broad spectrum of B-cell maturational stages (pre-B to plasma cells) provides multiple levels for HIV to alter the control of immunoglobulin production.

V. HIV and Monocytes/Macrophages

The observations of Levy et al. (152) demonstrated that the cellular host range of HIV is not limited to helper T lymphocytes. Monocytes can not only be attacked by HIV but can also be productively infected (95,96,156). Isolates of HIV appear to vary considerably in their respective tropisms for either $CD4^+$ T cells or macrophages (96). Clearly what still needs to be resolved is how HIV infects these cells and what, if any, direct alterations occur in their many immunologic support functions.

A. Effects of HIV Infection of Monocyte/Macrophages

Virus Infection

The process of infecting the monocyte/macrophage most probably occurs through one of two mechanisms. First, the virus may enter the monocyte/macrophage via a phagocytic process. Phagocytosis of infected cells or other materials containing HIV may permit entry of the virus into the intracellular environment of monocytes and macrophages. Phagocytosis of virus may also occur by Fc receptor-mediated internalization of HIV coated with anti-HIV antibodies. In vitro data demonstrate, however, that the virus can penetrate the cell in the absence of antiviral antibodies. Electron-micrographic analysis has detected viral particles in cytoplasmic vesicles as early as 10 min after in vitro exposure (95,96). The presence of HIV particles in these vesicles illustrates that phagocytosis, a normal physiologic function of monocytes and macrophages, may lead to the internalization of these particles. At present the fate of HIV particles after phagolysosome formation is not clear. Treatment of infected monocytes with inhibitors of phagolysosome fusion, however, has no apparent effect on virus production in monocyte/macrophage cultures (95). This finding indicates that either the virus is resistant to the enzymes within the lysosome or that another mechanism of penetration is more likely. The latter explanation is probably the case since phagocytic vesicles of granulocytes also can contain virus particles but apparently yield no infectious HIV (95).

The major mechanism for HIV penetration of cells of the monocyte lineage is via the CD4 antigen. Expression of this antigen on the surface of both monocytes and macrophages has been documented (152,157). Viral attachment to the CD4 antigen would presumably permit entry into the monocyte/macrophage in the same manner as with lymphocytes. Blocking studies using the OKT4A monoclonal antibody produced "substantial although not total" inhibition of HIV binding (95). Conversely, pretreatment of $CD4^+$ cells with HIV was capable of blocking the binding of these cells to the antibody, OKT4A.

Phenotypical Changes

Lymphocytes that are infected with HIV progressively lose the CD4 surface antigen after infection (59). Presumably the same situation would occur with the CD4 antigens on the surface of monocytes in vivo. A decrease in CD4 expression after HIV infection of the monocyte tumor cell line U937 has been reported (152). This has also been observed indirectly with decreased CD4 expression on monocytes from AIDS patients (158,159). Only 2-10% of the monocytes from AIDS patients expressed detectable amounts of CD4 compared with 60-80% of the monocytes from healthy controls. Although this strongly suggests the active infection of monocytes via the CD4 receptor, no significant correlations have yet been reported between these changes in CD4 surface antigen expression and alterations in the functional capacity of these cells.

A significant reduction in the expression of class II major histocompatibility complex (MHC) HLA-DR on monocytes from AIDS patients has been reported (160). Monocytes from three of four PGL patients in the same study were found to have HLA-DR expression that was higher than that of the control population. The progressive loss of immune function often observed after HIV infection suggests that there should be a corresponding decay in HLA-DR expression. This simple relationship is apparently not the case. Instead, there appears to be a biphasic response in the host that begins with an initial increase in HLA-DR-positive monocytes followed by a decline. This observation suggests two different hypotheses. First, this increase in the proportion of HLA-DR-positive monocytes after HIV infection could be a protective host response reflecting activation or recruitment of effector monocytes. The surface expression of class II MHC antigens on monocytes is associated with the ability of these cells to support both T- and B-cell activities (161,162). Alternatively, the reduced proportion of HLA-DR-positive monocytes might reflect an inability to sustain macrophage activation. Similar reductions in HLA-DR surface expression of monocytes have been observed with worsening immune responses in tuberculosis (163). These two hypotheses are not mutually exclusive.

Alteration of Monocyte/Macrophage Function

Abnormalities in monocyte/macrophage functions have also been reported in HIV infections, but their contribution to pathogenesis is not known. Smith et al. (164) noted a marked decrease in monocyte chemotactic response in AIDS patients. In contrast, it has also been reported that no significant difference exists in the ability of monocytes from either control or AIDS patients to phagocytize or kill fungi (165). This conflict may be related to the differentiation status of the cells tested. Important differences may exist in the susceptibility of subpopulations of macrophages and monocytes to infection with HIV. Murray and colleagues (166) found that neither peripheral blood monocytes nor alveolar macrophages from infected patients were significantly different from control cells in the ability to manifest oxidative or antimicrobial activity. Macrophages from HIV infected subjects were also capable of responding to γ-interferon to the same degree as control macrophages. It is possible that functional abnormalities and cytopathology induced by HIV may not only be due to the tropism of the HIV strain tested but also to the state of activation of the cells infected.

We are now aware that the immunodeficiencies caused by HIV infection can just as easily originate from monocyte/macrophage abnormalities as they can from T-lymphocyte defects. It is distinctly possible that the immune defects that lead to serious clinical sequealae result from damage to both of these cell populations and their functions. Therapeutic strategies that involve selective targeting of antiviral agents and/or cytokines to macrophages or T-cell subsets may be useful in repairing some of these defects.

VI. NK Cells

Natural killer cells are cytotoxic lymphocytes functionally defined by their ability to lyse a variety of tumor cells, virally infected cells, and other normal tissue cells (167). The mechanism by which they recognize target cells is unknown, but T-cell antigen receptor (T_3T_i) and MHC restriction are not involved. Many circulating NK cells (about 5-10% of total mononuclear cells) appear as large granular lymphocytes and display IgG Fc receptors. Various monoclonal antibodies exist which detect subpopulations of NK cells and also recognize some other types of cells which do not mediate NK cell function. These include anti-HNK-1 (Leu 7), CD16 anti-Fc receptor (Leu 11) and anti-NKH-1 or Leu 19 (168). Cytotoxicity by NK cells is augmented by IL-2 directly and indirectly by most interferons which are also induced by IL-2 (169).

Analysis of surface markers for NK cells such as NKH-1, HNK (Leu 7), or FcR (CD16) in HIV-infected individuals has given variable results. Some investigators find elevated numbers of Leu 7 or HNK-bearing cells (170), which could be explained in part by striking increases of $CD8^+$ Leu 7^+ cells as reported by our laboratory (13,14). One study (171) showed striking decreases in Leu 7^+ cells in lymph nodes from ARC and AIDS patients. Baron et al. (113) reported an increase in the *percentage* of Leu 11^+ (CD16) cells in AIDS but not in ARC. The absolute numbers of NK cells were unchanged in AIDS and decreased in ARC patients. When an index of target cell lysis per NK effector cell was calculated, both AIDS and ARC patients were defective in NK function.

Some studies with peripheral blood from HIV-infected individuals at various stages of health have found decreased NK cell function (113,172-174). Killing of ^{51}CR-labeled K562 tumor cells, an NK-sensitive cell line, has generally been used to assay NK function. Several laboratories, however, have reported normal or nearly normal NK function in similar patients (175, 176). Although unexplained, these discrepancies are likely duc to technical variations in the assay or heterogeneity among patient populations studied. Subpopulations of T cells may also kill NK-sensitive target cells as well (167).

The mechanism of diminished NK cell activity has been investigated by several groups. Bonavida et al. (174) showed no alterations in frequency of NK cells defined functionally, nor binding to target cells. However, bound target cells were not lysed, presumably due to failure of release of NK cell cytotoxic factors. Exogenous IL-2 was able to partially reverse this in vitro defect. In a study in hemophiliacs infected with HIV, Katzmann and Lederman (177) found similar defects in binding and "postbinding" or lytic events. Normal recycling of NK cells to attack multiple targets was noted as was absence of suppressor cells for NK activity. Creemers et al. (175) suggested plasma from HIV seropositives contained factors which could interrupt NK cytotoxicity. Although in vitro studies have shown augmentation by IL-2 or interferon of NK activity in normals and individuals with HIV disease (77, 172,174,170,178,179), the clinical significance remains moot. This fact may be due to the lack of convincing evidence of in vivo effectiveness of NK cells in immunity in general.

VII. Interleukin 2 and Other Cytokines

Interleukin 2 is a 15,500 mol wt protein produced by mature T cells when stimulated by antigen and interleukin 1 (IL-1) released by macrophages (77-81). The interaction of IL-2 with its specific receptor, which is induced by antigen or immunologically committed T cells themselves, eventually results in their proliferation. In addition, IL-2 augments cytotoxicity by NK cells by direct interaction with the IL-2 receptor and indirectly by γIFN released from stimulated cytotoxic or helper T cells (180,181).

Defects in the IL-2 system could be at the level of IL-2 production, IL-2 receptor expression, and IL-2 responsiveness. Nearly all studies have shown decreased in vitro production of IL-2 in AIDS and related conditions (79, 182-184). Some data suggest decreases in IL-2 production in association with the progression of HIV-related disease. Other investigators (81,183-185), in contrast, found no decrease in IL-2 production but rather decrease in IL-2 receptor expression. This discrepancy and others may relate to the stage of disease studied or to differences in culture methods used either for assay or generation of IL-2. Furthermore, functional assays for IL-2 ultimately depend on other factors such as the integrity of macrophage activation, production of IL-1 and particularly optimal kinetics. The majority of studies fail to normalize T-cell populations to compensate for severe alterations in helper and suppressor subsets that result from HIV infection. It is possible that IL-2 defects are mainly due to loss of cell populations which produce and respond to IL-2 rather than any intrinsic biochemical defect in remaining lymphocytes. In support of this hypothesis Arya and Gallo (123) have shown normal IL-2 gene transcription in HIV-infected cells. Several studies have demonstrated serum (186,187) or in vitro (182) factors which block IL-2 production. Neither the mechanism of action nor the chemical identity of these factors is fully established, but they do not appear to be antibodies to IL-2 or the IL-2 receptor. In one study (186), recombinant IL-2 was able to partially restore IL-2 responses in the presence of a serum inhibitory factor. Results from our laboratory (70) demonstrate that IL-2 is able to overcome the inhibitory effects of HIV gp120 in vitro.

In many studies exogenously added IL-2 partially restored proliferation or cytotoxic activity induced by mitogen or antigens (70,77,80,188-190).

Ebert and colleagues (183) differentiated the ability of IL-2 to restore responses in ARC but not AIDS patients due to failure of IL-2 receptor expression in the latter group. Particularly striking is the repeated observation of improved NK cytotoxicity that can be induced by IL-2 in vitro (77,80,190, 191). Tsang and colleagues (78) have reported improved IL-2 production and IL-2 receptor expression by in vitro addition of the immunostimulatory agent, isoprinosine. In general, therapy with IL-2, even at very large doses, has been disappointing in restoration of either immunological or clinical function in HIV-infected individuals (192).

Defects in the production of γIFN, and tumor necrosis factor-α and -β have been reported in patients with AIDS and ARC (81,193). Defects in responses to IL-1 but not in its production have also been found (80). The reasons for abnormal production or responses to IL-2 and other cytokines in HIV infections are not clear. Depletion of CD4 cells due to direct lytic effects of HIV is certainly involved in these deficiencies. It is also likely that proteins and genetic regulatory elements of HIV also directly or indirectly affect the production and effects of cytokines.

VIII. Autoimmunity Associated with HIV Infection

The association between viral infections and the development of various autoimmune phenomena has been suspected for some time. It should not be surprising then to find autoimmune phenomena associated with a virus which interferes with normal immunoregulatory mechanisms at many levels (194). It is not presently known whether or not the autoimmune events that have been documented contribute to the progression of the disease. This question is perhaps the most critical one in delineating the relationship between HIV infection and the development of autoimmune phenomena. Obviously the presence of autoimmunity does the host little good at a time that the immune response system needs to be fully marshalled to control the virus infection. A clear connection, however, between disease progression and autoimmunity could have major implications in terms of both therapeutic approaches and vaccine considerations.

A. Autoreactive Antibodies and HIV Infection

The existence of autoreactive antibodies in the sera and tissues in AIDS patients and other HIV-infected individuals has been clearly documented (Table 6). The specific host antigens responsible for inducing autoimmunity are not known in most cases. Various tissues have been observed to be targets for autoantibodies (195-204). These include lymphocytes, red blood cells, neutrophils, platelets, nerve tissue, and phospholipids. The pathogenic relevance of

Table 6 Autoantibodies in HIV-Infected Individuals

Tissue reactivity	Immunoglobulin isotype	Reference
Thymic epithelium	IgG, A, M	195
Platelets	IgG, M	196-198
RBC	IgG	199
Lymphocytes		
T	IgG	200,201
B	IgM	202
Myelin	IgG, M	203

autoantibodies in HIV-infections is suggested by the studies of Miller and colleagues (204) who showed that four of six patients with severe neurological impairment, presumably due to neurophilic autoantibodies, improved clinically during a course of plasmapheresis. In these HIV-related autoimmune phenomena, either a common antigen is being recognized inappropriately or a number of different host antigens are involved. Resolution of this question requires the elucidation of specific antigens.

B. Induction of Autoimmunity After HIV Infection

One leading hypothesis on the mechanism of autoimmunity in HIV-infected people involves the recognition system used by the virus to penetrate CD4-bearing cells. The molecular interactions of the antigen receptor (T_3T_i) *and* CD4 molecules of antiviral responder T cells with class II MHC antigen of the presenting macrophages are essential components of the process of $CD4^+$ lymphocyte activation. Since CD4 and class II MHC closely interact during this process, one could suggest that there is some similarity between the class II MHC molecules and a component of HIV (Figure 5).

This possibility has been documented to some degree. Auffray (205) identified a tetrapeptide present on the amino-terminal end of the β-chain for class II MHC molecules that is shared with the p27 of HIV. This tetrapeptide may function as an anchor for binding of HIV to the CD4 molecule. Jameson et al. (206) have suggested that there are regions of the HIV envelope protein that have a high potential for amino acid sequence overlap with the α-chain sulfhydral loop of class II MHC.

Antibodies are produced in infected individuals against a variety of antigens on HIV and recent data (118-120) indicate that cytotoxic T cells also respond to the virus (206). Any mimicry of host proteins by recognizable HIV antigens could result in the development of ''self''-reactive immunity, humoral, cellular, or both. Cross-reactivity with class II MHC molecules

1. Some antibodies and sensitized T cells that recognize the envelope protein of the AIDS-retrovirus cross-react with class II HLA-bearing cells.

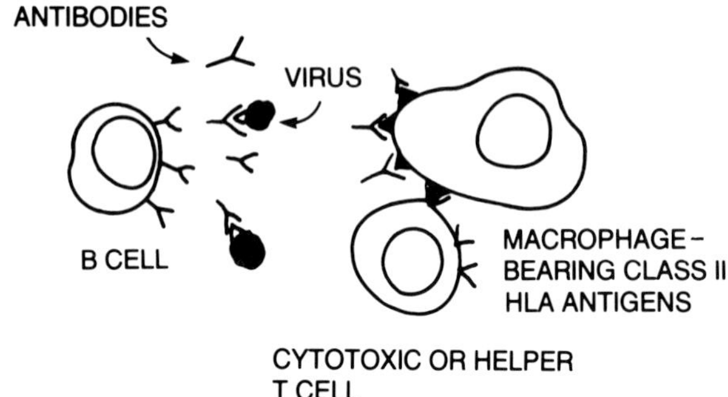

2. In addition to an autoimmune response to class II HLA antigens, anti-idiotypic antibodies or T cells may cross-react with CD-4-bearing cells.

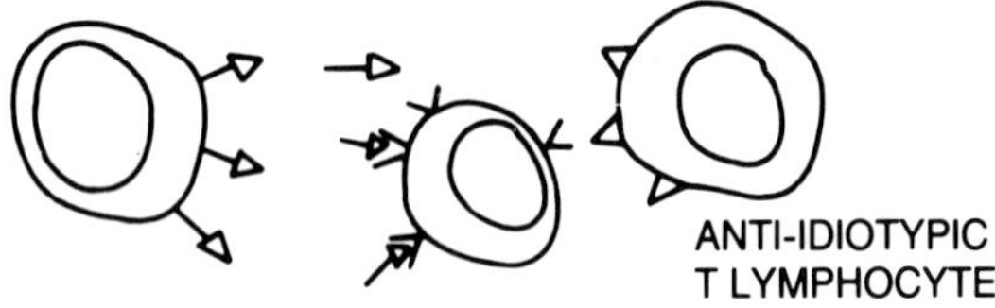

3. The net effect is a blockade of communication between CD4 lymphocytes and class II-bearing cells.

Figure 5 The combined effects of both humoral and cellular-mediated autoimmunity after HIV infection can potentially interrupt protective host responses.

could produce autoimmune events in a wide variety of tissues and block potentially protective immune responses to HIV antigens.

Limited cross-reactivity between virus and host could be possible even without direct nucleotide sequence homology between host and viral genome. This finding could occur by viral modification of host proteins. Phelan et al. (207) presented preliminary data demonstrating the presence of modified host HLA antigens on the surface of HIV. Immunogold staining with electron microscopy detected these modified HLA molecules at the same density on HIV membrane as they are on the host membrane. Such molecules could

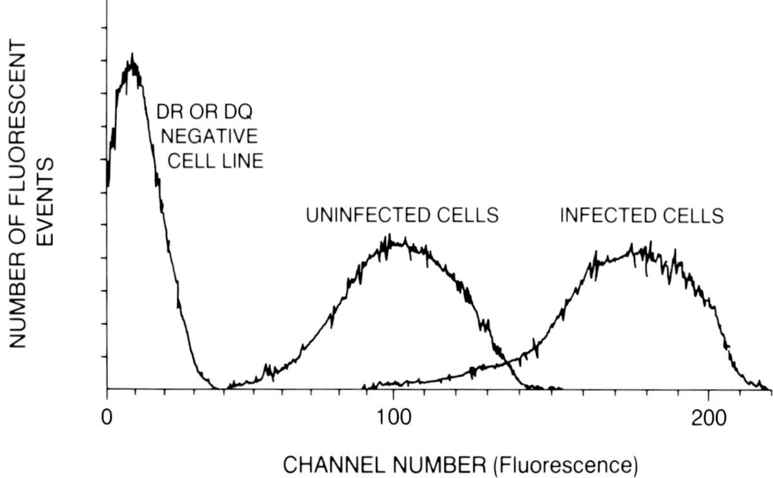

Figure 6 Flow cytometry analysis of class II MHC antigen changes on T cells after infection with HIV. Infected cells increase the relative density (X-axis, fluorescence intensity) of HLA-DR as well as HLA-DQ expression on H9 or HUT 78 cells.

mimic class II or other self antigens, thereby promoting autoreactivity. The immunoregulatory effects of class II MHC molecules which may be incorporated into HIV particles during the process of viral budding require further elucidation.

A second theory on autoimmunity in HIV infection involves IFN production and class II MHC antigens. Bottazzo et al. (208) proposed that viruses were capable of inducing the production of γIFN and that this event results in the expression of class II MHC antigens of the surface of stimulated cells. Indirect evidence to support this concept has been obtained from in vitro infection studies (Figure 6). Infection of HUT 78 cells with the HIV_{SF2} strain of HIV (45) results in a rapid and profound increase in the relative density of class II MHC antigens expressed on the cell surface. No concomitant enhancement in the expansion of either class I or known mature T cell antigens was observed. It is possible that this strong expression of class II MHC antigens can overcome normal tolerance to autoantigens (208). The potential for the development of autoantibodies directed against "self" HLA-DR components would then be greatly increased. Anti-HLA-DR antibodies are potent immunosuppressive signals capable of blocking antigen-reactive T cells from responding to the virus infection (209,210).

Aside from this concept of overcoming normal tolerance, there is some evidence that indicates that γIFN alone may contribute to autoimmunity.

This event can occur by stimulation of lymphocytes with IL-2 that is inducible with γIFN. This process in turn stimulates lymphokine activated killer cells to attack autologous noninfected, nontransformed lymphocytes (211). This effect may be a minor consideration when the host undergoes an acute viral infection but the significance could be profound in a state of chronic infection.

The interest in autoimmunity and HIV is not strictly a theoretical concern. There is genuine fear that inadequate understanding of the actual disease process caused by HIV may lead to erroneous applications of immunoaugmentative therapies with tragic consequences. For instance, design of vaccines needs to carefully consider cross-reactivity of HIV and HLA to avoid induction of autoimmunity in vaccine recipients.

IX. Summary and Conclusions

Infection with HIV causes many profound changes in the host's immune system. Prominent among these is a decrease in $CD4^+$, helper/inducer T cells especially because the receptor for HIV is the CD4 molecule itself. Subsequent fusion into giant cells and cytolysis results in reduction in helper T-cell function. Immunosuppressive properties of HIV gp120 may also impair immune responses. Functional attributes of T cells that include response to mitogens, antigen, clonal expansion, interaction with macrophages, and cytotoxic responses are all decreased to various degrees. Much of this reduction can be attributed to loss of $CD4^+$ helper T-cell function including IL-2 production which fosters these crucial immune responses. Clearly, there is a progressive loss in $CD4^+$ T-cell function and numbers as HIV disease progresses. Nevertheless, considerable variability in these parameters is present from individual to individual.

The $CD8^+$ or suppressor-cytotoxic subset of T cells increases both in percentage and absolute number in HIV infection. Many of these cells also coexpress the HNK (Leu 7) marker. This finding, in addition to the fact that they do not express the CD11b (Leu 15) marker, suggests that many of the cells may be cytotoxic rather than suppressive. However, convincing functional studies to prove this point are lacking. In addition, many of the $CD8^+$ cells bear MHC class II antigens, suggesting that they are activated or immature cells. Overall cytotoxic function for allogeneic cells or for lectin-coated target cells appears reduced, probably as a result of defective helper cell cooperation. Recently, $CD8^+$ cells have been shown to suppress viral replication in infected CD4 cells by an undefined mechanism (128). Many of the studies performed on T-cell numbers and function in HIV infections suffer from being done at a single point in time. Using these data for precise prognostic implications is therefore problematic.

Important abnormalities also occur in B cells, some of which are the result of indirect effects from disorders in the T-helper cell network but others appear to reflect direct effects of HIV, particularly those of polyclonal B-cell activation. Both EBV and HIV appear to be polyclonal activators of B cells. These viruses are likely to be involved in the increased serum immunoglobulins seen in HIV infection. In contrast, the ability of HIV-infected individuals to produce specific antibodies appears to be reduced. The presence, however, of anti-HIV antibodies in virtually all infected subjects indicates some degree of T-helper cell-B cell interactions. Under certain conditions B cells can be infected with HIV but this event does not appear to be directly related to the development of B-cell lymphomas which are increased in this population of individuals. Many B cells from HIV-infected individuals also coexpress CD5 (Leu 1) that has been related to autoantibody production (Table 5).

The monocyte/macrophage lineage can also be infected with HIV either directly through phagocytic mechanisms or through the CD4 antigen expressed on this cell population. These cells may represent an important reservoir for latent infection with HIV. Functional changes occur in this population after infection including reduced chemotaxis and decreased MHC class II expression. The latter possibly interferes with macrophage/lymphocyte interaction in the antigen-presenting function of macrophages. Natural killer cells appear to be increased in numbers in many HIV infected individuals. However, the functional capacity of these cells to kill NK-"sensitive" targets is reduced due to the failure of cytotoxic mechanisms at the killer-target cell interface. Production and receptor expression of IL-2 on T lymphocytes is almost uniformly reduced in HIV-infected individuals. Addition of IL-2 in vitro can positively correct this abnormality but clinical therapeutic trials with recombinant IL-2 have been relatively disappointing.

Although there is a large body of data on the immunological effects in HIV infection, some critical points remain unclear. Perhaps the most important is the nature of the host response to HIV itself. Antibodies are produced and T cells are probably involved in this reaction. However, direct evidence for T-cell activation by virus or viral antigens is not clearly established. The precise relationship between the immune response to HIV and protection or, alternatively, progression of the infection to disease remains one of the most important unanswered problems. The precise mechanisms of pathogenesis of the immunodeficiency in HIV infections are also not fully elucidated. The possible role of autoimmunity both at the humoral or cellular level in reducing T-helper cell or other effector mechanisms further must be considered. Fuller understanding of both the immune pathogenesis as well as the immune response is critical for the development of rational and effective therapeutic and prophylactic approaches to this devastating disease.

X. Recent Developments

Studies by Lasky et al. have identified a region of HIV gp120 that is critical for interaction with the CD4 receptor (214). In this study, deletion by in vitro mutagenesis of genes encoding 12 amino acids at positions 410 to 421 of HIV-1 gp120 abrogated its ability to bind CD4. Kowalski et al. also demonstrated that mutations at amino acid position 419 of HIV gp120 as well as mutations at positions 363 and 473 inhibited its ability to bind CD4 (215). These investigators also identified mutations that affect the anchorage of the envelope glycoprotein in the membrane, syncytia formation, the interaction of the gp120 and gp41 envelope glycoproteins, and the posttranslational processing of these proteins. In related studies, soluble forms of CD4 have been shown to block HIV infection or syncytia formation in vitro and are now being considered for use in HIV-infected patients (216). In contrast to HIV's inhibitory effects on immune responses, adaptive responses of T cells to HIV proteins and peptide subunits have been observed (217).

The levels of CTL are greatly increased in HIV-infected individuals (Table 4) but their role(s) in controlling HIV are still obscure. Walker et al. have demonstrated cytolytic activity mediated by CD8+ T cells from HIV-infected individuals against autologous target cells infected with recombinant vaccinia virus containing the HIV-1 reverse transcriptase (218). Moreover, using a novel system, Zarling et al. have demonstrated that CD4+ lymphocytes can be specifically focused to lyse HIV-infected cells using monoclonal antibody heteroconjugates that consist of anti-CD3 cross-linked to anti-HIV gp 120 (219).

Monocytes/macrophages can be infected by HIV (95,96) but the phenotypical characteristics of these cells are relatively normal in HIV-infected individuals (13,220). Functional impairment of monocytes by HIV may decrease their ability to serve as accessory cells for T-cell proliferation (63, 221).

Natural killer cells may also play a role in controlling HIV infection. Recent reports have demonstrated that NK-like cells can lyse HIV-infected or gp120-coated target cells by antibody-dependent or -independent mechanisms (219,222). These NK and related cell types may benefit HIV-infected individuals by killing HIV-infected cells or may contribute to depletion of uninfected helper T cells that have passively bound HIV gp120.

Finally, basic and clinical research programs are currently analyzing the antiviral, antitumor, and immunomodulatory effects of cytokines in HIV infections (see Section VII). Rinaldo et al. have demonstrated recently that IL2 can augment γIFN production in response to HIV antigens in vitro (223). The administration of IL-2 to AIDS patients, however, has not resulted in improvement of the patients' immunological status (224). Granulocyte-macrophage colony-stimulating factor (GM-CSF) has been shown to restrict HIV expression in vitro and to increase the levels of circulating leukocytes in leukopenic AIDS patients (225). However, this cytokine may increase HIV production (226).

Acknowledgments

Support for our studies was provided by grants from the California State AIDS Task Force, the National Institutes of Health, and the Giannini Foundation of the Bank of America. We are grateful to L. Wilhelm, J. Wang, S. Jain, T. McHugh, M. Sharp, and S. Richards for technical assistance in the execution of our studies. Charlene Anderson provided outstanding assistance in preparing the manuscript. The assistance of Dr. Harry Hollander, Tom Johnson, and Susan Stringari of the Adult Immunodeficiencies Clinic (University of California, San Francisco) was extremely valuable. We are also indebted to our colleagues at the Chiron Corporation (Emeryville, Calif.), particularly K. Steimer, C. George-Nascimento, P. Barr, and A. Gyenes for their assistance. Antigens of HIV, CMV, and *C. albicans* were generously provided by Drs. J. Yamamoto (University of California Davis, Davis), J. Mills (San Francisco General Hospital), and R. Morelli (San Francisco State University), respectively for our studies. We are particularly grateful to our study subjects for their continued cooperation.

References

1. Centers for Disease Control. Revision of the CDC surveillance case definition for acquired immunodeficiency syndrome. MMWR 1987; 36:1-15.
2. Redfield RR, Wright DC, Tramont EC. The Walter Reed staging classification for HTLV-III/LAV infection. N Engl J Med 1986; 314:131-2.
3. Singer A, Hodes RJ. Mechanisms of T cell-B cell interaction. Annu Rev Immunol 1983; 1:211-41.
4. Schwartz RH. The role of gene products of the major histocompatibility complex in T cell activation and cellular interactions. In: Paul, WE, ed. Fundamental immunology. New York: Raven Press, 1984:379-439.
5. Reinherz EL, Haynes BF, Nadler LM, Bernstein ID, eds. Leukocyte typing II. Vol. 1 New York: Springer-Verlag, 1986.
6. Shaw S. Characterization of human leukocyte differentiation antigens. Immunol Today 1987: 8:1-3.
7. Weir DM, ed. Handbook of experimental immunology. London: Blackwell Scientific, 1978.
8. Gottlieb MS, Schanker HM, Fan PT, Saxon A, Weisman JD, Pozalski I. *Pneumocystis* pneumonia—Los Angeles. MMWR 1981; 30:250-2.
9. Gottlieb MS, Schroff R, Schanker HM, et al. *Pneumocystis carinii* pneumonia and mucosal candidiasis in previously healthy homosexual men. N Engl J Med 1981; 305:1425-31.
10. Mildvan D, Mathur U, Enlow RW, et al. Opportunistic infections and immune deficiency in homosexual men. Ann Intern Med 1982; 96:700-4.
11. Mildvan D, Mathur U, Enlow R, et al. Persistent generalized lymphadenopathy among homosexual males. MMWR 1982; 31:249-51.

12. Stahl RE, Friedman-Kien A, Dubin R, Marmor M, Zolla-Pazner S. Immunologic abnormalities in homosexual men. Am J Med 1982; 73:171-8.
13. Stites DP, Casavant CH, McHugh T, et al. Flow cytometric analysis of lymphocyte phenotypes in AIDS using monoclonal antibodies and simultaneous dual immunofluorescence. Clin Immunol Immunopathol 1986; 38:161-77.
14. Krowka JF, Stites DP, Moss AR, et al. Interrelations of lymphocyte subset values, human immunodeficiency virus (HIV) antibodies and HIV antigen levels of homosexual males in San Francisco (submitted).
15. Nicholson JK, McDougal JS, Jaffe HW, et al. Exposure to human T-lymphotropic virus type III/lymphadenopathy-associated virus and immunologic abnormalities in asymptomatic homosexual men. Ann Intern Med 1985; 103:37-42.
16. Boyko WJ, Schechter MT, Jeffries E, Douglas B, Maynard M, O'Shaughnessy M. The Vancouver lymphadenopathy-AIDS study: 3. Relation of HTLV-III seropositivity, immune status and lymphadenopathy. Can Med Assoc J 1985; 133:28-32.
17. Dobozin BS, Judson FN, Cohn DL, et al. The relationship of abnormalities of cellular immunity to antibodies to HTLV-III in homosexual men. Cell Immunol 1986; 98:156-71.
18. Modlin RL, Meyer PR, Hofman FM, et al. T-lymphocyte subsets in lymph nodes from homosexual men. JAMA 1983; 250:1302-5.
19. Modlin RL, Hofman FM, Meyer PR, et al. Altered distribution of B and T lymphocytes in lymph nodes from homosexual men with Kaposi's sarcoma. Lancet 1983; i:768-71.
20. Mangkornkanok-Mark M, Mark AS, Dong J. Immunoperoxidase evaluation of lymph nodes from acquired immune deficiency patients. Clin Exp Immunol 1984; 55:581-6.
21. Wood GS, Burns BF, Dorman RF, Warnke RA. In situ quantitation of lymph node helper, suppressor, and cytotoxic T cell subsets in AIDS. Blood 1986; 67: 596-603.
22. Rodgers VD, Fassett R, Kagnoff MF. Abnormalities in intestinal mucosal T cells in homosexual populations including those with the lymphadenopathy syndrome and acquired immunodeficiency syndrome. Gastroenterology 1986; 90: 552-8.
23. Schwartz K, Visscher BR, Detels R, Taylor J, Nishanian P, Fahey JL. Immunological changes in lymphadenopathy virus positive and negative symptomless male homosexuals: two years of observation. Lancet 1985; i:831-2.
24. Nicholson JK, McDougal JS, Spira TJ, Cross GD, Jones BM, Reinherz EL. Immunoregulatory subsets of the T helper and T suppressor cell populations in homosexual men with chronic unexplained lymphadenopathy. J Clin Invest 1984; 73:191-201.
25. Nicholson JK, McDougal JS, Spira TJ. Alterations of functional subsets of T helper and T suppressor cell populations in acquired immunodeficiency syndrome (AIDS) and chronic unexplained lymphadenopathy. J Clin Immunol 1985; 5:269-74.
26. Cooper DA, Mcclean P, Finlayson R, et al. Acute AIDS retrovirus infection. Lancet 1985; i:537-40.

27. Tucker J, Ludlam CA, Craig A, et al. HTLV-III infection associated with glandular-fever-like illness in a haemophiliac. Lancet 1985; i:585.
28. Francis DP, Feorino PM, Broderson JR, et al. Infection of chimpanzees with lymphadenopathy-associated virus. Lancet 1984; ii:1276-7.
29. Carney WP, Rubin RH, Hoffman RA, Hansen P, Healey K, Hirsch MS. Analysis of T lymphocyte subsets in cytomegalovirus mononucleosis. J Immunol 1981; 126:2114-6.
30. Crawford DH, Brickell DH, Tidman N, McConnell I, Hoffbrand AV, Janossy G. Increased numbers of cells with suppressor T cell phenotype in the peripheral blood of patients with infectious mononucleosis. Clin Exp Immunol 1981; 43: 291-7.
31. Sheridan JF, Donnenberg AD, Aurelian L, Elpern DJ. Immunity to herpes simplex virus type 2: IV. Impaired lymphokine production during recredescence correlates with an imbalance in T lymphocyte subsets. J Immunol 1982; 129: 326-31.
32. Thomas HC, Brown D, Routhier G, et al. Inducer and suppressor T-cells in hepatitis B virus-induced liver disease. Hepatology 1982; 2:202-4.
33. Blomberg RS, Schooley RT. Lymphocyte markers in infectious diseases. Semin Hematol 1985; 22:81-114.
34. Casavant CH, Dixit RB, Stites DP, et al. Effects of acute infection with cytomegalovirus on lymphocyte phenotypes of homosexual males with or without infection with the human immunodeficiency virus. 1988 (submitted).
35. Reinherz E, Morimoto C, Fitzgerald KA, Hussey JF, Daley JF, Schlossman SF. Heterogeneity of human T4+ inducer T cells defined by a monoclonal antibody that delineates two functional subpopulations. J Immunol 1982; 128:463-8.
36. Gatenby PA, Kansos GS, Xian CY, Evans RL, Engleman EG. Dissection of immunoregulatory subpopulations of T lymphocytes within the helper and suppressor sublineages and man. J Immunol 1982; 129:1997-2000.
37. Gupta S. Subpopulations of CD4+ (T4+) cells in homosexual/bisexual men with persistent generalized lymphadenopathy. Clin Exp Immunol 1987; 68:1-4.
38. Tedder TF, Crain MJ, Kubagawa H, Clement LT, Cooper MD. Evaluation of lymphocyte differentiation in primary and secondary immunodeficiency diseases. J Immunol 1985; 135:1786-91.
39. Lederman MM, Ratnoff OD, Scillian JJ, Jones PK, Schachter B. Impaired cell-mediated immunity in patients with classic hemophilia. N Engl J Med 1983; 308: 79-83.
40. Menitove JE, Aster RH, Casper JT, et al. T lymphocyte subpopulations in patients with classic hemophilia treated with cryoprecipitate and lyophilized concentrates. N Engl J Med 1983; 308:83-6.
41. Pahwa S, Fikrig S, Kaplan M, Kahn E, Pahwa R. Expressions of HTLV-III in a pediatric population. In: Gupta S, ed. AIDS-associated syndromes. New York: Plenum Press, 1984:45-51.
42. Ammann AJ, Levy JA. Laboratory investigation of pediatric acquired immunodeficiency syndrome. Clin Immunol Immunopathol 1986; 40:122-7.
43. Barre-Sinoussi F, Chermann JC, Rey F, et al. Isolation of a T-lymphotropic retrovirus from a patient at risk for acquired immune deficiency syndrome (AIDS). Science 1983; 220:868-71.

44. Gallo RC, Salahuddin SZ, Popovic M, et al. Frequent detection and isolation of cytopathic retroviruses (HTLV-III) from patients with AIDS and at risk for AIDS. Science 1984; 224:500-3.
45. Levy JA, Hoffman AD, Kramer SM, Landis JA, Shimabukuro JM, Oshiro LS. Isolation of lymphocytopathic retroviruses from San Francisco patients with AIDS. Science 1984; 225:840-2.
46. Brun-Vezinet F, Rouzioux C, Barre-Sinoussi F, et al. Detection of IgG antibodies to lymphadenopathy-associated virus in patients with AIDS or lymphadenopathy syndrome. Lancet 1984; i:1253-6.
47. Safai B, Sarngadharan MG, Groopman JE. Seropeidemiological studies of human T-lymphotropic retrovirus type III in acquired immunodeficiency syndrome. Lancet 1984; i:1438-40.
48. Kaminsky LS, McHugh T, Stites DP, et al. High prevalence of antibodies to AIDS-associated retrovirus (ARV) in acquired immunodeficiency syndrome and related conditions and not in other disease states. Proc Natl Acad Sci USA 1985; 82:5535-9.
49. Popovic M, Sarngadharan MG, Read E, Gallo RC. Detection, isolation, and continuous production of cytopathic retroviruses (HTLV-III) from patients with AIDS and pre-AIDS. Science 1984; 224:497-500.
50. Kaltzmann D, Barre-Sinoussi F, Mugeyre MT, et al. Selective tropism of lymphadenopathy associated virus (LAV) for helper-inducer T lymphocytes. Science 1984; 225:59-63.
51. Dalgleish AG, Beverley PC, Clapham PR, Crawford DH, Greaves MF, Weiss RA. The CD4 (T4) antigen is an essential component of the receptor for the AIDS retrovirus. Nature 1984; 312:763-7.
52. Klatzmann D, Champagne E, Chamaret S, et al. T-lymphocyte T4 molecule behaves as the receptor for human retrovirus LAV. Nature 1984; 312:767-8.
53. McDougal JS, Kennedy MS, Sligh JM, Cort SP, Mawle A, Nicholson JKA. Binding of HTLV-III/LAV to T4+ T cells by a complex of the 110 K viral protein and the T4 molecule. Science 1986; 231:382-5.
54. Mcdougal JS, Nicholson JK, Cross GD, Cort SP, Kennedy MS, Mawle AC. Binding of the human retrovirus HTLV-III/LAV/ARV/HIV to the CD4 (T4) molecule: conformation dependence, epitope mapping, antibody inhibition, and potential for idiotypic mimicry. J Immunol 1986; 137:2937-44.
55. Lifson JD, Reyes GR, McGrath MS, Stein BS, Engleman EG. AIDS retrovirus induced cytopathology: giant cell formation and involvement of CD4 antigen. Science 1986; 232:1123-7.
56. Sodroski J, Goh WC, Rosen C, Campell K, Haseltine WA. Role of the HTLV-III/LAV envelope in syncytium formation and cytopathicity. Nature 1986; 322: 470-4.
57. Sattentau QJ, Dalgleish AG, Weiss RA, Beverley PC. Epitopes of the CD4 antigen and HIV infection. Science 1986; 234:1120-3.
58. Pert CB, Hill JM, Roff MR, et al. Octapeptides deduced from the neuropeptide receptor-like pattern of antigen T4 in brain potently inhibit human immunodeficiency virus receptor binding and T-cell infectivity. Proc Natl Acad Sci USA 1986; 83:9254-8.

59. McDougal JS, Mawle A, Cort SP, et al. Cellular tropism of the human retrovirus HTLV-III/LAV: I. Role of T cell activation and expression of the T4 antigen. J Immunol 1985; 135:3151-62.
60. Hoxie JA, Alpers JD, Rackowski, et al. Alterations in T4 (CD4) protein and mRNA synthesis in cells infected with HIV. Science 1986; 234:1123-7.
61. Friedman-Kien AE, Laubenstein LJ, Rubenstein P, et al. Disseminated Kaposi's sarcoma in homosexual men. Ann Intern Med 1982; 96:693-700.
62. Lane HC, Masur H, Edgar LC, Whalen G, Rook AH, Fauci AS. Abnormalities of B-cell activation and immunoregulation in patients with the acquired immunodeficiency syndrome. N Engl J Med 1983; 309:453-8.
63. Shannon K, Cowan MJ, Ball E, Abrams D, Volberding P, Ammann AJ. Impaired mononuclear-cell proliferation in patients with the acquired immune deficiency syndrome results from abnormalities of both T lymphocytes and adherent mononuclear cells. J Clin Immunol 1985; 5:239-45.
64. Lane HC, Depper JM, Greene WC, Whalen G, Waldmann TA, Fauci AS. Qualitative analysis of immune function in patients with the acquired immunodeficiency syndrome: evidence for a selective defect in soluble antigen recognition. N Engl J Med 1985; 313:79-84.
65. Gluckman JC, Klatmann D, Cavaille-Ceoll M, et al. Is there correlation of T cell proliferative functions and surface marker phenotypes in patients with acquired immune deficiency syndrome or lymphadenopathy syndrome? Clin Exp Immunol 1985; 60:8-16.
66. Krohn K, Ranki A, Antonen J, et al. Immune functions in homosexual men with antibodies to HTLV-III in Finland. Clin Exp Immunol 1985; 60:17-24.
67. Engleman EG, Benike CJ, Grumet FC, Evans RL. Activation of human T lymphocyte subsets: helper and suppressor/cytotoxic T cells recognize and respond to distinct histocompatibility antigens. J Immunol 1981; 127:2124-9.
68. Frederick WR, Epstein JS, Gelman EP, et al. Viral infections and cell-mediated immunity in immunodeficient homosexual men with Kaposi's sarcoma treated with human lymphoblastoid interferon. J Infect Dis 1985; 152:162-70.
69. Waner JL, Bodnick JE. Blastogenic response of human lymphocytes to human cytomegalovirus. Clin Exp Immunol 1977; 30:44-9.
70. Krowka JF, Stites DP, Mills J, et al. Effects of interleukin 2 and large envelope glycoprotein (gp120) of human immunodeficiency virus on lymphocyte proliferative responses to cytomegalovirus. Clin Exp Immunol 1988 (in press).
71. Blackwith DG, Halstead DC, Alpaugh A, Schweder D, Blouret-Fronefield, Toth K. Comparison of latex agglutination tests with five other methods for determining the presence of antibody against cytomegalovirus. J Clin Microbiol 1985; 21:328-31.
72. Pahwa S, Pahwa R, Saxinger C, Gallo RC, Good RA. Influence of the human T-lymphotropic virus/lymphadenopathy-associated virus on functions of human lymphocytes: evidence for immunosuppressive effects and polyclonal B-cell activation by banded viral preparations. Proc Natl Acad Sci USA 1985; 82: 8198-202.
73. Schnittman SM, Lane HC, Higgins SE, Folks T, Fauci AJ. Direct polyclonal activation of human B lymphocytes by the acquired immune deficiency syndrome virus. Science 1986; 233:1084-6.

74. Rosen A, Gergely P, Jondal M, Klein G, Britton S. Polyclonal Ig production after Epstein-Barr virus infection of human lymphocytes in vitro. Nature 1977; 267:52-4.
75. Yasukawa M, Zarling JM. Human cytotoxic T cell clones directed against herpes simplex virus-infected cells: I. Lysis restricted by HLA Class II MB and DR antigens. J Immunol 1984; 133:422-7.
76. Tucker MJ, Bretscher PA. T cells cooperating in the induction of delayed-type hypersensitivity act via the linked recognition of antigen determinants. J Exp Med 1982; 155:1037-41.
77. Rook AH, Masur H, Lane HC, et al. Interleukin-2 enhances the depressed natural killer and cytomegalovirus-specific cytotoxic activities of lymphocytes from patients with the acquired immune deficiency syndrome. J Clin Invest 1983; 72: 398-403.
78. Tsang KY, Fudenberg HH, Galbraith GM, Donnelly RP, Bishop LR, Koopman WR. Partial restoration of impaired interleukin-2 production and tac antigen (putative interleukin-2 receptor) expression in patients with acquired immune deficiency syndrome by isoprinosine treatment in vitro. J Clin Invest 1985; 75: 1538-44.
79. Murray HW, Welte K, Jacobs JL, Rubin BY, Mettelsmann R, Roberts RB. Production of an in vitro response to interleukin 2 in the acquired immunodeficiency syndrome. J Clin Invest 1985; 76:1959-64.
80. Alcocer-Verela J, Alarcon-Segovia D, Abud-mendoza C. Immunoregulatory circuits in the acquired immune deficiency syndrome and related complex: production of and response to interleukins 1 and 2, NK function and its enhancement by interleukin-2 and kinetics of the autologous mixed lymphocyte reaction. Clin Exp Immunol 1985; 60:31-8.
81. Murray JL, Hersh EM, Reuben JM, Munn CG, Mansell PW. Abnormal lymphocyte response to exogenous interleukin-2 in homosexuals with the acquired immune deficiency syndrome (AIDS) and AIDS related complex (ARC). Clin Exp Immunol 1985; 60:25-30.
82. Margolick JB, Volkman DJ, Lane HC, Fauci AS. Clonal analysis of T lymphocytes in the acquired immunodeficiency syndrome: evidence for abnormality affecting individual helper and suppressor T cells. J Clin Invest 1985; 76:709-15.
83. Lunardi-Iskandor Y, Georgoulias V, Rozenbaum W, et al. Abnormal in vitro proliferation and differentiation of T colony-forming cells in patients with lymphadenopathy syndrome. Blood 1986; 67:1063-9.
84. Sandstrom EG, Andrews C, Schooley RT, Byington R, Hirsch MS. Suppression of Concanavalin A-induced blastogenesis by HTLV-III infected H9 cells. Clin Immunol Immunopathol 1986; 40:253-8.
85. Margloick JB, Volkman DJ, Folks TM, Fauci AS. Amplification of HTLV-III/LAV infection by antigen-induced activation of T cells and direct suppression by virus of lymphocyte responses. J Immunol 1987; 138:1719-23.
86. Mann DL, Lasane F, Popovic M, et al. HTLV-III large envelope protein (gp120) suppresses PHA-induced lymphocyte blastogenesis. J Immunol 1987; 138: 2640-4.
87. Shalaby MR, Krowka JF, Gregory TJ, et al. The effects of human immunodeficiency virus recombinant envelope glycoprotein on immune cell functions in vitro. Cell Immunol 1987; 110:140-8.

88. Biddison WE, Rao PE, Talle MA, Goldstein G, Shaw S. Possible involvement of the OKT4 molecule in T cell recognition of class II HLA antigens: evidence from studies of cytotoxic T lymphocytes specific for SB antigens. J Exp Med 1982; 156:1065-76.
89. Romain PL, Schlossman SF, Reinherz EL. Surface molecules involved in self-recognition and T cell activation in the autologous mixed lymphocyte reaction. J Immunol 1984; 133:1093-100.
90. Flesicher B, Schrezenmeier H, Wagner H. Function of the CD4 and CD8 molecules in human cytotoxic T lymphocytes regulation of T cell triggering. J Immunol 1986; 136:1625-8.
91. Gelderblom HR, Reupke H, Pauli G. Loss of envelope antigens of HTLV III/LAV, a factor in AIDS pathogenesis. Lancet 1985; ii:1016-7.
92. Bicker U. Role of HTLV III/LAV envelope protein. Nature 1986; 324:307.
93. Weigent DA, Hoeprich PD, Bost KL, Brunck TK, Reiher WE, Blalock JE. The HTLV-III envelope protein contains a hexapeptide homologous to a region of interleukin-2 that binds to the interleukin-2 receptor. Biochem Biophys Res Commun 1986; 139:367-74.
94. Reiher WE, Blalock JE, Brunck TK. Sequence homology between acquired immunodeficiency syndrome virus envelope protein and interleukin 2. Proc Natl Acad Sci USA 1986; 83:9188-92.
95. Nicholson JK, Cross GD, Callaway CS, McDougal JS. In vitro infection of human monocytes with human T lymphotropic virus type III/lymphadenopathy-associated virus (HTLV-III/LAV). J Immunol 1986; 137:323-8.
96. Gartner S, Markovits P, Markovitz DM, Kaplan MH, Gallo RC, Popovic M. The role of mononuclear phagocytes in HTLV-III/LAV infection. Science 1986; 233:215-9.
97. Laurence J, Gottlieb AB, Kunkel HG. Soluble suppressor factors in patients with acquired immune deficiency syndrome and its prodrome. Elaboration in vitro by T lymphocyte-adherent cell interactions. J Clin Invest 1983; 72:2072-81.
98. Claman HN, Chaparon EA, Triplett RF. Thymus-marrow cell combinations. Synergism in antibody production. Proc Soc Exp Biol Med 1966; 122:1167-71.
99. Pilarski LM. A requirement for antigen-specific helper T cells in the generation of cytotoxic T cells from thymocyte precursors. J Exp Med 1977; 145: 109-15.
100. Bryant ML, Yamamoto J, Luciw P, et al. Molecular comparison of retroviruses associated with human and simian AIDS. Hematol Oncol 1985; 3:248-56.
101. Wahren B, Morfeldt-Mansson L, Biberfeld G, et al. Impaired specific cellular response to HTLV-III before other immune defects in patients with HTLV-III infection. N Engl J Med 1986; 315:393-4.
102. Steimer KS, Van Nest G, Dina D, Barr PJ, Luciw PA, Miller ET. Genetically engineered human immunodeficiency virus envelope glycoprotein gp120 produced in yeast is the target of neutralizing antibodies. In: Chanock RM, ed. Vaccines '87. New York: Cold Spring Harbor Laboratory, 1987:236-41.
103. Barr PJ, Steimer KS, Sabin EA, et al. Antigenicity and immunogenicity of domains of the human immunodeficiency virus (HIV) envelope polypeptide expressed in the yeast *Saccharomyces cerevesiae.* Vaccine 1987; 5:90-101.

104. Steimer KS, Puma JP, Power MD, et al. Differential antibody responses of individuals infected with AIDS-associated retroviruses surveyed using the viral core antigen p25^{gag} expressed in bacteria. Virology 1986; 150:283-90.
105. Gillis S, Smith KA. Long term culture of tumour-specific cytotoxic T cells. Nature 1977; 268:154-6.
106. Moretta A. Frequency and surface phenotype of human T lymphocytes producing interleukin 2. Analysis by limiting dilution and cell cloning. Eur J Immunol 1985; 15:148-55.
107. Zarling JM, Morton W, Moran PA, McClure J, Kosowski SG, Hu SL. T-cell responses to human AIDS virus in macaques immunized with recombinant vaccinia viruses. Nature 1986; 323:344-6.
108. Cupps TR, Bergin JL, Purcell RH, Goldsmith PK, Fauci AS. In vitro antigen-induced antibody responses to hepatitis B surface antigen in man: kinetic and cellular requirements. J Clin Invest 1984; 74:1204-13.
109. Lewis DE, Puck JM, Babcok GF, Rich RR. Disproportionate expansion of a minor T cell subset in patients with lymphadenopathy syndrome and acquired immunodeficiency syndrome. J Infect Dis 1985; 151:555-8.
110. Landay A, Gartland GL, Clement LT. Characterization of a phenotypically distinct subpopulation of Leu-2+ cells that suppress T cell proliferative responses. J Immunol 1983; 131:2757-61.
111. Sharma B, Gupta S. Antigen-specific primary cytotoxic T lymphocyte (CTL) responses in acquired immune deficiency syndrome (AIDS) and AIDS-related complexes (ARC). Clin Exp Immunol 1985; 62:296-303.
112. Salazar-Golzalez JF, Moody DJ, Giorgi JV, Martinez-Maza O, Mitsuyasu RT, Fahey JL. Reduced ecto-5′-nucleotidase activity and enhanced OKT10 and HLA-DR expression on CD8 (T suppressor/cytotoxic) lymphocytes in the acquired immune deficiency syndrome: evidence of CD8 cell immaturity. J Immunol 1985; 135:1778-85.
113. Baron GC, Klimas NG, Fischl MA, Fletcher MA. Decreased natural cell-mediated cytotoxicity per effector cell in acquired immunodeficiency syndrome. Diagn Immunol 1985; 3:197-204.
114. Shearer GM, Payne SM, Joseph LJ, Biddison WE. Functional T lymphocyte immune deficiency in a population of homosexual men who do not exhibit symptoms of acquired immune deficiency syndrome. J Clin Invest 1984; 74: 496-506.
115. Shearer GM, Salahuddin SZ, Markham PD, et al. Prospective study of cytotoxic T lymphocyte responses to influenza and antibodies to human T lymphotropic virus-III in homosexual men. J Clin Invest 1985; 76:1699-704.
116. Gerstorft J, Dickmeiss E, Mathiesen L. Cytotoxic capabilities of lymphocytes from patients with the acquired immunodeficiency syndrome. Scand J Immunol 1985; 22:463-70.
117. Veronese FD, De Vico AL, Copeland TD, Oroszlan S, Gallo RC, Sarngadharan MG. Characterization of gp41 as the transmembrane protein coded by the HTLV-III/LAV envelope gene. Science 1985; 229:1402-5.
118. Walker BD, Chakrabarti S, Moss B, et al. HIV-specific cytotoxic T lymphocytes in seropositive individuals. Nature 1987; 328:345-8.

119. Plata F, Autran B, Martins LP, et al. AIDS virus-specific cytotoxic T lymphocytes in lung disorders. Nature 1987; 328:348-51.
120. Zarling JM, Eichberg JW, Moran PA, McClure J, Sridhar P, Hu S-L. Proliferative and cytotoxic T cells to AIDS virus glycoproteins in chimpanzees immunized with a recombinant vaccinia virus expressing AIDS virus envelope glycoproteins. J Immunol 1987; 139:988-90.
121. Holt CA, Osorio K, Lilly F. Friend virus-specific cytotoxic T lymphocytes recognize both *gag* and *env* gene-encoded specificities. J Exp Med 1986; 164: 211-26.
122. Morris AG, Lin YL, Askonas BA. Immune interferon release when a cloned cytotoxic T-cell line meets its correct influenza-infected target. Nature 1982; 295:105-2.
123. Arya SK, Gallo RC. Human T-cell growth factor (interleukin 2) and γ-interferon genes: expression in human T-lymphotropic virus type III- and type I-infected cells. Proc Natl Acad Sci USA 1985; 82:8691-5.
124. Ruscetti FW, Mikovits JA, Kalyannasaman VS, et al. Analysis of effector mechanisms against HTLV-I and HTLV-III/LAV-infected lymphoid cells. J Immunol 1986; 136:3619-24.
125. Townsend AR, Rothbard J, Gotch FM, Bahadur G, Wraith D, McMichael AJ. Epitopes of influenza nucleoprotein can be recognized by cytotoxic T lymphocytes can by defined with short synthetic peptides. Cell 1986; 44:959-68.
126. Morrison LA, Lukacher AE, Braciole VL, Fan DP, Braciale TJ. Differences in antigen presentation to MHC Class I- and Class II-restricted influenza virus-specific cytotoxic T lymphocyte clones. J Exp Med 1986; 163:903-21.
127. Hersh EM, Mansell PW, Reuben JM, et al. Suppressor cell activity among the peripheral blood leukocytes of selected homosexual subjects. Cancer Res 1983; 43:1905-9.
128. Hoffman B, Odum N, Jakobsen BK, et al. Immunological studies in the acquired immunodeficiency syndrome: II. Active suppression or intrinsic defect investigated by mixing AIDS cells with HLA-DR identical normal cells. Scand J Immunol 1986; 23:669-78.
129. Walker CM, Moody DJ, Stites DP, Levy JA. CD8+ lymphocytes can control HIV infection in vitro by suppressing virus replication. Science 1986; 234: 1563-6.
130. Polk BF, Fox R, Brookmeyer R, et al. Predictors of the acquired immunodeficiency syndrome developing in a cohort of seropositive homosexual men. N Engl J Med 1987; 316:61-6.
131. Geedert JJ, Biggar RJ, Melbye M, et al. Effect of T4 count and cofactors on the incidence of AIDS in homosexual men infected with human immunodeficiency virus. JAMA 1987; 257:331-4.
132. Lang W, Anderson RE, Perkins H, et al. Clinical, immunologic and serologic findings in men at risk for acquired immunodeficiency syndrome. JAMA 1987; 257:326-30.
133. Murray HW, Hillman JK, Rubin BY, et al. Patients at risk for the AIDS-related opportunistic infections: clinical manifestations and impaired gamma interferon production. N Engl J Med 1985; 313:1504-10.

134. Jaffe HW, Feorino PM, Darrow WW, et al. Persistent infection with human T-lymphotropic virus type III/lymphadenopathy-associated virus in apparently healthy homosexual men. Ann Intern Med 1985; 102:627-8.
135. Vadhan-Raj S, Wong G, Gnecco C, et al. Immunological variables as predictors of prognosis in patients with Kaposi's sarcoma and the acquired immunodeficiency syndrome. Cancer Res 1986; 46:417-25.
136. Taylor J, Afrasiabi R, Fahey JL, Weaver M, Mitsuyosu R. Prognostically significant classification of immune changes in AIDS with Kaposi's sarcoma. Blood 1986; 67:666-71.
137. Lasky LA, Groopman JE, Fennie CW, et al. Neutralization of the AIDS retrovirus by antibodies to a recombinant envelope glycoprotein. Science 1986; 233:209-12.
138. Putney JD, Matthews TJ, Robey WG, et al. HTLV-III/LAV-neutralizing antibodies to an *E. coli*-producing fragment of the virus envelope. Science 1986; 234:1392-5.
139. Ballieux RE, Heijnen CJ. Immunoregulatory T cell subpopulations in man: dissection by monoclonal Ab and Fc receptors. Immunol Rev 1983; 74:5-28.
140. Morimoto C, Letvin NL, Boyd AW, Hogan M, Brown HM, Kornacki NM, Schlossman SF. The isolation and characterization of the human helper inducer T cell subset. J Immunol 1985; 134:3762-69.
141. Morimoto C, Letvin NL, Distaso JA, Aldrich WR, Schlossman SF. The isolation and characterization of the human suppressor inducer T cell subset. J Immunol 1985; 1508-15.
142. Fauci AS, Macher AB, Longo DL, Lane HC, Rook AH, Masur H, Gilman EP. Acquired immunodeficiency syndrome: epidemiologic, clinical, immunologic, and therapeutic considerations. Ann Intern Med 1984; 100:92-106.
143. Birx DL, Redfield RR, Tosato G. Defective regulation of Epstein-Barr virus infection in patients with acquired immunodeficiency syndrome (AIDS) or AIDS-related disorders. N Engl J Med 1986; 314:874-9.
144. Tosato G, Magiath IT, Blasse RM. T cell mediated immunoregulation of Epstein-Barr virus (EBV) induced B lymphocyte activation in EBV-seropositive and EBV-seronegative individuals. J Immunol 1982; 128:575-9.
145. Charpentier B, Michelson S, Martin B. Definition of human cytomegalovirus specific target antigens recognized by cytotoxic T cells generated in vitro by using an autologous system. J Immunol 1986; 137:330-36.
146. Ioachim HL, Cooper MC, Hellman GC. Lymphomas in men at high risk for acquired immune deficiency syndrome (AIDS). A study of 21 cases. Cancer 1985; 56:2831-42.
147. Groopman JE, Sullivan JL, Mulder C, Ginsburg D, Orkin SH, O'Hara CJ, Falchuk K, Wong-Staal F, Gallo RC. Pathogenesis of B cell lymphoma in a patient with AIDS. Blood 1986; 67:612-5.
148. Archibald DW, Lon L, Groopman JE, McLare MF, Essex M. Antibodies in human T-lymphotropic virus type III (HTLV-III) in saliva of acquired immunodeficiency syndrome (AIDS) patients and in persons at risk for AIDS. Blood 1986; 67:831-4.
149. Robert-Guroff M, Brown M, Gallo RC. HTLV-III neutralizing antibodies in patients with AIDS and AIDS-related complex. Nature 1984; 316:72-4.

150. Ammann AJ, Schiffman G, Abrams D, Volberding P, Ziegler J, Conant M. B cell immunodeficiency in acquired immune deficiency syndrome. JAMA 1984; 251:1447-9.
151. Montagnier L, Gruest J, Chamaret S, Daugnet C, Axler C, Guetard D, Mugeyne MT, Barre-Sinoussi F, Chermann J, Brumet JB, Klatzmann D, Gluckman JC. Adaptation of lymphadenopathy associated virus (LAV) to replication in EBV-transformed B lymphoblastoid cell lines. Science 1984; 225:63-6.
152. Levy JA, Shimabukuro J, McHugh TM, Casavant CH, Stites DP, Oshiro L. AIDS-associated retrovirus (ARV) can productively infect other cells besides human T helper cells. Virology 1985; 147:441-8.
153. Ewing EP, Chandler FW, Spira TJ, Brynes RK, Chan WC. Primary lymph node pathology in AIDS and AIDS-related lymphadenopathy. Arch Pathol Lab Med 1985; 109:977-81.
154. Hayalawa K, Hardy RR, Honda M, Herzenberg LA, Steinberg AD, Herzenberg LA. Ly-1 B cells: functionally distinct lymphocyte that secretes IgMg autoantibodies. Proc Natl Acad Sci USA 1984; 81:2494-9.
155. Antin JH, Emerson SG, Martin P, Gadot N, Ault KA. Leu-1+ (CD5+) B cells. A major lymphoid subpopulation in human fetal spleen: phenotypic and functional studies. J Immunol 1986; 136:505-10.
156. Ho DD, Rota TR, Hirsch MS. Infection of monocyte/macrophages by human T lymphotropic virus type III. J Clin Invest 1986; 77:1712-4.
157. Wood GS, Warner NL, Warnke RA. Anti-Leu 3/T4 antibodies reacting with cells of monocyte/macrophage and Langerhans lineage. J Immunol 1983; 131: 212-6.
158. Rieber P, Riethmuller G. Loss of circulating T4+ monocytes in patients infected with HTLV-III. Lancet 1986; i:270.
159. Salahuddin SZ, Rose RM, Groopman JE, Markham PD, Gallo RC. Human T lymphotropic virus type III infection of human alveolar macrophages. Blood 1986; 68:281-4.
160. Heagy W, Kelly VE, Strom TB, Mayer K, Shapiro HM, Mandel R, Finberg R. Decreased expression of human class II antigens on monocytes from patients with acquired immune deficiency syndrome. Increased expression with interferon-γ. J Clin Invest 1984; 74:2089-96.
161. Taskalos ND, Lachman LB, Newhouse YG, Whisler RL. Lysopolysaccharide (LPS) modulation of human monocytes accessory cell function in promoting T-cell colonies: inability of LPS and IL-2 to abrogate the need for monocytes with high HLA-DR expression. Cell Immunol 1984; 83:229-41.
162. Whisler RL, Newhouse YG, Lachman LB. Differential abilities of human peripheral blood monocytes quantitatively or qualitatively differing in HLA-DR and HLA-DS expression to support B cell activation in liquid and semisolid cultures. Transplantation 1985; 40:57-61.
163. Tweardy DJ, Schacter BZ, Ellner JJ. Association of altered dynamics of monocyte surface expression of human leukocyte antigen DR with immunosuppression in tuberculosis. J Infect Dis 1984; 149:31-7.
164. Smith PD, Ohura K, Masur H, Lane HC, Fauci RS, Wahl SM. Monocyte function in acquired immune deficiency syndrome. Defective chemotaxis. J Clin Invest 1984; 74:2121-8.

165. Washburn RG, Tuazon CU, Bennet JE. Phagocytic and fungicidal activity of monocytes from patients with acquired immunodeficiency syndrome. J Infect Dis 1985; 151:565-2.
166. Murray HW, Gellene RA, Libby DM, Rothermel CD, Rubin BY. Activation of tissue macrophages from AIDS patients: in vitro response of AIDS alveolar macrophages to lymphokines and interferon-γ. J Immunol 1985; 135:2374-7.
167. Lanier LL, Phillips JH, Hackett J, Tutt M, Kumar V. Opinion: Natural killer cells: Definition of a cell type rather than a function. J Immunol 1986; 137: 2735-9.
168. Lanier LL, Phillips JH. Evidence for three types of human cytotoxic lymphocyte. Immunol Today 1986; 7:132-34.
169. Ortaldo JR, Herberman RB. Natural killer cells. Annu Rev Immunol 1984; 2: 359-71.
170. Poli G, Introna M, Zanaboni F, Peri G, Carbonari M, Aiuti F, Lazzarin A, Moroni M, Mantovani A. Natural killer cells in intravenous drug abusers with lymphadenopathy syndrome. Clin Exp Immunol 1985; 62:128-35.
171. Jothy S, Gilmore N, El Gabalawy H, Prchal J. Decreased population of Leu 7+ NK cells in lymph nodes of homosexual men with AIDS-related persistent lymphadenopathy. Can Med Assoc J 1985; 132:141-4.
172. Hersh EM, Gutterman JU, Spector S, Friedman H, Greenberg SB, Reuben JM, LaPushin R, Matza M, Mansell PWA. Impaired in vitro blastogenic and natural killer cell responses to viral stimulation in AIDS. Cancer Res 1985; 45: 406-10.
173. Wisecarver J, Bechtold T, Lipscomb H, Davis J, Collins M, Purtillo D. Comparison of ADCC and NK activities of peripheral blood mononuclear cells from patients at risk for AIDS. AIDS Rev 1984; 1:347-52.
174. Bonavida B, Katz J, Gottlieb M. Mechanism of defective NK cell activity in patients with AIDS and ARC. J Immunol 1986; 137:1157-63.
175. Creemers PC, Stark DF, Boyko WJ. Evaluation of natural killer cell activity in patients with persistent generalized lymphadenopathy and AIDS. Clin Immunol Immunopathol 1985; 36:141-50.
176. Schroff RW, Gottlieb MS, Prince HE, Chai LL, Fahey JL. Immunologic studies of homosexual men with immunodeficiency and Kaposi's sarcoma. Clin Immunol Immunopathol 1982; 27:300-14.
177. Katzman M, Lederman MM. Defective post-binding lysis underlies the impaired natural killer activity in Factor VIII-treated HTLV-III serpositive hemophiliacs. J Clin Invest 1986; 77:1057-62.
178. Kabelitz D, Kirchner H, Amerding D, Wagner H. Recombinant IL-2 rapidly augments human natural killer cell activity. Cell Immunol 1985; 93:38-45.
179. Lew F, Tsang P, Solomon S, Selikoff IJ, Bekesi JG. Natural killer cell function and modulation by αIFN and IL-2 in AIDS patients and prodromal subjects. J Lab Clin Immunol 1984; 14:115-21.
180. Smith KA. Interleukin 2. Annu Rev Immunol 1984; 4:33-46.
181. Oppenheim JJ, Ruscetti FW, Steeg PS. Interleukin and interferons. In: Stites DP, et al., eds. Basic and clinical immunology. Los Altos, CA: Lange Medical Publications, 1984:86-103.

182. Kirkpatrick CH, Davis KC, Horsburgh CR, Cohn DL, Pentky K, Judson FN. IL-2 production by persons with the generalized lymphadenopathy syndrome in AIDS. J Clin Immunol 1985; 5:31-7.
183. Ebert EC, Stoll DB, Cassens BJ, Lipshutz WH, Hauptman SP. Diminished interleukin 2 production and receptor generation characterize the acquired immunodeficiency syndrome. Clin Immunol Immunopathol 1985; 37:283-97.
184. Gupta S. Study of Activated T cells in man. Clin Immunol Immunopathol 1986; 38:93-100.
185. Prince HE, Kermani-Arab V, Fahey JL. Depressed interleukin 2 receptor expression in acquired immune deficiency and lymphadenopathy syndromes. J Immunol 1984; 133:1313-7.
186. Siegel JP, Djeu JY, Stocks NI, Masur H, Geimann EP, Quinnan GV. Sera from patients with the acquired immunodeficiency syndrome inhibit production of interleukin-2 by normal lymphocytes. J Clin Invest 1985; 75:1957-64.
187. Farmer JL, Gottlieb AA, Nishihara T. Inhibition of interleukin 2 production and expression of the interleukin 2 receptor by plasma from acquired immune deficiency syndrome patients. Clin Immunol Immunopathol 1986; 38:235-43.
188. Ciobanu N, Welte K, Kruger G, Venuta S, Gold J, Feldman SP, Wang CY, Koziner B, Moore MAS, Safai B, Mertelsmann R. Defective T-cell response to PHA and mitogenic monoclonal antibodies in male homosexuals with acquired immunodeficiency syndrome and its in vitro correction by interleukin 2. J Clin Immunol 1983; 3:332-40.
189. Sheridan JF, Aurelian L, Donnenberg AD, Quinn TC. Cell-mediated immunity to cytomegalovirus (CMV) and herpes simplex virus (HSV) antigens in the acquired immune deficiency syndrome: interleukin-2 and interleukin-2 modify in vitro responses. J Clin Immunol 1984; 4:304-12.
190. Lifson JD, Benike CJ, Mark DF, Koths K, Engleman EG. Human recombinant interleukin-2 partly reconstitutes deficient in-vitro immune responses of lymphocytes from patients with AIDS. Lancet 1984; i:698-702.
191. Reddy MM, Pinyavat N, Grieco MH. Interleukin 2 augmentation of natural killer cell activity in homosexual men with acquired immune deficiency syndrome. Infect Immun 1984; 44:339-43.
192. Ernest M, Kern P, Flad H-D, Ulmer AJ. Effects of systemic in vivo interleukin-2 (IL-2) reconstitution in patients with acquired immune deficiency syndrome (AIDS) and AIDS-related complex (ARC) on phenotypes and functions of peripheral blood mononuclear cells (PBMC). J Clin Immunol 1986; 6:170-81.
193. Ammann Aj, Palladino MA, Volberding P, Abrams D, Martin NL, Conant M. Tumor necrosis factors alpha and beta in acquired immunodeficiency syndrome and AIDS related complex. J Clin Immunol 1987; 7:481-5.
194. Ziegler JL, Stites DP. Hypothesis: AIDS is an autoimmune disease directed at the immune system and triggered by a lymphotropic retrovirus. Clin Immunol Immunopathol 1986; 41:305-13.
195. Savino W, Dardenne M, March C, et al. Thymic epithelium in AIDS: An immunologic study. Am J Pathol 1986; 122:302-7.
196. Daugherty H, Chorba TL, Personette DW, et al. Immunoglobulin bound to platelets as immune complexes or specific antibody in specimens from acquired

immunodeficiency syndrome and immune thrombocytopenic purpura. Diagn Immunol 1985; 3:205-14.
197. Walsh CR, Nardi MA, Kerpatkin S. On the mechanism of thrombocytopenic purpura in sexually active homosexual men. N Engl J Med 1984; 311:635-9.
198. Stricker RB, Abrams DI, Corash L, Shuman MA. Target platelet antigen in homosexual men with immune thrombocytopenia. N Engl J Med 1985; 313: 1375-80.
199. Toy PI, Reid ME, Burns M. Positive direct antiglobulin test associated with hyperglobulinemia in acquired immunodeficiency syndrome (AIDS). Am J Hematol 1985; 19:145-50.
200. Dorsett B, Cronin W, Churna V, Iochim HL. Anti-lymphocyte antibodies in patients with the acquired immune deficiency syndrome. Am J Med 1985; 78:621-6.
201. Stricker RB, McHugh TM, Moody DJ, et al. Autoimmunity and AIDS: An AIDS-related cytotoxic autoantibody reacts with a specific antigen on stimulated helper/inducer T cells. Nature 1987; 327:710-3.
202. Pruyanski W, Jacobs H, Laing LP. Lymphocytotoxic antibodies against peripheral blood B and T lymphocytes in homosexuals with AIDS and ARC. AIDS Res 1984; 1:211-20.
203. Kiprov DD, Pfaeffle W, Parry G, et al. Antibody-mediated peripheral neuropathies associated with ARC and AIDS: successful treatment with plasma phoresis. J Clin Apheresis 1987; in press.
204. Miller RG, Parry G, Long W, Lippert R, Kiprov D. AIDS-related polyradiculoneuropathy: Prediction of response to plasma exchange with electrophysiologic testing. Muscle Nerve 1985; 8:626-31.
205. Auffray C. A molecular model of interaction between the T4 antigen and HLA class II antigens on the AIDS virus. Abstract. International Conference on AIDS, Paris, 1986.
206. Jameson BA, Guertler L, Gelderblom H, Wolf H. Priming of anti-HIV neutralizing antibodies with ENV-derived synthetic peptide. In: Chanock R, et al., eds. Vaccines '87. Cold Spring Harbor, NY: Cold Spring Harbor Press, 1986.
207. Phelan M, Gerrad TL, Quinnan GV, Epstein JS. A protease-resistant glycoprotein (PrGP) closely associated with HTLV-III/LAV particles as a class II HLA antigen. Abstract. International Conference on AIDS, Paris, 1986.
208. Botazzo GF, Pujol-Borrell R, Hanafusa T, Feldman M. Role of aberrant HLA-DR expression and antigen presentation in induction of endocrine autoimmunity. Lancet 1983; ii:1115-8.
209. Muchmore AV, Decker JM, Mann DL. Evidence that antisera that react with products of the human HLA-DR locus may block in vitro antigen-induced proliferation by inducing suppression. J Immunol 1982; 128:2063-6.
210. Kruisbeek A, Titus JA, Stephany DA, Gause BL, Longo DL. In vivo treatment with monoclonal anti-Ia antibodies: disappearance of splenic antigen-presenting cell function concomitant with modulation of splenic cell surface IA and IE antigens. J Immunol 1985; 134:3605-14.
211. Sondel PM, Hank JA, Kohler PC, Chen BP, Meinkoff DZ, Molenda JA. Destruction of autologous human lymphocytes by interleukin 2 activated cytotoxic cells. J Immunol 1986; 137:502-11.

212. Wong G, et al. J Immunol 1988; 140:120.
213. Moss A, et al. Br Med J 1988; 296:745.
214. Lasky LA, Nakamura G, Smith DH, et al. Delineation of a region of the human immunodeficiency virus type 1 gp120 glycoprotein critical for interaction with the CD4 receptor. Cell 1987; 50:975-85.
215. Kowalski M, Potz J, Basiripoor L, et al. Functional regions of the envelope glycoprotein of human immunodeficiency virus type 1. Science 1987; 237:1351-5.
216. Weiss RA. Receptor molecule blocks HIV. Nature 1988; 331:15.
217. Krowka JF, Stites DP, Jain S, et al. Lymphocyte proliferative responses to human immunodeficiency virus antigens *in vitro*: Enhanced immunogenicity of liposome-coupled synthetic peptide antigens (submitted).
218. Walker BD, Flexner C, Paradis TJ, et al. HIV-1 reverse transcriptase is a target for cytotoxic T lymphocytes in infected individuals. Science 1988; 240:64-6.
219. Zarling JM, Moran PA, Grosmaire LS, McClure J, Shriver K, Ledbetter JA. Lysis of cells infected with HIV-1 by human lymphocytes targeted with monoclonal antibody heteroconjugates. J Immunol 1988; 140:2609-13.
220. Haas JG, Riethmuller G, Ziegler-Heitbrock HW. Monocyte phenotype and function in patients with the acquired immunodeficiency syndrome (AIDS) and AIDS-related disorders. Scand J Immunol 1987; 26:371-9.
221. Petit AJ, Tersmette M, Terpstra FG, De Goede RE, Van Lier AW, Miedema F. Decreased accessory cell function by human monocytic cells after infection with HIV. J Immunol 1988; 140:1485-9.
222. Ojo-Amaize EA, Nishanian P, Keith DE, et al. Antibodies to human immunodeficiency virus in human sera induce cell-mediated lysis of human-immunodeficiency virus-infected cells. J Immunol 1987; 139:2458-63.
223. Rinaldo C, Piazza P, Wang Y, et al. HIV-1 specific production of IFN-γ and modulation by recombinant IL-2 during early HIV-1 infection. J Immunol 1988; 140:3389-93.
224. Volberding P, Moody DJ, Beardslee D, Bradley EL, Wofsy CB. Therapy of acquired immune deficiency syndrome with recombinant interleukin-2. AIDS Res Human Retroviruses 1987; 3:115-24.
225. Hammer SM, Gillis JM, Groopman JE, Rose RM. *In vitro* modification of human immunodeficiency virus infection by granulocyte-macrophage colony-stimulating factor and γ interferon. Proc Natl Acad Sci USA 1986; 83:8734-8.
226. Folks TM, Justement J, Kinter A, Dinarello CA, Fauci AS. Cytokine-induced expression of HIV-1 in a chronically infected promonocyte cell line. Science 1987; 238:800-2.

11
Pathology of AIDS

Michael B. Cohen* and Jay H. Beckstead
School of Medicine
University of California
San Francisco, California

I. Introduction

The pathological manifestations of the acquired immunodeficiency syndrome (AIDS) are protean. Any organ may be involved with disseminated disease, which includes a large variety of infections and several malignancies. In some of the organs, characteristic primary abnormalities may be identified.

In this chapter, we hope to give a brief overview of these diseases (see Table 1). The chapter is divided into two sections. The first section is a discussion of those organs most commonly biopsied antemortem, including the skin, bone marrow, liver and gastrointestinal tract, lung, and lymph nodes. The second section provides a summary of the pathology of organs that are usually examined at autopsy. Selected examples of more unusual microscopic pathology in AIDS have also been included. A discussion of pathology of the central nervous system can be found in Chapter 15. The references cited have focused on those within the pathology literature and are by no means exhaustive. Several general reviews concerning the surgical and autopsy pathology of AIDS have been published and are recommended for those seeking more detailed descriptions (1-9).

**Current affiliation*: College of Physicians and Surgeons of Columbia University, New York, New York.

Table 1 Common Pathological Findings of AIDS by Organ System

Organ	Infection	Neoplasm	Other pathology
Skin	CMV	KS	Seborrheic dermatitis
	Herpes simplex virus		Drug reaction
	Cryptococcus		
	MAI		
Bone marrow	Fungi	ML	
	MAI		
Liver	CMV	KS	Kupffer cell hyperplasia
	Fungi	ML	Steatosis
	MAI		
Oral cavity	EBV		Hairy leukoplakia
	HPV		
GI tract	CMV	KS	
	Herpes	ML	
	HPV	SCC	
	Fungi		
	MAI		
	Giardia		
	Cryptosporidia		
Lung	PC	KS	Diffuse alveolar damage
	CMV	ML	Lymphoid interstitial pneumonia
	Fungi		
	MAI		
Lymph Nodes	*Cryptococcus*	ML	Spectrum of reactive changes
	MAI	KS	
Adrenal	CMV	KS	Lipid depletion
Heart	CMV	KS	Marantic endocarditis
	Toxoplasmosis		
Spleen	Fungi	ML	
	MAI	KS	
Reproductive System	CMV		Atrophic changes
Thymus	CMV		Lymphoid depletion
			Epithelial destruction

Abbreviations: CMV, cytomegalovirus; KS, Kaposi's sarcoma; MAI, *Mycobacterium avium-intracellulare*; ML, malignant lymphoma; SCC, squamous cell carcinoma; HPV, human papillomavirus; EBV, Epstein-Barr virus; PC, *Pneumocystis carinii*.

II. Organs Commonly Biopsied Before Death

A. Skin

The most dramatic skin manifestation of AIDS is Kaposi's sarcoma (KS), but other entities have been described. These include a variety of lesions associated with infections, adverse reactions to trimethoprim-sulfamethoxazole, and more recently, a seborrheic-like dermatitis.

The characteristic clinical stages of KS (patch, plaque, nodular) can be correlated histologically. However, the diagnosis of KS is being made earlier both clinically and pathologically. Classic KS has two microscopic patterns (inflammatory and angiomatous), but in AIDS, the angiomatous form of the disease is seen almost exclusively. Histologically, there is a characteristic spindle cell infiltrate that forms ill-defined vascular channels, which dissect through collagen with a tendency to "hug" adnexal structures (10,11). Other useful features include red blood cell extravasation, inflammation with a prominent plasma cell component, and eosinophilic globules. The main differential diagnosis histologically includes dermatofibroma, hemangioma, and scar formation (12). Beckstead et al. (13), using a variety of enzyme histochemical and immunohistochemical markers, have shown that KS may originate from lymphatic endothelium. Jones and colleagues (14) have recently confirmed these observations. The etiology of KS is undetermined.

A variety of infections may also involve the skin as a result of disseminated disease. These most commonly include cytomegalovirus (CMV), which is especially noted in the perianal region, herpes simplex virus (HSV), and herpes zoster, as well as *Cryptococcus neoformans* and *Mycobacterium avium-intracellulare* (MAI). The histological features of the viral infections are characteristic. They typically produce intranuclear inclusions which may be eosinophilic (CMV) or "steel gray" (herpes) in hematoxylin and eosin-stained sections. Frequently CMV also produces inclusions in the cytoplasm. Disseminated fungal and mycobacterial infections require special stains to demonstrate the organisms. The granulomatous inflammation is often atypical, but with a silver or Fite stain the organism may be identified.

Recently, a seborrheic dermatitis-like eruption has been described (15). Although it closely resembles seborrheic dermatitis, it does have several unique histological features in patients with AIDS. These features include scattered keratinocytic necrosis, leukoexocytosis, and a superficial perivascular infiltrate of plasma cells. This entity, at present, is poorly understood but serves as a useful indicator of AIDS and its related syndromes.

A characteristic erythematous maculopapular rash, involving the whole body, has been found with increasing frequency in patients with AIDS treated for *Pneumocystis carinii* pneumonia (PCP) with trimethoprim-sulfamethoxazole (16). No distinctive histological features are present, but this entity should be kept in mind for the differential diagnosis of disorders of the skin in AIDS. A more detailed review covering the skin manifestations of AIDS, including histopathology, has recently been published (17).

B. Bone Marrow

The bone marrow is very often affected in patients with AIDS (18-22). However, there is considerable variation in both the type and degree of involvement. Generally, the bone marrow is normo- to hypercellular and has a normal to slightly increased myeloid-erythroid ratio, with normal maturation of both cell lines, and adequate megakaryocytes. A large number of nonspecific features have also been described in the marrow. Those most often observed are plasmacytosis, lymphocytosis, nonparatrabecular lymphoid aggregates, eosinophilia, serous atrophy, increased reticulin staining, increased iron staining, and hemophagocytosis.

Atypical lymphohistiocytic infiltrates are not uncommon and may indicate infection or tumor. The poor tendency of these patients to form granulomas has been well described and probably reflects their immunological disorder (22,23). In most series, granulomas in the marrow have been seen in the minority of patients and are often nonspecific.

Malignant lymphoma may involve the marrow and is characterized by paratrabecular collections of atypical lymphoid cells. Comparison with other tissue(s) and marker studies have been useful in establishing the diagnosis. Schneider and Picker (24) have reported on eight patients with myelodysplasia in AIDS, but these results have not been confirmed by others. In our own experience at the University of California, San Francisco, we have seen mild dysplastic changes in occasional marrows, primarily in the myeloid cell line. However, we have not encountered substantial numbers of clear cut myelodysplasias nor have we seen progression to acute leukemia. Kaposi's sarcoma, as a rule, does not involve the bone marrow.

The most common infection to involve the marrow is MAI and it rarely yields a prominent host response. Often, there is subtle and diffuse histiocytic infiltrate within the marrow. Routine staining for mycobacterial organisms is therefore necessary in the examination of all bone marrow specimens. Fungal involvement, however, in the marrow usually has some histological features that lead the pathologist to perform the special stains necessary to demonstrate the organism. Rarely, viral infections may also involve the bone marrow and, of these, CMV is the most common.

C. Liver

Primary liver pathology is rare in AIDS (25-27). Hepatotropic viruses produce a spectrum of inflammatory lesions that have been well described, but are not unique to this disease. Similarly, disseminated CMV, mycobacterial, and fungal infections may involve this organ. The liver is also a common site for metastatic KS and malignant lymphoma.

A number of nonspecific findings have been described similar to those in the bone marrow that are characteristic of any organ forming part of the mononuclear phagocyte system. These most commonly include Kupffer cell hyperplasia, erythrophagocytosis, and macrovesicular steatosis. Czapar et al. (28) have described two patients with peliosis hepatitis of the liver, a rare, diffuse, angiomatoid change.

D. Gastrointestinal Tract

The gastrointestinal (GI) tract and the lung are probably the two most commonly biopsied organs in AIDS. The GI tract is the site of many infections and neoplastic processes (29,30).

Numerous bacterial infections may involve this organ system, including *Neisseria gonorrhoeae*, meningococcus, *Treponema pallidum*, lymphogranuloma venereum (LGV), *Shigella* and *Salmonella*, and *Campylobacter*. Viral infections most commonly include CMV, HSV, and human papillomavirus (HPV). Parasitic infections include *Giardia lamblia*, *Entamoeba*, *Cryptosporidia*, *Isospora*, and pinworm. Mycobacterial infections, most commonly MAI, may also involve the gastrointestinal tract. The neoplasms most commonly found are KS, non-Hodgkin's lymphoma, and squamous cell carcinoma of the mouth and rectum.

The pathologist can rarely make a diagnosis of a specific bacterial infection. Certain histological features are suggestive of some of the organisms, especially LGV and enteric pathogens, but biopsies are rarely made for these conditions. CMV infection of the GI tract, although more common at the proximal and distal ends of the GI tract, may involve its entire length. The characteristic intranuclear and cytoplasmic inclusions are readily identified, often affecting endothelial cells and fibroblasts. Similarly HSV infection is most commonly found in the esophagus and the rectum, and the characteristic intranuclear inclusions are usually found within degenerating epithelial cells. Fungal infection most commonly includes *Candida* and *Cryptococcus* organisms. *Candida* is usually found in the esophagus, while *Cryptococcus* may involve any portion of the GI tract, since it is a manifestation of disseminated disease.

Protozoal infection can readily be identified by the pathologist. Giardiasis most often involves the small bowel and can lead to blunting or thickening of villi with a mixed inflammatory infiltrate. The trophozoites are found on the lumenal surface. A number of entamoebal species may involve the GI tract and the ascending colon is most commonly involved, followed by the sigmoid and rectum. Amebic ulcers have a relative paucity of inflammatory infiltration and do not tend to penetrate the bowel wall. Cryptosporidiosis

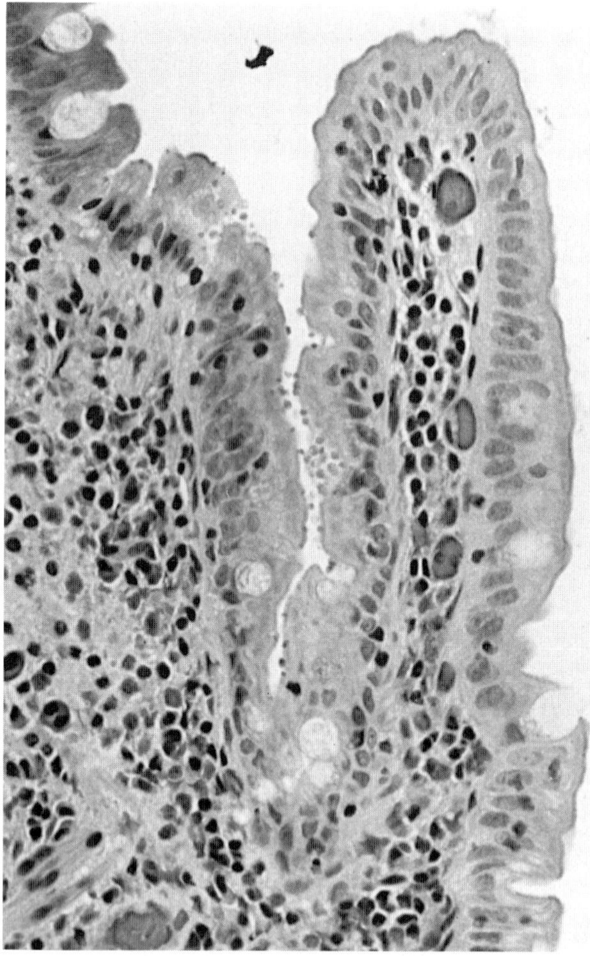

Figure 1 Small intestinal biopsy showing cryptosporidiosis. Numerous organisms are found along the luminal surface (×250).

produces a minimal inflammatory infiltrate (Figure 1), and like *Giardia*, is found on the luminal surface of the small bowel, and rarely, the gall bladder. MAI infection rarely produces granulomatous inflammation, but more commonly produces a histiocytic infiltrate within the lamina propria (Figure 2). This lesion was originally confused with Whipple's disease. Special stains are necessary to make this diagnosis. In the tongue, a distinctive lesion, termed "hairy leukoplakia," has been identified (31,32). This form of leukoplakia is often found on the lateral aspects of the tongue and clinically has a "hairy" surface. Histologically, this lesion resembles a flat wart with fine keratin projection, koilocytosis, and a minimal subepithelial inflammatory infiltrate (Figure 3). Greenspan et al. (32) have recently observed Epstein-Barr virus (EBV) and perhaps HPV within the same affected cells (32).

Kaposi's sarcoma often involves the GI tract when it disseminates (33). Large tumor nodules are found within the bowel wall and have a histological

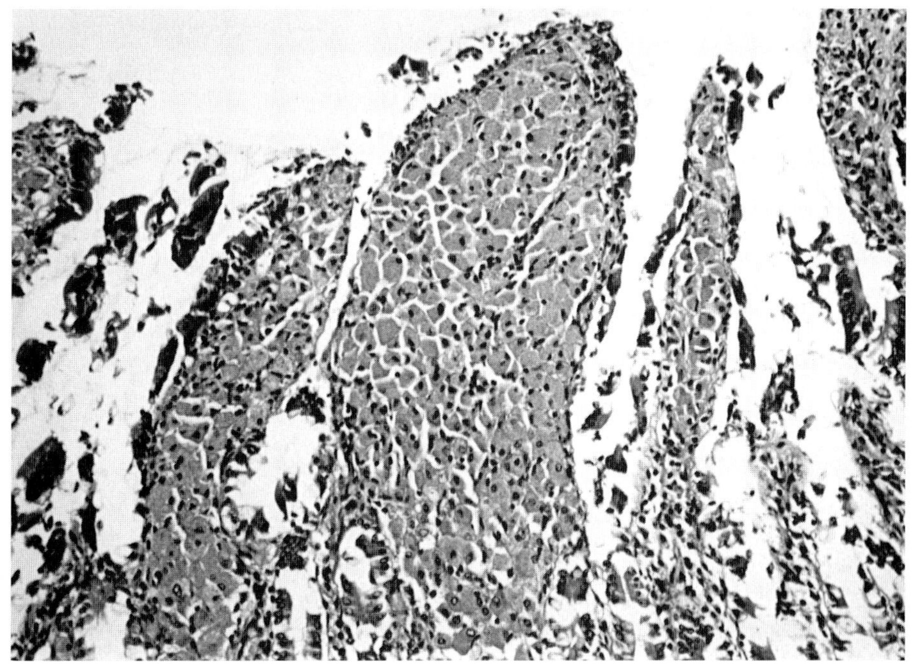

Figure 2 An MAI infection in the small bowel, reminiscent of Whipple's disease. The lamina propria is filled with mononuclear cells stuffed with organisms (× 100).

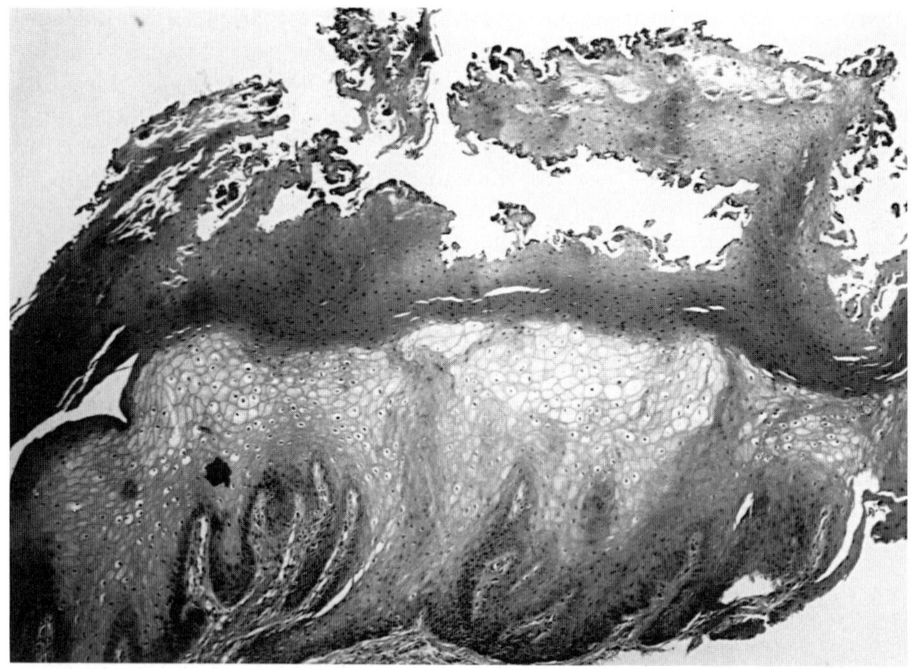

Figure 3 A case of "hairy leukoplakia." Note the fine keratin projections and koilocytosis (×25).

picture similar to that seen in the skin. Malignant lymphomas may also involve the GI tract, not uncommonly as the initial site of presentation. Patients with AIDS also have a higher incidence of rectal carcinoma, which is usually of squamous cell type, or less commonly of apparent cloacogenic origin (34,35). The histological features are similar to those seen in non-AIDS patients. Recently, precancerous lesions have been identified in the anal mucosa (36).

E. Lung

The lung is almost always affected at some stage of the disease in patients with AIDS (37,38). Furthermore, there are usually multiple processes taking place and respiratory problems are the primary cause of death (39). Infectious processes are more often found than neoplastic ones. Both pre- and postmortem, PCP is the most common infection (see Chapter 16). Histologically, there is a typical foamy eosinophilic exudate in the alveolar spaces

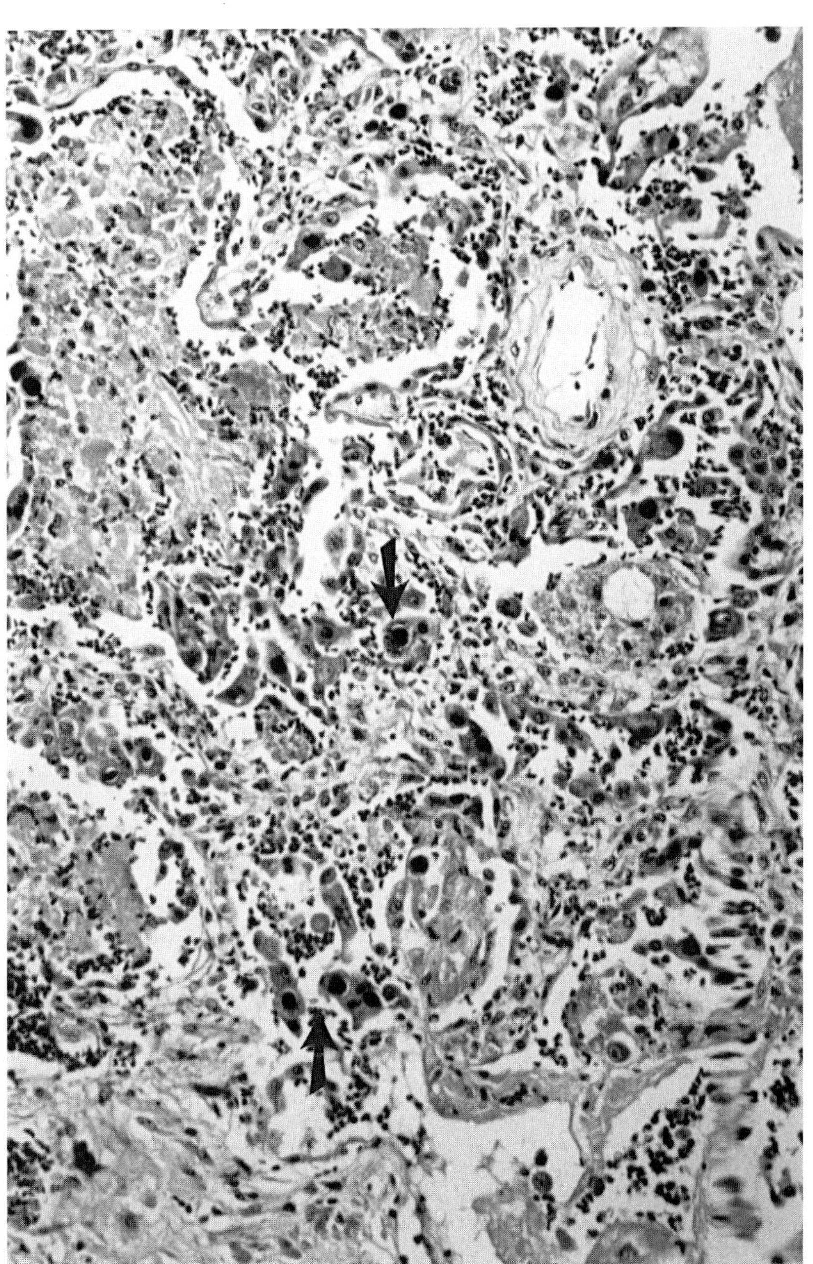

Figure 4 Extensive CMV infection involving the lung. There are many large cells with prominent intranuclear inclusions (*arrow*) (×40).

within which the organisms of PCP may be identified with a silver stain. There may be an accompanying chronic inflammatory cell infiltrate within the alveolar septae, and not uncommonly, there may be evidence of diffuse alveolar damage (DAD, clinically known as adult respiratory distress syndrome [ARDS]) (40). Mycobacterial infection of the lung may also be observed, and is characteristically composed of a diffuse histiocytic infiltrate containing the organisms, without granulomatous inflammation, and rarely leads to tissue destruction. A large number of fungal organisms, particularly *Candida*, *Cryptococcus*, *Aspergillus*, and *Histoplasma*, may involve the lung; CMV infection of the lung is the single most common infectious virus identified (Figure 4). Involvement tends to be extensive and severe, and is also commonly associated with DAD. Other viral infections, such as HSV, are observed less often.

Lung involvement by KS is usually interstitial and may produce both linear as well as nodular tumor aggregates. The linear type of involvement follows the path of the alveolar walls as well as the bronchovascular sheath.

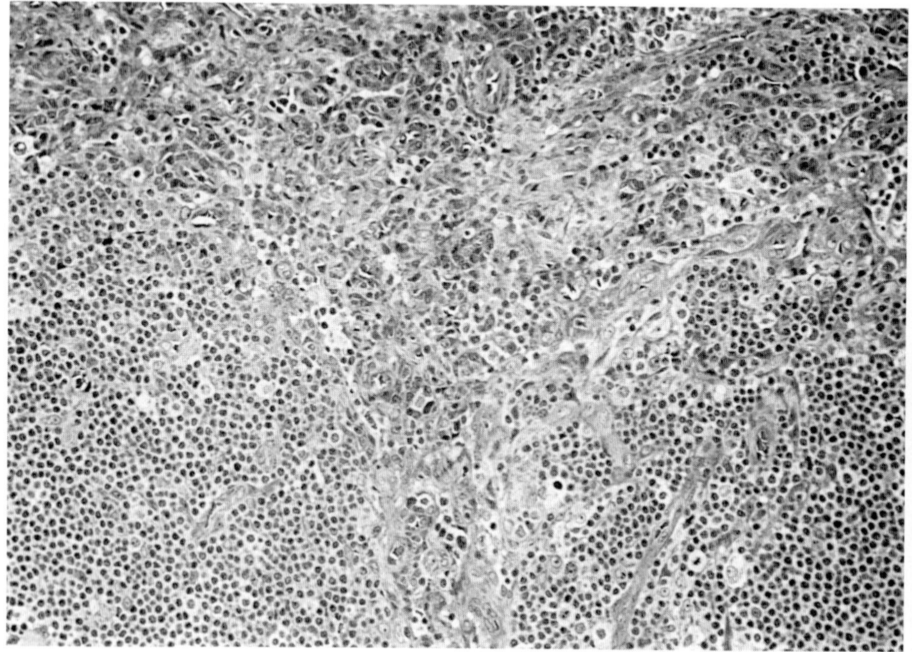

Figure 5 High-grade malignant lymphoma. The lymph node is replaced by a monotonous population of small noncleaved lymphocytes (×100).

Nodular involvement by KS is usually along larger airways and vessels. Both may lead to fatal pulmonary hemorrhage. Malignant lymphomas may also involve the lung, but the lung is rarely the primary site.

In children, the diagnosis of AIDS may be made with the identification of lymphoid interstitial pneumonia (LIP) (41,42). In this poorly understood entity, one finds diffuse infiltration of the septae and peribronchial areas with lymphocytes, plasma cells, and immunoblasts. There may be some nodular aggregates and rare germinal centers may be identified. No viral inclusions or mycobacterial or fungal organisms are identifiable. The etiology of LIP is uncertain, but may be related to primary infection with HIV.

F. Lymph Nodes

Lymph node involvement with AIDS and its related syndromes is a prominent feature and may take one of several different appearances histologically (43-47). Most common is a characteristic florid follicular hyperplasia typically observed in patients with persistent lymphadenopathy syndrome (see Chapter 12). This pattern includes marked expansion of the follicles with

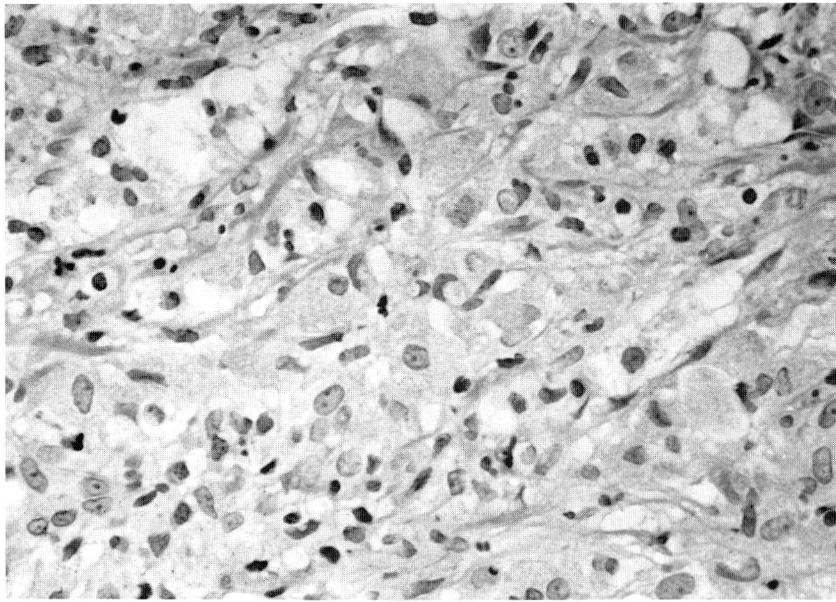

Figure 6 Kaposi's sarcoma involving lymph node. Numerous abnormal vascular channels are present (×40).

compression of interfollicular tissue. The cell population within the follicles is heterogeneous. Absence of lymphocytic mantles is not uncommonly observed. At times, there may be a prominent interfollicular proliferation of small- to medium-sized lymphocytes, histiocytes, plasma cells, as well as increased numbers of small vessels. Terminally, and postmortem, there is often a prominent lymphocytic depletion of the lymph nodes with overall lymph node hypocellularity featuring small or absent follicular centers. Hyalinization may be a prominent feature.

A variety of intermediate and high-grade malignant lymphomas have also been observed with increasing frequency (Figure 5). Recent evidence indicates these are of B-cell origin (48-51,68). There may also be an increase in Hodgkin's disease (45,52). Moreover, the lymph node may be the site of "metastatic spread" of Kaposi's sarcoma or involvement with so-called lymphadenopathic KS (10,53). In the lymph nodes, the subcapsular sinus is almost invariably involved, with extension into the main portion of the lymph

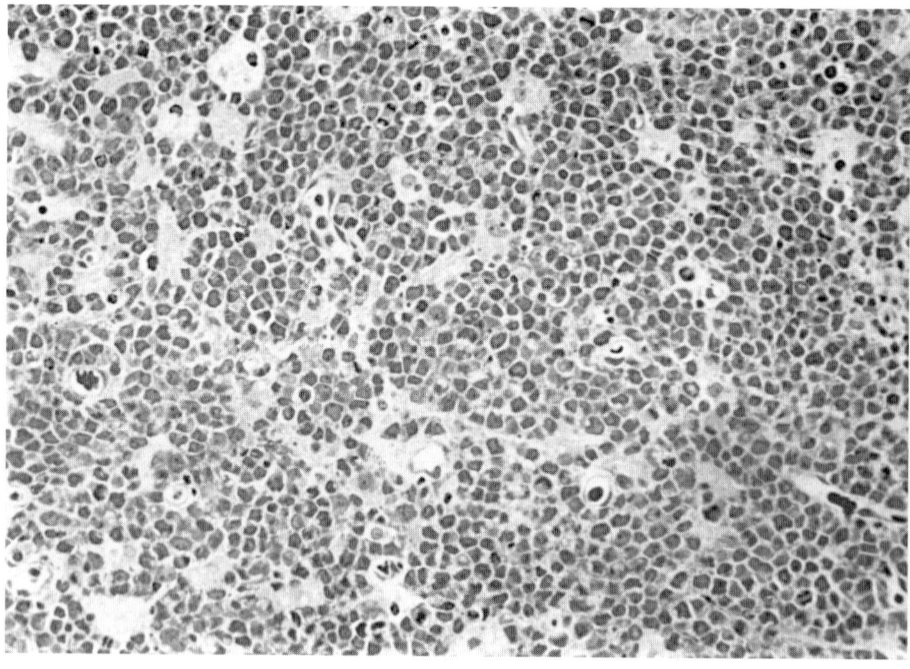

Figure 7 An MAI infection involving a lymph node. The node is replaced by foamy macrophages with numerous organisms (×100).

node along fibrous septae (Figure 6). Not uncommonly, there is an associated inflammatory component.

Numerous infections, all representing disseminated disease, may involve the lymph node. The most frequently encountered are MAI (Figure 7) and *Cryptococcus*. Involvement of the lymph node with CMV is not often observed.

III. Organs at Autopsy

A. Adrenal

Clinical features of adrenal steroid deficiency are not uncommon in patients with AIDS (64). The adrenal has not been biopsied antemortem, but is very often involved with disseminated diseases at autopsy (54). Most commonly, these are CMV and KS. Involvement by CMV may be focal or diffuse, and the medulla is most severely affected. There is a minimal inflammatory response, but necrosis can be extensive and appears to be related to the extent of involvement. Additionally, CMV infection has been documented in other endocrine organs, including the pancreas, parathyroid, and thyroid.

Metastatic KS is the most common neoplasm involving the adrenal, but it spreads to this organ considerably less often than to lymph nodes or the GI tract.

In a review of 41 patients, Glasgow et al. (54) found lipid depletion of the adrenal gland often focal in all AIDS cases. Only two cases of Waterhouse-Friderichsen's syndrome have been recognized at autopsy (3).

B. Heart

The heart is rarely involved, but primary cardiac pathology most commonly includes marantic endocarditis and pericarditis (55,56). Reports of disseminated infections (toxoplasmosis, CMV) and metastatic KS have also been published. Because most patients with AIDS have been young, cardiac disease has been a rare cause of death. In the series of 36 patients reported by Welch et al. (6) acute myocardial infarction was found in only two patients, and six additional patients had focal interstitial fibrosis (6). Similar findings were reported in the series by Cammarosano and Lewis (55).

C. Reproductive System

Testicular involvement with CMV and KS has been observed. A variable spermatic maturation arrest and tubular fibrosis has been noted, probably accounting for the hypospermia. These findings, however, are nonspecific. The prostate has similarly been the site of disseminated disease, but primary pathology has not been described.

D. Spleen

Involvement of the spleen in AIDS mimics involvement in lymph nodes. Primary diseases affecting the spleen include lymphoma. Kaposi's sarcoma may secondarily involve this organ. Numerous infections may be found in the spleen, usually with overwhelming dissemination of the responsible microbiological agent.

E. Thymus

The thymus is rarely involved with disseminated infection or neoplasm, and when it is, it is usually by infection with CMV. All reports, however, have indicated severe disease in this organ in AIDS, possibly by the direct effect of HIV (57-59).

Marked involution is the rule with a decrease in weight, lymphoid and epithelial elements, and an increase in fat. The severe lymphoid depletion results in the loss of normal architecture with absent lobules and ill-defined corticomedullary junctions. A variable, nonspecific plasma cell infiltrate is also commonly observed. Recent evidence indicates that there is also marked epithelial cell destruction contributing to the abnormal architecture and manifested by rare or absent Hassall's corpuscles. Growdy et al. (58) have also described nonspecific vascular changes, including hyalinization and onion-skinning.

In a report of four children, Joshi and colleagues (57) found similar changes in the thymus, but vascular changes were not observed.

F. Miscellaneous

Involvement of the eye is most usually due to CMV choreoretinitis, but reports of ocular toxoplasmosis and PCP have been published (60,65,66). The involvement of KS in the eye is very rarely observed. In some patients, a perivasculitis has been observed that was unrelated to CMV or KS (66). A peculiar sialadenitis has been observed clinically. Pathological examination, however, is limited. Some of these appear to be related to hyperreactive lymph nodes within the salivary glands and disseminated CMV infections (8,61). Recently a Sjögren's syndrome-like illness has been recognized (62). A number of organ-specific renal abnormalities have been described in AIDS patients (63,67), including: acute tubular necrosis, interstitial nephritis, proliferative glomerulonephritis, and HIV-associated nephropathy.

References

1. Millard PR. AIDS: histopathological aspects. J Pathol 1984; 143:223-39.
2. Amberson JB, DeCarlo EF, Metroka CE, Koizumi JH, Momadrian JA. Diagnostic pathology in the acquired immunodeficiency syndrome. Arch Pathol Lab Med 1985; 109:345-51.

3. Reichert CM, O'Leary TJ, Levens DL, Simrell CR, Macher AM. Autopsy pathology in the acquired immune deficiency syndrome. Am J Pathol 1983; 112: 357-82.
4. Guarda LA, Luna MA, Smith JL, Mansell PWA, Gyorkey F, Roca AN. Acquired immune deficiency syndrome: postmortem findings. Am J Clin Pathol 1984; 81:549-57.
5. Hui An, Koss MN, Meyer PR. Necropsy findings in acquired immunodeficiency syndrome: a comparison of premortem diagnoses with postmortem findings. Hum Pathol 1984; 15:670-6.
6. Welch K, Finkbeiner W, Alpers CE, Blumenfeld W, Davis RL, Smuckler EA, Beckstead JH. Autopsy findings in the acquired immune deficiency syndrome. JAMA 1984; 252:1152-9.
7. Urmacher C, Nielsen S. The histopathology of the acquired immune deficiency syndrome. Pathol Annu 1985; 20:197-220.
8. Mobley K, Rotterdam HZ, Lerner CW, Tapper ML. Autopsy findings in the acquired immune deficiency syndrome. Pathol Annu 1985; 20:45-65.
9. Niedt GW, Schinella RA. Acquired immunodeficiency syndrome: clinicopathologic study of 56 autopsies. Arch Pathol Lab Med 1985; 109:727-34.
10. Finkbeiner WE, Egbert BM, Groundwater JR, Sagebiel RW. Kaposi's sarcoma in young homosexual men: a histopathologic study with particular reference to lymph node involvement. Arch Pathol Lab Med 1982; 106:261-4.
11. Francis ND, Parkin JM, Weber J, Boylston AW. Kaposi's sarcoma in acquired immune deficiency syndrome (AIDS). J Clin Pathol 1986; 39:469-74.
12. Blumenfeld W, Egbert BM, Sagebiel RW. Differential diagnosis of Kaposi's sarcoma. Arch Pathol Lab Med 1985; 109:123-7.
13. Beckstead JH, Wood GS, Fletcher V. Evidence for the origin of Kaposi's sarcoma from lymphatic epithelium. Am J Pathol 1985; 119:294-300.
14. Jones RR, Spaull J, Spry C, Jones EW. Histogenesis of Kaposi's sarcoma in patients with and without acquired immune deficiency syndrome (AIDS). J Clin Pathol 1986; 39:742-9.
15. Soeprono FF, Schinella RA, Cockerell CJ, Comite SL. Seborrheic-like dermatitis of acquired immunodeficiency syndrome. J Am Acad Dermatol 1986; 14: 242-8.
16. Gordin FM, Simon GL, Wofsy CB, Mills J. Adverse reactions to trimethoprim-sulfamethoxazole in patients with the acquired immunodeficiency syndrome. Ann Intern Med 1984; 100:495-9.
17. Warner LC, Fisher BK. Cutaneous manifestations of the acquired immunodeficiency syndrome. Int J Dermatol 1986; 25:337-50.
18. Spivak JL, Bender BS, Quinn TC. Hematologic abnormalities in the acquired immune deficiency syndrome. Am J Med 1984; 77:224-8.
19. Osborne BM, Guarda LA, Butler JJ. Bone marrow biopsies in patients with the acquired immunodeficiency syndrome. Hum Pathol 1984; 15:1048-53.
20. Abrams DI, Chinn EK, Lewis BJ, Volberding P, Conant MA, Townsend RM. Hematologic manifestations in homosexual men with Kaposi's sarcoma. Am J Clin Pathol 1984; 81:13-8.
21. Geller SA, Muller R, Greenberg ML, Siegal FP. Acquired immunodeficiency syndrome: distinctive features of bone marrow biopsies. Arch Pathol Lab Med 1985; 109:138-41.

22. Castella A, Croxson TS, Mildvan D, Witt DH, Zalusky R. The bone marrow in AIDS: a histologic, hematologic, and microbiologic study. Am J Clin Pathol 1985; 84:425-32.
23. Jagadha V, Andavolu RH, Huang CT. Granulomatous inflammation in the acquired immune deficiency syndrome. Am J Clin Pathol 1985; 84:598-602.
24. Schneider DR, Picker LJ. Myelodysplasia in the acquired immune deficiency syndrome. Am J Clin Pathol 1985; 84:144-52.
25. Glasgow BJ, Anders K, Layfield LJ, Steinsapir KD, Gitnick GL, Lewin KJ. Clinical and pathologic findings of the liver in the acquired immune deficiency syndrome (AIDS). Am J Clin Pathol 1985; 83:582-8.
26. Lebovics E, Thung SN, Schaffner F, Radensky PW. The liver in the acquired immunodeficiency syndrome: a clinical and histologic study. Hepatology 1985; 5:293-8.
27. Orenstein MS, Tavitian A, Yonk B, Dincsoy HP, Zerega J, Iyer SK, Straus EW. Granulomatous involvement of the liver in patients with AIDS. Gut 1985; 26: 1220-5.
28. Czapar CA, Weldon-Linne CM, Moore DM, Rhone DP. Peliosis hepatitis in the acquired immunodeficiency syndrome. Arch Pathol Lab Med 1986; 110:611-3.
29. Baker RW, Peppercorn MA. Gastrointestinal ailments of homosexual men. Medicine 1982; 61:390-405.
30. Rotterdam H, Sommers SC. Alimentary tract biopsy lesions in the acquired immune deficiency syndrome. Pathology 1985; 17:181-92.
31. Greenspan D, Conant M, Silverman S, Greenspan JS, Petersen V, DeSouza Y. Oral "hairy" leucoplakia in male homosexuals: evidence of association with both papillomavirus and a Herpes-group virus. Lancet 1984; 2:831-4.
32. Greenspan JS, Greenspan D, Lennette ET, Abrams DI, Conant MA, Petersen V, Freese UK. Replication of Epstein-Barr virus within the epithelial cells of oral "hairy" leukoplakia, an AIDS-associated lesion. N Engl J Med 1985; 313: 1564-71.
33. Friedman SL, Wright TL, Altman DF. Gastrointestinal Kaposi's sarcoma in patients with acquired immunodeficiency syndrome: endoscopic and autopsy findings. Gastroenterology 1985; 89:102-8.
34. Li FP, Osborn D, Cronin CM. Anorectal squamous carcinoma in two homosexual men. Lancet 1982; 2:391.
35. Cooper HS, Patchefsky AS, Marks G. Cloacogenic carcinoma of the anorectum in homosexual men. Dis Colon Rectum 1979; 22:557-8.
36. Nash G, Allen W, Nash S. Atypical lesions of the anal mucosa in homosexual men. JAMA 1986; 256:873-6.
37. Nash G, Fligiel S. Pathologic features of the lung in the acquired immune deficiency syndrome (AIDS): an autopsy study of seventeen homosexual males. Am J Clin Pathol 1984; 81:6-12.
38. Marchevsky A, Rosen MJ, Chrystal G, Kleinerman J. Pulmonary complications of the acquired immunodeficiency syndrome: a clinicopathologic study of 70 cases. Hum Pathol 1985; 16:659-70.
39. Moskowitz L, Hensley GT, Chan JC, Adams K. Immediate causes of death in acquired immunodeficiency syndrome. Arch Pathol Lab Med 1985; 109:735-8.

40. Ramaswamy G, Jagadha V, Tchertkoff V. Diffuse alveolar damage and interstitial fibrosis in acquired immunodeficiency syndrome patients without concurrent pulmonary infection. Arch Pathol Lab Med 1985; 109:408-12.
41. Oleske J, Minnefor A, Cooper R, Thomas K, delaCruz A, Ahdieh M, Guerrero I, Joshi VV, Desposito F. Immune deficiency syndrome in children. JAMA 1983; 249:2345-9.
42. Joshi VV, Oleske JM, Minnefor AB, Saad S, Klein KM, Singh R, Zabala M, Dadzie C, Simpser M, Rapkin RH. Pathologic pulmonary findings in children with the acquired immunodeficiency syndrome: a study of ten cases. Hum Pathol 1985; 16:241-6.
43. Ioachim HL, Lerner CW, Tapper ML. The lymphoid lesions associated with the acquired immunodeficiency syndrome. Am J Surg Pathol 1983; 7:543-53.
44. Meyer PR, Yanagihara ET, Parker JW, Lukes RJ. A distinctive follicular hyperplasia in the acquired immune deficiency syndrome (AIDS) and the AIDS related complex. Hematol Oncol 1984; 2:319-47.
45. Burns BF, Wood GS, Dorfman RF. The varied histopathology of lymphadenopathy in the homosexual male. Am J Surg Pathol 1985; 9:287-97.
46. Ewing EP, Chandler FW, Spira TJ, Brynes RK, Chan WC. Primary lymph node pathology in AIDS and AIDS-related lymphadenopathy. Arch Pathol Lab Med 1985; 109:977-81.
47. Raphael M, Pouletty P, Cavaille-Coll M, Rozenbaum W, Homond A, Nonnenmacher L, Delcourt A, Gluckman JC, Debre P. Lymphadenopathy in patients at risk for acquired immunodeficiency syndrome: Histopathology and histochemistry. Arch Pathol Lab Med 1985; 109:128-32.
48. Editorial. Malignant lymphomas in homosexuals. Lancet 1986; 1:193-94.
49. Ziegler JL, Beckstead JH, Volberding PA, Abrams DI, Levine AM, Lukes RJ, Gill PS, Burkes RL, Meyer PR, Metroka GE, Mouradian J, Moore A, Riggs SA, Butler JJ, Cabanillas FC, Hersh E, Newell GR, Laubenstein LJ, Knowles D, Odajnyk C, Raphael B, Koziner B, Urmacher C, Clarkson BD. Non-Hodgkin's lymphoma in 90 homosexual men: Relation to generalized lymphadenopathy and the acquired immunodeficiency syndrome. N Engl J Med 1984; 311: 565-70.
50. Kalter SP, Riggs SA, Cabanillas F, Butler JJ, Hagemeister FB, Mansell PW, Newell GR, Velasquez WS, Salvador P, Barlogie B, Rios A, Hersh EM. Aggressive non-Hodgkin's lymphomas in immunocompromised homosexual males. Blood 1985; 66:655-9.
51. Ioachim HL, Cooper MC, Hellman GC. Lymphomas in men at high risk for acquired immune deficiency syndrome (AIDS): a study of 21 cases. Cancer 1985; 56:2831-42.
52. Unger PD, Strauchen JA. Hodgkin's disease in AIDS complex patients. Cancer 1986; 58:821-5.
53. Moskowitz LB, Hensley GT, Gould EW, Weiss SD. Frequency and anatomic distribution of lymphadenopathic Kaposi's sarcoma in the acquired immunodeficiency syndrome: an autopsy series. Hum Pathol 1985; 16:447-56.
54. Glasgow BJ, Steinsapir KD, Anders K, Layfield LJ. Adrenal pathology in the acquired immune deficiency syndrome. Am J Clin Pathol 1985; 84:594-7.

55. Cammarosano C, Lewis W. Cardiac lesions in acquired immune deficiency syndrome (AIDS). J Am Coll Cardiol 1985; 5:703-6.
56. Roldan EO, Moskowitz L, Hensley GT. Pathology of the heart in acquired immunodeficiency syndrome. Arch Pathol Lab Med 1987; 111:943-6.
57. Joshi VV, Oleske JM. Pathologic appraisal of the thymus gland in acquired immunodeficiency syndrome in children: a study of four cases and a review of the literature. Arch Pathol Lab Med 1985; 109:142-6.
58. Grody WW, Fligiel S, Naeim F. Thymus involution in the acquired immunodeficiency syndrome. Am J Clin Pathol 1985; 84:85-95.
59. Savino WM, Dardenne M, Marche C, Trophilme D, Dupuy J-M, Pekovic D, LaPointe N, Bach J-F. Thymic epithelium in AIDS: an immunohistologic study. Am J Pathol 1986; 122:302-7.
60. Friedman AH. The retinal lesions of the acquired immune deficiency syndrome. Trans Am Ophthalmol Soc 1984; 82:480-91.
61. Ryan JR, Ioachim HL, Marmer J, Loubeau JM. Acquired immune deficiency syndrome-related lymphadenopathies presenting in the salivary gland lymph nodes. Arch Otolaryngol 1985; 111:554-6.
62. Ulirsch RC, Jaffe ES. Sjögren's syndrome-like illness associated with the acquired immunodeficiency syndrome-related complex. Hum Pathol 1987; 18: 1063-8.
63. Rao TKS, Friedman EA, Nicastri AD. The types of renal disease in the acquired immunodeficiency syndrome. N Engl J Med 1987; 316:1062-8.
64. Membreno L, Irony I, Dere W, et al. Adrenocortical function in acquired immunodeficiency syndrome. J Clin Endocrinol & Metab 1987; 65:482-7.
65. Khadem M, Kalish SB, Goldsmith J, et al. Ophthalmologic findings in acquired immune deficiency syndrome (AIDS). Arch Ophthalmol 1984; 102:201-6.
66. Kestelyn P, Van de Perre P, Rouvroy D, et al. A prospective study of the ophthalmologic findings in the acquired immune deficiency syndrome in Africa. Am J Ophthalmol 1985; 100:230-8.
67. Cohen AH, Nast CC. HIV-associated nephropathy. Mod Pathol 1988; 1:87-97.
68. Kaplan MH, Susin M, Pahwa SG, et al. Neoplastic complications of HTLV-III infection: Lymphomas and solid tumors. Am J Med 1987; 82:389-96.

12

The Persistent Lymphadenopathy Syndrome and Immune Thrombocytopenic Purpura in HIV-Infected Individuals

Donald I. Abrams

Cancer Research Institute
School of Medicine
University of California
and San Francisco General Hospital
San Francisco, California

I. Introduction

Two years before the acquired immunodeficiency syndrome (AIDS) was first described in the medical literature, clinical conditions now known to be "AIDS-related" had caught the attention of physicians caring for large numbers of homosexual men in New York and California. In 1979, these physicians noticed an increased incidence of generalized lymphadenopathy with constitutional symptoms among their male homosexual patients. No clues to the etiology of the adenopathy were obtained from serological testing or lymph node biopsies, which revealed only benign reactive changes. The patients were advised to diminish immune system stimulation by modifying their life-styles.

By mid-1981, when the first formal definitions of the acquired immunodeficiency syndrome were published (1-3), a high incidence of generalized lymphadenopathy was noted on physical examination in patients with the opportunistic infections and unusual malignancies characteristic of this syndrome (4). The question arose: were those homosexual men seen two years previously with persistent generalized lymphadenopathy now the ones developing the life-threatening diseases associated with AIDS? And if the two phenomena were connected, how should the generalized lymphadenopathy be defined in relation to acquired immunodeficiency, and what should it be called?

Investigators soon became convinced that these syndromes were indeed connected and terms to describe the generalized lymphadenopathy proliferated in the literature. Names included persistent generalized lymphadenopathy (PGL), chronic lymphadenopathy syndrome, extended lymphadenopathy syndrome, chronic polyadenopathy, chronic unexplained lymphadenopathy, and "lesser AIDS." The terms "pre-AIDS" and "AIDS prodrome" arose after publication of observations of the natural history of cohorts of patients with lymphadenopathy which indicated that some were at risk for developing the more life-threatening manifestations of AIDS. All of these terms described overlapping subsets of patients, yet the sheer abundance of names and the lack of a commonly held definition of the conditions they designated were confusing and a potential stumbling block to epidemiological and clinical research.

In an effort to establish a more workable definition and to assure uniformity of the subsets of patients being followed in various prospective studies and therapeutic intervention trials, an extramural AIDS working group of the National Institutes of Health convened by telephone conference call on June 10, 1983. During this conversation, the term "AIDS-related complex" (ARC) was first proposed as an umbrella term to cover patients with symptomatology indicative of acquired immunodeficiency but without the opportunistic infections or malignancies diagnostic of AIDS. The working group came up with a definition of ARC based on clinical signs, symptoms, and laboratory abnormalities. The definition required a risk group patient to have at least two of the following clinical signs and symptoms listed in Table 1 that lasted for three or more months.

Unfortunately, this definition was not published until recently (5), and the acronym ARC entered the medical vocabulary as an ambiguous umbrella term that probably has caused more confusion than it has alleviated.

The term ARC, like AIDS, embraces a large number of clinical diagnoses. The former includes patients with the PGL syndrome, as well as those with or without lymphadenopathy with marked constitutional symptoms and laboratory features highly suggestive of an "AIDS prodrome."

Table 1 AIDS-Related Complex: Definition[a]

ARC: At least two from column A and two from column B	
Column A: Clinical	Column B: Laboratory
Fever >100°, ⩾ 3 months	Depressed helper T cells
Weight loss 10% or ⩾ 15 lbs	Depressed H/S ratio
Lymphadenopathy	Depressed blastogenesis
Diarrhea, ⩾ 3 months	Abnormal skin tests
Fatigue	Elevated serum globulins
Night sweats, ⩾ 3 months	At least one of:
	Anemia
	Leukopenia
	Thrombocytopenia
	Absolute lymphopenia

[a]NCI/NIAID Extramural AIDS Working Group: Correspondence 1983.

The acronym also has come to stand for "AIDS-related condition," an interpretation which brings under the ARC umbrella patients with immune thrombocytopenic purpura (ITP) and other diagnoses not recognized as AIDS by the Centers for Disease Control (CDC).

Several investigators noted that patients with ARC may progress to diseases categorized in the definition for AIDS (6-11). Until the retrovirus responsible for the underlying immunodeficiency was identified, however, AIDS and ARC were thought to be related, but distinct, nonoverlapping syndromes. Once a probable causative agent for the immune deficiency was found, it became more logical to conceive of AIDS, ARC, and the other unnamed manifestations as stages in a continuum of host response to the retroviral infection. At one extreme of this gradient are entirely healthy asymptomatic, antibody seropositives; at the other are patients with severely impaired immunity and life-threatening opportunistic infections. The large subset of patients between these two extremes fall into the category of ARC.

Because of the ambiguity and perceived lack of precision in the definition of the term ARC, many investigators believe it would be worthwhile to eliminate it from the working vocabulary of the AIDS researcher and clinician. The CDC's recent reformulation of a staging system for AIDS retroviral infection may provide the needed impetus to do this (12). Even if the term falls into disuse, however, persistent generalized lymphadenopathy (PGL) and immune thrombocytopenic purpura (ITP), two of the most frequent ARC diagnoses, remain an important part of the spectrum of AIDS-related disorders. These syndromes will be discussed with regard to the clinical problems they raise in diagnosis and management, their natural history, and prognostic implications.

II. Persistent Generalized Lymphadenopathy

The causes of peripheral lymphadenopathy in individuals at risk for developing AIDS remain unclear. Insofar as the human immunodeficiency virus (HIV) targets lymphocytes, causing substantial disturbances of function, it is not surprising that peripheral lymphadenopathy may result. It is uncertain, however, whether lymphadenopathy is a primary response to HIV infection or secondary to reactivation of an underlying virus infection, for example, a herpesvirus.

Individuals with peripheral lymphadenopathy may have one of a number of neoplasms or opportunistic infections associated with AIDS, but generally will have other signs or symptoms suggestive of the pertinent underlying disorder. Among the miscellaneous causes of lymphadenopathy reported in this subset of patients are angioimmunoblastic lymphadenopathy and angiofollicular hyperplasia (13,14). The most frequent cause of peripheral lymphadenopathy, however, is the PGL syndrome (6,15).

Persistent generalized lymphadenopathy is classified under group III in the CDC's staging schema for HIV infection. The CDC defines PGL as palpable lymphadenopathy (lymph node enlargement of 1 cm or greater) at two or more extrainguinal sites persisting for more than three months in the absence of concurrent illness or conditions other than HIV to explain the findings (12).

First recognized among homosexual men in the late 1970s, PGL subsequently has been identified among heterosexuals at risk for AIDS, including Haitians (16), intravenous drug users (17), hemophiliacs (18), female sexual partners of men with AIDS (19), and prison inmates (20). Because PGL is not a reportable condition at this time, its true incidence is unknown. Estimates suggest that the lymphadenopathy syndrome may currently occur 10-20 times more frequently as a response to HIV infection than the "full-blown" manifestations of AIDS.

A. Clinical and Laboratory Features

Descriptions of the clinical features of PGL have been remarkably similar in studies by numerous clinicians at different institutions. The clinical characteristics of our cohort are summarized in Table 2. In one-third of patients

Table 2 Persistent Generalized Lymphadenopathy Patient Characteristics

n = 200 homosexual men enrolled 1981-1983
Nodes for 6 months, two or more extrainguinal sites, 1 cm
Mean age at initial evalatuion = 32.5 years (19-43)
Onset PGL after 1979
33% of patients describe antecedant flulike illness
70% with intermittent mild-moderate constitutional symptoms

with PGL in the San Francisco General Hospital cohort, onset of the lymphadenopathy syndrome was noted one to two months after illness with fever, upper respiratory symptoms, and frequently diarrhea—all symptoms of the acute HIV retroviral infection (21). After developing of lymphadenopathy, one-third of our patients experience no other associated symptoms. The majority, however, report some combination of fatigue, low-grade intermittent fever, night sweats, or weight changes. These symptoms usually are not severe and may diminish over time. In addition to constitutional symptoms, patients with PGL may suffer from frequent, often recurrent episodes of infectious processes involving the skin, respiratory tract, and gastrointestinal tract. Rarely, a patient with lymphadenopathy syndrome will have symptoms consistent with a distal sensory neuropathy (22).

Headaches frequently accompany the lymphadenopathy syndrome. Neurologic evaluation of 50 PGL patients with headaches found that the majority were secondary to tension or vascular in origin. Examination of cerebrospinal fluid from a small subset of patients with severe and persistent headaches, however, revealed a mild lymphocytic pleocytosis. This finding most probably constitutes evidence of acute HIV infection of the central nervous system (23,24) (see Chapter 15).

Almost all patients with diffuse lymphadenopathy syndrome are found on examination to have involvement of the axillary and inguinal nodes. Approximately 85% of patients have posterior cervical adenopathy. Preauricular, postauricular, and epitrocheal nodes are involved in adenopathy of at least 50% of patients at our institution. Supraclavicular nodes are generally not involved. In addition to peripheral lymphadenopathy, patients with PGL often have increased numbers of normal-sized retroperitoneal lymph nodes. Abdominal computed tomography scans in our patients repeatedly demonstrated a triad of findings including splenomegaly, increased retroperitoneal lymphadenopathy, and thickening of the rectal mucosa consistent with a chronic proctitis (25). In patients with clinical evidence of subdiaphragmatic lymphadenopathy, routine chest x-rays usually do not reveal hilar or mediastinal nodes (26). Further investigation should be pursued in such cases to rule out an occult opportunistic infection or malignancy.

Laboratory evaluation of patients with lymphadenopathy syndrome is useful not only to assess clinical status but also to obtain some indication of the risk of progression to the more life-threatening manifestations of retroviral infection. In its classification system for HIV infection, the CDC notes that results of hematological or immunological laboratory studies, or both, may be used as a basis for subclassification of patients in group III, PGL if "results are abnormal in a manner consistent with the effects" of HIV infection (12).

The presence of HIV antibodies in patients with PGL has been reported in most published series; however, in a small group of patients in these cohorts, no HIV antibodies have been detected (27). These patients may have been inappropriately classified as having HIV-related lymphadenopathy, or they may have had active viremia without antibody production at the time of the studies. Conceivably, antibody production may be masked by a heavy virus (antigen) load. The majority of patients with PGL syndrome demonstrate the classic depletion of T-helper lymphocytes and reversal of the helper/suppressor ratio of T lymphocytes observed in of HIV infection. In addition, the majority of these patients demonstrate hypergammaglobulineamia with a polyclonal pattern on serum protein electrophoresis. This finding reflects the hypertrophy in B-lymphocyte follicular and germinal center areas that may be seen on histological examination of lymph nodes.

Hematological and immunological laboratory studies useful in evaluating a patient's risk of progressing to more severe manifestations of HIV infection are discussed in the following section on the natural history of PGL.

B. Natural History of PGL

In the early 1980s, numerous prospective studies of cohorts of patients with HIV-related PGL syndrome were established to ascertain the natural history of this syndrome (6,10,15,28). To date, these studies all demonstrate a persistent risk of progression from group III, PGL, to the more symptomatic, life-threatening conditions of group IV. Although the percentage of patients who progress varies among these studies, the range is from 10% to 30% with up to five years of followup reported in some of the cohorts. In an ongoing prospective study of 200 patients at San Francisco General Hospital (Table 2), more than 25% of patients have now progressed to AIDS diagnoses after

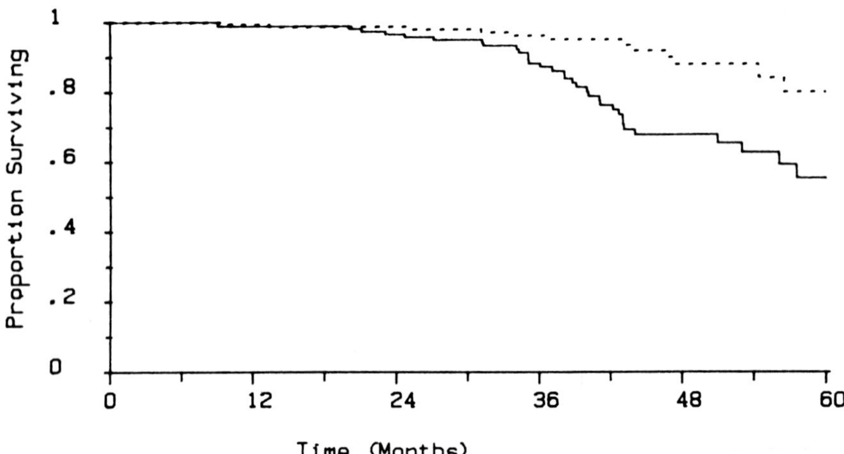

Figure 1 Lymphadenopathy syndrome—time to AIDS diagnosis. —— AIDS. ——— Death.

four and a half years of followup. The mean duration of adenopathy prior to an AIDS diagnosis has been 30 months. A Kaplan-Meier projection of outcome predicts 50% of the cohort will evolve to AIDS diagnoses with 60 months of followup (see Figure 1).

In a separate, retrospective review of 303 charts of patients with PGL at our institution, a Kaplan-Meier statistical analysis was used to estimate the probabilities of progression from PGL to AIDS. The likelihood that a patient with PGL would remain clinically stable for longer than five years was estimated to be only 34% (29). As yet, there appears to be no safe period of time after which the risk of progression from PGL to AIDS declines. Continued followup of established prospective natural history cohorts of PGL patients is needed to confirm the accuracy of this assessment.

Several features distinguish patients with PGL who progress to AIDS. The majority of PGL patients who develop AIDS have constitutional symptoms at the time of initial evaluation or during the course of their followup. Patients with shrinking nodes may be more likely to develop the opportunistic infections associated with AIDS. A tendency for lymph nodes to disappear in patients with lymphadenopathy has been observed (11,30). This phenomenon seems to support the hypothesis that lymphadenopathy represents an appropriate initial adaptive response to HIV infection, but when the immune system ultimately becomes exhausted and the lymph nodes disappear, AIDS supervenes.

Analysis of the first 14 patients who progressed from PGL to AIDS in the San Francisco General Hospital natural history cohort suggests some clinical and laboratory features that may be of value in predicting which patients will be more likely to progress (Table 3) (8). The relative risk of developing bona fide AIDS is increased by a factor of 54 in patients with lympha-

Table 3 Frequency of Clinical and Laboratory Features in PGL Patients Who Progressed to AIDS

Feature	Frequency in AIDS patients	Frequency in cohort (%)[c]	Statistical significance[a]
Antecedent thrush/ leukoplakia	10 of 12	10	<0.0001
Elevated ESR[b]	7 of 12	14	0.00081
Mild thrombocytopenia	5 of 14	8	0.0019
Leukopenia	5 of 14	6	0.0022
Anemia	3 of 14	5	0.043
History of herpes zoster	3 of 14	3	0.015

[a]Calculated by one-sided P value.
[b]ESR, erythrocyte sedimentation rate.
[c]Compared with remainder of 200-patient cohort at San Francisco General Hospital.
Source: Adapted from Ref. 8.

denopathy and antecedent oral thrush or hairy leukoplakia (5,7,8). An elevated erythrocyte sedimentation rate is an important laboratory indicator of the likelihood of disease progression. Moreover, patients with normal complete blood counts appear to have a more favorable prognosis compared with those with anemia, leukopenia, lymphopenia, or thrombocytopenia. Similar observations have been made in studies of other large patient cohorts (10,11,28,30).

Some investigators suggest that the total number of helper T-lymphocytes also may indicate increased risk of evolving to AIDS. A University of California, Los Angeles study found that patients who had helper T-cell counts of less than 400/mm^3 were at greatest risk for progression to AIDS (10). Whether depletion of the T-helper lymphocyte population will ultimately occur in all PGL patients in time can only be answered through close followup of the cohorts already under prospective evaluation.

Other laboratory findings possibly predictive of increased risk of progression to AIDS include a pattern of follicular involution or a reversed helper/suppressor lymphocyte ratio within the lymph node specimen itself (6,31-33), the presence of HLA-DR5 (34), and the presence of circulating acid-labile alpha interferon (35).

C. Treatment of Persistent Lymphadenopathy

With the appreciation that with time the transition from PGL to AIDS is continuing to occur in increasing numbers of patients, additional theoretical rationale for therapeutic intervention in patients with PGL has mounted. Whereas patients with AIDS already manifest the endpoint of HIV destruction of the immune system, PGL patients demonstrate more intact immunity, as well as possibly more retroviral activity to target with therapy. If one postulates that the immune system of an AIDS patient is too depleted to improve with immunomodulatory therapy, perhaps such immune augmentation may be more beneficial in the subset of patients with AIDS-related conditions. Certainly there would be more of the immune system to save through attempting to abort the viral infection in patients with PGL than in those with full-blown AIDS.

Despite the theoretical advantages to early intervention with immunomodulatory and antiretroviral therapy, there have been some drawbacks as well. Evidence suggests that HIV preferentially infects stimulated lymphocytes. Therefore the use of immunomodulatory agent that may stimulate CD4 cells may, in fact, make them more susceptible to infection with previously dormant virus. Some investigators suggest that immune augmenting therapy should only be used in conjunction with an antiviral agent. The difficulty with this suggestion, however, is that, to date, antiviral agents have not proven to be particularly effective against HIV or generally well tolerated without undue toxicities. To take patients with PGL and subject them to experimental agents about which little is known puts them at risk for unknown toxicities and potential detriment in the short run. However, as the natural history of PGL unfolds, patients with the syndrome are more willing to take the risk, acknowledging that the ultimate outcome may, in fact, be the development of life-threatening AIDS.

To this end, a number of studies of various agents have been employed in patients with PGL (5). The most rational approach in this patient population with a variable natural history depending upon length of time since infection has been the placebo-controlled trials. At San Francisco General Hospital, alpha interferon, isoprinosine, and ribiviran have been evaluated in placebo controlled trials in patients with PGL (5,36). Eligibility for these protocols has usually mandated that patients have, in addition to PGL, other evidence that they are at greater risk to evolve to full-blown AIDS, including the presence of thrush, and/or hairy leukoplakia, low helper lymphocyte number, and/or other cytopenias, thereby suggesting greater risk of progression. To date, none of these placebo controlled studies have demonstrated any true efficacy of the therapeutic intervention over placebo.

A trial of the reverse transcriptase inhibitor suramin in patients with AIDS-related lymphadenopathy was also performed at San Francisco General Hospital as part of a multicenter evaluation of this potential antiretroviral agent (5,37). In the eight PGL patients treated in our cohort, no evidence of clinical improvement, protection from opportunistic infection, or symptomatic improvement was noted. In fact, there was some suggestion that hepatotoxicity secondary to this intervention led to the early death of two of the PGL participants who had antecedent histories of chronic hepatitis.

Recent analysis of the multicenter trial of azidothymidine in patients with AIDS-related conditions suggest that this agent may offer an advantage to patients treated (38). In a placebo-controlled study, which evaluated 60 patients with PGL and constitutional symptoms treated with azidothymidine compared to an equal number of patients on placebo, analysis of data reported after a mean of four months demonstrated a trend towards increased helper T-lymphocytes and decreased opportunistic infections in patients treated with azidothymidine. This, in part, has led to the recent approval and licensing of azidothymidine for patients with evidence of HIV infection and less than 200 T-helper lymphocytes even in the absence of an AIDS diagnosis. The hope is that earlier intervention with this agent may protect the immune system and forestall the progression to life-threatening infections and malignancies.

To date, no truly effective therapy exists for the retroviral infection and immune impairment demonstrated in patients with PGL. Further well-monitored, carefully controlled clinical trials will be necessary to evaluate the impact of future therapeutic interventions in this AIDS-related condition.

III. Immune Thrombocytopenic Purpura

Immune thrombocytopenic purpura (ITP) has been observed in association with all of the major clinical manifestations of HIV infection and has been reported in many patients with confirmed AIDS diagnoses (39). The disorder was first recognized as an AIDS-related condition in 1982, when Morris and colleagues (40) described a cluster of 11 cases in male homosexuals in New York City. The demographic and immunological characteristics of these patients closely resembled those features that had been described in patients with AIDS. Isolated thrombocytopenia has been reported in narcotics addicts (41) and hemophiliacs (42,43). In our cohort of patients with PGL at San Francisco General Hospital, mild platelet count depression has been observed in 5-10% of patients. As reported above, thrombocytopenia in combination with lymphadenopathy syndrome appears to be associated with increased risk of progression to bona fide AIDS.

This AIDS-related thrombocytopenia may be an as yet unexplained response to HIV infection, similar to peripheral lymphadenopathy, or it may result from drug therapy or immune system processes that are not yet well understood. Patients with Kaposi's sarcoma and AIDS-related lymphoma frequently have thrombocytopenia at the time of diagnosis or during therapy with various cytotoxic or experimental drugs. In patients with *Pneumocystis carinii* pneumonia (PCP), thrombocytopenia may be detected at diagnosis, but more commonly, platelet counts drop off dramatically during treatment of the opportunistic infection (44). Although the fall in platelets during treatment is generally thought to be drug-induced, it is also possible that thrombocytopenia may be secondary to clearance of a previously blocked reticuloendothelial system.

A. Mechanism of ITP

The mechanism of AIDS-related ITP remains a matter of controversy. Two hypotheses have been investigated. Walsh and colleagues (45) at New York University have postulated that the mechanism of thrombocytopenia in a cohort of 24 homosexual men with AIDS-related ITP differs from that in classic autoimmune thrombocytopenia. In contrast to patients with classic ITP, their patients had higher levels of platelet-associated immunoglobulin and platelet complement. Although platelet eluates from the majority of patients with classic ITP were capable of binding to platelets from other patients, only 1 in 10 platelet eluates from their homosexual patients had this capability. Elevated levels of circulating immune complexes were reported in 21 of 24 patients with AIDS-related ITP, but none of five patients with classic ITP tested showed immune complexes. The homosexual patients had neither serum IgG nor platelet IgG capable of binding to normal platelets, but 79% of the circulating immune complexes detected in these patients were capable of binding to normal platelets.

Walsh and colleagues (45) hypothesized that, in contrast to classic ITP in which an antiplatelet IgG is directed against platelet antigenic determinants, AIDS-related ITP appears to result from the deposition of immune complexes and complement on platelets.

They postulated that the immune complex deposition occurs on platelet Fc receptors. Monocytes or macrophages would then bind to free Fc domains of exposed IgG molecules or to platelet-bound complement by their C3B receptors. Thus, they concluded that ITP in homosexual men may be an epiphenomenon related to the presence of circulating immune complexes rather than a true autoimmune disorder.

Data from studies by other investigators support an alternative hypothesis that AIDS-related thrombocytopenia may result from an autoimmune process associated with an effective clearance of a previously blocked reticuloendothelial system. Stricker et al. (46) evaluated 30 homosexual men with ITP in our San Francisco cohort. Twenty-nine of these patients were found to have a serum antibody that bound to a target platelet antigen of 25,000 daltons. This antibody was not detectable in patients with classic ITP or in patients with thrombocytopenia secondary to nonimmune processes. The 25-kD antigen was found to be integrated into the platelet membrane rather than an adsorbed antigen, since it resisted trypsin hydrolysis and thrombin stimulation of platelets. The serum antibody was shown to bind to the antigen through the $F(ab)_2$ portion of the molecule: this binding indicated that it was a true antibody and not an immune complex as Walsh and colleagues had hypothesized. The presence of elevated circulating immune complexes in only 7 to 11 of the patients with AIDS-related ITP tested by Stricker and colleagues further reduced the likelihood of an immune complex mediated mechanism.

In a control group of 16 patients with AIDS-related lymphadenopathy or bona fide AIDS but without thrombocytopenia, the unique antibody to the 25 kD antigen was detected in 15 of 16 patients studied. Platelet-associated IgG was detected in five of five patients studied.

Why some patients with PGL or AIDS have normal platelet counts in the presence of platelet-associated IgG and the antibody to the 25-kD antigen remains an unanswered question. One attractive hypothesis is that Fc receptor-mediated clearance is defective in patients with AIDS as it is in other patients with hypergammaglobulinemia and chronic infectious diseases (47-49). Defective reticuloendothelial system clearance in the presence of antibody-coated platelets results paradoxically in a normal platelet count. In patients whose reticuloendothelial function is relatively "unblocked," immunoglobulin-coated platelets may be removed and thrombocytopenia may result.

Clinical observations of our patient cohort at San Francisco General Hospital support this hypothesis (50,51). For example, one patient whose thrombocytopenia was not corrected by splenectomy maintained a low platelet count in the 30,000/mm^3 range. During an acute hepatitis-like illness, characterized by low-grade fever, malaise, and minimal right upper quadrant tenderness, his platelet count rose to normal levels. As his symptoms resolved, thrombocytopenia recurred. Two other patients with untreated AIDS-related thrombocytopenia maintained average platelet counts of between 20,000 and 30,000/mm^3 for two years. Both patients ultimately progressed to *Pneumocystis carinii* pneumonia. At the time of diagnosis with PCP, one patient presented with a normal platelet count. The other patient, who had experienced some prodromal symptoms, mild anemia, and elevated sedimentation rate one month earlier, presented with a platelet count of 400,000/mm^3. A third ITP patient had been treated briefly with steroids eight months prior to hospitalization for treatment of cryptococcal meningitis. When he was hospitalized, he had a platelet count of 150,000/mm^3 but during therapy with amphotericin B and 5-FU, the platelet count dropped rapidly to his previous 20,000/mm^3 range. Although in this case the mechanism of thrombocytopenia was thought to be drug-induced, in fact the recurrent thrombocytopenia may have reflected "unblocking" of the reticuloendothelial system following clearance of the cryptococcal infection. Thus ITP may reflect a healthier state in HIV infected individuals than a normal platelet count (see below).

B. Clinical and Laboratory Features of ITP

AIDS-related thrombocytopenia occurs both as an isolated phenomenon and in combination with other manifestations of HIV infection. Remarkably similar clinical and laboratory findings emerged from studies of patient cohorts with isolated thrombocytopenia conducted at New York University and at San Francisco General Hospital. The clinical status of 37 homosexual men with isolated thrombocytopenia studied at San Francisco General Hospital has been reported previously (50,51). Their clinical status is summarized in Table 4. In general, patients with isolated thrombocytopenia were found to be clinically "healthier" than the majority of patients with AIDS or

Table 4 Clinical Status of Patients with ITP[a]

Mean age at ITP diagnosis (yr)	33.6 (range 23-47)
Peripheral lymphadenopathy (n)	20
Palpable splenomegaly (n)	6
Oral *Candida* at diagnosis (n)	2
Bleeding other than petechiae (n)	6
Hospitalized during course of disease (n)	14
Central nervous system hemorrhage (n)	0
Significant gastrointestinal blood loss (n)	0

[a]n = 37 homosexual men (33 white, 4 Hispanic); San Francisco study (50,51,53).

related conditions presenting at our clinic. This fact is not surprising considering the findings noted above on more effective reticuloendothelial system clearance. The most common clinical manifestations of thrombocytopenia were easy bruising and petechiae reported in more than 50% of patients. Epistaxis, gingival bleeding, rectal bleeding, and blood in ejaculate were each reported by a few patients, but no major bleeding complications have been observed despite often marked lowering of platelet counts. No gastrointestinal or central nervous system bleed has occurred during the course of followup. Six patients denied any bleeding antecedent to their diagnosis of ITP. Mean duration from onset of symptoms to the diagnosis of ITP was one month in our cohort. The cohort has been evaluated for a mean of 36 months.

On physical examination, the majority of patients with ITP showed evidence of mucosal bleeding with cutaneous or palatal petechiae or ecchymoses. Varying degrees of peripheral lymphadenopathy were present in 20 of 35 patients in our series, a finding demonstrating again that there is considerable overlap between this group of patients and those with the other common AIDS-related condition, PGL. Minimal splenomegaly was found on palpation in six patients. Oral *Candida* was present in two patients at initial evaluation.

Although mild anemia was present in 4 of 35 patients with "isolated" thrombocytopenia, in general, anemia, leukopenia, or both, were absent in these patients. Table 5 summarizes initial laboratory findings in this cohort revealed a mean platelet count of 21,000/mm^3 (range 3000-69,000/mm^3). Platelet-associated immunoglobulin G was detected by fluorescence-activated cytometric assay in all 30 patients tested. Bone marrow aspirates and biopsies performed on 25 patients revealed adequate to increased megakaryocytes and findings consistent with peripheral destruction.

Table 5 Laboratory Findings in Patients with ITP at Time of Diagnosis[a]

Initial platelet count (/mm^3)	21,000 (3,000-69,000)
Mild anemia (hematocrit: 37-39%) (n)	4
Mean leukocyte count (/mm^3)	6,600
Lymphocytes (/mm^3)	1,700 (800-3,100)
CD4$^+$ (/mm^3)	390 (70-750)
CD8$^+$ (/mm^3)	1,200 (600-2,800)
CD4$^+$ (%)	18 (8-29)
CD8$^+$ (%)	51 (19-71)
H/S ratio	0.45 (0.1-0.8)
HIV antibody positive (%)	100
Platelet associated IgG or anti-25 kD antibody (%)	100
Circulating immune complexes	6/11

[a]n = 35; San Francisco Study (50,51,53).

In general, patients with autoimmune phenomena usually are found to have increased levels of helper T cells and consequently elevated T-lymphocyte helper/suppressor ratios. Patients with AIDS-related ITP demonstrate the same inversion of the helper/suppressor ratio seen in patients with AIDS and related conditions (40,51). In our group of 35 ITP patients (Table 5), the mean number of helper T cells present was decreased to 390 per mm^3 and the mean number of suppressor T cells was 1200/mm^3, yielding a helper/suppressor T-lymphocyte ratio of 0.45 (range 0.1-0.8).

The inversion of the helper/suppressor ratio has been explained as a consequence of HIV infection of T-helper lymphocytes. Antibodies to HIV were detected by the ELISA assay in 21 of 25 patients with ITP in our study; results were borderline in four cases, but subsequent analysis of these by immunoblot assay confirmed that they were positive. In the New York University series, HIV antibodies were detected in sera from 13 of 14 thrombocytopenia patients evaluated by indirect immunofluorescence assay (52). This high prevalence of HIV antibody seropositivity in these patients supports the clinically based inference that isolated thrombocytopenia in itself can be an AIDS-related condition. Finally, studies on recovery of infectious HIV from the blood of ITP patients have indicated a lower frequency of detection than other HIV-infected individuals (53). In our series, only 2 of 16 patients showed presence of HIV compared with more than 50% of other HIV-infected individuals (52,58). This finding may also reflect a somewhat healthier state of these patients resulting from an intact immune system (see Chapters 8, 10).

C. Natural History of ITP

Serial followup of patients with ITP in San Francisco and New York has demonstrated that, with time, increasing numbers of these patients do progress along the gradient of infection to AIDS regardless of whether they had treatment or no treatment (50-52). Combining the experience from New York and San Francisco, 11 of 68 ITP patients (16%) are reported to have developed bona fide AIDS. The mean time from initial diagnosis of ITP to the development of AIDS in the five San Francisco General Hospital patients was 26 months, compared with a mean of 20 ± 2 months for the patients in the New York cohort. This number and time course is virtually identical to the observed rate of progression to AIDS in patients with PGL. Figure 1 is a projected Kaplan-Meier analysis of the risk of developing AIDS as a function of time from initial ITP diagnosis from the San Francisco cohort data.

Two San Francisco patients without prior treatment for thrombocytopenia have developed AIDS. In both patients, platelet counts returned to normal just before or conincidentally with the development of an AIDS-related opportunistic infection. Again, this finding may be evidence that thrombocytopenic AIDS-related conditions may be associated with normal reticuloendothelial function. As blocking of the reticuloendothelial system increased in association with the development of an AIDS-related opportunistic infection, patients may become unable to clear antibody-coated platelets from the circulation. Paradoxically, then, the platelet count was seen to increase as AIDS developed—this situation, therefore, resembles to some extent the shrinkage or disappearance of adenopathy observed in patients with PGL who have progressed to AIDS.

D. Treatment of ITP

The use of steroid therapy and splenectomy to treat thrombocytopenia at first seemed problematic because of their possible adverse consequences on an already depressed immune system. At this time, however, data accumulated on each of these treatments provide no real evidence of further immune suppression as a consequence of these interventions (50).

Although lack of a standard measure of response to steroid therapy in patients with AIDS-related ITP has hampered assessment of its effectiveness, reports of studies at New York University and San Francisco General Hospital indicate that steroids have some utility in treating AIDS-related ITP. Walsh and colleagues (52) at New York University reported that 8 of 17 patients with thrombocytopenia achieved an "excellent" response to prednisone treatment, and another 8 patients had a moderate response. When steroids were tapered, however, platelet counts in 13 of the treated patients fell to their pretreatment levels or lower. Only two patients maintained normal platelet counts after steroid therapy was completed (52). Similarly, at San Francisco General Hospital, 19 of 24 patients initially started on daily prednisone (1 mg/kg orally) responded favorably, but only 2 patients maintained normal platelet counts after the steroids were tapered (51).

The mean duration of steroid therapy in the 24 patients in our cohort was 10 months (range 3 weeks to 36 months). The median duration was 5 months, a discrepancy that reflects the tendency toward more protracted trials of steroid therapy in patients who were treated more recently.

None of the patients treated in either series developed an opportunistic infection or malignancy during steroid therapy. However, some complications of treatment did occur. Weight gain, moon facies, steroid acne, and reactivation of herpes labialis were observed in over one-half of the patients with AIDS-related thrombocytopenia treated at San Francisco General Hospital. Fourteen of 24 treated patients developed oral *Candida* while on therapy, and 10 patients experienced marked dysphoria. More severe side effects of prednisone therapy included proximal myopathy of the lower extremities (one patient) and severe distal-sensory neuropathy (one patient).

A noteworthy observation was made when steroids were used in our patients with both ITP and diffuse lymphadenopathy. While these patients were treated with prednisone, their lymph nodes shrank to the point of disappearance, and as the steroids were tapered, the generalized lymphadenopathy again became appreciable. This shrinking adenopathy in the face of a therapeutic intervention contrasts with the poor prognosis of spontaneously disappearing nodes in PGL patients.

Splenectomy has produced higher platelet counts in treated patients in New York and San Francisco. A combined overall response rate of 80% was observed among these patients. All 10 of the New York patients who underwent surgery achieved normal postsplenectomy counts and experienced no postoperative complications. In all 10 of these patients, surgery was performed after initial steroid treatment had failed. The mean time of surgery was 3.6 ± 0.7 months after diagnosis of thrombocytopenia.

Fifteen patients in the San Francisco cohort underwent splenectomy within the first six months of their diagnosis with ITP; two patients had splenectomy as the initial therapy. Ten of these patients sustained complete remissions with normal platelet counts following surgery. Patients experienced minimal postoperative complications and no postoperative mortality. This finding contrasts with our experience in performing splenectomies on patients with AIDS, which often has been associated with substantially increased morbidity and occasional mortality. A postoperative lymphocytosis was appreciated in patients serially studied with concomitant increases on both T-helper and T-suppressor populations yielding no overall change in this ratio.

Other treatments have been employed in an effort to avoid possible further immune system suppression from steroids or splenectomy. According to two reports, high-dose intravenous gamma-globulin has produced transient responses in some patients with AIDS-related ITP (54-56). Presumedly, this therapy works by blocking the reticuloendothelial system. This intervention may be most useful preoperatively as a means of increasing platelets to safe levels in patients who will undergo splenectomy. The necessity of this intervention depends on the expertise of the general surgeon.

Danazol in a daily dosage of 800 mg orally was reported to be effective in raising platelet counts after three months of therapy in four of six patients with AIDS-related thrombocytopenia (57). Normal T-lymphocyte ratios were achieved in two patients. A similar number of patients in our San Francisco cohort were treated with Danazol at the same dosage and for the same duration in conjunction with their initial course of prednisone therapy. No substantial response was noted either in platelet counts or T-lymphocyte helper/suppressor ratios (5).

Regardless of the treatment modality, sustained remissions occur infrequently in patients with AIDS-related ITP. Many of our patients are reluctant to undergo splenectomy. Because no serious bleeding complications have been observed in our patient cohort, no therapy has been recommended to most of our recently diagnosed patients. Even patients with initial platelet counts as low as $8000/mm^3$ who chose no treatment have done well when closely monitored over the past two and one-half years. Patients should be advised of the risks and benefits of treatment versus no treatment for AIDS-related ITP and encouraged to participate in decision-making about the wisdom of opting for therapy or careful observation.

IV. Conclusion

Persistent generalized lymphadenopathy and immune thrombocytopenic purpura are two frequently recognized "AIDS-related" diagnoses classified midway along the spectrum of HIV infection. Both conditions challenge the clinician's skill in patient management and psychosocial counseling and the patient's ability to cope with the consequences of suppressed immune function and the prospect of an uncertain future. Because of our rather brief experience with these disorders, our knowledge about optimal therapies and ultimate prognosis remains incomplete. They both appear to represent expression of a host in a somewhat healthier state than other HIV-infected individuals. What can be done to maintain this condition requires further study. It is hoped that ongoing prospective investigation will help us to identify the subset of patients at greatest risk for developing AIDS and that treatments will be found that will halt the progression of disease.

Acknowledgments

Donald I. Abrams is a recipient of an American Cancer Socity Career Development Award. The author thanks Karen Heller for valuable editorial assistance.

References

1. Centers for Disease Control. Kaposi's sarcoma and pneumocystis pneumonia among homosexual men—New York City and California. MMWR 1981; 30: 305-8.
2. Gottlieb MS, Schroff R, Schanker H, Weisman JD, Peng TF, Wolf RA, Saxon A. *Pneumocystis carinii* pneumonia and mucosal candidiasis in previously healthy homosexual men: evidence of a new acquired cellular immunodeficiency. N Engl J Med 1981; 305:1425-31.
3. Masur H, Michelis MA, Greene JB, Onorato I, Vande Stouwe RA, Holzman RS, Wormser G, Brettman L, Lange M, Murray HW, Cunningham-Rundles S. An outbreak of community-acquired *Pneumocystis carinii* pneumonia: initial manifestation of cellular immune dysfunction. N Engl J Med 1981; 305:1431-8.
4. Centers for Disease Control. Epidemiological aspects of the current outbreak of Kaposi's sarcoma and opportunistic infections. N Engl J Med 1982; 306:248-52.
5. Abrams DI. AIDS-related conditions. Clin Immunol Allergy 1986; 6:581-99.
6. Metroka CE, Cunningham-Rundles S, Pollack MS, Sonnabend JA, Davis JM, Gordon B, Fernandez RD, Mouradian J. Persistent generalized lymphadenopathy in homosexual men. Ann Intern Med 1983; 99:585-91.
7. Abrams DI. Lymphadenopathy syndrome in male homosexuals. In: Gallin JI, Fauci AS, eds. Advances in host defense mechanisms. Vol. 5. New York: Raven Press, 1985:75-97.
8. Abrams DI. Lymphadenopathy related to the acquired immunodeficiency syndrome in homosexual men. Med Clin North Am 1986; 70:693-706.
9. Abrams DI, Mess T, Volberding P. Lymphadenopathy: endpoint or prodrome? Update of a 36-month prospective study. In: Gupta S, ed. AIDS associated syndromes. New York: Plenum Press, 1985:73-84.
10. Gottlieb MS, Wolfe PR, Fahey JL, Knight S, Hardy D, Eppolito L, Ashida E, Patel A, Beall GN, Sun N. The syndrome of persistent generalized lymphadenopathy: experience with 101 patients. In: Gupta S, ed. AIDS associated syndromes. New York: Plenum Press, 1985:85-92.
11. Mathur-Wagh U, Mildvan D, Spigland I, Brun-Vezinet F, Barre-Sinousi F, Montagnier L, Chermann J-C. Longitudinal assessment of persistent generalized lymphadenopathy (PGL) in homosexual men. In: Gupta S, ed. AIDS associated syndromes. New York: Plenum Press, 1985:93-6.
12. Centers for Disease Control. Classification system for human T-lymphotropic virus type III/lymphadenopathy-associated virus infection. MMWR 1986; 35: 344-9.
13. Blumenfeld W, Beckstead JH. Angioimmunoblastic lymphadenopathy with dysproteinuria in homosexual men with acquired immune deficiency syndrome. Arch Pathol Lab Med 1983; 107:567-9.

14. Lachant NA, Leung LA, Sun NCJ, Oseas RS. Angiofollicular lymph node hyperplasia (Castleman's disease) and Kaposi's sarcoma in 2 homosexual males with AIDS (abstr.). Blood 1983; 62 (Suppl. 1):113a.
15. Abrams DI, Lewis BJ, Beckstead JH, Casavant CA, Drew WL. Persistent diffuse lymphadenopathy in homosexual men: endpoint or prodrome? Ann Intern Med 1984; 100:801-8.
16. Pitchenik AE, Fischl MA, Dickinson GM, Becker DM, Fournier AM, O'Connell MT, Colton RM, Spira TJ. Opportunistic infections and Kaposi's sarcoma among Haitians: evidence of a new acquired immunodeficiency state. Ann Intern Med 1983; 98:277-84.
17. Metroka C, Cunningham-Rundles S, Mouradian J, Moore A. Generalized lymphadenopathy in intravenous drug users (abstr.). Blood 1983; 62 (Suppl. 1):114a.
18. Andes WA, DeShazo RD, Reed RJ, Harkin JC, Wang N. Hemophilic lymphadenopathy: clinical, histologic, cytologic and chromosomal changes in patients with immune deficiency (abstr.). Blood 1983; 62 (Suppl. 1):108a.
19. Harris C, Small CB, Klein RS, Friedland GH, Moll B, Emeson EE, Spigland I, Steigbigel NH. Immunodeficiency in female sexual partners of men with the acquired immunodeficiency syndrome. N Engl J Med 1983; 308:1181-4.
20. Han T, Barcos M, Takeuchi J, Ozer H, Poiesz B, Pollard C, Sandberg AA. Prison-acquired lymphoproliferative syndrome (PALS) with special reference to AIDS: immunohistopathology and cytogenetics of lymphadenopathy (abstr.). Blood 1983; 62 (Suppl. 1):110a.
21. Cooper DA, Gold J, Maclean P, Donovan B, Finlayson R, Barnes TG, Michelmore HM, Brooke P, Penny R. Acute AIDS retrovirus infection. Lancet 1985; 1:537-40.
22. Lipkin WI, Parry G, Kiprov D, Abrams D. Inflammatory neuropathy in homosexual men with lymphadenopathy. Neurology 1985; 35:1479-83.
23. Levy JA, Hollander H, Shimabukuro J, Mills J, Kaminsky L. Isolation of AIDS-associated retroviruses from cerebrospinal fluid and brain of patients with neurological symptoms. Lancet 1985; 2:586-8.
24. Levy RM, Bredesen DE, Rosenblum ML. Neurological manifestations of the acquired immunodeficiency syndrome (AIDS): experience at UCSF and review of the literature. J Neurosurg 1985; 62:475-95.
25. Moon KL, Federle MP, Abrams DI, Lewis BJ, Volberding PA. Abdominal computed tomography in Kaposi's sarcoma and lymphadenopathy syndrome: limitations of the technique. Radiology 1984; 150:479-83.
26. Stern RG, Gamsu G, Golden JA, Hirji M, Webb WR, Abrams DI. Intrathoracic adenopathy: differential feature of AIDS and diffuse lymphadenopathy syndrome. AJR 1984; 142:689-92.
27. Kaminsky LS, McHugh T, Stites D, Volberding P, Henle G, Henle W, Levy JA. High prevalence of antibodies to AIDS associated retrovirus (ARV) in acquired immunodeficiency syndrome and related conditions and not in other disease states. Proc Natl Acad Sci USA 1985; 82:5535-9.
28. Mathur-Wagh U, Enlow RW, Spigland R, Winchester RJ, Sacks SHS, Romat E, Yancovitz SF, Mildvan D, William DC. Longitudinal study of persistent generalized lymphadenopathy in homosexual men: relation to acquired immunodeficiency syndrome. Lancet 1984; 1:1033-8.

29. Senechek DR, Abrams DI. Status of lymphadenopathy syndrome: a retrospective chart review of 303 patients (abstr.). Proceedings of the Second International Conference on AIDS, Paris, France. 1986:43.
30. Metroka CE, Cunningham-Rundles S, Krim M, Pollack MS, Sonnabend JA, Gunby TC, Alonso ML, Davis JM, Mouradian J, Witkin SS. Generalized lymphadenopathy in homosexual men: an update of the New York experience. Ann NY Acad Sci 1984; 407:400-11.
31. Fernandez R, Mouradian J, Metroka C, Davis J. The prognostic value of histopathology in persistent generalized lymphadenopathy in homosexual men (lett.). N Engl J Med 1983; 309:185-6.
32. Modlin RL, Meyer PR, Hofman FM, Mehlmaver M, Levy NB, Lukes RJ, Parker JW, Ammann AJ, Conant MA, Rea TH, Taylor CR. T-lymphocyte subsets in lymph nodes from homosexual men. JAMA 1983; 250:1302-5.
33. Ewing EP, Chandler FW, Spira JJ. Primary lymph node pathology in AIDS and AIDS-related lymphadenopathy. Arch Pathol Lab Med 1985; 109:977-81.
34. Enlow RW, Nunez-Roldan A, Lo Galbo P, Mildvan D, Mathur U, Winchester RJ. Increased frequency of HLA-DR5 in lymphadenopathy stage of AIDS. Lancet 1983; 2:51.
35. Eyster ME, Goedert JJ, Man-Chiu P, Preble OT. Acid-labile alpha interferon: a possible preclinical marker for the acquired immunodeficiency syndrome in hemophilia. N Engl J Med 1983; 309:583.
36. Abrams DI, Andes WA, Kisner DL, Golando JP, Volberding PA. A trial of alpha-2 interferon in a benign reactive lymphadenopathic syndrome (abstr.). Proceedings of the Second International Conference on AIDS, Paris, France. 1986:34.
37. Kaplan LD, Wolfe PR, Volberding PA, Feorino P, Levy JA, Abrams DI, Kiprov D, Wong R, Kaufman L, Gottlieb M. Lack of response to suramin in patients with AIDS and AIDS-related complex. Am J Med 1987; 82:615-20.
38. AZT Collaborative Working Group. The efficacy of azidothymidine in treatment of patients with AIDS and AIDS-related complex: a double-blind placebo-controlled trial (abstr.). Proceedings of the Third International Conference on AIDS, Washington, D.C. 1987:101.
39. Abrams DI, Chinn EK, Lewis BJ, Volbnerding PA, Conant MA, Townsend RM. Hematologic manifestations in homosexual men with Kaposi's sarcoma. Am J Clin Pathol 1984; 81:13-8.
40. Morris L, Distenfeld A, Amorosi E, Karpatkin S. Autoimmune thrombocytopenic purpura in homosexual men. Ann Intern Med 1982; 96:714-7.
41. Savona S, Nardi M, Lennette ET, Karpatkin S. Thrombocytopenic purpura in narcotic addicts. Ann Intern Med 1985; 102:737-41.
42. Ratnoff OD, Menitove JE, Aster RH, Lederman MM. Coincident classic hemophilia and "idiopathic" thrombocytopenic purpura in patients under treatment with concentrates of anti-hemophilic factor (factor VIII). N Engl J Med 1983; 308:439-42.
43. Zeitlhuber U, Haschke F, Puspok R, Lechner K, Knapp W, Imbach P. Hemophilia and thrombocytopenia in a patient with impared cellular immunity. Blut 1984; 48:393-5.

44. Jaffe HS, Abrams DI, Ammann AJ, Lewis BJ, Golden JA. Complications of co-trimoxazole in treatment of AIDS-associated Pneumocystis carinii pneumonia in homosexual men. Lancet 1983; 2:1109-11.
45. Walsh CM, Nardi MA, Karpatkin S. On the mechanism of thrombocytopenic purpura in sexually active homosexual men. N Engl J Med 1984; 311:635-6.
46. Stricker RB, Abrams DI, Corash L, Shuman MA. Target platelet antigen in homosexual men with immune thrombocytopenia. N Engl J Med 1985; 313: 1375-80.
47. Frank MM, Hamburger MI, Lawley TJ, Kimberly RP, Plotz PH. Defective reticuloendothelial system Fc-receptor function in systemic lupus erythematosus. N Engl J Med 1979; 300:518-23.
48. Bender BS, Frank MM, Lawley TJ, Smith WJ, Brickman CM, Quinn TC. Defective reticuloendothelial system Fc-receptor in patients with acquired immunodeficiency syndrome. J Infect Dis 1985; 152:409-12.
49. Kelton JG, Carter CJ, Rodger C, Bebenek G, Gauldie J, Sheridan D, Kassam YB, Kean WF, Buchanan WW, Rooney PJ, Bianchi F, Denburg J. The relationship among platelet-associated IgG, platelet lifespan, and reticuloendothelial cell function. Blood 1984; 63:1434-8.
50. Abrams DI, Kiprov DD, Volberding PA. Isolated thrombocytopenia in homosexual men—longitudinal follow-up. In: Gupta S, ed. AIDS associated syndromes. New York: Plenum Press, 1985:117-22.
51. Abrams DI, Kiprov DD, Goedert JJ, Sarngadharan MG, Gallo RC, Volberding PA. Antibodies to human T-lymphotropic virus type III and development of the acquired immunodeficiency syndrome in homosexual men presenting with immune thrombocytopenia. Ann Intern Med 1986; 104:47-50.
52. Walsh C, Krigal R, Lennette E, Karpatkin S. Thrombocytopenia in homosexual patients. Ann Intern Med 1985; 103:542-5.
53. Abrams DI, French D, Feigal DW, Levy JA. AIDS-related immune thrombocytopenia: HIV expression and progression to AIDS. Proceedings of the Third International Conference on AIDS, Washington, D.C. 1987:69.
54. Delfraissy JF, Tertian G, Dreyfus M, Tchernia G. Intravenous gammaglobulin, thrombocytopenia, and the acquired immunodeficiency syndrome. Ann Intern Med 1985; 103:478.
55. Imbach P, Beck EA, Frei F, Tonz O, Entacher-Zeitlhuber U. IVIG treatment in patients with HIV infection and ITP. Vox Sang 1986; 52:7.
56. Tertian G, Boue F, Lebras P, Laurian Y, Dreyfus M, Delfraissy JF, Tchernia G. Thrombocytopenia in ARC: management with high-dose IVIG. Vox Sang 1986; 52:9.
57. Fischl MA, Ahn YS, Limas N, Harrington WJ, Fletcher MA. Use of danazol in autoimmune thrombocytopenia associated with the acquired immunodeficiency syndrome (abstr.). Blood 1984; 64 (Suppl. 1):236a.
58. Levy JA, Shimabukuro J. Recovery of AIDS-associated retroviruses from patients with AIDS or AIDS-related conditions, and from clinically healthy individuals. J Infect Dis 1985; 152:734-8.

13
Kaposi's Sarcoma in AIDS

Paul A. Volberding
School of Medicine
University of California
and San Francisco General Hospital
San Francisco, California

I. Introduction

In the spring of 1981, Kaposi's sarcoma, a rare and often misunderstood cancer, suddenly began coming to the attention of health professionals and medical personnel on both the East and West coasts of the United States. An unprecedented incidence of Kaposi's sarcoma was appearing in previously healthy young adults, predominately homosexual males. Surveillance was initiated by the Centers for Disease Control (CDC) in June, 1981. Reports published by the CDC that year indicated a significant and increasing number of cases of Kaposi's sarcoma and of *Pneumocystis carinii* pneumonia in this population (1,2). In addition, all patients tested showed a marked deficiency in cell-mediated immunity. Clearly, a new disease had originated (1,3).

Kaposi's sarcoma, one of the earliest recognized sequelae of AIDS, has continued to be a crucial agent for the surveillance of the disease and a determinative focus for clinical therapy trials. It is the purpose of this chapter to facilitate clinical decision-making for treatment of AIDS-related Kaposi's sarcoma patients. We will begin by presenting clinical features and symptoms of the disease and by differentiating the Kaposi's sarcoma subgroup of the current AIDS population. A review of incidence of Kaposi's sarcoma in non-AIDS patients will follow. Clinical features and diagnosis will be discussed as well as the staging system in common usage (4,47). With this background, conventional and experimental therapies will be reviewed with recommendations for application.

II. Epidemiology of Kaposi's Sarcoma in AIDS Patients

A. Distinguishing Clinical Features

Non-AIDS-related Kaposi's sarcoma in the United States has traditionally affected patients over 70 years of age. Current figures for AIDS-associated Kaposi's sarcoma reveal a median age at onset of 35 years. In addition, patients with AIDS-related Kaposi's sarcoma tend to have a much more actively disseminating form of the malignancy often resulting in the presence of widespread tumor at time of diagnosis. Lymph nodes and visceral structures as well as the skin are often affected. In this respect, AIDS-related Kaposi's sarcoma behaves in a pattern more similar to the aggressive lymphadenopathic variety found in black African children (5) than to the malignancy present in aging patients.

B. Diagnosis of AIDS-Related Kaposi's Sarcoma

Diagnosis of Kaposi's sarcoma is rarely difficult. The gay community, particularly in urban areas, has been highly effective in communicating and educating the gay population about AIDS and Kaposi's sarcoma. Prevention, warning signals, and care are topics of primary concern in the gay media. Kaposi's sarcoma lesions are readily identifiable by alert homosexual men and immediate medical attention is generally sought. Early cutaneous lesions [Figure 1 (for Figures 1-7, see Plates I to III, after page 356)] are usually the first symptom to be observed by the individual. Generally they are palpable (Figure 2) but rarely exophytic. Red or violaceous, they do not blanch upon application of pressure. Although generally painless at onset, as the disease advances, lesions can become painful, particularly in the feet and lower extremities (Figure 3). Very frequently, the oral cavity will also be affected by the disease at the time of original diagnosis. This is particularly true of the hard palate, which is affected by the cancer in up to one third of all cases (Figure 4) (6). In addition, gingival mucosa may also be involved (Figure 5). Lymph node involvement is seen in half of all AIDS-associated Kaposi's sarcoma patients.

As the disease progresses, plaques of coalesced lesions are common particularly over the thigh (Figure 6). Tumors tend to be circular although linear lesions are not uncommon, especially in the area of the neck and back where they may appear to follow cutaneous lymphatics.

Although not necessarily the most threatening to the patient's health, Kaposi's sarcoma lesions are the most visible of all manifestations of AIDS. The sociological implications of this cannot be ignored. The uninformed public's fear of AIDS and the concomitant severe social reactions Kaposi's sarcoma patients experience can often be more painful and deleterious than the early stages of the malignancy.

C. Visceral and Pulmonary Involvement

Although gastrointestinal Kaposi's sarcoma (Figure 7) is extremely common (7-9), it is frequently silent clinically. Gastrointestinal bleeding is extremely rare. Endoscopic biopsies of gastrointestinal Kaposi's sarcoma lesions are often negative. This is thought to occur because the tumor is submucosal beyond the depth of biopsy achieved by endoscopy.

Although less common than gastrointestinal Kaposi's sarcoma, pulmonary Kaposi's sarcoma is clinically more significant. Caution should be exercised not to confuse pulmonary Kaposi's sarcoma with *Pneumocystis carinii* pneumonia. In the absence of concurrent pulmonary infections, a pulmonary gallium scan should give negative results. In addition, pleural effusions are more commonly seen with pulmonary Kaposi's sarcoma (10-12). Another important but uncommon site of Kaposi's sarcoma is the eye where conjunctival lesions are occasionally seen (Figure 8).

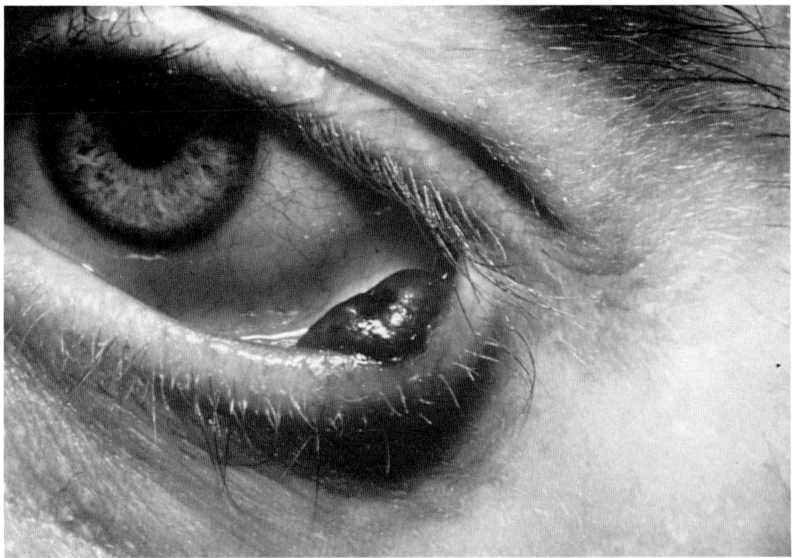

Figure 8 Ocular conjunctival Kaposi's sarcoma. These lesions can progress to involve the globe.

D. Histological Diagnosis of Kaposi's Sarcoma

A biopsy should be performed to provide histological confirmation of Kaposi's sarcoma even though clinical information might seem sufficient. A small punch biopsy of affected skin is generally the most convenient, although enlarged peripheral lymph nodes can also be biopsied and may be the only site of the cancer.

Generally, a biopsy of AIDS-related Kaposi's sarcoma will show the same features (6) as does the malignancy in other populations (Figure 9). An infiltration of spindle-shaped cells is seen with an often dramatic proliferation of small, incompletely formed, blood vessels lined by unusually large cells with the histological characteristics of endothelium. Extravasated erythrocytes are also common.

III. Prevalence of Kaposi's Sarcoma in AIDS Risk Groups

In addition to homosexual men, members of several other groups have a significantly higher risk of HIV infection than the general population. Among these are intravenous drug users (13), Haitians (14), hemophiliacs (15-17), sexual partners of HIV-infected individuals (18), and infants born to infected women (19,20) (see Chapter 1).

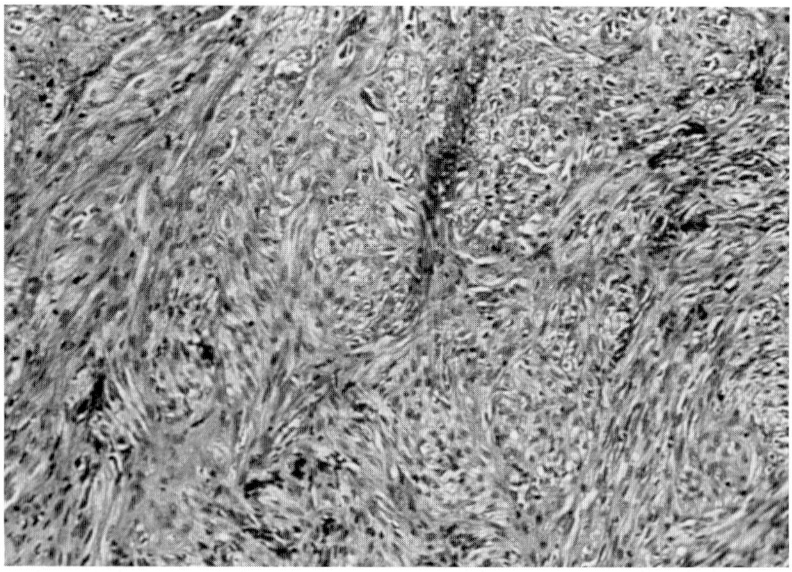

Figure 9 Skin biopsy of Kaposi's sarcoma in AIDS demonstrating vascular proliferation, infiltration of spindle-shaped cells, and extravasation of erythrocytes.

Kaposi's sarcoma, for uncertain reasons, appears much more frequently in homosexual men than in members of other AIDS risk groups (21). The previous popularity of nitrite inhalants among male homosexuals to increase sexual stimulation and facilitate anal intercourse (22,23) might be an important variable. These or other recreational drugs could be a factor in the development of Kaposi's sarcoma particularly in combination with HIV-induced immunodeficiency (24).

It has also been postulated that the frequency of receptive anal-genital intercourse among male homosexuals has allowed for co-infection with cytomegalovirus. This agent or other sexually transmitted viruses may play a role in the development of Kaposi's sarcoma (25,26) (see Chapter 19). In this regard, recently the prevalence of Kaposi's sarcoma in homosexual AIDS patients has declined concomitant with a decrease in CMV transmission (48). This observation may reflect the changes in sexual practice.

IV. Kaposi's Sarcoma in Non-AIDS Patients

Kaposi's sarcoma has been previously observed in several non-AIDS populations. In these settings Kaposi's sarcoma has clinical characteristics that distinguish it from its behavior in AIDS patients (Table 1).

First described in 1872, Kaposi's sarcoma was an extremely rare malignancy for over a century in the United States and Europe (27,28). Elderly men, particularly of Mediterranean or Jewish descent, would occasionally develop this cancer. Clinically it appeared most frequently as an indolent cutaneous tumor of the feet and lower extremities (27). It was not accompanied by immune depression beyond the expected immunological attrition of aging. Systemic chemotherapy was rarely necessary.

In the early 1960s, studies in Uganda sponsored by the National Cancer Institute (29) indicated that Kaposi's sarcoma was a common cancer (up to 9% of all cancer cases). Again, no associated immunodeficiency was determined

Table 1 "Traditional" Kaposi's Sarcoma: Clinical Features

Group	Disease features	Response to therapy
1. Elderly men especially Jewish	Indolent, skin of legs, feet	Local radiation, good control
2. Black Africans	Variable:	Systemic chemotherapy
	Children-aggressive	poor
	Adults-indolent	excellent
	No underlying immune deficiency	
3. Renal transplant recipients	Aggressive, visceral involvement	Controlled by stopping immunosuppressive medications

although reports of particularly aggressive cases (often in the young) were recorded. Due to political difficulties, long-term followup studies on treatment were not possible, but special agents were definitely active in helping control the cancer.

A third population that developed Kaposi's sarcoma offers significant clinical parallels to current AIDS-related cases. These patients developed Kaposi's sarcoma as a result of receiving immunosuppressive therapy following renal allografts (30,31). As with many AIDS patients, their cancer was often aggressive and these patients frequently contracted opportunistic infections. Of particular relevance was the finding that the Kaposi's sarcoma in renal allograft patients often regressed completely after the withdrawal of immunosuppressing drugs.

V. Staging of AIDS-Related Kaposi's Sarcoma

Krigel et al., in 1983, developed a staging system for AIDS-related Kaposi's sarcoma using conventional measures of tumor extent (Table 2) (4). Here, four stages are utilized to group patients. Although in common use, application is seriously limited in two aspects. Most AIDS-associated Kaposi's sarcoma patients are already in stage 3 or 4 at time of diagnosis. In addition, the degree of underlying immune deficiency now known to be an important prognostic variable in HIV infection (32-34) is not part of the staging system. Nevertheless, no other widely accepted system has been developed.

To improve upon the assessment of prognosis and treatment, symptoms other than Kaposi's lesions, lymph node, or visceral involvement must be taken into account. Awareness of "B" symptoms offers further information for predicting the clinical course of Kaposi's sarcoma and establishing the patient's correct staging position. The B symptoms include unexplained fever, unexplained weight loss greater than 10 pounds, and drenching night sweats lasting longer than several weeks. By subdividing each of the four

Table 2 Clinical Staging of Epidemic Kaposi's Sarcoma

Stage I - cutaneous, locally indolent
Stage II - cutaneous, locally aggressive with or without regional lymph nodes
Stage III - generalized mucocutaneous and/or lymph node involvement
Stage IV - visceral

Subtypes

A. No systemic signs or symptoms
B. Systemic signs: 10% weight loss or fevers unrelated to an identifiable source of infection lasting more than 2 weeks

Source: Refs. 8, 34.

clinical tumor stages as to the presence or absence of B symptoms, prognosis can be better estimated. Recent articles have considered these factors in reviewing the staging criteria (47,49,50).

VI. Experimental Treatments for AIDS-Related Kaposi's Sarcoma

The use of immune modulators or antiviral drugs in Kaposi's sarcoma remains experimental and trials should be conducted within carefully defined research environments. To date, drugs tested for their ability to expand the number of T-helper lymphocytes include interferons both alpha and gamma (35-37), isoprinosine, cimetidine, thymic hormones, and interleukin-2. All are either inactive or still being tested except for alpha interferon which has activity comparable to that of the chemotherapy drug vinblastine in AIDS/Kaposi's sarcoma. The antiviral drug zidovudine (retrovir) shown to prolong survival in AIDS, is also being tested in early Kaposi's sarcoma.

VII. Conventional Therapy of Kaposi's Sarcoma: Chemotherapy

In approaching clinical treatment of AIDS-related Kaposi's sarcome, considerable difficulty and uncertainty can occur because of the clinical differences between AIDS and non-AIDS populations (Table 3). In the absence of any treatment capable of correcting the underlying immunological suppression, we must choose that therapy most likely to control the tumor without exacerbating underlying immune dysfunction (50,51). Further refining of staging will be of crucial importance to more effectively interpreting clinical trials results.

Trials of cytotoxic chemotherapeutic agents in treating AIDS-related Kaposi's sarcoma have been conducted in several centers in the United States (Table 4). These studies were initially conducted largely within the guidelines

Table 3 AIDS/Kaposi's Sarcoma: Therapeutic Problems

1. Natural history and clinical staging essentially unknown
2. Trials of Kaposi's sarcoma in other populations not reliable
3. Nature of lesions (number, nodularity, pigmentation) make response assessment somewhat subjective
4. Disease occurs in setting of variably severe immune deficiency
   Treatment may exacerbate deficiency
   Selection biases in treatment groups may affect outcome

Table 4 Chemotherapy of Kaposi's Sarcoma

Agent	Regimen	Response Rate
VP-16-213	150 mg/m^2 IV qd x 3 q 28 d	75% PR & CR
Vinblastine	4-8 mg/week IV	25% PR 50% Stable
Vincristine	1.4-2 mg/week IV	25-50% PR
Vinblastine/Vincristine	Doses as above. Drugs used individually on alternate-week basis	25-50% PR

PR, partial response (>50% reduction in tumor burden); CR, complete response (no visible lesions); IV, intravenous.

suggested at the September 1981 National Institutes of Health workshop on the therapy of AIDS-related Kaposi's sarcoma (38). Patients in earlier stages of the cancer were treated with single agents to best determine activity and toxicity. Drugs found to be active in Kaposi's sarcoma include vinblastine (39), vincristine (40), and etoposide (VP-16-213) (41). These are in common clinical use. Trials with vinzolidine (42), ICRF-159 (43), and mitoxantrone have shown considerably less activity. Tests are currently being conducted with additional agents such as adriamycin, bleomycin, and methotrexate alone and in combination with other drugs (51).

A. Vinblastine Therapy

Vinblastine has been shown to be effective in treatment of non-AIDS-related Kaposi's sarcoma and is also a useful therapy for Kaposi's sarcoma patients with AIDS. Trials conducted at the University of California, San Francisco and the San Francisco General Hospital included weekly vinblastine treatment of 38 evaluable patients. All patients were homosexual or bisexual, with a median age of 33.8 years. Patients had a median helper/suppressor T-lymphocyte subset ratio of 0.5. Prior opportunistic infections had occurred in three of the patients studied, whereas 29 of the 38 had prior B symptoms. Tumor extent varied significantly. Cutaneous disease was seldom limited to one anatomic region of the body: 30 patients had clinically enlarged lymph nodes, and five patients had visceral Kaposi's sarcoma. All patients received vinblastine as a weekly intravenous bolus beginning at a total dose of 4 mg with dosage increasing in gradual increments to maintain a total leukocyte count of 2500-3000 cells/mm^3.

Vinblastine therapy resulted in an objective response rate of 27% with an additional 50% of patients showing stable disease (39). Vinblastine was relatively nontoxic, easily administered, and minimally immunosuppressing. Not rapidly active in AIDS-related Kaposi's sarcoma, treatment should be continued for six to eight weeks before being considered ineffective.

B. Vincristine

Early trials with vincristine therapy show that it is active in Kaposi's sarcoma. Results of one study reported in 1985 show a response rate of 60% with minimal toxicity (40). Trials conducted at the University of California, San Francisco and San Francisco General Hospital, however, showed that vincristine when used as a single agent in a weekly 1.4-2.0-mg intravenous bolus caused frequent and severe peripheral neuropathy.

Vincristine therapy should be utilized with extreme caution especially in patients with prior AIDS-related neurological problems. This therapy may be appropriate, however, for Kaposi's sarcoma patients with severe neutropenia or thrombocytopenia. Furthermore, alternating vincristine with vinblastine in weekly, single-agent therapy has shown as much activity as vinblastine alone with less toxicity than when either drug is used as a single agent.

C. Etoposide (VP-16-213)

Initial reports on etoposide therapy indicate it may be more active in Kaposi's sarcoma than either vinblastine or vincristine. In a study conducted by investigators at New York University (44), etoposide as a single agent had a 75% objective response rate. The 32 evaluable patients received 150 mg of VP-16/m^2 body surface area intravenously for three days every three to four weeks. A complete response was reported in 38% of patients, while 41% showed a partial response. The remaining 21% showed either minimal response or progressive disease. Toxicity levels were acceptable. Objective toxicities were generally limited to alopecia, while myelosuppression and stomatitis were minimal. It is important to note, however, that patients selected for this study did not have any history of prior opportunistic infections or B symptoms. Response rates to etoposide therapy may not be as high in patients in later stages of Kaposi's sarcoma or in patients exhibiting other symptoms.

D. Alpha-Interferon

A variety of clinical trials have shown that alpha-interferon when used in a high-dose regimen (usually more than 10-20 million units daily) is effective against Kaposi's sarcoma. Alpha-interferon has the theoretical advantage of less immunosuppressive activity than some chemotherapeutic agents. However, the need for frequent parenteral administration is a liability as well as the fevers and flulike toxicity that are commonly seen with this drug.

Table 5 Guidelines for Chemotherapy in Kaposi's Sarcoma

Group	Recommendations
Minimal KS No infection or B symptoms	Experimental immune modulators and/or antiviral drugs Vinblastine or other single-agent chemotherapy Expectant observation
Minimal KS History of infections and/or B symptoms	Vinblastine or other single-agent chemotherapy
Advanced cutaneous KS or pulmonary KS	VP-16-213 or other single-agent chemotherapy
KS with severe neutropenia or thrombocytopenia	Vincristine or bleomycin

Abbreviation: KS, Kaposi's sarcoma.

E. Radiation Therapy

Kaposi's sarcoma is radiation responsive; however, radiation is a palliative rather than curative treatment due to the systemic nature of the cancer. Large erosive oral lesions, painful lesions of the feet, and areas of the face or lower extremities where extensive Kaposi's sarcoma has caused lymphedema often respond well to radiation therapy in doses between 1800 and 3000 rads (45,46).

VIII. Guidelines for Therapy of AIDS-Related Kaposi's Sarcoma

Because the progression of AIDS can vary so widely, the decision as to when to initiate therapy and whether to use single agents or drug combinations is often problematic. Frequently patients in early stages of Kaposi's sarcoma with minimal B symptoms and no history of opportunistic disease can function well without treatment for months or years. In others, the disease will progress rapidly and death will occur as a direct result of Kaposi's sarcoma or of AIDS-related disease. However, mortality statistics show that only 23% of patients with Kaposi's sarcoma who do not have other major opportunistic infections die direclty from Kaposi's sarcoma (2). Recommendations for therapy are therefore to be considered extremely general until such time as sufficient additional clinical trials can be completed and evaluated (Table 5).

A. Early Kaposi's Sarcoma and Absence of Poor Prognostic Factors

Patients in this category will exhibit few cutaneous lesions and no ''B'' symptoms, and will have no history of prior serious infections. These patients are ideal candiates for experimental therapies such as immune modulators, or antiviral drugs. If unavailable, the patient may be observed until disease progression is documented, or chemotherapy can be initiated immediately. Vinblastine or alternating use of this drug with vincristine is recommended as it offers both convenience and minimal toxicity. Single-agent adriamycin in a frequent low-dose schedule can also be considered. Alpha-interferon may be especially useful as well in this patient group.

B. Advanced Kaposi's Sarcoma or Presence of Poor Prognostic Factors

Patients in this category generally exhibit extensive and actively progressing Kaposi's sarcoma or a history of prior infection or B symptoms. Chemotherapy is generally more appropriate than experimental therapies unless these can be combined with cytotoxic agents. Vinblastine is often recommended if the Kaposi's sarcoma is less advanced but etoposide or adriamycin (in low, frequent doses) may be a better choice in cases where the disease is extensive or rapidly progressing.

C. Pulmonary Kaposi's Sarcoma

Diffuse pulmonary Kaposi's sarcoma is the most fatal form of Kaposi's sarcoma. Progression of the disease is generally extremely active and rapid. Radiation therapy or chemotherapy should be initiated at once, and more aggressive agents such as etoposide or adriamycin should be considered. Initial trials of radiation therapy have occasionally been effective in treating pulmonary Kaposi's sarcoma, but it is not known whether chemotherapy or radiation therapy is more beneficial.

IX. Summary

Because Kaposi's sarcoma is a highly visible disease and one readily confirmed histologically, it continues to play an important role in the clinical spectrum of AIDS. At this time, it can not be confirmed whether AIDS-related Kaposi's sarcoma is caused by an initial viral infection, whether the development of an immune deficiency predisposes patients to develop this malignancy, or whether viral or other cofactors may be involved.

Evaluation of therapies for AIDS-related Kaposi's sarcoma is made more difficult by the lack of natural history information. In addition, available drugs are often immunosuppressing and investigators have considerable concern in utilizing these therapies to treat Kaposi's sarcoma, a cancer that is intimately associated with immune deficiency. Extensive research continues on single-agent trials of cytotoxic agents as well as immune modulators and antiviral agents.

Although considerable progress has been made in the treatment of AIDS-related Kaposi's sarcoma, therapeutic decision-making is extremely difficult.

It is expected that additional trials and experimental agents will ımprove our ability to provide effective treatment.

References

1. Centers for Disease Control. Kaposi's sarcoma and *Pneumocystis* pneumonia among homosexual men—New York City and California. MMWR 1981; 30:305-8.
2. Centers for Disease Control. Follow-up on Kaposi's sarcoma and *Pneumocystis* pneumonia. MMWR 1981; 30:409-10.
3. Hymes KB, Cheung TL, Greene JB, et al. Kaposi's sarcoma in homosexual men: A report of eight cases. Lancet 1981; 2:598.
4. Krigel R, Laubenstein L, Muggia F. Kaposi's sarcoma: A new staging classification. Cancer Treat Rep 1983; 67:531-4.
5. Templeton AC, Bhana D. Prognosis in Kaposi's sarcoma. J NCI 1975; 55:1301-4.
6. Losada F. Personal communication. 1983.
7. Hui AN, Koss MN, Meyer PR. Necropsy findings in acquired immunodeficiency syndrome: a comparison of premorten diagnoses with postmortem findings. Hum Pathol 1984; 15:670-6.
8. Krigel RL, Laubenstein LJ, Muggia FM. Kaposi's sarcoma: a new staging classification. Cancer Treat Rep 1983; 67:531-4.
9. Friedman SL, Wright TL, Altman DF. Gastrointestinal Kaposi's sarcoma in patients with acquired immune deficiency syndrome—endoscopic and autopsy findings. Gastroenterology 1985; 890:102-8.
10. Pitchenik AE, Fischl MA, Saldana MJ. Kaposi's sarcoma of the tracheobronchial tree: clinical bronchoscopic and pathologic features. Chest 1985; 87:122-4.
11. Kornfeld A, Axelrod JL. Pulmonary presentation of Kaposi's sarcoma in a homosexual patient. Am Rev Resp Dis 1983; 127:248-9.
12. Ognibene FP, Steis RG, Macher AM, et al. Kaposi's sarcoma causing pulmonary infiltrates and respiratory failure in the acquired immunodeficiency syndrome. Ann Intern Med 1985; 102:471-5.
13. Small CB, Klein RS, Friedland GH, Moll B, Emeson EE, Spigland I. Community-acquired opportunistic infections and defective cellular immunity in heterosexual drug users and homosexual men. Am J Med 1983; 74:433-41.
14. Pitchenik AE, Fischl MA, Dickinson GM, Becker AM, Fournier M, O'Connell MT, et al. Opportunistic infections and Kaposi's sarcoma among Haitians: evidence of a new acquired immunodeficiency state. Ann Intern Med 1983; 98: 277-84.
15. Centers for Disease Control. *Pneumocystis carinii* pneumonia among persons with hemophilia A. MMWR 1982; 31:365-7.
16. Centers for Disease Control. Update on acquired immunodeficiency syndrome (AIDS) among patients with hemophilia. MMWR 1982; 31:644-52.
17. Jett JR, Kuritsky JN, Katzmann JA, Homburger HA. Acquired immunodeficiency syndrome associated with bloodproduct transfusions. Ann Intern Med 1983; 99:621-4.
18. Harris C, Small CB, Klein RS, Friedland GH, Moll B, Meson EE, et al. Immunodeficiency in female sexual partners of men with the acquired immunodeficiency syndrome. N Engl J Med 1983; 308:1181-4.
19. Oleski J, Minnefor A, Cooper R, Thomas K, Dela Crus A, Andieh H, et al. Immune deficiency syndrome in children. JAMA 1983; 249:2345-9.

Plate I

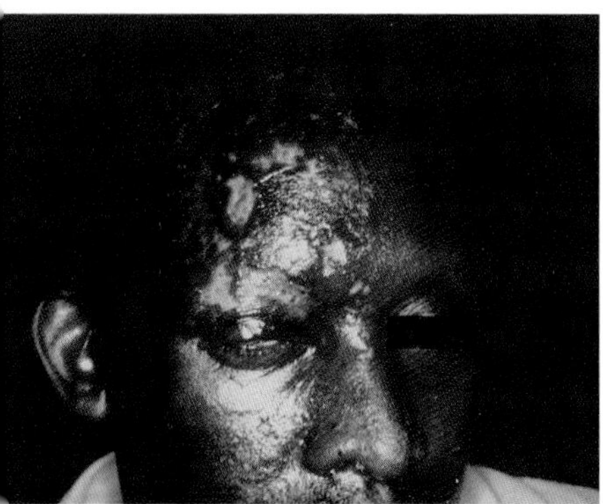

'igure 2.1 Extended facial herpes zoster ıfection in an African patient with ARC. Courtesy of Professor Achten, St. Pierre Jniversity Hospital, Brussels, Belgium.)

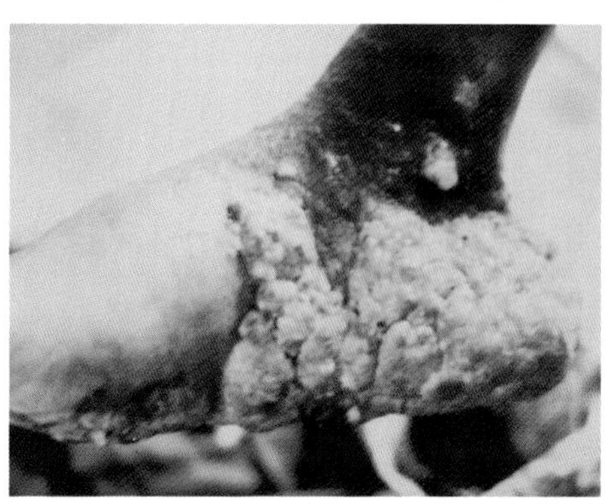

Figure 2.2 Classical form of Kaposi's sarcoma. (Courtesy of Dr. Gigase, Institute of Tropical Medicine, Antwerp, Belgium.)

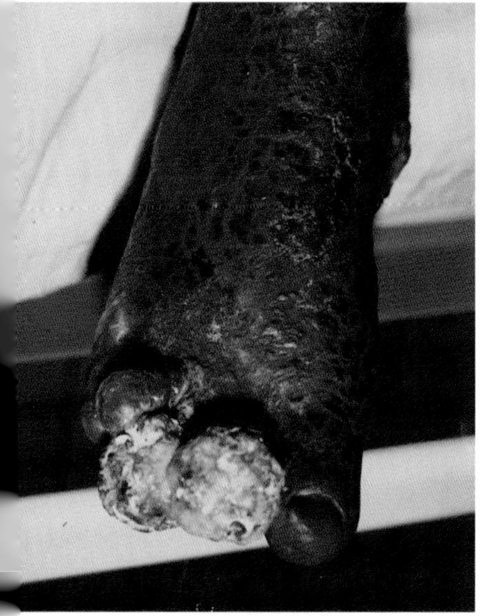

gure 2.4 Aggressive form of Kaposi's rcoma of the limb in an African case of DS.

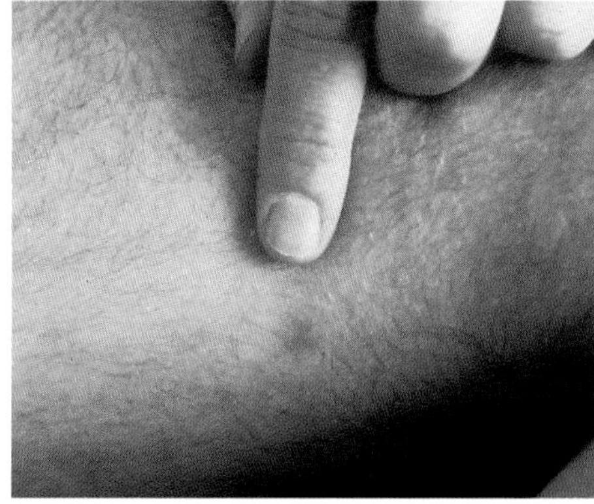

Figure 13.1 Early cutaneous Kaposi's sarcoma lesion in an AIDS patient on the medial aspect of the right thigh.

Plate II

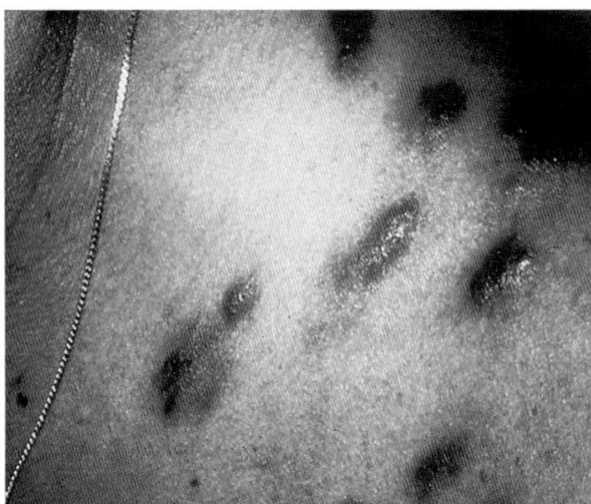

Figure 13.2 Cutaneous lesions of Kaposi's showing nodularity and linear characteristics.

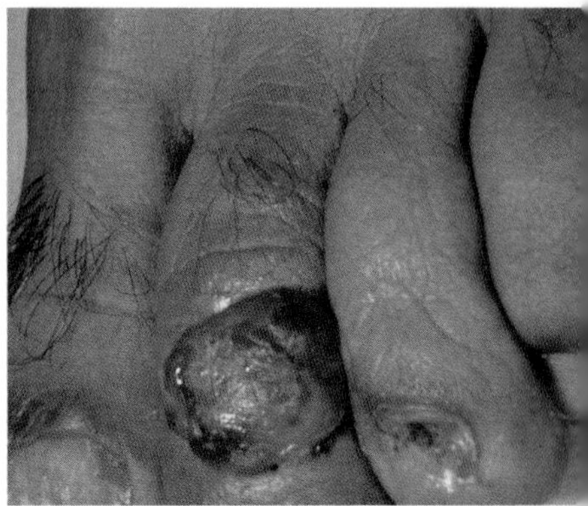

Figure 13.3 Necrotic painful lesions of Kaposi's sarcoma on the toe of a patient with AIDS.

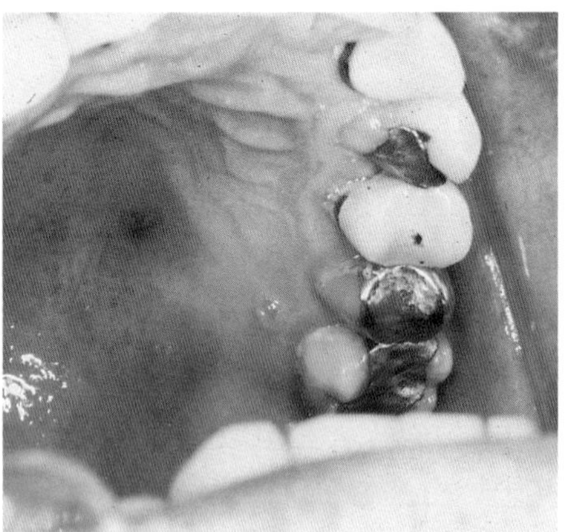

Figure 13.4 Kaposi's sarcoma involving the hard palate.

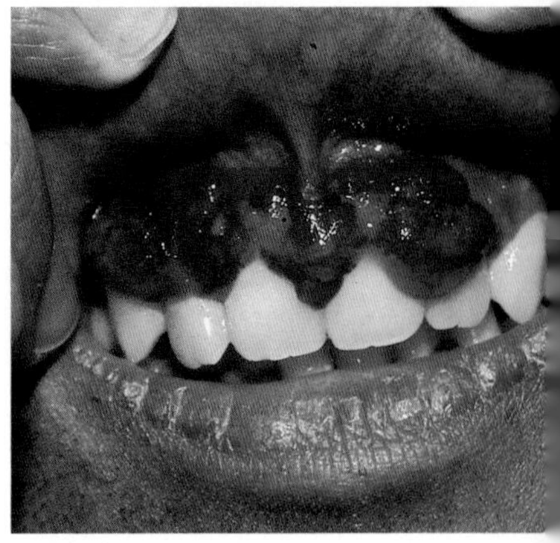

Figure 13.5 Gingival involvement with Kaposi's sarcoma.

Plate III

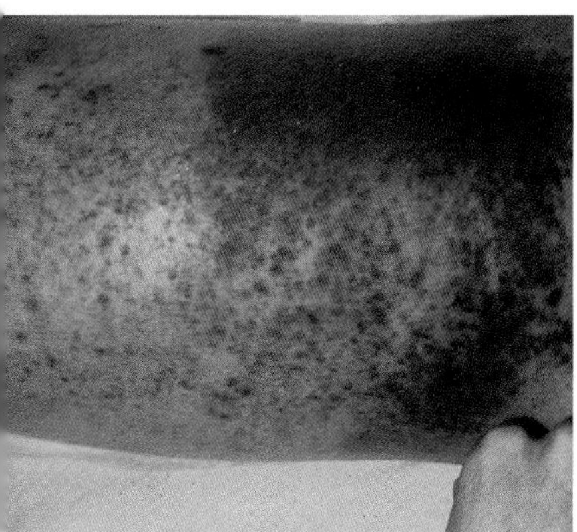

igure 13.6 Nodular cutaneous lesions Kaposi's sarcoma on the thigh of an AIDS tient which have progressed to a coalescent aque of tumor with underlying lymphema.

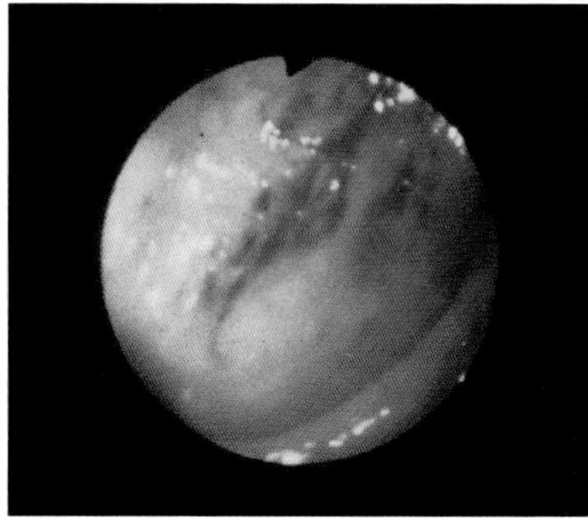

Figure 13.7 Endoscopic view of asymptomatic Kaposi's sarcoma lesions in the sigmoid colon.

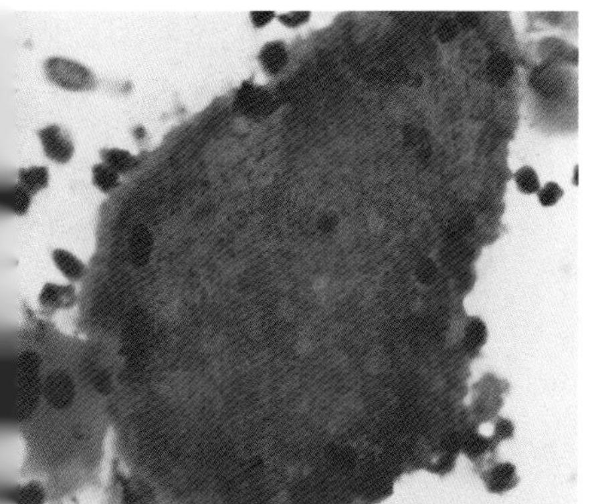

gure 16.1C Lung pathology of *P. carii* pneumonia. Giemsa stain revealing troozoite forms within the alveolar exudate.

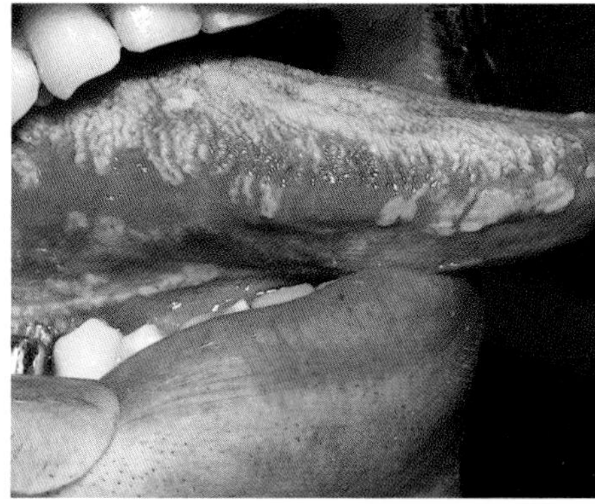

Figure 17.1 Hairy leukoplakia—moderate involvement.

Plate IV

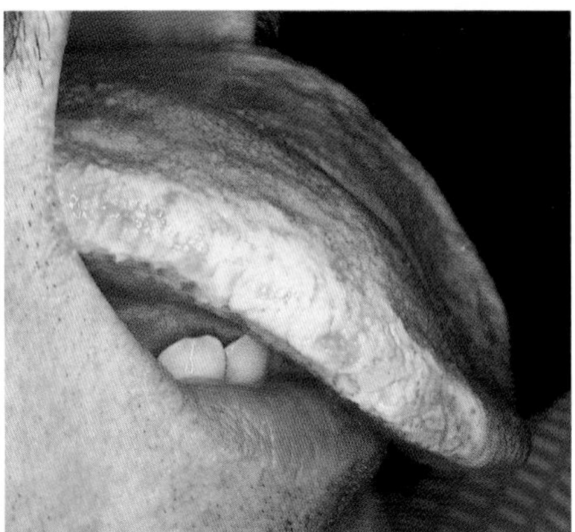

Figure 17.2 Hairy leukoplakia—extensive lesion.

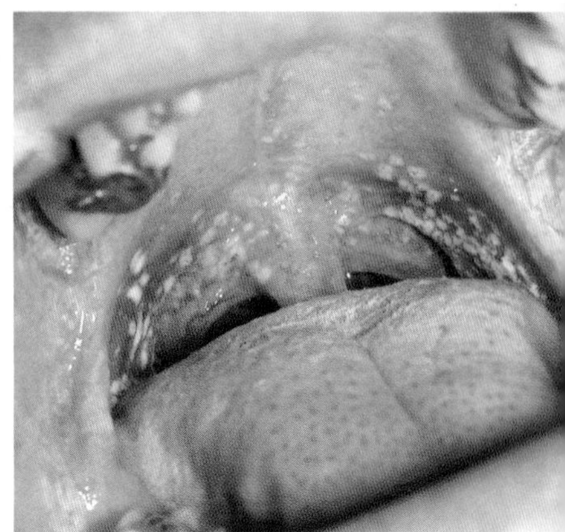

Figure 17.8 Pseudomembranous candidiasis.

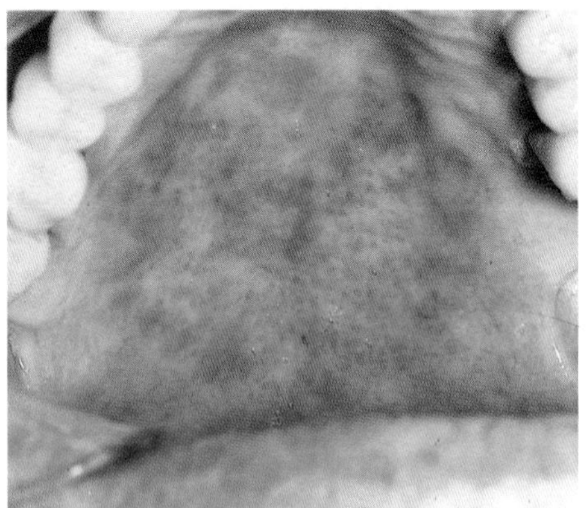

Figure 17.9 Atrophic candidiasis.

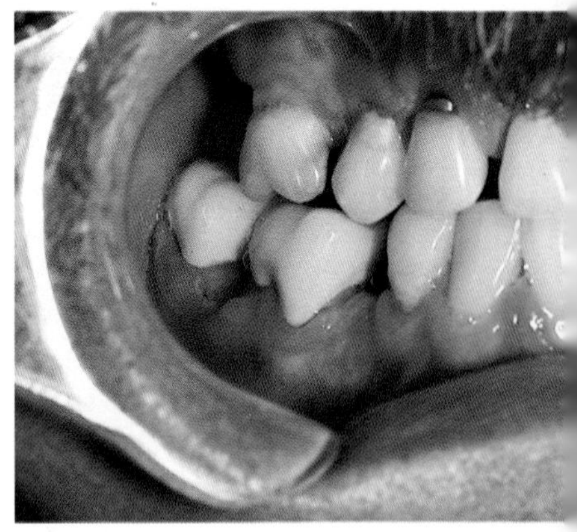

Figure 17.10 HIV-associated periodontitis.

20. Rubenstein A, Sicklick M, Gupta A, Bernstein L, Klein N, Rubenstein E, et al. Acquired immunodeficiency with reversed T4/T8 ratios in infants born to promiscuous and drug-addicted mothers. JAMA 1983; 249:2350-6.
21. Ziegler JL, Templeton AC, Vogel CL. Kaposi's sarcoma: a comparison of classical endemic and epidemic forms. Semin Oncol 1984; 11:47-52.
22. Marmor M. Friedman-Klein AE, Laubenstein L, Byrum RD, Williams DC, D'Onofrio S, et al. Risk factors for Kaposi's sarcoma in homosexual men. Lancet 1982; 1:1089-7.
23. Jaffe HW, Choi K, Thomas PA, Haverkos HW, Auerback DM, Guinan ME, et al. National case-control study of Kaposi's sarcoma and *Pneumocystis carinii* pneumonia in homosexual men: 1. Epidemiologic results. Ann Intern Med 1983; 99:145-51.
24. Quinto I. Mutagencity of alkyl nitrites in the *Salmonella* test. Boll Soc Ital Biol Sper 1980; 56:816-20.
25. Giraldo G, Beth E, Kourilsky FM, et al. Antibody patterns to herpes viruses in Kaposi's sarcoma: serologic association of European Kaposi's sarcoma with cytomegalovirus. Int J Cancer 1975; 15:839-48.
26. Drew WL, Miner RC, Ziegler JL, et al. Cytomegalovirus and Kaposi's sarcoma in young homosexual men. Lancet 1982; 2:125-7.
27. Safai B, Good RA. Kaposi's sarcoma: a review and recent developments. Clin Bull 1980; 10:62-9.
28. Biggar RJ, Horm J, Fraumeni JF Jr, Greene MH, Goedert JJ. The incidence of Kaposi's sarcoma in the United States and Puerto Rico, 1973-81, JNCI (in press).
29. Volberding P, Conant MA, Strickler RB, Lewis BJ. Chemotherapy in advanced Kaposi's sarcoma: implications for current cases in homosexual men. Am J Med 1983; 74:652-6.
30. Harwood AR, Osoba D, Hofstader SL, et al. Kaposi's sarcoma in recipients of renal transplants. Am J Med 1979; 64:759-65.
31. Myers BD, Kessler E, Levi J, et al. Kaposi's sarcoma in kidney transplant patients. Arch Intern Med 1974; 133:307-11.
32. Volberding P, Kaslow K, Bilk M, et al. Prognostic factors in staging Kaposi's sarcoma in the acquired immunodeficiency syndrome (abstr.). Proc Am Soc Clin Oncol Annu Meet 1984; 3:51.
33. Moss AR, McCallum G, Volberding PA, et al. Mortality associated with mode of presentation in the acquired immunodeficiency syndrome. JNCI 1984; 78: 1281-4.
34. Krigel R, Ostreicher F, LaFleur L, et al. Epidemic Kaposi's sarcoma (EKS): identification of a subset of patients with a good prognosis (abstr.) Proc Am Soc Clin Oncol Annu Meet 1985; 4:4.
35. Krown SE, Real FX, Cunningham-Rundles S, et al. Preliminary observations on the effect of recombinant leukocyte A interferon in homosexual men with Kaposi's sarcoma. N Engl J Med 1083; 308:1071-6.
36. Groopman JE, Gottlieb MS, Goodman J, et al. Recombinant alpha-2 interferon therapy for Kaposi's sarcoma associated with the acquired immunodeficiency syndrome. Ann Intern Med 1984; 100:671-6.
37. Rios A, Mansell PWA, Newell GR, et al. Treatment of acquired immunodeficiency syndrome-related Kaposi's sarcoma with lymphoblastoid interferon. J Clin Oncol 1985; 2:506-12.

38. DeWys WD, Curran J, Henle W, Johnson G. Workshop on Kaposi's sarcoma: meeting report. Cancer Treat Rep 1982; 66:1387-90.
39. Volberding PA, Abrams DI, Conant M, et al. Vinblastine therapy for Kaposi's sarcoma in the acquired immunodeficiency syndrome. Ann Intern Med 1985; 103:335-38.
40. Mintzer DM, Real FX, Jovino L, Krown SE. Treatment of Kaposi's sarcoma and thrombocytopenia with vincristine in patients with the acquired immunodeficiency syndrome. Ann Intern Med 1985; 102:200-2.
41. Leubenstein LJ, Krigel RL, Odajnyk CM. Treatment of epidemic Kaposi's sarcoma with etoposide or a combination of doxorubicin, bleomycin, and vinblastine. J Clin Oncol 1984; 2:1115-20.
42. Sarna G, Mitsuyasu R, Figlin R, et al. Oral vinzolidine as therapy for Kaposi's sarcoma and carcinomas of lung, breast, colon and rectum. Cancer Chemother Pharmacol 1985; 14:12-4.
43. Volberding P, Abrams D, Kaplan L, et al. Therapy of AIDS-related Kaposi's sarcoma with ICRF-159 (abstr.). Proc Am Soc Clin Oncol Annu Meet 1985; 4:4.
44. Laubenstein L, Krigel R, Himes K, Mugin F. Treatment of epidemic Kaposi's sarcoma with VP-16-213 (etoposide) and a combination of doxorubin, bleomycin and vinblastine (ABV). Proc Am Soc Clin Oncol Annu Meet 1983; 2:228.
45. Cooper JS, Fried PR, Laubenstein LJ. Initial observations of the effect of radiotherapy on epidemic Kaposi's sarcoma. JAMA 1984; 252:934-5.
46. Harris JW, Reed TA. Kaposi's sarcoma in AIDS: the role of radiation therapy. Fron Radiat Ther Oncol 1985; 19:126-32.
47. Mitsuyasu RT. Clinical variants and staging of Kaposi's sarcoma. Sem Oncol 1987; 44:13-8.
48. Drew WL, Mills J, Hauer LB, Miner RC, Rutherford, GW. Declining prevalence of Kaposi's sarcoma in homosexual AIDS patients paralleled by fall in cytomegalovirus transmission. Lancet 1988; 1:66.
49. Volberding PA. Clinical features and staging. In: Ziegler, JL, Dorfman RF, eds. Kaposi's Sarcoma: Pathophysiology and Clinical Management. New York: Marcel Dekker, 1988:169-88.
50. Krown SE. AIDS-associated Kaposi's sarcoma: Pathogenesis, clinical course, and treatment. AIDS 1988; 2:71-80.
51. Volberding PA. Chemotherapy. In: Ziegler JL, Dorfman RF, eds. Kaposi's Sarcoma: Pathophysiology and Clinical Management. New York: Marcel Dekker, 1988:249-60.

14

Lymphomas and Other Neoplasms Associated with AIDS

John L. Ziegler
Veterans Administration Medical Center
and School of Medicine
University of California
San Francisco, California

I. Introduction

The association of neoplasia and, in particular, the lymphoproliferative malignancies with congenital and acquired immunodeficiency disorders is well known (1). The finding of a large incidence of Kaposi's sarcoma and non-Hodgkin's lymphoma (NHL) among acquired immunodeficiency syndrome (AIDS) patients strengthens the association and provides additional avenues of research into pathogenesis and treatment. This chapter will review the incidence, etiology, and management of AIDS-associated NHL, and discuss briefly other neoplasms that may be associated with human immunodeficiency virus (HIV) infection.

II. Epidemiology

Several months after the AIDS epidemic was recognized in San Francisco, we noted an unusual presentation of Burkitt-like NHL in four homosexual men (2). These four patients developed high-grade undifferentiated NHL of B-cell origin and two of these lymphomas contained Epstein-Barr virus genomes. A review of NHL in young (20-45 years of age), never-married men in the San Francisco Bay Area disclosed a threefold increase in the early 1980s, and 19 cases were characterized as high-grade, aggressive lymphomas (3). At the San Francisco General Hospital, the number of AIDS-associated cases of NHL has doubled between 1986 and 1987.

III. Clinical Features

An analysis of 90 cases collected from five medical centers was published in 1984 and established a relationship between NHL in homosexual men and AIDS and AIDS-related complex (ARC) (4). The age distribution coincided with that of AIDS (Figure 1). One-third of the cases had chronic lymphadenopathy, and one-half had AIDS before lymphoma was diagnosed. After the diagnosis of NHL, another 25% developed AIDS (Table 1). All lymphomas

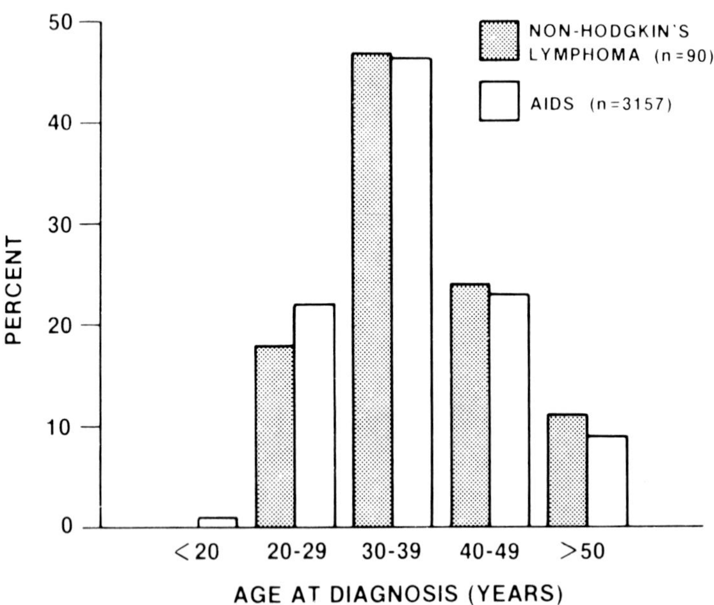

Figure 1 Age distribution (percentage of total) of 90 homosexual men with non-Hodgkin's lymphoma, as compared with that of 3157 cases of AIDS reported to the Centers for Disease Control as of January 1984. (Data obtained courtesy of the Centers for Disease Control, Atlanta.) (From Ref. 4.)

Table 1 Prodromal Manifestations According to Diagnosis of NHL

	Diagnosis of NHL (no. of patients)	
	At autopsy	Antemortem
Prodrome		
None		15
Generalized lymphadenopathy		33
Total		48 (53%)
AIDS		
Opportunistic infection	8	15
Kaposi's sarcoma	1	9
Kaposi's sarcoma and opportunistic infection	4	5
Total	13 (14%)	29 (32%)

Source: Ref. 4.

Table 2 Extranodal Sites of NHL in 88 Patients

Site	No. of patients*
Central nervous system	
Brain mass	21
Meninges	14
Cranial/peripheral nerves	5
Paraspinal	5
Total	38
Bone marrow	30
Skin/mucosa	
Intraoral	4
Anorectal	3
Thigh	3
Popliteal fossa	1
Ear lobes	1
Cutaneous nodules	1
Scalp	1
Total	14
Bowel	15
Lung	8
Liver	8
Kidney	2
Orbit	2
Pericardium	1
Bone	1
Gallbladder	1

*Some patients had lymphoma at more than one site.
Source: Ref. 4.

were consistent with B-cell origin and were clinically aggressive. Often the NHL would appear in atypical sites such as the orbit, mouth, rectum, or skin. One-third of patients had bone marrow involvement and 40% had NHL in the central nervous system (Table 2). Therapy varied but the response rates were poorer than expected, and mortality bore a close relationship to either ARC or AIDS.

Primary lymphoma of the central nervous system (CNS) developed in 21 (23%) patients in this series and has been noted by other investigators as a sign of AIDS (5,6). These tumors usually present as intracranial mass lesions (headache, altered mental status, cranial nerve palsy, seizures) and are predominately immunoblastic on histological examination. Meningeal involvement is uncommon. Tumors tend to be multicentric in the brain parenchyma, but spread to extracranial sites is rare (5). The major tumor deposits are in the cerebral hemispheres and cortical structures, with posterior fossa involvement less common. The differential diagnosis includes other causes of intracranial mass lesions, such as brain abscess, toxoplasmosis, and hemorrhage. Nuclear magnetic resonance imaging is a very useful technique in evaluation. Cerebrospinal fluid (CSF) is abnormal but nonspecific, showing elevated CSF pressure and protein levels, and mild mononuclear pleocytosis with usually negative cytology (5). The mainstays of treatment are surgical excision or radiotherapy, but the majority of patients die of tumor relapse or opportunistic infections within one year of diagnosis.

IV. Pathogenesis

Many investigations have pointed to immunodysregulation as a key element in lymphomagenesis (6,7). The immune system is equiped uniquely with the ability to respond to antigens and mitogens by autocrine and paracrine mechanisms. Thus, the stimulated T cell will produce interleukin 2 (IL-2) and, as a consequence, upregulate the expression of the IL-2 receptor (8). The B-cell system also responds to specific lymphokines that promote activation, proliferation, differentiation, and immunoglobulin production. These activation events are opposed by both cellular (e.g., T-suppressor cells) and humoral (e.g., anti-idiotypic antibodies) restraints that eventually modulate the immune response. An impairment in normal immunoregulatory circuits would be expected to result in uncontrolled lymphoproliferation (9).

In addition to dysregulation, the immune system can be provoked into perpetual activity by a constant barrage of foreign antigens such as may occur in recipients of blood products, intravenous drug abusers, or patients with chronic infection or neoplasia. Finally, an array of viruses, most notably the human T-cell leukemia virus, type 1 (HTLV-1) retrovirus, and the B-cell-tropic Epstein-Barr virus (EBV) can potentially cause their respective target lymphocytes to proliferate indefinitely (8,10).

Certain rare T-cell malignancies (e.g., adult T-cell leukemia, Sezary syndrome) have been associated with HTLV-I infection wherein the viral genome codes for excessive production of IL-2. Only a rare individual infected with HTLV-I (which is endemic in parts of Japan and the Caribbean) will develop T-cell lymphoma, a phenomenon that clearly implicates etiological cofactors.

Burkitt's lymphoma in Africa has long been associated with EBV, but the majority of sporadic Burkitt-like lymphomas in the United States lack EBV-DNA in the tumor cells (11). In the immunocompromised host, reactivation of EBV is common, and a variety of lymphoproliferative disorders develop in this population (1,12,13).

There is now evidence in immunosuppressed patients of stepwise progression from benign lymphadenopathy to polyclonal lymphoblastic lymphoma to monoclonal malignant lymphoma (14). Studies of lymphomagenesis have been aided recently by identification of immunoglobulin or T-cell receptor gene rearrangement disclosing clonal excess in lymphoproliferative tissues, leading eventually to mono- or biclonal lymphomas (15,16). Most important, the discovery of cellular oncogenes has opened up new avenues of research to explore the multistep process toward neoplasia (17).

Briefly, oncogenes were recognized first as cellular analogues of acute transforming genes of oncogenic retroviruses (18). Transfection experiments that introduce DNA from malignant cells into a "primed" or initiated cell line (NIH 3T3 cells) also identified cell-transforming oncogenes. These highly conserved genes have a presumed role in normal physiological processes such as embryogenesis, differentiation, and tissue repair. There are now two separable "families" of oncogenes, one whose protein product acts on the nucleus and another whose product affects the cytoplasm (17). These gene products induce an array of cellular events ranging from cell proliferation to the coding of growth factors or their receptors to activation of postreceptor signals. Nuclear-acting oncogenes are derived from chromosome translocational and dysregulatory events, whereas cytoplasm-acting oncogenes appear to occur as a result of somatic point mutations. Just how these genes become activated and how their products induce phenotypic changes are unknown. Since oncogenesis is a multistep process, and in most cases malignant transformation of a normal cell will not occur under the influence of a single oncogene, current theories propose a sequence of cell-perturbing events that involve cooperating families of oncogenes.

Burkitt's lymphoma provides an instructive though speculative example of such a process. Epstein-Barr virus infection probably starts in the nasopharynx, and secondarily infects B cells in Waldeyer's ring (19). Both B cells and epithelial cells harbor virus in the latent state, but when T-cell control of EBV falters (such as may occur in malaria, X-linked immune deficiency, or AIDS), EBV reactivation results in B-cell proliferation. This event is now linked to the induction of the *fgr* oncogene (20). The immortalized B cells also produce immunoglobulin, causing active rearrangement of Ig genes. By accident, the long arms of chromosome 8 (containing the c-*myc* oncogene) and chromosome 14 (containing the immunoglobulin heavy chain gene) translocate, moving the transcriptionally inactive *myc* segment into a region of excessive promotional activity. The *myc* gene product then contributes additional proliferative stimulus to the EBV infected lymphocytes rendering them immortal, but B-cell growth factor dependent (21). By further mutational (mutation rates perhaps rising in proportion to cell turnover) or epigenetic accident, another oncogene becomes activated, this time possibly B-*lym*, whose gene product resembles transferrin and is analogous to the transforming oncogene in lymphoma of chickens (22). These events give rise to a single clone with overwhelming growth potential and its progeny emerge as a monoclonal, malignant B-cell lymphoma. Proliferation is doubtless enhanced

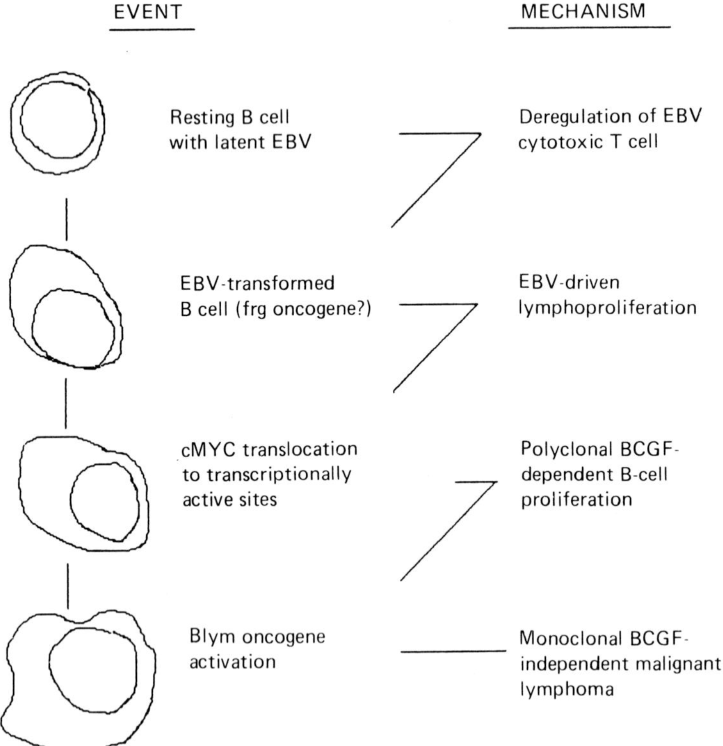

Figure 2 Hypothetical pathogenesis of lymphoma in AIDS (see text).

by a more permissive environment where normal regulatory restraints are lacking. Thus B-cell lymphomas are found commonly in immunologically "privileged" extranodal sites, particularly the brain, or in sites where cellular growth is generally promoted (e.g., bone marrow, gastrointestinal tract). These events are summarized in Figure 2.

While the foregoing proposal is speculative, current observations in AIDS patients disclose the major landmarks: T-cell immunodeficiency, elevated titers of EBV antibodies, evidence of EBV reactivation, evidence of B-cell proliferation, and presence of EBV and typical translocations involving the long arm of chromosome 8 in AIDS-associated lymphomas. A diligent search for HIV in lymphomas has not revealed retrovirus in the tumor cells. It is likely that the polyclonal B-cell lymphoproliferation in AIDS is a complex result of EBV infection, HIV antigenic stimulation, and T-cell-dependent HIV activation (23).

At the University of California San Francisco, we are examining the hypothesis that the lymphoma-forming clone is stimulated exogenously by HTLV envelope glycoprotein, analogous to the situation in retroviral-associated murine lymphoma (24). Preliminary data (McGrath MS, personal communication) suggest that sera from up to 75% of patients with AIDS-associated NHL react with the envelope glycoprotein of HTLV-I, and that the surface immunoglobulin of an AIDS-NHL cell line binds to retroviral glycoprotein. Thus, dysregulation, viral activation, and exogenous stimulation by a co-infecting retrovirus may conspire to enhance lymphomagenesis in AIDS.

V. Treatment

Successful management of systemic AIDS-associated NHL depends on prompt diagnosis, effective chemotherapy, and control of infectious complications. Although patients with high-grade, advanced stage NHL that arise *de novo* have a probability of cure of 40-60%, patients with AIDS-associated NHL fare poorly. This fact is due largely to a diminished primary response to chemotherapy, high relapse rate, and complicating infections. Poor bone marrow reserve and leukopenia compromise effective doses and schedules of commonly employed cytotoxic agents. A high frequency of meningeal relapse demands aggressive prophylaxis and treatment. Finally, progressive immunodeficiency, aggravated by neoplasia and cytotoxic drugs, gives rise to fatal opportunistic infections (25-29).

At the University of California, San Francisco, we have adopted an NHL treatment regimen that delivers cytotoxic therapy tailored to the special requirements of the AIDS patients: a weekly outpatient regimen, effective meningeal prophylaxis, minimal bone marrow and immune depression,

Table 3 Chemotherapy of AIDS-Associated NHL at University of California, San Francisco

Drug	Dose	Route	Schedule
Cyclophosphamide	1400 mg/m^2	IV push	Day 1
Vincristine	1.4 mg/m^2	IV push	Day 1
Methotrexate	500 mg	IV over 6h	Day 8
Leukovorin rescue	25 mg	p.o. q 6hx6	Day 9
Etoposide	200 mg/m^2	IV push	Day 15
Cytosar	3000 mg/m^2	IV push	Day 15
Methotrexate	12.5 mg	IT	Day 1, 8, 15

Abbreviations: IT, intrathecal; IV, intravenous.
Repeat entire course at day 21 (delay one week for neutrophil count $<1000/mm^3$).

prophylaxis of *Pneumocystis carinii* pneumonia, and delivery of effective NHL cytotoxic drugs in a frequent, alternating manner (Table 3).

VI. Other Neoplasms

It is not possible as yet to determine whether Hodgkin's disease (HD) occurs in increased frequency in association with AIDS, since this neoplasm is most common in the same age groups at risk for AIDS. It is clear, however, that HD in gay men who have some of the clinical features of ARC and AIDS has a poor prognosis (30,31). In collaboration with workers at Stanford University, we identified 19 gay men with HD in the San Francisco Bay Area. Unusual tumor presentations included three in the CNS, two in the skin, and one each with endobronchial, mesenteric, and bone marrow involvement. Kaposi's sarcoma developed in eight and was associated with a poor survival (30,31).

Early in the AIDS epidemic, attention directed to oral manifestations led to the discovery of an EBV (and possibly papillomavirus)-related leukoplakia, called "oral hairy leukoplakia" (see Chapter 17). In association with this lesion nine nonsmoking gay men developed squamous carcinoma of the tongue (32, and Silverman S, personal communication). This finding is an intriguing observation noted also by others (33), and begins to fit into a growing pattern of virus-cancer associations in AIDS. Epithelial carcinomas of the head and neck and anogenital regions are associated increasingly with herpesvirus and/or papilloma virus, the latter having two particularly oncogenic serotypes, 16 and 18 (34). Cloacogenic carcinoma of the anus is more prevalent in homosexual men and has been associated with HPV infection (34,35). While it is not the purpose of this chapter to review the virus-cancer link, it is evident that AIDS, with its attendant deregulation of latent

Table 4 DNA Viruses Associated with Cancer

Virus	Cancer	Link[a]
Epstein-Barr (EBV)	African Burkitt's lymphoma	+ + +
	Nasopharyngeal carcinoma	+ + +
	Thymic carcinoma	+
Hepatitis B (HBV)	Hepatocellular carcinoma	+ + +
Herpes simplex (HSV)	Cervical carcinoma	+ +
	Head and neck cancer	+ +
Cytomegalovirus (CMV)	Kaposi's sarcoma	+ +
	Carcinoma of the colon	+
Human papilloma (HPV)	Laryngeal papillomatosis and cancer	+ + +
	Cervical carcinoma	+ +
	Cloacogenic carcinoma	+ +

[a]Degree of association: + + + = very strong association (9]% of cases); + + = moderate association (25-50% of cases); + = weak association (insufficient numbers of cases studied).

herpesviruses, may increase susceptibility to epithelial neoplasms. As noted in Chapter 13, Kaposi's sarcoma is associated with cytomegalovirus, adding yet another virus-associated cancer to neoplasms in AIDS. The only missing tumors (which may yet appear if predisposing cofactors are provided) are hepatocellular carcinoma (associated with hepatitis B virus, 36) and nasopharyngeal carcinoma (associated with EBV in Orientals, 24). Table 4 summarizes these relationships. Because of a longer tumor doubling time, the development of epithelial cancer in immunodeficient patients takes longer than the hematopoietic malignancies (1). If AIDS patients survive long enough, we may witness an increase in DNA-virus associated tumors in patients infected with HIV.

Sporadic reports of other tumors in AIDS patients do not substantiate an etiological association. These include embryonal cell carcinoma, small cell carcinoma of the lung, carcinoid, and adenocarcinoma of the colon. Benign angiolipomas have also been observed in excess among gay men (33, 37-39). Only additional surveillance of AIDS risk groups will determine whether these tumors are more prevalent than in the general population.

In conclusion, the immune dysregulation in AIDS has "uncovered" a variety of virus-associated neoplasms. The epidemic thus provides an unprecedented opportunity to discover occult virus association (e.g., Hodgkin's disease) in these patients. Such associations will undoubtedly disclose important cofactors that promote the progress toward neoplastic transformation.

References

1. Penn I. Depressed immunity and the development of cancer. Clin Exp Immunol 1981; 46:459-74.
2. Ziegler JL, Drew WL, Miner RC, et al. Outbreak of Burkitt's-like lymphoma in homosexual men. Lancet 1982; 2:631-3.
3. Zeigler JL, Bragg K, Abrams D, et al. High-grade non-Hodgkin's lymphomas in patients with AIDS. Ann NY Acad Sci 1985; 437:412-7.
4. Ziegler JL, Beckstead JA, Volberding PA, et al. Non-Hodgkin's lymphoma in 90 homosexual men. N Engl J Med 1984; 311:565-70.
5. Levy RM, Bredesen DE, Rosenblum ML. Neurological manifestations of the acquired immunodeficiency syndrome (AIDS): experience at UCSF and review of the literature. J Neurosurg 1985; 62:475-98.
6. Louie S, Daoust PT, Schwartz RS. Immunodeficiency and the pathogenesis of non-Hodgkin's lymphoma. Semin Oncol 1980; 7:267-84.
7. Hanto DW, Gajl-Peczalska G, Frizzera G, et al. Epstein-Barr virus (eBV) induced polyclonal and nonoclonal B-cell lymphoproliferative diseases occuring after renal transplantation. Ann Surg 1983; 198:356-69.
8. Waldmann TA. The structure, function, and expression of interleukin-2 receptors on normal and malignant lymphocytes. Science 1986; 232:727-32.
9. Schwartz RS. Immunoregulation, oncogenic viruses, and malignant lymphomas. Lancet 1972; 1:1266-9.
10. Kieff E, Dambaugh T, Hummel M, Heller M. Epstein-Barr virus transformation and replication. Adv Viral Oncol 1983; 3:133-82.
11. Ziegler JL, Anderson M, Klein G, Henle W. Detection of Epstein-Barr virus DNA in American Burkitt's lymphoma. Int J Cancer 1976; 17:701-6.
12. Hanto DW, Frizzera G, Purtilo DT, et al. Clinical spectrum of lymphoproliferative disorders in renal transplant recipients and evidence for the role of Epstein-Barr virus. Cancer Res 1981; 41:4253-61.
13. Birx DL, Redfield RR, Tosato G. Defective regulation of Epstein-Barr virus infection in patients with acquired immunodeficiency syndrome (AIDS) or AIDS-related disorders. N Engl J Med 1986; 314:874-9.
14. Klein G. The role of gene dosage and genetic transpositions in carcinogenesis. Nature 1981; 294:313-8.
15. Arnold A, Cossman J, Bakhashi BM, et al. Immunoglobulin gene rearrangements as unique clonal markers in human lymphoid neoplasms. N Engl J Med 1983; 309:1593-9.
16. Aisenberg AC, Krontiris TG, Mak TW, Wilkes BM. Rearrangement of the gene for the beta chain of the T-cell receptor in T-cell chronic lymphocytic leukemia and related disorders. N Engl J Med 1985; 313:529-33.
17. Weinberg RA. The action of oncogenes in the cytoplasm and nucleus. Science 1985; 230:770-6.
18. Bishop JM. Cancer genes come of age. Cell 1983; 32:1018-20.
19. Yough LS, Sixbey JW, Clark D, Rickinson AB. Epstein-Barr receptors on human pharyngeal epithelia. Lancet 1986; 1:240-2.

20. Cheah MSC, Ley TJ, Tronik SR, Robbins KC. Fgr proto-oncogene mRNA induced in B lymphocytes by Epstein-Barr virus infection. Nature 1986; 319:238-40.
21. Klein G, Klein E. Evolution of tumors and the impact of molecular oncology. Nature 1985; 315:190-7.
22. Diamond A, Cooper GM, Ritz J, Lance MA. Identification and molecular cloning of the human Blym transforming gene activated in Burkitt's lymphomas. Nature 1983; 305:112-6.
23. Yarchoan R, Redfield RR, Broder S. Mechanisms of B-cell activation in patients with acquired immunodeficiency syndrome and related disorders. J Clin Invest 1986; 78:439-47.
24. McGrath MS, Weissman IL. AKR leukemogenesis: identification and biological significance of thymic lymphoma receptors for AKR retroviruses. Cell 1979: 65-73.
25. Gottlieb MS, Groopman JE, Weinstein WM, Fahey JL, Detels R. The acquired immunodeficiency syndrome. Ann Intern Med 1983; 99:208-20.
26. Levine AM, Meyer PR, Begandy MK, et al. Development of B-cell lymphoma in homosexual men. Ann Intern Med 1984; 100:7-13.
27. Ioachim HL, Cooper MC, Hellman GC. Lymphomas in men at high risk for acquired immune deficiency syndrome. Cancer 1985; 56:2831-42.
28. Ciobanu N, Andreeff M, Safai B, Koziner B, Mertelsman R. Lymphoblastic neoplasia in homosexual patient with Kaposi's sarcoma. Ann Intern Med 1983; 98:151-55.
29. Chaganti RSK, Jhanwar SC, Koziner B, Mertelsman R, Clarkson BD. Specific translocations characterize Burkitt's-like lymphoma of homosexual men with the acquired immunodeficiency syndrome. Blood 1983; 61:1269-72.
30. Schoeppel S, Hoppe R, Abrams D, et al. Hodgkin's disease in nonsexual men: the San Francisco experience (abstr.). Proc Am Soc Clin Oncol Annu Meet 1986; 5:3.
31. Ioachim HL, Cooper MC, Hellman GC. Hodgkin's disease and the acquired immunodeficiency syndrome (lett.). Ann Intern Med 1984; 101:876.
32. Lozada F, Silverman S, Conant M. New outbreak of oral tumors, malignancies and infectious diseases strikes young male homosexuals. Calif Dent J 1982; 10: 39-42.
33. Groopman JE, Mayer K, Zipoli T, Wallach S, Fallon B, Clark J. Unusual neoplasms associated with HTLV-III infection (abstr.). Proc Am Soc Clin Oncol Annu Meet 1986; 5:4.
34. Editorial. Human papillomaviruses and neoplasia. Lancet 1983; 2:435-6.
35. Daling JR, Weiss NS, Klopfenstern LL, Cochran LE, Chow WH, Daifuku R. Correlates of homosexual behavior and the incidence of anal cancer. JAMA 1982; 247:1988-90.
36. Blumberg BS, London WT. Hepatitis B virus and the prevention of primary cancer of the liver. JNCI 1985; 74:267-73.
37. Weldon-Linne CM, Rhone DP, Blatt D, Moore D, Montiz M. Angiolipomas in homosexual men (lett.). N Engl J Med 1984; 310:1193-4.

38. Moser RJ, Tenholder MF, Ridemour R. Oat cell carcinoma in transfusion associated acquired immune deficiency syndrome. Ann Intern Med 1985; 103:478.
39. Nasbaum NJ. Metastatic small cell carcinoma of the lung in a patient with AIDS. N Engl J Med 1985; 312:1706.

15

Central Nervous System Disorders in AIDS

Robert M. Levy
Northwestern University Medical School
Chicago, Illinois

Dale E. Bredesen, Mark L. Rosenblum, and Richard L. Davis
School of Medicine
University of California
San Francisco, California

I. Introduction

From the beginning of the acquired immunodeficiency syndrome (AIDS) epidemic, reports of neurological dysfunction in AIDS patients have appeared (1, 2). Only recently, however, have the frequency and breadth of the neurological manifestations of AIDS become apparent (3). Of great importance has been the demonstration that these neurological illnesses arise not only from opportunistic processes that affect the nervous system but that the human immunodeficiency virus (HIV) may also primarily infect the nervous system (4-99). Thus, HIV has as a target both the immune and the nervous systems; primary infection with HIV can produce a number of previously unknown neurological diseases. As the AIDS epidemic spreads and the number of patients increases dramatically, it is imperative for physicians to become familiar with the spectrum of the neurological manifestations of AIDS.

II. Incidence of AIDS-Related CNS Illness

Our data base includes 1286 patients with AIDS or AIDS-related complex (ARC) who have been treated at the University of California San Francisco (UCSF) Affiliated Hospitals. Of these, 482 patients were identified with significant neurological complaints or neurological illness (37%). In these 482 patients, 553 neurological diseases were identified, with 474 affecting the central nervous system (CNS) and 79 affecting the peripheral nervous system; 65 patients had multiple neurological illnesses.

The annual incidence of AIDS-related neurological illness at UCSF has at least doubled over each of the 6 years that we have evaluated patients with AIDS. Of interest is the observation that one-third of all neurologically symptomatic patients with AIDS presented with these neurological complaints as their initial manifestation of AIDS. Thus, 10% of all AIDS patients first presented with symptoms of neurological illness.

The incidence data derived from our experience at UCSF appears to be corroborated by the experience of others. Data derived from cases reported to the Centers for Disease Control (CDC) (10) reveal that 7.5% of AIDS patients have reliably diagnosed neurological illness at the time of their presentation with AIDS. This number does not include patients presenting with peripheral neurological illness or those illnesses associated with primary HIV infection of the brain. Snider and co-workers (1) found that 50 of 160 AIDS patients developed neurological complications (31%), while Koppel et al. (11) identified 28 neurologically symptomatic patients from their population of 121 AIDS patients (23%).

Our initial investigation suggested that the incidence of AIDS-related nervous system illness may be underestimated. We frequently encountered patients in whom neurological symptoms were not appreciated due to their subtlety, the physician's lack of interest in pursuing an evaluation of these symptoms, or the fact that these complaints were overshadowed by overwhelming systemic illnesses. In an attempt to more accurately determine the scope of nervous system disease associated with AIDS, we undertook an unselected postmortem study of 104 patients with AIDS. On postmortem examination, the incidence of nervous system involvement was 75%. Neuropathological abnormalities were identified in 70 of 94 brains. In 20 of the 70 abnormal brains (29%), more than one pathological entity was identified. The most common of these pathologies was viral encephalitis or encephalomyelitis (48%), while infarction was noted with an unusual frequency in this

Table 1 Symptoms Related to Central Neurological Illness in AIDS

Headache
Altered mental status
Motor weakness
Sensory loss
Paresthesias
Pain
Seizures
Aphasia
Dizziness
Visual disturbances
Disordered gait

young patient population (19%). In two other reported series, the incidence of neuropathological abnormalities was similar to that observed at UCSF (12, 13).

III. AIDS-Related Central Neurological Syndromes

Central neurological syndromes associated with AIDS or ARC may arise from primary HIV infection or secondary opportunistic processes. Neurological disease may occur as part of a diffuse systemic or an isolated illness. These processes may manifest neurological illness by virtue of nonfocal, diffuse CNS involvement, focal involvement by a space-occupying lesion, or the production of obstructive hydrocephalus. Central neurological syndromes include focal or diffuse encephalopathy, myelopathy, meningitis, cranial neuropathy, and retinopathy.

The specific symptoms of AIDS-associated central neurological illness include virtually all those related to nervous system dysfunction (Table 1). Disorders of cognition are most common, evident in 68% of 482 neurologically symptomatic patients we examined. Headaches are only slightly less frequent; they are major complaints in 55% of these patients. Also common are complaints of focal weakness (18%), incoordination (18%), and seizures (17%). Less frequently, patients present with aphasia (12%), incontinence (10%), cranial neuropathies (9%), sensory loss (8%), and visual disturbances (8%). Such symptoms as stiff neck, photophobia, nausea, and vomiting occur frequently in patients with cryptococcal or viral meningitis but are rare in patients with encephalitis or myelitis.

IV. AIDS-Related Central Nervous System Diseases

The spectrum of diseases known to affect the central nervous system in AIDS is presented in Table 2; the clinical signs and symptoms of these diseases are listed in Table 3.

Table 2 Illness Affecting the Central Nervous System in AIDS

Primary viral (HIV)
subacute encephalopathy
atypical aseptic meningitis
vacuolar myelopathy
Secondary viral (encephalitis, retinitis, vasculitis, myelitis)
cytomegalovirus
herpes simplex virus I and II
papovavirus (progressive multifocal leukoencephalopathy)
Nonviral infections (encephalitis, meningitis, abscess)
Toxoplasma gondii
Cryptococcus neoformans
Candida albicans
Coccidioides immitis
Histoplasma capsulatum
Aspergillus funigatus
Mycobacterium avium intracellulare
Mycobacterirum tuberculosis hominis
Listeria monocytogenes
Nocardia asteroides
Neoplasms
primary CNS lymphoma
metastatic systemic lymphoma
metastatic Kaposi's sarcoma
Cerebrovascular
infarction
hemorrhage
vasculitis
Complications of systemic AIDS therapy

A. Primary Viral Infection

AIDS Encephalopathy

The most common central neurological illness associated with AIDS is also one that is unique to this syndrome. First reported by Snider et al. (1) as subacute encephalitis, this invariably fatal dementing illness has also been called AIDS encephalopathy and the AIDS dementia complex.

The first step toward understanding the pathogenesis of this illness was made by Shaw and co-workers (4), who demonstrated the presence of viral RNA in the brains of demented AIDS patients using in situ hybridization techniques. Subsequently, Levy and co-workers (5) reported the isolation of the infectious AIDS retrovirus from the brains and cerebrospinal fluid (CSF) of neurologically symptomatic AIDS patients. Ho and co-workers (6) also isolated

HIV from the CSF and neural tissues of patients with AIDS-related neurological syndromes. This latter study included 16 patients with AIDS-related dementia; in 10 of these patients, HIV was isolated from the brains, CSF, or both. At the same time, Resnick and colleagues (7) demonstrated the intra-blood-brain-barrier synthesis of HIV-specific IgG in 10 of 11 patients with AIDS-related mental status alterations. Sharer and co-workers (8) later reported the presence of multinucleated giant cells and HIV in patients with AIDS encephalopathy. More recently, Wiley et al. (14) and Koenig et al. (15) detected HIV within macrophages in brain tissue from patients with AIDS encephalopathy. Thus, it appears that AIDS encephalopathy results from primary infection of the brain by HIV. The major cells replicating this virus appear to be of macrophage origin, but other cell types—particularly capillary endothelial cells (14), astrocytes, and oligodendrocytes (14, 17)—may also be infected.

The subsequent pathobiology of HIV-related dementia remains largely a matter of conjecture. The regional distribution of HIV brain infection is noteworthy. The brunt of the disease is borne by subcortical white matter, deep hemispheric nuclei including the basal ganglia, and the thalamus and brain stem. In light of these findings, possible mechanisms for the production of dementia by HIV brain infection can be proposed. If the primary target of the virus is the neuron, the virus—which is known to be cytotoxic—might produce dementia by destroying those brain cells that ultimately subserve intellectual and motor functions. If the site of infection is primarily the glial cells, HIV might have its effect by depriving neurons of their glial-derived nutritional elements or by preventing glial cells from myelinating neurons. Thus, neurons might function abnormally or die secondarily of a metabolic "starvation," or the complex communications between neurons necessary for higher level intellectual functioning might be slowed to such a degree that dementia results. Finally, if the target of HIV brain infection is the monocyte or multinucleated giant cell, HIV might result in the production of neurotoxic substances, perhaps already known cytokines (see Chapter 10), or might initiate an autoimmune phenomenon that would then result in dysfunction and cell death.

Price and his co-workers have carefully studied the clinical profile of patients with AIDS-related dementia and coined the term *AIDS dementia complex,* or ADC. ADC may be the presenting or sole manifestation of HIV infection (18, 19) or may occur in the setting of other AIDS-related illnesses. All patients with ADC initially present with cognitive impairment. The syndrome is characterized by a progressive dementia, first appearing as a confusional state, often accompanied by fever or mild metabolic derangement. Less commonly, patients demonstrate motor weakness (34%), personality change (38%), or transient dysarthrias or movement disorders (7%). Brain

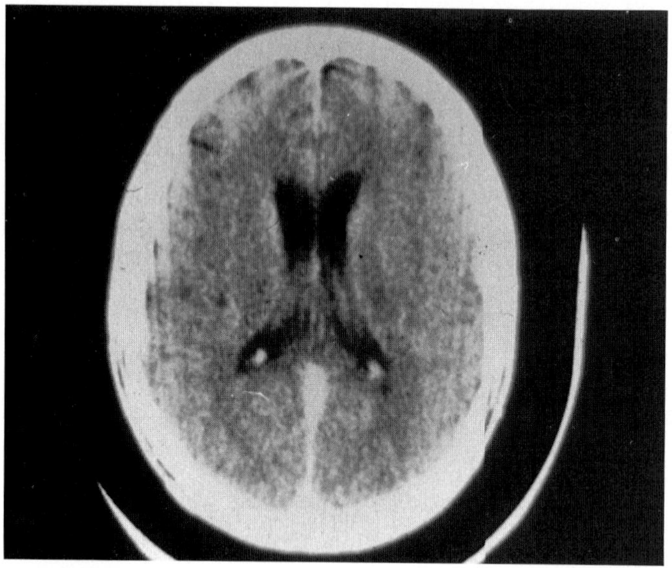

Figure 1 CT scan of an AIDS patient with HIV encephalopathy. Note the diffuse cerebral atrophy without other accompanying abnormalities.

atrophy and white matter changes can be evident on computerized tomographic (CT) scans or magnetic resonance imaging (MRI) (20) (Figures 1 and 2). Neuropathological studies reveal diffuse white matter changes and multinucleated cell and macrophage infiltrates (18-20); HIV can be isolated from blood, brain, or CSF (21). The reported frequency of HIV encephalopathy varies from series to series, but Price and co-workers indicate that as many as 90% of their patients with AIDS have some degree of dementia; two-thirds of AIDS patients had moderate to substantial dementia, while an additional one-quarter had subclinical or mild dementia.

At UCSF, 100 patients with AIDS encephalopathy were seen from 1979 until mid 1986. The mean age of these patients was 38.8 years; all but one male child were homosexual or bisexual males. In only three patients was AIDS encephalopathy the presenting illness that led to the diagnosis of AIDS. Rather than suggest that this illness is infrequently the initial manifestation of AIDS, we feel that this observation reflects more the subtlety of the initial dementia that accompanies AIDS encephalopathy and the difficulty in establishing the diagnosis. In three patients, this dementing illness ultimately led to the diagnosis of AIDS. Eighty-seven patients had AIDS at the time of their neurological presentation. The remaining 13 patients had ARC; with the newer CDC criteria for AIDS, these patients as well would be considered to have AIDS encephalopathy as their initial manifestation of AIDS.

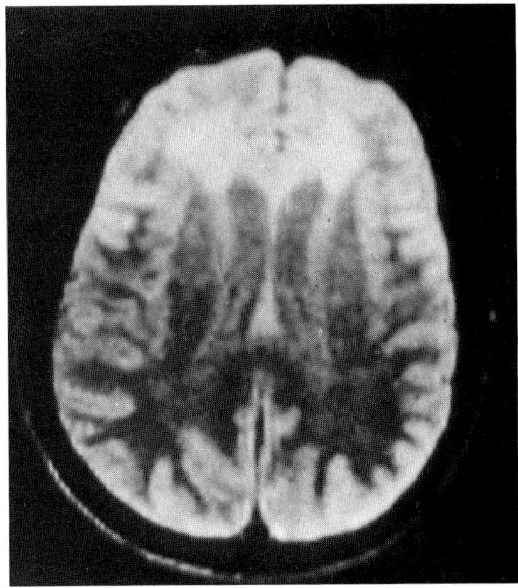

Figure 2 MRI of an AIDS patient with HIV encephalopathy. This is the same patient as in Figure 1. Note the diffuse cerebral atrophy as well as the bifrontal high-signal intensity in the subcortical white matter. Biopsy and autopsy revealed HIV encephalitis.

Thus, 16% of patients with AIDS encephalopathy had their dementia as the initial manifestation of AIDS.

Disorders of consciousness or cognition, by definition, are the most common presenting symptoms of AIDS encephalopathy. Ninety percent of these 100 patients had cognitive deficits. These problems ranged from subtle alterations in memory to frank confusion and disorientation, hallucinations, and psychotic behavior, and, in the most extreme cases, stupor and coma. Also frequent were presenting complaints of headache (39%), incoordination and gait disturbances (18%), and aphasia (17%). Less common complaints included seizures (12%), incontinence (9%), hemiparesis (9%), visual disturbances (including nystagmus and gaze palsies) (5%), and hemisensory loss (3%). Other reported neurological signs included hyperreflexia (9%), upgoing toes (8%), anisocoria or unreactive pupils (5%), increased muscle tone (3%), and facial nerve palsy (3%). Two patients had evidence of meningitis.

Disordered consciousness or cognition had been present for a mean of 48 days prior to the diagnosis of AIDS encephalopathy. Headaches had been present for a mean of 43 days prior to diagnosis, and hemiparesis for a mean of 36 days. Aphasia, when detected, was present for 11 days prior to diagnosis.

Radiologic evaluation of these patients demonstrated that of 86 patients in whom CT scans were obtained, 38 (44%) were within normal limits. Forty-one (48%) patients had diffuse cerebral atrophy only on CT scans. Three patients were felt to have hydrocephalus, which may represent an ex vacuo phenomenon reflecting focal atrophy. Four patients (5%) had focal lesions identified on CT scans; these were located throughout the brain. Magnetic resonance imaging has been used in only 10 patients; three patients had normal MR scans. In the seven patients with focal findings on MRI, five had diffuse white matter lesions, one had focal calcification, and one had multiple bilateral lesions throughout the brain.

Cerebrospinal fluid evaluation in these patients was only of specific diagnosis value in ruling out other neurological illnesses. Of the 78 patients in whom data from lumbar punctures were available, 36 were reported only as "normal." In the remaining 42 patients, the mean CSF protein was 62 mg/dl, the mean glucose was 53 mg/dl, and the mean white blood cell count per cubic milliliter was 3; all of these cells were in the monocyte/lymphocyte line. All toxoplasma, cryptococcus, and viral titers and cultures were negative. Several patients had HIV cultured from the CSF (21). Recent evidence suggests that pleocytosis can be a common feature in acute HIV infection even without neurological findings; this acute pleocytosis subsequently resolves (R. Johnson, personal communication).

What is clinically AIDS encephalopathy may in fact have a number of different pathological substrates. As noted above, CT scans frequently reveal diffuse cerebral atrophy and regions of hypodensity within the subcortical white matter and brain stem. At autopsy, there is usually no gross change, except perhaps for some atrophy, within areas of low density on CT. Even at the microscopic level, there may be no obvious changes. In some cases, there is a clear, though usually mild, degree of demyelination associated with the presence of macrophages, some multinucleate giant cells, a mild gliosis. The macrophages and giant cells are present in the perivascular spaces and in the white matter, but they do not form true granulomas, and necrosis is not a feature of this condition (Figure 3).

As noted, both peroxidase-antiperoxidase (PAP) methods and in situ hybridization have shown the presence of HIV in these cells, and electron microscopy has shown budding virus of appropriate morphology to be present in both macrophages and multinucleate giant cells (14-16). Viral particles have also been identified in astrocytes, and HIV has been grown in cultured astrocytes (22, 23). Reports of HIV identification in cells resembling oligodendrocytes have appeared (17, 23); this observation needs further confirmation.

At present, there is no therapy proven effective for AIDS encephalopathy, and the mean survival of these patients is very short. Azidothymidine

(AZT) may prove to be helpful in some cases (24a). Of 56 patients treated at UCSF for whom there is good follow-up data, 47 patients are dead; the mean length of life after diagnosis was 71 days. In the remaining living patients, mean length of survival is 212 days. Forty-four patients have been lost to follow-up.

The prototype patient with AIDS encephalopathy treated at UCSF is a 39-year-old homosexual male. He presents with complaints referable to diminished intellectual function, and his neurological examination is nonfocal; the only significant finding is progressive dementia that has been present for seven to eight weeks. The disease is rapidly progressive and invariably fatal; his mean survival is a little over 3 months.

Atypical Aseptic Meningitis

In 1983, we first reported 15 homosexual patients with an aseptic meningitis (2). We have now documented 26 such cases, made atypical by their chronic and recurrent nature and often accompanying cranial neuropathies involving those of the fifth, seventh, and eighth cranial nerves. Several patients had evidence of elevated intracranial pressure; all by definition had CSF pleocytosis. Cerebrospinal fluid profiles were otherwise similar to those of patients with AIDS-related encephalopathy. Prior to the availability of culture techniques for HIV, the etiology of this syndrome was unclear. One patient had CMV cultured from the CSF. It now appears that *atypical aseptic meningitis* is something of a misnomer. Recent studies have demonstrated that HIV can be cultured from the CSF in the majority of these patients (6, 21, 25). Thus, this syndrome might better be named *acute relapsing HIV meningitis.*

Aseptic meningitis presents clinically in an entirely different manner from AIDS-related encephalopathy. Common features include headache, fever, and meningeal signs. The clinical course is also different, being self-limited or recurrent rather than progressive. In some, the acute syndrome can be followed for over 2 years with no recurrent signs of neurological disease. The occurrence of either AIDS-related encephalopathy or atypical meningitis as a manifestation of HIV infection may reflect different degrees of immunosuppression (1, 26), although both illnesses have been seen in otherwise asymptomatic patients (18). Autopsy findings, however, indicate a remarkable similarity between these clinical entities.

Spinal Vacuolar Myelopathy

Vacuolar myelopathy, reported by Snider et al. (1) and Goldstick et al. (27), and characterized by Petito and co-workers (28), appears to be a third, unique AIDS-related central neurological syndrome. Petito et al. reported a vacuolar myelopathy, most severe in the lateral and posterior columns of the thoracic spinal cord, in 20 of 89 patients with AIDS undergoing autopsy (22%). Pathologically, this syndrome was reported to resemble closely the

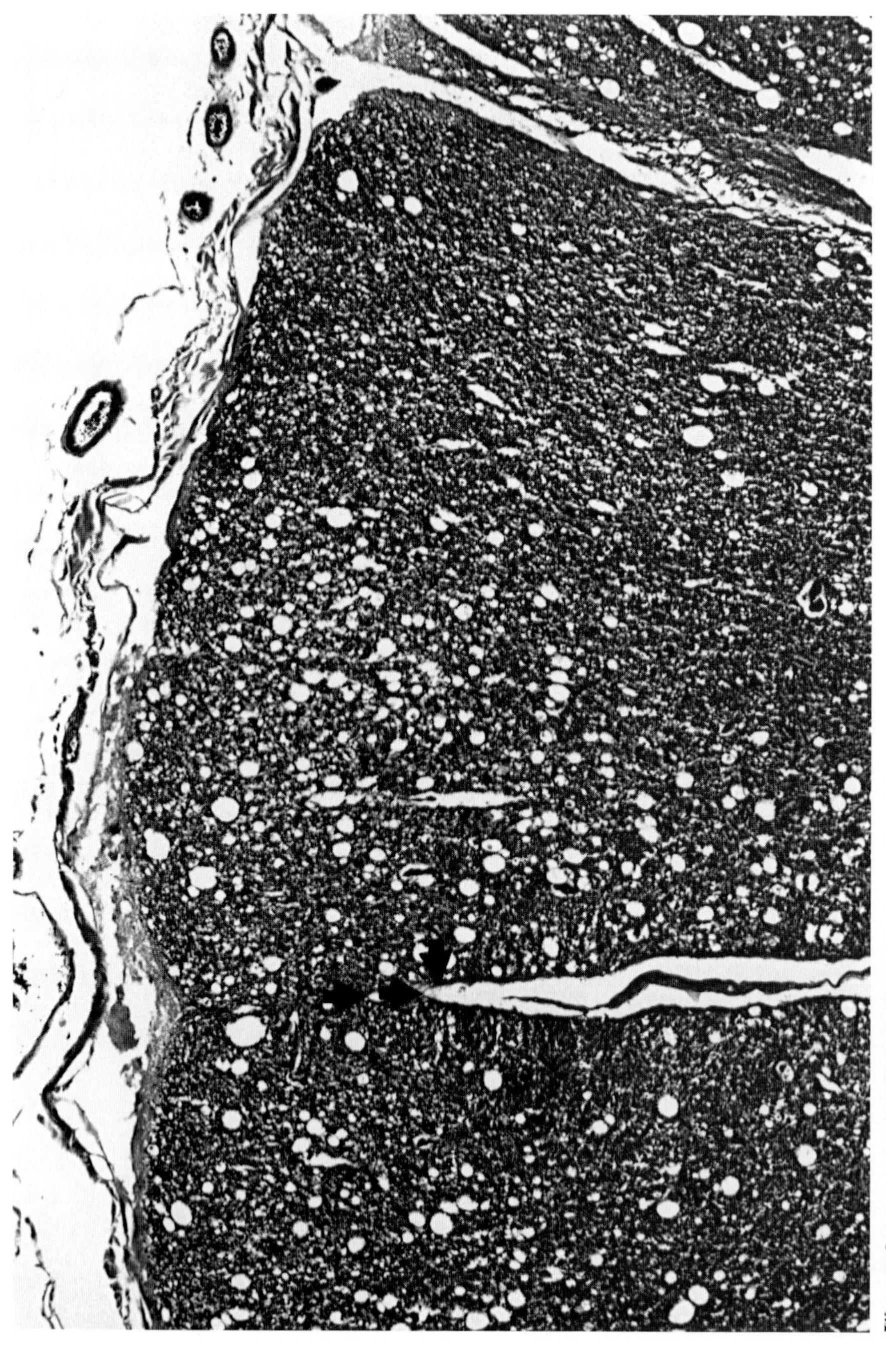

subacute combined degeneration of vitamin B^{12} deficiency, with loss of myelin and spongy degeneration of the cord substance (Figure 3).

The initial reports of this syndrome emphasized this close resemblance of vacuolar myelopathy to the subacute combined degeneration of the B^{12} deficiency type. However, further study of a greater number of cases had suggested that, although the demyelination is concentrated in the posterior columns and the corticospinal pathways, it is not by any means confined to these areas. In fact, the entire spinal white matter may be more or less severely involved. This disease, like that seen in association with the dementia of AIDS, seems to be pathologically primarily demyelinative, yet the mechanism for the demyelination is unclear.

HIV has been cultured from the spinal cord in many such cases (6, 17, 21), and in situ hybridization has shown HIV in macrophages (14, 15) and cells resembling oligodendrocytes (17). While the resulting pathogenic processes are not well defined, it appears that HIV infection is required for the development of this clinical syndrome. Immunosupression, on the other hand, does not appear to be necessary; at least one patient without evidence of immunosuppression and a near normal helper:suppressor ratio (1.2) has been reported (17).

Pathologically, the demyelination is manifest by the vacuolated appearance of the white matter of the spinal cord, concentrated especially in the posterior and lateral white columns. With careful examination, residual axons can be seen in the vacuoles, and macrophages can be visualized in the residual empty myelin tubes. There is usually a mild but definite gliosis in the adjacent tissues, but there is most often no inflammatory response and so far the evidence for significant oligodendroglial nuclear decrease is absent (Figure 4). There is need for additional careful study to determine if HIV infection of spinal cord elements is always present in this illness, what specific cellular elements are involved, and what the actual mechanism of the demyelinative process is.

The most common symptoms associated with vacuolar myelopathy include leg weakness and incontinence (28,29). Neurological examination often reveals paraparesis, spasticity, and ataxia. Berger and Resnick (29) note that hyperreflexia and extensor plantar responses may be detected in the absense of weakness. They note that muscle stretch reflexes may occasionally be absent presumably due to concomitant peripheral neuropathy. Petito and coworkers (28) noted that neurological findings were present more frequently in

Figure 3 Photomicrograph of high thoracic spinal cord showing "spongiform myelopathy," with demyelination in the gracile columns, and less involvement of the adjacent cuneate columns. Midline dorsal median fissure is indicated by arrowheads. ($\times 10$. Luxol fast blue stain for myelin.)

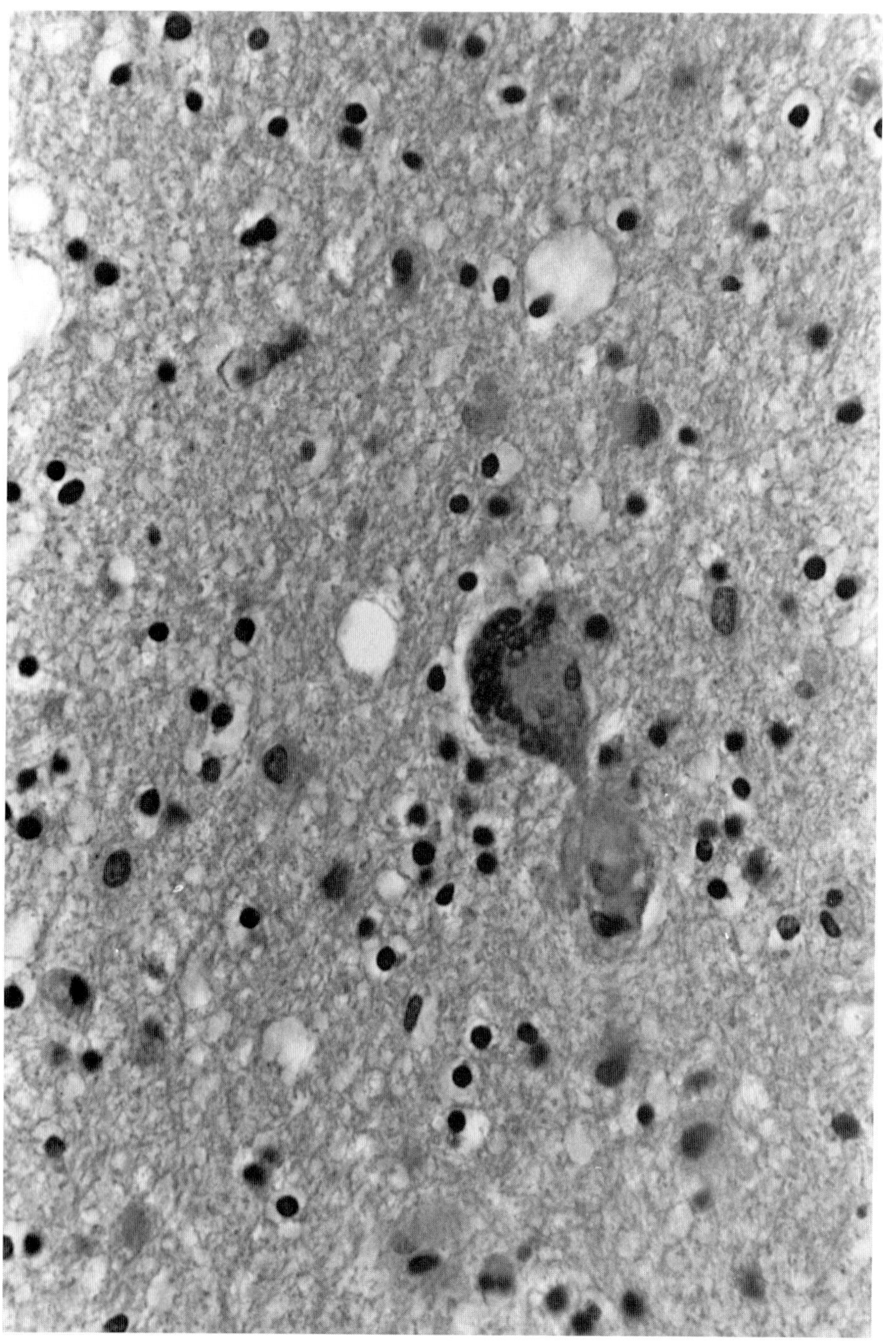

Figure 4

those patients with more severe pathological changes and occurred in 12 of the 20 patients examined. Interestingly, 14 of these patients (70%) also had dementia.

B. Opportunistic Viral Infections

The spectrum of opportunistic infections in AIDS can be predicted on the basis of the known immunodeficiency; the types of viral infection are not dissimilar to those seen in immunosuppressed transplant patients (30).

Progressive Multifocal Leukoencephalopathy

Progressive multifocal leukoencephalopathy (PLM) is an unusual infectious central demyelinating disease caused by the papovavirus JC (31). Affected patients present with mental status alterations, blindness, aphasia, hemiparesis, ataxia, and other focal deficits, which slowly progress until death (32). The characteristic CT finding is that of low-density lesions without contrast enhancement, mass effect, or associated edema. Autopsy findings reveal focal myelin loss with sparing of axis cylinders and the presence of bizarre astrocytes and enlarged oligodendrocytes containing eosinophilic intranuclear inclusions surrounding these areas of demyelination (33).

The first report of PML occurring in association with AIDS was that by Miller et al. (34). They described a male homosexual with a T-cell immune deficiency, progressive brainstem dysfunction, and a lucent cerebellar lesion demonstrated by CT; biopsy of this lesion demonstrated PML. Later, Bedri and co-workers (35) reported the electron microscopic demonstration of papovavirus virions in an AIDS patient with PML. In a published series of these patients, Krupp and co-workers (36) detailed seven cases of PML; four of these patients also had AIDS. Of note was that CT abnormalities were disproportionately less abnormal than clinical findings.

As of February 1987, 184 cases of AIDS-related PML had been reported to the CDC. Eight of these patients with AIDS and PML have been diagnosed at UCSF. Clinically, PML in the AIDS patient appears to behave in a fashion similar to PML in other immunocompromised patients. Survival after diagnosis of PML is extremely short. Several patients died within 1 month of diagnosis; the longest survivor survived for 5 months after biopsy. No effective therapy exists for PML. The early suggestion by Snider et al. (1) that cytarabine therapy may be effective in these patients has not been confirmed (36).

Figure 4 Photomicrograph of cerebral white matter showing HIV encephalopathy, with mild demyelination, astrogliosis, and the presence of both macrophages and multinucleate giant cells. (X100. Hematoxylin and eosin.)

Other Opportunistic Viral Infections

The ubiquity of the herpes viruses as well as the specific defect in cellular immunity associated with AIDS suggests that these viruses should represent a significant cause of opportunistic infection in the AIDS patient population. In fact, infection with cytomegalovirus (CMV), herpes simplex viruses types 1 and 2 (HSV-1 and HSV-2), and varicella zoster virus (HVZ) is a major source of neurological disease in AIDS patients.

Several reports of AIDS-related central nervous system infection with herpes simplex virus (2, 37, 38) or herpes simplex virus combined with cytomegalovirus (39, 40) have recently appeared. We initially reported eight AIDS patients with HSV encephalitis. These patients fell into four groups, with the rapidity of disease progression and the severity of inflammation being roughly proportional to the degree of immune competence (26).

Cytomegalovirus meningoencephalitis has also been reported in patients with AIDS (41-43). In a study of 10 patients with CMV encephalitis, Post et al. (44) noted that CMV infection of the central nervous system was the cause of death in six patients, was superimposed on systemic infection in two patients, and was not clinically evident in two patient. Diffuse cerebral atrophy was evident on CT scans in all cases, although CT significantly underestimated the degree of CNS involvement and frequently failed to demonstrate focal abnormalities when they were present at autopsy. In a series of patients studied by in situ hybridization, Nelson et al. (45) found a high percentage of cases showing both CMV and HIV infection, at times in the same cell.

Herpes varicella-zoster virus is also a major opportunistic central nervous system pathogen in AIDS patients (26, 46). Ryder et al. (47) reported the case of a patient with AIDS who developed progressive, ultimately fatal neurological deficits 12 weeks after a course of cutaneous zoster. Autopsy revealed a diffuse herpes zoster encephalomyelitis.

While viruses other than papovaviruses or herpes viruses are potential opportunistsic central nervous system pathogens in patients with AIDS, very few such cases have been reported. West and co-workers (48) reported a single patient with AIDS and adenovirus type 2 encephalitis.

At UCSF, 28 patients have presented with AIDS-related opportunistic viral infections of the CNS. The presence of opportunistic CNS viral infection was associated with a poor prognosis, despite the availability of acyclovir for the treatment of herpes viral infections and anti-CMV agents such as DHPG.

C. Opportunistic Nonviral Infections

Toxoplasma gondii

Toxoplasmosis, an infection caused by the obligate intracellular protozoan *Toxoplasma gondii*, is one of the most common infections of animals and man (49). In immunocompetent patients, infection of the central nervous system with *T. gondii* produces acute focal of diffuse meningoencephalitis with cellular necrosis, microglial nodules, and perivascular mononuclear inflammation associated with both intra- and extracellular trophozoites (50). Thrombosis of blood vessels causing large areas of coagulation necrosis may produce mass lesions in the brain. In immunodeficient hosts, the lack of cell-mediated immunity may result in a "persistent acute" infection with severe necrotizing lesions. Pathological analysis of biopsy specimens from AIDS patients reveals necrotizing granulomas, usually within thin capsules, and little inflammation (51). Encysted *T. gondii* and tachyzoites are usually present.

The first report of cerebral toxoplasmosis in a patient with AIDS was by Rutsaert et al. (52). Several series of such patients have since appeared (53-56) and have emphasized the increased risk of toxoplasmosis in the Haitian AIDS patient, the frequency of multiple deep ring-enhancing lesions of CT scans, and the common clinical findings of lethargy, seizures, and weakness. Toxoplasmosis is commonly seen in African AIDS patients (see Chapter 2). In general, early aggressive diagnosis and therapy with pyrimethamine and sulfadiazine have resulted in a dramatic clinical and radiographic response, although most reported patients died from other AIDS-related illnesses.

Several groups have recommended the routine biopsy of all patients with presumed cerebral toxoplasmosis (57, 58). The remarkable sensitivity of biopsy techniques for the diagnosis of toxoplasmosis was addressed by Chan et al. (59). The morbidity of biopsy techniques, however small, and the sheer number of affected patients have led some groups to suggest that empiric therapy be initiated prior to biopsy (60). We agree that in stable patients with strong clinical and radiologic evidence for cerebral toxoplasmosis, an empiric trial of pyrimethamine and sulfadiazine may establish the diagnosis without the need for cerebral biopsy.

By February 1987, 766 cases of cerebral toxoplasmosis had been reported to the Centers for Disease Control. The incidence of cerebral toxoplasmosis ranges between 2 and 13%, depending on patient risk group and geographic location. Epidemiological studies suggest that Haitian AIDS patients and AIDS patients living in Florida are at greatest risk of contracting toxoplasmosis.

At the University of California, San Francisco, 53 patients with AIDS and proven cerebral toxoplasmosis have been treated; these patients are summarized in Tables 3 and 4. The diagnosis of toxoplasmosis was made in 4.1% of patients with AIDS treated by UCSF. The prototype patient with AIDS and cerebral toxoplasmosis in San Francisco is a 40-year-old homosexual male who presents with a 2- to 3-week history of headaches and altered mental status. CT scan reveals multiple bilateral enhancing intracerebral lesions, and cerebrospinal fluid analysis reveals a mildly elevated protein and few lymphocytes.

Table 3 AIDS-Related CNS Disease: Signs and Symptoms

	Overall	HIV	Other virus	PML[a,b]	Toxo[c].	Crypto.[d]	CNS Lymphoma
Headaches	55	39	50	75	45	85	40
Altered mental status	68	90	50	75	70	42	64
Incoordination	18	18	21	0	21	10	32
Aphasia	12	17	17	0	8	5	16
Seizures	17	12	17	0	24	13	32
Incontinence	10	9	4	0	13	3	32
Hemiparesis	18	9	21	50	38	3	44
Hemisensory loss	8	3	13	25	11	3	16
Visual disturbances	8	5	0	25	8	6	20
Cranial neuropathies	9	3	21	0	11	6	20
Pain	1	0	0	0	4	2	0

[a]Data from three patients.
[b]Progressive multifocal leukoencephalopathy.
[c]Toxoplasmosis.
[d]Cryptococcal meningitis.

Data are expressed as percentage of patients with a given diagnosis demonstrating a given symptom.

Therapy with pyrimethamine and sulfadiazine is quite effective in controlling this illness; meaningful survival for as long as 1 year after diagnosis has been reported.

Cryptococcus neoformans

Cryptococcus neoformans, a common soil fungus, usually infects via the respiratory tract and results in the most common fungal infection of the central nervous system. Despite appropriate treatment with amphotericin B, the mortality rate of CNS cryptococcal infection in immunocompetent hosts is 40%. Pathologically, cryptococcal meningitis results in a granulomatous meningitis with additional granulomas and cysts that form within the cerebral cortex and deeper brain structures (61).

Seventy-nine cases of cryptococcal meningitis have been reported by various authors in patients with AIDS (1, 26, 62). Kovacs and co-workers (62) reported 27 patients with AIDS and cryptococcal meningitis. This was the initial manifestation of AIDS in seven of these patients (26%). Meningitis was the most common clinical feature (67%). Blood cultures and serum crypt-

Table 4 CSF Findings in Patients with AIDS-Related CNS Disease

	Protein (mg/dl)	Mean CSF glucose (mg/dl)	WBC/cm^3
HIV encephalopathy	62	53	3
Viral encephalitis	95	63	64
PML	69	46	4
Toxoplasmosis	97	58	6
Cryptococcosis	82	43	49
Primary CNS lymphoma	81	57	9
Normal values	60	40-60	0

ococcal antigen were frequently positive. Studies of CSF frequently revealed no pleocytosis and normal protein and glucose concentrations; CSF India ink test was positive in 82% of cases while cryptococcal antigen and cultures were positive in 100% of cases. In their series, only 10 of 24 patients had no evidence of continued cryptococcal infection after the completion of therapy; six of these 10 had either clinical or autopsy-demonstrated relapses. The authors concluded, somewhat contrary to our experience, that standard therapy with amphotericin B, with or without additional 5-fluorocytosine, was ineffective.

By February 1987, 1388 cases of AIDS-related cryptococcal meningitis had been reported to the Centers for Disease Control. This number, reflecting best the incidence of cryptococcosis at presentation with AIDS, represents an overall incidence of approximately 5% of all patients with AIDS. At particular risk are AIDS patients from New Jersey and those who are black or intravenous (IV) drug users. These risk factors may increase the risk of contracting cryptococcal meningitis to as high as 10% (7). Cryptococcal meningitis is also common in African AIDS patients (see Chapter 2).

At the University of California, San Francisco, 121 reliably diagnosed cases of AIDS-related cryptococcal meningitis were recorded as of May 1988. This number represents an institutional incidence of 5.5%. The prototype AIDS patient with cryptococcal meningitis in San Francisco is a 38-year-old homosexual man who already carries the diagnosis of AIDS. He has had 20 days of decreasing mental status, 10 days of headache, and 5 days of meningismus. Cranial CT scan is normal; the diagnosis of cryptococcosis is made by CSF examination. He responds well initially to antibiotic therapy but his survival is still limited; mean survival is 2 to 3 months. Recurrent cryptococcal meningitis is a significant problem; thus, continued treatment at weekly intervals is recommended. Ommaya reservoirs have been used in some cases during initial treatment but have not been shown to improve outcome.

Candida albicans

Candidiasis, usually associated with diabetes, leukemia, lymphoma, and intravenous drug abuse, is a relatively rare central nervous system pathogen (63). Nine cases of cerebral candidiasis have been reported in patients with AIDS. In consideration of the frequency of oral candidiasis in these patients, it is perhaps surprising that so few cases of intracerebral candidiasis have been observed. Three patients with AIDS and CNS candidiasis have been treated at UCSF. Surgical abscess excision followed by amphotericin B appears to be the only effective therapy.

Aspergillus fumigatus

Infections with the mold *Aspergillus fumigatus* are uncommon, even in immunocompromised patients. Aspergillosis affecting the central nervous system may present as meningitis, encephalitis, or abscess. Four cases of AIDS-related central nervous system aspergillosis have been reported.

Coccidioides immitis

Meningeal infection occurs in nearly one-half of all cases of disseminated coccidioidomycosis. Although in immunocompetent patients the majority of cases have a subclinical or chronic, relapsing meningitis, coccidioidal meningitis can present as a rapid, fulminant illness in the immunocompromised patient. Treatment involves the long-term administration of intrathecal amphotericin B; frequently this therapy requires the placement of an Ommaya reservoir.

We have treated two cases of coccidioidomycosis in patients with AIDS at UCSF. One of these presented with coccidioidal meningitis; the other, with disseminated coccidioidal infection, was found to harbor multiple coccidioidal microabscesses throughout the cerebellum. A few other cases of AIDS-related central nervous system infection with *Coccidioides immitis* have been reported (64).

Miscellaneous Fungal Infections

We have treated one child with AIDS and cerebral mucormycosis. Micozzi et al. (65) have reported five cases of mucormycosis in intravenous drug users; these cases may well be AIDS-related. Two cases of cerebral infection with *Rhizopus species* and one case of cerebral infection with *Acremonium alabamensis* have been reported (66); these patients also probably had AIDS. There are also scattered case reports of intracranial infection with *Histoplasma capsulatum* (64).

Mycobacterial Infections

Mycobacterium tuberculosis: The pathology and presentation of *Mycobacterium tuberculosis* meningitis have been well described (62). Mycobacterial infection can result in meningitis, encephalitis, or brain abscess formation. Fifteen patients with AIDS and *M. tuberculosis* infections of the central nervous system have appeared in the literature (67). These patients were uniformly either Haitians or intravenous drug abusers; these reports are consistent with the endemic nature of tuberculosis in the Caribbean basin and with the endemiological data that indicate that Haitians are at a higher overall risk of contracting AIDS-related neurological illnesses (see Chapter 3). The clinical profiles of these patients have not been fully reported; of note is that roughly two-thirds presented with CNS mass lesions while one-third presented with signs and symptoms of meningitis only. Of nearly 1300 HIV-infected patients treated at UCSF, we have seen only one case of tuberculous meningitis.

Mycobacterium avium intracellulare: While *Mycobacterium avium intracellulare* (MAI) infection is extremely common in the AIDS patient population, central nervous system infection with MAI is rare. Fourteen such cases have been reported (68). Four patients with AIDS and MAI infections of the nervous system have been treated at UCSF. In contrast to CNS *M. tuberculosis* infection, there does not appear to be a Haitian predilection for AIDS-related CNS MAI infection. Of patients reported in the literature, most had disseminated systemic MAI infection prior to their neurological presentation with diffuse encephalitis. Meningitis, facial cranial neuropathy, and peripheral neuropathy have also been reported in association with MAI infection of the CNS, although whether MAI was etiological in these syndromes is unclear. Survival after contracting CNS MAI infection is extremely limited; results with both standard tuberculosis chemotherapeutic agents and experimental regimens have been uniformly poor (69).

One patient with AIDS and CNS infection with *Mycobacterium kansasii* has been reported (70).

Bacterial Infections

Reports of AIDS-related CNS complications from common bacterial pathogens have been conspicuously absent from the literature. None of the patients in the series presented by Snider et al. (1) or Levy and Bredesen (26) had bacterial infections of the CNS. Nervous system infections with opportunistic bacterial pathogens in patients with AIDS have rarely been reported. Thus, the immunological defect initiated by HIV infection does not appear to place the AIDS patient at increased risk for contracting common bacterial infections of the CNS.

Listeria monocytogenes: *Listeria*, the most common cause of bacterial meningitis in immunocompromised patients, has only rarely been the cause of AIDS-related neurological disease. We have treated three patients with AIDS and *Listeria* infections of the CNS at UCSF. Penicillin is the treatment of choice.

Nocardia asteroides: Nocardia infection of the CNS usually accompanies pulmonary infection in immunosuppressed patients; like *Listeria, Nocardia* CNS infection in the AIDS patient population is extremely rare. Sharer and Kapila (71) reported a single case of *Nocardia* brain abscess in a 34-year-old female intravenous drug abuser with AIDS.

Other bacterial infections: Central nervous system infection with common bacterial pathogens is extremely rare in the AIDS patient population. One case each of AIDS-related *Escherichia coli* meningitis and meningoencephalitis has been reported (64, 72); the clinical profiles of these patients are lacking. Syphilitic meningoencephalitis has been reported in patients with HIV infection (72, 73).

D. Neoplasms

Primary CNS Lymphoma

Primary malignant lymphomas are rare tumors of the CNS, representing less than 1.5% of primary brain tumors (74). While systemic lymphoma frequently invades the meninges (75), primary CNS lymphomas more frequently involve the brain parenchyma (76). These neoplasms are commonly seen in immunosuppressed patients, particularly renal and cardiac allograft recipients (77). Histochemical studies indicate that CNS lymphomas are ATPase-positive and can thus be distinguished from systemic lymphomas (78).

The risk of developing CNS lymphoma in the general population has been estimated at 0.0001% (73). In immunosuppressed patients, this risk increases to 0.2%; in the population of patients with AIDS, the risk is roughly 2%. The annual incidence of primary CNS lymphoma in the United States prior to the AIDS epidemic was approximately 225 cases; in 1986, an estimated 240 cases were reported, and by 1991, projections suggest that over 1800 cases will occur. Thus, primary CNS lymphoma is becoming a disease predominantly affecting the AIDS patient population.

Three large series of patients with AIDS-related primary CNS lymphomas have been studied, summarizing the experience of UCSF (58, 78) and at the University of Southern California (79, 80). One hundred seventy-two cases of AIDS-related primary CNS lymphoma had been reported to the Centers for Disease Control by August 1986. This represents an incidence at presentation of 0.74%. At the University of California, San Francisco, 25 (1.9%) patients with AIDS-related primary CNS lymphomas have been treated. The prototype San Francisco AIDS patient with primary CNS lymphoma is a 37-year-old homosexual man. He presents with a subacute onset of altered mental status, headaches, and hemiparesis. His CT scan reveals multiple enhancing intracranial lesions, and cerebrospinal fluid examination is remarkable only for a mild lymphocytic pleocytosis. CSF cytology is usually negative. Empiric therapy with pyrimethamine and sulfadiazine for toxoplasmosis fails, and the diagnosis of primary CNS lymphoma is made by biopsy. Until recently, such a patient has tended to survive for less than 2 months; his death has been related to his CNS neoplasm. Our recent experience with a protocol for the aggressive early treatment of these patients with radiation therapy (81) suggests that these tumors are radiation-sensitive and that radiation therapy may have a small but significant effect on survival.

Systemic Lymphoma with CNS Involvement

Systemic lymphoma most frequently affects the central nervous system by invasion of the meninges. Ziegler and co-workers (82) first described the outbreak of a Burkitt's-like lymphoma in homosexual men; later reports firmly established the association of AIDS and systemic lymphomas. All the first four patients described had significant neurological complications, including epidural spinal cord compression, meningitis, and cranial neuropathies. Fernandez et al. (83) reported a similar series of six patients with neurological complications of systemic lymphomas. The review by Snider et al. (1) describes four patients with meningeal lymphoma and one each with epidural thoracic lymphoma and epidural thoracic plasmacytoma. We have seen an additional three patients with metastatic systemic non-Hodgkin's lymphoma.

Neurological manifestations of systemic lymphoma in these 19 patients included neoplastic meningitis in nine patients, five of whom also had cranial neuropathies. Three other patients had isolated cranial neuropathies, four patients had epidural spinal cord compression by metastatic lymphoma, two patients had intracerebral hemorrhage from metastasis, and one patient had brachial plexus invasion by tumor resulting in a brachial plexopathy. While transient improvement was noted in most cases following the institution of therapy, most patients were dead within 1 year after the onset of neurological symptoms.

Metastatic Kaposi's Sarcoma

Until the recent outbreak of AIDS, Kaposi's sarcoma was rarely documented in Europe or North America, with an annual incidence of 0.02 to 0.06% per 1000,000 population (84). This neoplasm most often affected elderly Italian and Ashkenazic Jewish men. It responded well to therapy, with a mean survival ranging from 8 to 13 years. Central nervous system involvement with Kaposi's sarcoma has been remarkably rare (85) (see Chapter 13).

The Kaposi's sarcoma associated with AIDS is characteristically much more aggressive that the classic form of the disease, being rapidly progressive and manifesting widespread visceral involvement. Although Kaposi's sarcoma has been a primary feature of AIDS, CNS presentation of this neoplasm has been remarkably rare. Reports of four patients with AIDS and Kaposi's sarcoma in the brain have appeared in the literature (86).

E. Cerebrovascular Complications

We have treated 20 patients with AIDS and documented cerebrovascular complications at UCSF (1.6% of all AIDS patients). Our recent neuropathological study (87, 87a) suggests this to be an extreme underestimate; in this series, 18 of 94 unselected patients with AIDS (19%) had cerebral infarctions. These infarcts varied from small multifocal infarctions to large infarcts, suggesting acute embolic phenomena. Of our 20 patients, six presented with transient ischemic attacks, four had hemorrhagic infarcts, five had ischemic cerebral infarcts, and four had multifocal small infarcts. One patient presented with a subdural hematoma.

Snider et al. (1) reported six of 50 patients with AIDS and cerebrovascular disease (12%). Three patients each had bland infarction or hemorrhagic infarction; two of the patients with intracerbral hemorrhage also had thrombocytopenia. Two patients had nonbacterial thrombotic endocarditis.

Most of the hemorrhages have been found in the setting of central nervous system neoplasia, with most bleeding occurring within tumors. The ischemic infarcts have been more difficult to explain. Marantic endocarditis was not present in the vast majority of these patients. While there have been occasional cases of cerebral vasculitis in AIDS (88), these appear to be uncommon and probably do not explain the large number of infarcts in the AIDS patient population. Circulating coagulation inhibitors have recently been isolated from some HIV-infected patients (89). The presence of such factors may explain the unusually high frequency of multifocal infarction in this young patient population.

F. CNS Complications as a Result of AIDS Therapy

Several groups have reported neurological symptoms arising as complications of AIDS therapy. Hollander and co-workers (90) reported the development of extrapyramidal motor symptoms in AIDS patients treated with low-dose antiemetic therapy. Bates et al. (91) have reported acute myelopathy following intrathecal chemotherapy for lymphoma in an AIDS patient. Antiviral therapy in AIDS patients resulting in startle myoclonus, dysphasia, and delirium has also been reported (92).

V. Multiple Intracranial Pathologies

The evaluation and treatment of the AIDS patient with neurological disease is complicated by the observation that multiple intracranial pathological processes may be present in patients with AIDS (10, 93, 94). Of 482 neurologically symptomatic patients with AIDS, 65 patients were identified with multiple intracranial pathological processes (13.5%). Reviewing biopsy and necropsy data, we identified 20 of 69 patients with nervous system illness (29%) who had more than one pathological process identified. These diseases were identified both within the same lesion and within spatially separated lesions, both sequentially and simultaneously. Thus, patients treated following biopsy or with a correct presumptive diagnosis may have other intracranial diseases that remain untreated.

VI. Diagnosis of AIDS-Related CNS Disease

As with any other neurological disease, the initial approach to the patient with AIDS-related neurological illness involves obtaining a careful history and physical examination. Cognitive assessment with neuropsychological testing can be extremely valuable in detecting early subclinical dementias. Radiologic and cerebrospinal fluid examinations are then required in the evaluation of the neurologically symptomatic AIDS patient. Serologic testing, unfortunately, is of little value in the differential diagnosis of AIDS-related CNS disease (95), as positive HIV titers indicate only exposure to HIV and not necessarily active disease.

Cerebrospinal fluid examination is critical for the evaluation and therapy of AIDS patients with CNS disease. The CSF examination may provide the definitive diagnosis in several of these processes, including HIV or other viral infections and cryptococcal meningitis. We have evaluated the CSF profiles of our AIDS patients with neurological illness to determine whether findings apart from the direct identification of organisms (by titers, stains, or cultures) can be of value in differential diagnosis (96).

The CSF profiles for these patients are listed in Table 4. The mean CSF protein ranged from 62 to 97 mg/dl, depending on the specific diagnosis; thus, all the studied AIDS-related CNS diseases produced a mild elevation in CSF protien. The mean CSF glucose concentrations ranged from 43 to 63 mg/dl and were not diagnostic. The concentration of cells within the CSF was normal in patients with HIV encephalopathy, PML, and toxoplasmosis. A mild pleocytosis was noted in patients with primary CNS lymphoma, while more marked CSF pleocytoses were noted in patients with cryptococcal meningitis and opportunistic viral infections. In all cases, these white blood cells were almost exclusively monocytes of lymphocytes. Thus, CSF studies can be diagnostic when organisms are directly seen or cultured. In addition, in patients with nonfocal radiologic studies and no CSF pleocytosis, the diagnosis of HIV encephalopathy is suggested. Finally, analysis of IgG profiles in the CSF may be helpful in establishing HIV infection in the brain (7).

Computerized tomographic (CT) brain scans are the most widely used radiologic examination in the neurologically symptomatic AIDS patient. In our review of 200 cases (96), CT scans were normal in about 40% of cases, revealed focal lesions in 25% of cases, and demonstrated diffuse cerebral atrophy in only 35% of cases. These findings were of some prognostic value: Patients with only diffuse cerebral atrophy were three times more likely than patients with normal CT scans to manifest neurological progression and subsequently demonstrate CNS pathology. Patients with focal abnormalities on CT scans have been subsequently shown to have toxoplasmosis in 50 to 70% of reported cases, primary CNS lymphoma in 10 to 25% of cases, and PML in 10 to 22% of cases. They had nondiagnostic biopsies in 10% of cases and other diseases in 9% of cases (88, 96).

In those patients with no focal CT abnormalities, cryptococcosis was by far the most frequent diagnosis (28%). While these studies report an incidence of CMV and HIV encephalitis in 11% and 3% of these patients, respectively, this probably reflects the difficulty in establishing these diagnoses rather than their true infrequency. Our experience would suggest that nearly one-half of neurologically symptomatic AIDS patients actually have HIV encephalitis.

The CT findings in our 482 patients with AIDS-related neurological illness were evaluated in an attempt to determine whether these findings could be of value in the specific differential diagnosis (Table 5). CT results identified two major groups of patients: those with normal scans or with diffuse cerebral atrophy only and those with focal lesions on CT. Nonfocal examinations were obtained in patients with HIV encephalopathy (92% of patients with HIV encephalopathy and nonfocal studies), opportunistic viral infection (82%), and cryptococcal meningitis (84%). Focal CT abnormalities were identified in patients with toxoplasmosis (88%), primary CNS lymphoma (86%), and PML (80%). Within this latter group, patients with low-density lesions that demonstrated little or no enhancement after the administration of iodinated contrast material tended to have PML or primary CNS lymphoma. Restriction of these lesions to the white matter suggested the diagnosis of PML, while the presence of mass effect tended to suggest lymphoma. The demonstration of ring-enhancing lesions, especially within the basal ganglia, suggested the diagnosis of toxoplasmosis. Unfortunately, there were many cases in which ring-enhancing lesions were proven to be primary CNS lymphomas and in which toxoplasma brain abcesses did not enhance. Thus, CT scans alone cannot provide a definitive diagnosis in AIDS-related CNS disease.

Our studies have demonstrated that magnetic resonance imaging (MRI) is more sensitive than CT to intracranial pathology in the patient with AIDS and neurological symptoms (97, 98). MRI also more accurately reflects the extent and distribution of histologically verified CNS disease. This increased sensitivity and accuracy has been demonstrated to have an important impact on the evaluation and therapy of patients with AIDS-related CNS illness. Interestingly, in all but one of our cases of histologically proven toxoplasmosis, MRI demonstrated multiple bilateral abnormalities. Thus, a single lesion on MRI probably reflects an illness other than toxoplasmosis. On the basis of these findings, we recommend that MRI, if available, be used as the initial radiologic imaging procedure in these patients.

VII. Summary and Conclusions

AIDS is no longer a rare disease affecting only a small segment of our population. It has now been observed throughout the United States and most other countries in the world. As the current data demonstrate, the effect of AIDS on the nervous system is profound and widespread. About 10% of all AIDS patients will first present with a neurological complaint. Evaluation of this complaint will then lead to the diagnosis of AIDS. Nearly 40% of all AIDS patients will develop major neurological symptoms during their lifetime; these symptoms may be related to primary HIV infection or secondarily to any of a number of opportunistic processes. At autopsy, 75% of AIDS patients will have neuropathological abnormalities.

The AIDS-related central neurological syndromes are many and varied, as are their associated signs and symptoms. As with radiologic and serologic examination, the findings resulting from clinical examination of the AIDS patient with neurological illness are nonspecific. While there are clinical findings that are suggestive of one or another class of AIDS-related neurological illness, there is such overlap in their presentations as to make specific CNS diagnosis on the basis of clinical examination virtually impossible.

The differential diagnosis of AIDS-related neurological illness is made even more difficult by the frequent observation of multiple CNS pathological processes in the same AIDS patient. Nearly one-third of all histologically examined AIDS cases had multiple intracranial pathologies. Multiple treatable pathological abnormalities have been identified both within the same intrcranial lesion and within different lesions, and both simultaneously and sequentially.

Thus, the evaluation and treatment of the AIDS patient with central neurological illness is a difficult challenge. Close attention must be paid to subtle neurological complaints, and careful neurological examination is warranted in all AIDS patients. Once the patient complains of neurological dysfunction or a neurological abnormality is identified on clinical examination, a careful workup including MRI or CT brain scanning and cerebrospinal fluid examination is indicated. Specific diagnosis must then be made on the basis of CSF findings, response to empiric therapy or biopsy.

Therapy for AIDS-related CNS diseases in not unlike that for the same disease in other patient populations (see Chapters 18 and 19). There is no cure for HIV encephalitis; azidothymidine (AZT) appears to cross the blood-brain barrier, and trials of AZT for the treatment of HIV encephalitis show early promise.

After obtaining a definitive diagnosis and beginning appropriate therapy, the physician must apply great diligence to evaluating the response to therapy; the very real possibility of multiple, treatable, intracranial pathological processes may necessitate a repetition of the patient's diagnostic evaluation and the institution of additional therapies. It is only with such an approach that we may optimally treat the patient with AIDS-related neurological illness.

References

1. Snider WD, Simpson DM, Nielsen S, et al. Neurological complications of acquired immune deficiency syndrome: analysis of 50 patients. Ann Neurol 1983; 14:403-18.
2. Bredesen DE, Messing R. Neurological syndromes heralding the acquired immune deficiency syndrome. Ann Neurol 1983; 14:141.
3. Levy RM, Bredesen DE, Rosenblum ML. Neurological manifestations of the acquired immunodeficiency syndrome (AIDS): Experience at UCSF and review of the literature. J Neurosurgery 1985; 62:475-95.
4. Shaw GM, Harper ME, Hahn BH et al. HTLV-III infection in brains of children and adults with AIDS encephalopathy. Science 1985; 227:177-82.
5. Levy JA, Shimabukuro J, Hollander H, et al. Isolation of AIDS associated retroviruses from cerebrospinal fluid and brain of patients with neurological symptoms. Lancet 1985; 2:586-8.
6. Ho DD, Rota TR, Schooley RT, et al. Isolation of HTLV-III from cerebrospinal fluid and neural tissues of patients with neurologic syndromes related to the acquired immunodeficiency syndrome. N Engl J Med 1985; 313:1493-7.
7. Resnick L, DiMarzo-Veronese F, Schupbach J, et al. Intra-blood-brain-barrier synthesis of HTLV-III-specific IgG in patients with neurologic symptoms associated with AIDS or AIDS-related complex. N Engl J Med 1985; 313:1498-504.
8. Sharer LR, Cho E-S, Epstein LG. Multinucleated giant cells and HTLV-III in AIDS encephalopathy. Hum Pathol 1985; 16:760.
9. Meyenhofer MF, Epstein LG, Cho E-K, Sharer LR. Ultrastructural morphology and intracellular production of human immunodeficiency virus (HIV) in brain. J Neuropathol Exp Neurol 1987; 46:474-84.

10. Levy RM, Janssen RS, Bush TJ, Rosenblum ML. Neuroepidemiology of acquired immunodeficiency syndrome. In: Rosemblun ML, Levy RM, Bredesen DE, eds. AIDS and The Nervous System. New York: Raven, 1987; 13-27.
11. Koppel KBS, Wormser GP, Tuchma AJ, et al. Central nervous system involvement in patients with acquired immune deficiency syndrome (AIDS). Acta Neurol Scand 1985; 71:337-51.
12. Urmacher C, Nielsen S. The histopathology of the acquired immune deficiency syndrome. Pathol Ann 1985; 20:197-220.
13. Moskowitz LB, Hensley GT, Chan JC, et al. The neuropathology of acquired immune deficiency syndrome. Arch Pathol Lab Med 1984; 108:867-72.
14. Wiley CA, Oldstone MBA, Nelson JA. Pathogenesis of AIDS encephalitis. J Neuropathol Exp Neurol 1987; 46:348.
15. Koenig S, Gendelman HE, Orenstein JM, et al. Detection of AIDS virus in macrophages in brain tissue from AIDS patients with encephalopathy. Science 1986; 233:1089-93.
16. Epstein LG, Sharer LR, Cho E-S, et al. HTLV-III/LAV-like retrovirus particles in the brains of patients with AIDS encephalopathy. AIDS Res 1984-1985; 1:447-54.
17. Levy JA, Cheng-Mayer C, Pan L-Z, et al. The biologic and molecular properties of the AIDS-associated retrovirus that affect antiviral therapy. Ann Inst Pasteur 1987; 138:101-11.
18. Navia BA, Price RW. The acquired immunodeficiency dementia complex as the presenting or sole manifestation of human immunodeficiency virus infection. Arch Neurol 1987; 44:65-9.
19. Navia BA, Jordan BD, Price RW. The AIDS dementia complex: I. clinical features. Ann Neurol 1986; 19:517-24.
20. Navia BA, Cho E-S, Petito CK, et al. The AIDS dementia complex: II. Neuropathology. Ann Neurol 1986; 19:525-35.
21. Levy JA. The biology of the human immunodeficiency virus and its role in neurological disease. In: Rosenblum ML, Levy RM, Bredesen DE, eds. AIDS and the Nervous System. New York: Raven, 1987; 327-45.
22. Cheng-Mayer C, Rutka JT, Rosenblum ML, et al. The human immunodeficiency virus (HIV) can productively infect cultured human glial cells. Proc Natl Acad Sci (USA) 1987; 84:3526-30.
23. Gyorkey F, Melnick JL, Gyorkey P, et al. Human immunodeficiency virus in brain biopsies of patients with AIDS and progressive encephalopathy. J Infect Dis 1987; 155:870-6.
24. Fischl MA, Richman DD, Grielo MH, et al. The efficacy of azidothymidine (AZT) in the treatment of patients with AIDS and AIDS related complex. N Engl J Med 1987; 185-91.
24a. Yarchoan R, Thomas RV, Grafam J, et al. Long-term administration of 3'-azido-2',3'-dideoxythymidine to patients with AIDS-related neurological disease. Ann Neurol 1988; 23(suppl):S82-7.
25. Levy RM, Bredesen DE, Rosenblum ML. Multiple coexistent intracranial pathologies in the acquired immunodeficiency syndrome (AIDS). 1987; Second International Conference on AIDS, Paris.

26. Levy RM, Bredesen DE. Central nervous system dysfunction in acquired immunodeficiency syndrome. In: Rosenblum ML, Levy RM, Bredesen DE, eds. AIDS and the Nervous System. New York: Raven, 1987; 29-63.
27. Goldstick L, Mandybur TI, Bode R. Spinal cord degeneration in AIDS. Neurology 1985; 35:103-6.
28. Petito CK, Navia BA, Eun-Sook C, et al. Vacuolar myelopathy pathologically resembling subacute combined degeneration in patients with the acquired immunodeficiency syndrome. N Engl J Med 1985; 874-9.
29. Berger JR, Resnick L. HTLV-III/LAV-related neurological disease. In: Broder S, ed. AIDS: Modern Concepts and Therapeutic Challenges. New York: Marcel Dekker, 1987:263-83.
30. Armstrong D, Wong B. Central nervous system infection in immunocompromised hosts Ann Rev Med 1982; 33:293-308.
31. Nayaran O, Penny JB, Johnson RT, et al. Etiology of progressive multifocal leukoencephalopathy. Identification of papovavirus. N Engl J Med 1973; 289:1278-82.
32. Astrom KE, Mancall EL, Richardson EP. Progressive multifocal leukoencephalopathy: A hitherto unrecognized complication of chronic lymphatic leukaemia and Hodgkin's disease. Brain 1958; 81:93-111.
33. ZuRhein GM. Association of papova-virions with a human demylinating disease (progresive multifocal leukoencephalopathy). Prog Med Virol 1969; 11:185-247.
34. Miller JR, Barrett RE, Britton CB, et al. Progressive multifocal leukoencephalopathy in a male homosexual with T-cell immune deficiency. N Engl J Med 1982; 307:1436-8.
35. Bedri J, Weinstein W, DeGregorio P. Progressive multifocal leukoencephalopathy in acquired immunodeficiency syndrome. N Engl J Med 1983; 309:492-3.
36. Krupp LB, Lipton RB, Swerdlow ML, et al. Progressive multifocal leukoecephalopathy: clinical and radiographic features. Ann Neurol 1985; 17:344-8.
37. Britton CB, Mesa-Tejeda R, Fenoglio CM, et al. A new complication of AIDS: thoracic myelitis caused by herpes simplex. Neurology 1985; 35:1071-4.
38. Dix RD, Bredesen DE, Erlich KS, Mills J. Recovery of herpesviruses from cerebrospinal fluid of immunodeficient homosexual men. Ann neurol 1985; 18:611-4.
39. Pepose JS, Hilborne LH, Cancilla PA, Foos RY. Concurrent herpes simplex and cytomegalovirus retinitis and encephalitis in the acquired immune deficiency syndrome (AIDS). Ophthalmology 1984; 91:1660-77.
40. Tucker T, Dix RD, Katzen C, et al. Cytomegalovirus and herpes simplex virus ascending myelitis in a patient with acquired immune deficiency syndrome. Ann Neurol 1985; 18:74-9.
41. Hawley DA, Schaefer JF, Schulz DM, Muller J. Cytomegalovirus encephalitis in acquired immunodeficiency syndrome. Am J Clin Pathol 1983; 80:874-7.
42. Vital C, Vital A, Vignoly B, et al. Cytomegalovirus encephalitis in a patient with acquired immunodeficiency syndrome. Arch Pathol Lab Med 1985; 109:105-6.
43. Edwards RH, Messing R, McKendall RR. Cytomegalovirus meningoencephalitis in a homosexual man with Kaposi's sarcoma: Isolation of CMV from CSF cells. Neurology 1985; 35:560-1.

44. Post MJD, Hensley GR, Moskowitz LB, Fischl M. Cytomegalic inclusion virus encephalitis in patients with AIDS: CT, clinical and pathologic correlation. Am J Neuroradiol 1986; 7:275-80.
45. Nelson JA, Reynolds-Kohler C, Oldstone MBA, Wiley C. HIV and CMV coinfect brain cells in patients with AIDS. Virology 1988. In press.
46. Cole EL, Meisler DM, Calabrese LH, et al. Herpes zoster ophthalmicus and acquired immune deficiency syndrome. Arch Ophthalmol 1984; 102:1027-9.
47. Ryder JW, Croen K, Kleinschmidt-DeMasters BK, et al. Progressive encephalitis three months after resolution of cutaneous zoster in a patient with AIDS. Ann Neurol 1986; 19:182-8.
48. West TE, Papsian CJ, Park BH, Parker SW. Adenovirus type-2 encephalitis and concurrent Epstein-Barr virus infection in an adult man. Arch Neurol 1985; 42:815-7.
49. Anderson S. Toxoplasma gondii. In: Mandell GL, Douglas RG Jr, Bennett JE, eds. Principles and Practice of Infectious Diseases. New York: Wiley, 1979; 2127-37.
50. Remington JS, Desmonts G. Toxoplasmosis. In: Remington JS, Klein JD, eds. Infectious Disease of the Fetus and Newborn Infant. Philadelphia: Saunders, 1976; 191-332.
51. Sher JH. Cerebral toxoplasmosis. Lancet 1983; 1:1225.
52. Rutsaert J, Melot C, Ectors M, et al. Complications infectieuses pulmonaires et neurologiques d'un sarcome de Kaposi. Annales d'Anatomie Pathologique 1980; 25:125-8.
53. Chan JC, Moskowitz LB, Olivella J, et al. Toxoplasma encephalitis in recent Haitian entrants. South Med J 1983; 76:1211-5.
54. Handler M, Ho KV, Whelan M, Budzilovich G. Intracerebral toxoplasmosis in patients with acquired immune deficiency syndrome. J Neurosurg 1983; 59:994-1001.
55. Post JD, Hensley GT, Sheldon JJ, et al. CNS disease in AIDS: a CT-MR pathologic correlation. Radiology 1984; 153:55-6.
56. Luft BJ, Conley F, Remington JS. Outbreak of central-nervous-system toxoplasmosis in Western Europe and North America. Lancet 1983; 1:781-3.
57. Levy RM, Pons VG, Rosemblum ML. Central nervous system mass lesions in the acquired immunodeficiency syndrome (AIDS). J Neurosurg 1984; 61:9-16.
58. Rodan BA, Cohen FL, Bean WJ. CT biospy of cerebral toxoplasmosis in AIDS. J Fla Med Assn 1984; 71:158-60.
59. Chan JC, Hensley GT, Moskowitz LB. Toxoplasmosis in the central nervous system. Ann Intern Med 1984; 100:615-6.
60. Wong B, Gold JWM, Brown AE, et al. Central-nervous-system toxoplasmosis in homosexual men and parenteral drug abusers. Ann Intern Med 1984; 100:36-42.
61. Adams RD, Victor M. Principles of Neurology. 2d ed New York: McGraw-Hill, 1981; 475-506.
62. Kovacs JA, Kovacs AA, Polis M, et al. Cryptococcosis in the acquired immunodeficiency syndrome. Ann Intern Med 1985; 103:533-8.
63. Thompson RA. Clinical features of central nervous system fungus infection. In: Thompson RA, Green JR, eds. Infectious Diseases of the Central Nervous System. Vol. 6 Advances in Neurology. New York: Raven, 1974:93-100.

64. Post JD, Kursunoglu SJ, Hensley GT, et al. Cranial CT in acquired immunodeficiency syndrome: spectrum of diseases and optimal contrast enchancement technique. Am J Neuroradiol 1985; 145:929-40.
65. Micozzi MS, Wetli CV. Intravenous amphetamine abuse, primary cerebral mucormycosis and acquired immunodeficiency. Forens Sci 1985; 30:504-10.
66. Wetli CV, Weiss SD, Cleary TJ, Gyori E. Fungal cerebritis from intravenous drug abuse. Forens Sci 1984; 29:260-8.
67. Bishburg E, Sunderam G, Reichman LB, Kapila R. Central nervous system tuberculosis with the acquired immunodeficiency syndrome and its related complex. Ann Intern Med 1986; 105:210-3.
68. Zakowski P, Fligiel S, Berlino GW, Johnson BL. Disseminated *Mycobacterium avium-intracellulare* in homosexual men dying of acquired immunodeficiency syndrome. JAMA 1982; 248:2980-2.
69. Hawkins C, Gold JM, Whimberg E, et al. *Mycobacterium avium* complex infections in patients with AIDS. Ann Intern Med 1986; 105:184-8.
70. Armstrong D, Gold JWM, Dryjanski J, et al. Treatment of infections in patients with the acquired immunodeficiency syndrome. Ann Intern Med 1985; 103:738-43.
71. Sharer LR, Kapila R. Neuropathologic observations in acquired immunodeficiency syndrome (AIDS). Acta Neuropathol 1985; 66:188-98.
72. Berger JR, Moskowitz L, Fischl M, Kelly RE. The neurologic complications of AIDS, frequently the initial manifestation. Neurology 1984; 34 (supp 1):134-5.
73. Berry CD, Hooton TM, Collier AC, Lukehart SA. Neurologic relapse after benzathine penicillin therapy for secondary syphilis in a patient with HIV infection. N Engl J Med 1987; 316:1587-9.
74. Henry JM, Heffiner RR, Dillard SH, et al. Primary malignant lymphomas of the central nervous system. Cancer 1974; 34:1293-302.
75. Griffin JW, Thompson RW, Mitchinson MJ, et al. Lymphomatous leptomeningitis. Am J Med 1971; 51:200-8.
76. Bunn PA, Schein PS, Banks PM, DeVita VT. Central nervous system complications in patients with diffuse histiocytic and undifferentiated lymphoma: Leukemia revisited. Blood 1976; 47:3-10.
77. Penn I. The incidence of malignancies in tranplant recipients. Transplant Proc 1975; 7:323-6.
78. So YT, Beckstead JH, Davis RL. Primary central nervous system lymphoma in acquired immune deficiency syndrome: A clinical and pathologic study. Ann Neurol 1986; 20:566-72.
79. Gill PS, Levine AM, Meyer PR, et al. Clinico-pathologic characteristics of primary central nervous system (CNS) lymphoma in patients with acquired immunodeficiency syndrome (AIDS). ASCO Abstracts. Vol 54. 1984.
80. Gill PS, Levine AM, Meyer PR, et al. Primary central nervous system lymphoma in homosexual men: Clinical, immunologic, and pathologic features. Am J Med 1985; 78:742-7.
81. Rosenblum ML, Levy RL, Bredesen DE, et al. Primary central nervous system lymphomas in patients with AIDS. Ann Neurol 1988; 23(suppl):S13-6.
82. Ziegler JL, Miner RC, Rosenbaum KE, et al. Outbreak of Burkitt's-like lymphoma in homosexual men. 1982; 2:631-3.

83. Fernandez R, Mouradian J, Moore A, Asch A. Malignant lymphoma with central nervous system involvement in six homosexual men with acquired immunodeficiency syndrome. Lab Invest 1983; 48:25A.
84. Rothman S. Remarks on sex, age and racial distribution of Kaposi's sarcoma nad on possible pathogenetic factors. Acta Un Int Cancer 1962; 18:326-9.
85. Rwomushana RJW, Bailey IC, Kyalwazi SK. Kaposi's sarcoma of the brain. Cancer 1975; 36:1127-31.
86. Gorin FA, Bale JF Jr, Hawks-Miller M, Schwartz RA. Kaposi's saracoma metastatic to the CNS. Arch Neurol 1985; 42:162-5.
87. Levy RM, Bredesen DE, Rosenblum ML, Davis Rl. Postmortem neuropathology of the acquired immunodeficiency syndrome (AIDS): 106 consecutive AIDS autopsies. Congress of Neurological Surgeons, 35th Annual Meeting, New Orleans 1986.
87a. Engstrom JW, Lowenstein DH, Bredesen DE. Cerebral infarctions and transient neurolgical deficits associated with AIDS. Neurol 1988; 38(suppl 1):241.
88. Yankner BY, Skolnick P, Shoukimas GM, et al. Cerebral granulomatous angiitis associated with acute HTLV-III infection of the central nervous system. Ann Neurol 1986; 20:362-4.
89. Cohen AJ, Phillips T, Keffler C. Circulating coagulation inhibitors in the acquired immune deficiency syndrome. Ann Intern Med 1986; 104:175-80.
90. Hollander H, Golden J, Mendelson T, Cortland D. Extrapyramidal symptoms in AIDS patients given low-dose metoclopramide or chlorpromazine. Lancet 1985; 2:1186.
91. Bates S, McKeever P, Masur H, et al. Myelopathy following intrethecal chemotherapy in a patient with extensive Burkitt's lymphoma and altered immune status. Am J Med 1985; 78:697-702.
92. Gold JWM, Leyland-Jones B, Urmacher C, Armstrong D. Pulmonary and neurologic complications of treatment with fiac (2'fluro-5-iodo-aracytosine) in patients with acquired immune deficiency syndrome (AIDS). 1984; 1:243-52.
93. Pitlik SD, Rios L, Hersh EM, et al. Polymicrobial brain abscess in a homosexual man with Kaposi's sarcoma. South Med J 1984; 77:271-2.
94. Fischl MA, Pitchenik AE, Spira TJ. Tuberculous brain abscess and Toxoplasma encephalitis in a patient with the acquired immunodeficiency syndrome. JAMA 1985; 253:3428-30.
95. Levy RM, Pons VG, Rosenblum ML. Intracerebral-mass lesions in the acquired immunodeficiency syndrome (AIDS). N Engl J Med 1983; 309:1454-5.
96. Levy RM, Rosenbloom S, Perrett L. Neuroradiologic findings in the acquired immunodeficiency syndrome: A report of 200 cases. Am J Radiol 1986; 7:833-9.
97. Delapaz R, Enzmann D. Neuroradiology of acquired immunodeficiency syndrome In: Rosenblum ML, Levy RM, Bredesen DE, eds. AIDS and the Nervous System. New York: Raven, 1987:121-53.
98. Levy RM, Mills C, Posin J, et al. The superiority of MR to CT in the detection of intracranial pathology in the acquired immunodeficiency syndrome (AIDS). 1986; Second International Conference on AIDS, Paris.
99. Price RW, Brew B, Sidtis J, et al. The brain in AIDS: Central nervous system HIV-1 infection and AIDS dementia complex. Science 1988; 586-92.

16

Pulmonary Complications of AIDS

Jeffrey A. Golden
School of Medicine
University of California
San Francisco, California

I. Introduction

With no laboratory test for the diagnosis of acquired immunodeficiency syndrome (AIDS), the manifestation of immune deficiency implied by the presence of opportunistic infections, tumors, and other pathological processes heralds the presence of this disease complex. *Pneumocystis carinii* pneumonia is the most common opportunistic infection afflicting patients with AIDS coming from areas outside of Africa. More than 60% of these AIDS patients will develop *P. carinii* pneumonia and 30-50% of these patients will develop recurrent *P. carinii* pneumonia within 12 months (1-3). In Africa, this disease may not be as frequent, but its diagnosis can be difficult there (see Chapter 2). In view of the epidemic nature of AIDS, physicians should be familiar with presenting clinical and laboratory characteristics that might suggest the presence of *P. carinii* pneumonia. Patients who are diagnosed and treated early are more likely to survive a particular episode of this pneumonia (4).

Table 1 Types and Frequency of Pulmonary Disorders in 441 Patients with AIDS

Pulmonary disorders	No. of patients
Pneumocystis carinii pneumonia	373
Without coexisting infection	255
With coexisting infection	118
Cytomegalovirus	50
Mycobacterium avium-intracellulare	37
Mycobacterium tuberculosis	15
Legionella	9
Cryptococcus	8
Other	3
Other pulmonary infections	93
M. avium-intracellulare	37
Cytomegalovirus	18
Cytomegalovirus/*M. avium-intracellulare*	5
Cytomegalovirus/cryptococcus	1
Pyogenic bacteria	11
Legionella	10
Fungi	6
M. tuberculosis	4
Herpes simplex	2
Toxoplasmosis	1
Kaposi's sarcoma	36

Source: Ref. 5. Reprinted by permission of the *New England Journal of Medicine* 1984; 310:1682-1688.

The spectrum of pulmonary complications related to AIDS is expanding. In the review of 1067 patients with AIDS who were evaluated at a workshop sponsored by the National Heart, Lung and Blood Institute (NHLBI), 41% (441 patients) had pulmonary complications (5). The specific pulmonary infections and their frequencies are listed in Table 1. Of the patients with pulmonary complications 85% had *P. carinii* pneumonia followed in frequency by infection with *Mycobacterium avium-intracellulare* and cytomegalovirus. It should be stressed that in the NHLBI series, besides *P. carinii*, other infecting agents, either with or without *P. carinii* pneumonia, were found in 48% (211) of the 441 patients making a precise diagnosis of specific infection mandatory (5,6).

This review will focus primarily on *P. carinii* pneumonia. The other important pulmonary problems associated with AIDS will be discussed with an emphasis on their presenting clinical and laboratory characteristics.

II. *Pneumocystis carinii* Pneumonia

A. The Organism

Pneumocystis carinii was first identified in Brazil by Carini in 1910 who felt the organism was the schizogonal form of *Trypanosoma lewisi* (7). In 1912, Delanoe identified the same organism as Carini in the lungs of Parisian sewer rats and gave the cystlike organisms the name *Pneumocystis*. In 1942, Van der Meer in the Netherlands identified *P. carinii* in human lungs and 10 years later in Czechoslovakia, Vanek showed that *P. carinii* was the cause of interstitial plasma cell pneumonitis among malnourished infants that occurred in epidemic form consequent to the socioeconomic collapse of post-World War II Europe. Subsequently, *P. carinii* pneumonia was diagnosed in immunosuppressed or immunodeficient patients and the first reports of *P. carinii* pneumonia in the United States were in 1956 (7).

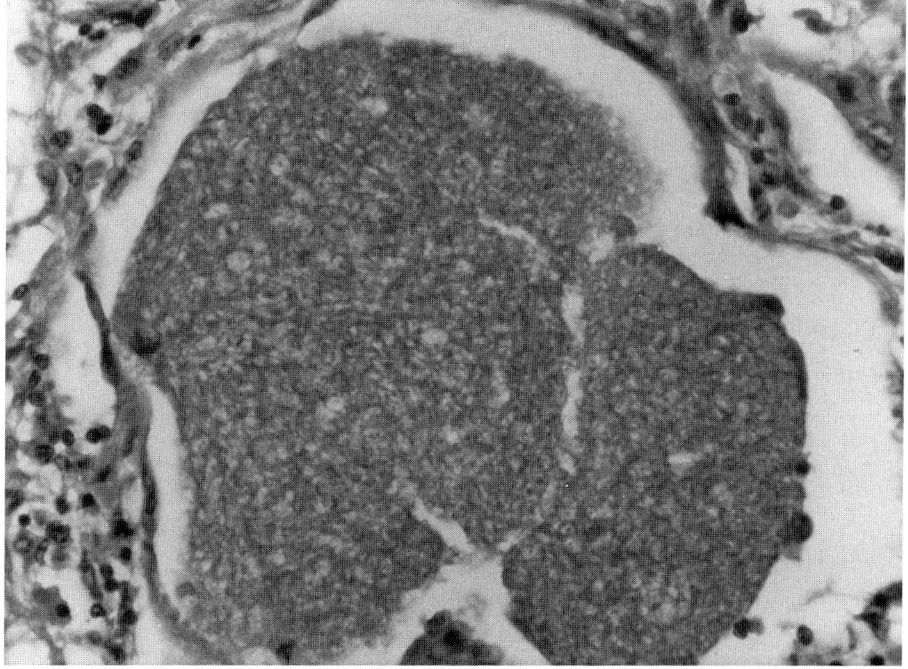

A

Figure 1 Lung pathology of *P. carinii* pneumonia. Hematoxylin and eosin stain showing eosinophilic foamy material filling the alveolar airspace (*A*); Gomori's methenamine silver stain of cysts (*B*) and Giemsa stain revealing trophozoite forms (*C*) within the alveolar exudate. (Figure 1C is reproduced in color in Plate III, after page 356.)

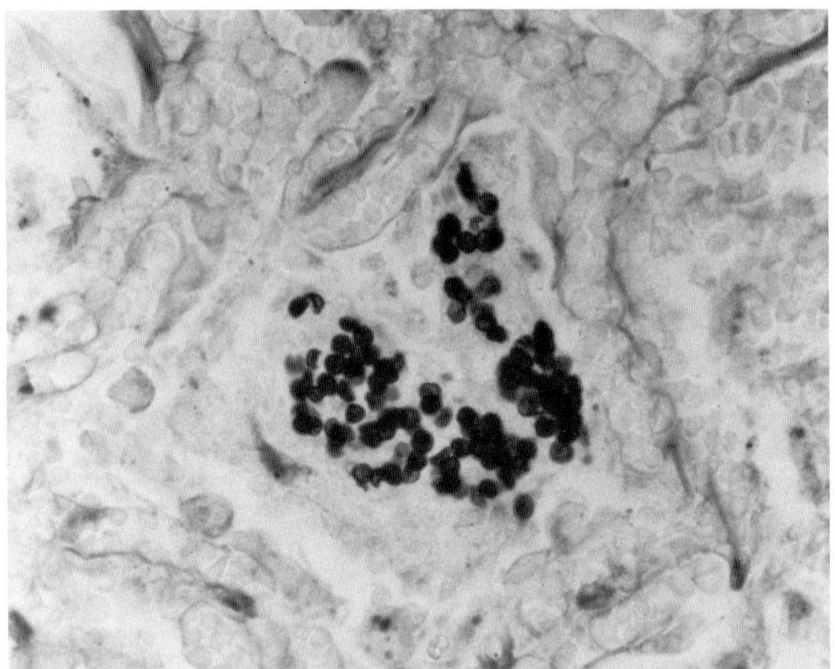

B

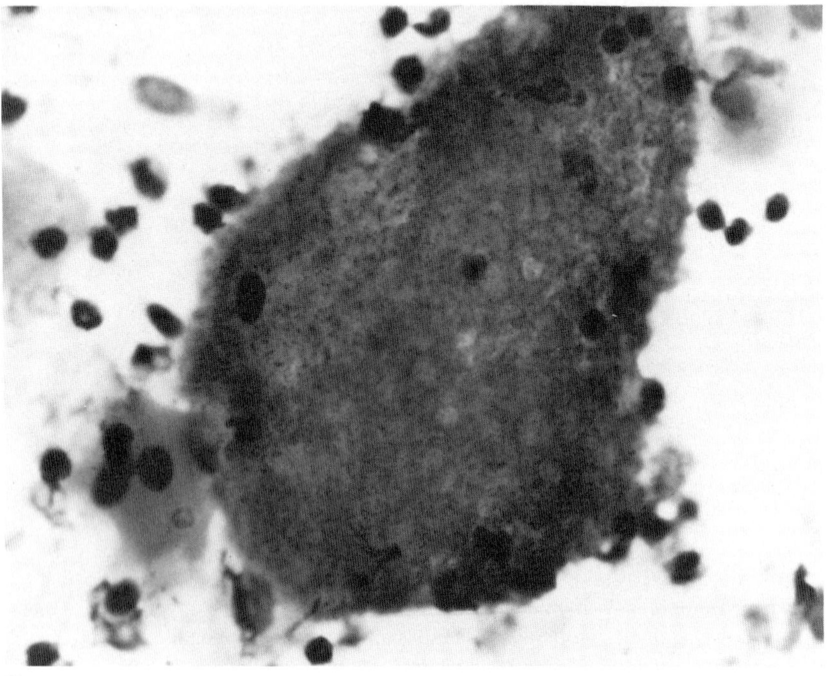

C

Figure 1 (continued)

The organism, *P. carinii* exists in cystic and extracystic forms (8). The oval cyst measures 4-6 μm in diameter and contains up to eight intracystic cells or sporozoites. The extracystic form, or trophozoite, is pleomorphic with a diameter of 2-5 μm. No form of the organism stains with hematoxylin and eosin. The cyst form is identified by Gomori's methenamine silver nitrate (Figure 1) or toluidine blue stains, neither of which stains the trophozoite. Conversely, sporozoite and trophozoite forms stain with Giemsa (Figure 1), Wright, Gram-Weigert, or methylene blue stains that do not stain the cyst wall (9).

The precise life cycle of *P. carinii* is unclear but speculation is afforded by cell culture techniques such as primary chicken embryo epithelial lung cell culture and certain human cell lines (7,10,11). During a 4-6-h period, a trophozoite develops into a thick-walled cyst inside of which sporozoites develop. Sporozoites are subsequently released and develop into trophozoites (8,10,12). The trophozoites develop filopodia which may (10) or may not (13) directly attach to alveolar-lining epithelial cells.

B. Epidemiology

The organism is ubiquitous; two-thirds of healthy children have serological evidence of prior *P. carinii* infection (14). Worldwide, most mammals have evidence of infection. On the basis of indirect immunofluorescent antibody studies, the antigenic characteristics of rat, mouse, and human *P. carinii* can be compared. The mouse and rat *P. carinii* appear to be more closely related antigenically to each other than to human *P. carinii*. Walzer suggests this observation supports the possibility of species or strain differences in the organism (15).

P. carinii rarely if ever causes disease without the presence of immune dysfunction (16-18). Treating Sprague-Dawley rats with steroids will result in *P. carinii* pneumonia, which is evidence that this pneumonia results from latent infection in the context of immune dysfunction (19). Nevertheless, contagion may play a role in the development of *P. carinii* pneumonia. Intranasal infection with *P. carinii* organisms in mice can result in *P. carinii* pneumonia, and other animal studies clearly demonstrate airborne environmental transmission of *P. carinii* (20,21). Further evidence of contagion is demonstrated by clusters of *P. carinii* pneumonia cases including nursery epidemics that were controlled by isolating patients with *P. carinii* pneumonia from other malnourished or immunosuppressed infants (22,23). Until the precise epidemiology of *P. carinii* pneumonia can better be defined, it has been suggested that patients with *P. carinii* pneumonia should be isolated (24).

C. Host Response

The specific host humoral and cellular immune response to *P. carinii* infection is poorly understood. In vitro, *P. carinii* adheres to the surface of alveolar macrophages. Only with the addition of antibody against *P. carinii* can each adherent trophozoite rapidly become engulfed or interiorized by the alveolar macrophage and killed (12). As noted above, steroids have clinical and experimental impact on the development of *P. carinii* pneumonia in the context of latent infection. Yet steroids have no effect on the ability of the alveolar macrophage to ingest the organism in the presence of anti-*Pneumocystis* antibody. Therefore, other investigators have suggested a role for the lymphocyte in combatting this disease (25). Thymus-derived or T lymphocytes from normal adults proliferate when exposed to *P. carinii*; this action is an acquired lymphocytic response as organisms do not stimulate lymphocytes from cord blood (26). In experimental animal studies, sensitization of the T lymphocyte and not the presence of serum antibody against *P. carinii* induces protection against the development of *P. carinii* pneumonia. Passive transfer of sensitized T lymphocytes and not immune serum is important in the recovery from *P. carinii* pneumonia (27). Steroids, which enhance the development of *P. carinii* pneumonia, have fundamental effects on T-lymphocyte function. This fact further emphasizes the lymphocyte as a key element in the protection of the host from this organism. Finally, given the increased presence of alveolar macrophages in the lungs of patients with *P. carinii* pneumonia, the alveolar macrophage, perhaps requiring the presence of sensitized T lymphocytes, may also be one of the principal host defense mechanisms in preventing the development of *P. carinii* pneumonia (25,27,28).

D. Pulmonary Pathology

There is a continuum of pulmonary pathological response to the presence of *P. carinii* (29). At autopsy there is subclinical or latent infection in less than 5% of patients dying with primary diseases or after therapy resulting in immunodeficiency (16,30-32). Scattered organisms alone are identified without clinical or histologic evidence of pneumonia. It is extremely unlikely to find organisms at autopsy in patients dying without impairment of their immune status.

The next pathological stage involves production of increased numbers of *P. carinii* organisms with desquamation of alveolar cells into the alveolar air space unassociated with alveolar wall thickening. Ultimately, with more extensive infection, the alveolar air spaces become filled with an eosinophilic foamy material that includes trophozoites, thick-walled cysts, and other debris that may or may not include alveolar macrophages (Figure 1) (33,34). Inflammatory infiltrates involve the alveolar septum to a variable extent but, unlike the epidemic infantile form of the pneumonitis, there is not an extensive interstitial plasma cell infiltration that greatly thickens the alveolar wall (7). Although infection is usually confined to the lungs, with severe infestation, organisms can be identified in spleen, liver, blood, lymph nodes, bone marrow, and retina—all evidence of systemic dissemination (35-37).

E. Clinical Presentation

The clinical features of *P. carinii* pneumonia are consistent but not sufficiently distinctive to differentiate this infection from other AIDS-related pulmonary problems. The classic symptoms of *P. carinii* pneumonia are dyspnea and nonproductive cough with or without temperature elevation (5). In contrast to non-AIDS patients with *P. carinii* pneumonia who present with symptoms over a four- or five-day period, AIDS patients with this pneumonia present with an insidious onset of dyspnea and cough with a mean duration of illness prior to diagnosis of approximately one month (range 2-10 weeks) (1,38). Even asymptomatic AIDS patients have been diagnosed with *P. carinii* pneumonia, because of an abnormal chest radiograph or pulmonary physiology (39,40).

Although râles on pulmonary auscultation are characteristically absent with pneumonia due to *P. carinii* (7), there are clinical findings that help identify which patients presenting with mild respiratory symptoms have *P. carinii* pneumonia in the context of AIDS. The history of possible exposure to the AIDS virus through sexual contact or blood is obviously fundamental. Further, clinical symptoms and signs characteristic of AIDS may suggest that even minimal shortness of breath is due to *P. carinii* pneumonia. Obviously a patient with the prior diagnosis of AIDS or AIDS-related complex (ARC) who presents with respiratory symptoms must be considered to have *P. carinii* pneumonia or other AIDS-related pulmonary problems. However, clinical evaluation, while helpful, cannot precisely determine the presence or absence of *P. carinii* pneumonia (Table 2).

Chest Radiograph

The clasic chest roentgenogram in *P. carinii* pneumonia reveals diffuse bilateral interstitial or ground glass infiltrates which unfortunately are nonspecific. Furthermore the chest roentgenogram is normal in 4-25% of cases or otherwise atypical revealing focal abnormalities or an upper lobe distribution simulating reactivation tuberculosis (5,41-43). Hilar or mediastinal adenopathy is not felt to be secondary to *P. carinii* pneumonia, and other processes such as Hodgkins or non-Hodgkins lymphoma, typical or atypical tuberculosis, cryptococcus as well as Kaposi's sarcoma should all be considered (42). Similarly, in our experience, chest roentgenogram evidence of adenopathy should not be ascribed to the lymphadenopathy syndrome. Finally, round nodular infiltrates and/or pleural effusions are more typical of pulmonary Kaposi's sarcoma than *P. carinii* pneumonia (44,45).

Routine Laboratory Data

As in the case of the clinical evaluation, presenting routine laboratory data do not clearly distinguish patients with *P. carinii* pneumonia from

Table 2 Presenting Clinical Characteristics of Patients with *P. carinii* Pneumonia Compared with Those of Patients with AIDS or Risk of AIDS and Respiratory Symptoms Not Due to *P. carinii* Pneumonia

	AIDS patients with *P. carinii* pneumonia			Patients without *P. carinii* pneumonia		
Symptoms	No. with abnormality	No. evaluated	Percent (abnormal)	No. with abnormality	No. evaluated	Percent (abnormal)
Dyspnea and/or cough	18	20	90	12	12	100
Fever	19	20	95	12	12	100
Weight loss	14	19	74	6	12	50
Diarrhea	5	20	25	4	12	33
Physical Examination						
Oral mucosal candidiasis	20	20	100	5	12	42
Increased temperature	14	20	70	9	12	75
Funduscopic abnormalities	6	20	30	2	12	17
Lymphadenopathy	10	11	91	8	12	67
Increased respiratory rate	14	14	100	9	12	75
Auscultatory rales	5	15	33	3	12	25

patients with AIDS or risk of AIDS with other respiratory problems (5,40). Anemia, lymphopenia, thrombocytopenia, and increased erythrocyte sedimentation rate, although frequently present, are not specific findings. However, in evaluating a patient with respiratory symptoms, the absence of thrush and a normal erythrocyte sedimentation rate would suggest withholding bronchoscopy and employing close followup of the patient instead.

Others have corroborated our finding of the frequent elevation of the serum lactate dehydrogenase (LDH) (40,46). Isomorphic elevation of this enzyme is felt to be a marker for pulmonary interstitial inflammation from *P. carinii* or lymphoid interstitial pneumonia. Elevated serum LDH levels were found to decline with clinical resolution of *P. carinii* pneumonia (46).

Arterial Blood Gases

Arterial blood gas analysis in the setting of *P. carinii* pneumonia classically reveals hypoxia, hypocarbia, and increased pH consistent with an uncompensated respiratory alkalosis and hyperventilation (7). In a study of patients with *P. carinii* pneumonia before the AIDS epidemic, arterial hypoxia was significantly related to intrapulmonary right to left shunt and not to the reduction of the diffusing capacity (47). Hypoxia and hyperventilation are nonspecific findings; thus the presence and degree of hypoxia cannot distinguish between patients with and without *P. carinii* pneumonia. Further, 10-30% of patients with *P. carinii* pneumonia have normal oxygen tension (PaO_2 greater than 80) (4,48). Even the sensitive assessment of the alveolar minus arterial partial pressure of oxygen difference at rest ($A\text{-}aDO_2$) can be normal (less than 15 mmHg) in 8% to 20% of patients (6,49). The sensitivity of arterial blood gas analysis in predicting which patients with respiratory symptoms at risk for AIDS have *P. carinii* pneumonia was improved by a practical exercise technique; a 19-gauge scalp vein needle provides arterial samples at rest and after one and a half minutes of Master's two-step exercise. All patients with *P. carinii* pneumonia had an increased $A\text{-}aDO_2$ between rest and exercise of at least 10 mmHg; normally the $A\text{-}aDO_2$ stays the same or actually improves (decreases) with exericse. Unfortunately, other processes such as pulmonary Kaposi's sarcoma can also cause an abnormal increase in the $A\text{-}aDO_2$ with exercise; thus this sensitive technique is not specific for *P. carinii* pneumonia (49).

F. Pulmonary Function

Like any peripheral infiltrative pulmonary process, *P. carinii* pneumonia may result in a restrictive ventilatory defect associated with a decreased diffusing capacity for carbon monoxide (6,47,49). Furthermore, air flow rates (particularly when corrected for lung volume) may be increased above normal even before lung volumes decrease. This effect presumably results from increased elastic recoil on airway caliber (50). Pulmonary function was assessed at the time of initial diagnosis of *P. carinii* pneumonia in 18 patients with AIDS (Figures 2 and 3). Although the lung volumes of patients with *P. carinii* pneumonia as a group were reduced or restricted significantly compared with normal controls, the majority of patients had lung volumes within 20% of their individually predicted values. Therefore, using lung volumes to detect the presence of *P. carinii* pneumonia may be insensitive.

In contrast, the single-breath diffusing capacity for carbon monoxide as well as air flow rates were both very accurate in predicting the presence of *P. carinii* pneumonia. Comparing the diffusing capacity for carbon monoxide

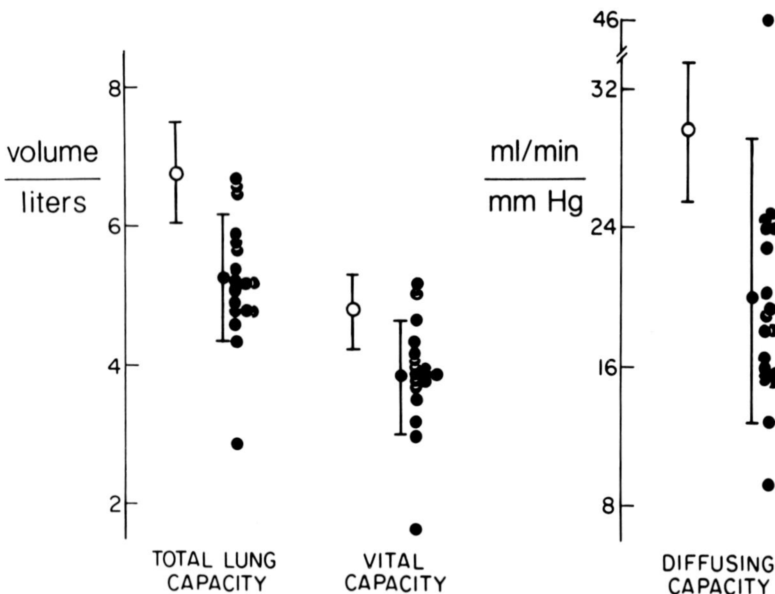

Figure 2 Lung volumes (total lung capacity and vital capacity) and single-breath carbon monoxide diffusing capacity ($D_L$co). Patients with *P. carinii* pneumonia mean ± 1 SD and individual data points. Predicted normal ± 1 SD. For patients with *P. carinii* pneumonia the mean vital capacity was 3.8 ± 0.8 and the mean total lung capacity was 5.24 ± 0.9 liters; predicted normal vital capacity and total lung capacity were 4.77 ± 0.52 and 6.76 ± 0.72 liters, respectively ($p < .001$). In patients with pneumonia, the mean $D_L$co was 20.1 ± 7.75 ml/mm × mmHg and was decreased significantly compared to the mean predicted $D_L$co in our laboratory (29.3 ± 4.3 ml/mm × mmHg, $p < .001$).

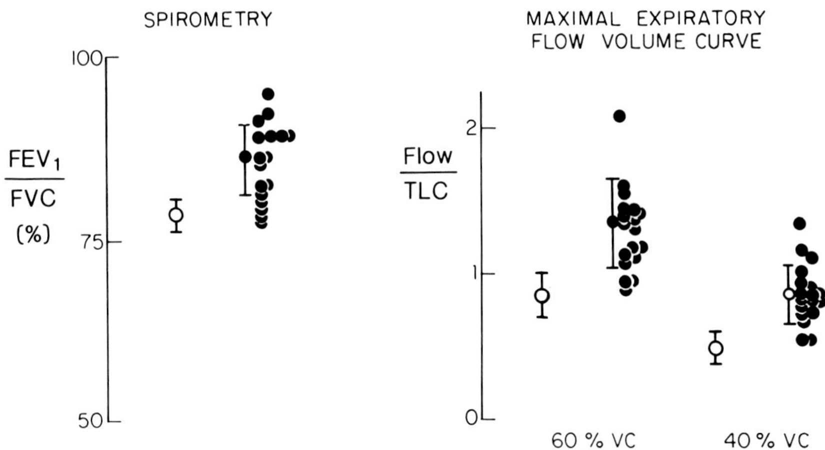

Figure 3 Spirometry (n = 17) and maximal expiratory flow-volume curve (n = 18). Same legend as for Figure 2. Patients with *P. carinii* pneumonia had a mean FEV_1/FVC of 86 ± 5.3% which was significantly increased ($p < .001$) above their predicted normal $FEV_1/FVC\%$ (78.1 ± 2.0). See text for details of correction of flow-rates by lung volumes (total lung capacity, TLC) for group analysis of maximal expiratory flow volume curve. Maximum expiratory flow-rates were analyzed at two lung volumes (60% and 40% of exhaled capacity). The volume corrected mean flows at 60% and 40% were 1.31 ± 0.29 and 0.84 ± 0.21 TLC/s, respectively. These flows were significantly increased ($p < 0.001$) when compared to healthy, nonsmoker controls in our laboratory at 60% and 40% of exhaled vital capacity (0.84 ± 0.21 and 0.5 ± 0.08 TLC/s, respectively).

for each patient with *P. carinii* pneumonia to his predicted diffusing capacity revealed that only 2 of 18 patients had a diffusing capacity measurement within 20% of their individually predicted values. One of these two patients with a normal diffusing capacity had asthma, a condition which may be associated with an increased diffusing capacity (51). On repeat testing eight days later, this particular patient experienced a decrease of his diffusing capacity to 42% of predicted. Sixteen of 18 patients (88%) had diffusing capacity for carbon monoxide less than 80% of their individually predicted values. As in the case of alveolar proteinosis, this reduction in the diffusing capacity among patients with *P. carinii* pneumonia is likely due to a true barrier to gas diffusion and not to abnormalities of the alveolar capillary bed itself.

In the usual outpatient setting, the diffusing capacity may be difficult to obtain. However, air flow rates (including spirometry and maximal expiratory flow-volume curves) may be obtained easily in the acute setting. In our experience, the finding of increased airflow rates was very helpful in selecting which patients with respiratory symptoms may in fact have *P. carinii* pneumonia (Figure 3). For 16 of 17 patients, the forced expired volume in 1 second as a percentage of the forced vital capacity (FEV_1/FVC%) was increased above their individually predicted values.

Similarly, air flow rates measured during the maximal flow-volume maneuver also revealed increased expiratory flow rates. To facilitate group comparison, flows at two midlung volumes, 60% and 40% of exhaled vital capacity, were normalized by dividing flow rates at these lung volumes by observed total lung capacity (TLC/s) (52). The volume-corrected flows at these two midlung volumes were increased in each of these 17 patients in comparison to their individually predicted values.

G. Pulmonary Function in Patients with Respiratory Symptoms with AIDS or Risk of AIDS without *P. carinii* Pneumonia

We also evaluated pulmonary function in 12 patients with AIDS or at risk for AIDS with respiratory symptoms found subsequently not to be caused by *P. carinii* pneumonia. In contrast to patients with *P. carinii* pneumonia, these patients as a group did not have significantly decreased lung volumes compared to predicted values ($p > 0.05$). In addition, the patients without *P. carinii* pneumonia did not have a significantly decreased diffusing capacity. Each of these patients without *P. carinii* pneumonia had a diffusing capacity within 20% of their predicted individual normal value. Further, as a group, patients without *P. carinii* pneumonia did not have a significantly increased FEV_1/FVC%. Finally, although there were individual patients with increased flows by spirometry or by maximal flow-volume maneuver, no patient without *P. carinii* pneumonia had the combination of an increased expiratory flow rate and a decreased diffusing capacity for carbon monoxide.

Before the AIDS epidemic the pulmonary physiology in patients with *P. carinii* pneumonia had been similarly characterized by the presence of small or restricted lung volumes, decreased diffusing capacity and increased flow rates (47). Also, other centers have reported that AIDS patients with *P. carinii* pneumonia have statistically significant differences in mean vital capacity, FEV_1/FVC% and diffusing capacity relative to patients without *P. carinii* pneumonia (6,49). Although, there is some overlap of pulmonary function findings between AIDS patients with and without *P. carinii* pneumonia, almost every patient with *P. carinii* pneumonia had a diffusing capacity less than 80% of predicted and usually less than 70% of predicted. Although sensitive to the presence of *P. carinii* pneumonia, a low diffusing capacity can result from other processes including Kaposi's sarcoma (49) or intravenous drug abuse itself (53). Furthermore, unlike children with hematological malignancy who resolve their pulmonary function tests after one month of therapy for *P. carinii* pneumonia (47), AIDS patients have persistent physiological abnormalities following successful therapy for *P. carinii* pneumonia (54). Therefore, after a prior episode of effectively treated *P. carinii* pneumonia, a persistently low diffusing capacity will not be necessarily predictive of recurrent *P. carinii* pneumonia.

H. Gallium Lung Scanning

Gallium lung scans have been used to document the presence of many different types of pulmonary processes (55,56). The use of gallium to detect the presence of *P. carinii* pneumonia is not new in the setting of a normal chest roentgenogram in or out of the context of AIDS (56-60). The resolution of a positive gallium lung scan after successful *P. carinii* pneumonia therapy has also been reported (5,48,56,61). Although sensitive, gallium lung scanning is expensive, not acutely available and generally nonspecific. However, in our experience the specificity for *P. carinii* pneumonia in the context of AIDS is enhanced by employing a grading system for assessing gallium lung scan activity: 1, normal pulmonary activity, less than or equal to adjacent soft tissue gallium uptake; 2, appreciably greater lung uptake than adjacent soft tissue, but less than liver; 3, equal to liver; and 4, greater than liver lung uptake of gallium (55). We obtained gallium lung scans at the time of initial presentation in 14 patients with *P. carinii* pneumonia, the gallium lung scan was diffusely positive even among 5 of these 14 patients (42%) in whom the PaO_2 and/or chest roentgenogram were normal. All 14 scans were grade 3 or 4 diffuse uptake (55).

Although potentially nonspecific, especially if a graded system of interpretation is not employed, the fact that gallium lung scans were diffusely positive grade 3 or 4 in all of our patients with *P. carinii* pneumonia was very helpful. In our patients with respiratory symptoms not attributed to *P. carinii* pneumonia, none had a diffusely positive gallium lung scan above grade 2. Therefore, at either end of the scale, gallium lung scanning provides useful information.

The mechanism of abnormal gallium uptake is unknown. There is some evidence that at sites of inflammation in the lung, gallium is taken up by neutrophils, lymphocytes, and/or activated alveolar macrophages (61a). Recent data suggest that gallium accumulation in the lung is due to a protein leak secondary to increase vascular permeability. After intravenous injection, almost all gallium is bound in the serum to transferrin. Presumably, gallium bound to transferrin leaks out of the vascular compartment and into the alveolar space (61b).

In patients at risk for AIDS with minimal but persistent symptoms and signs of pneumonia, a diffusely positive gallium lung scan associated with

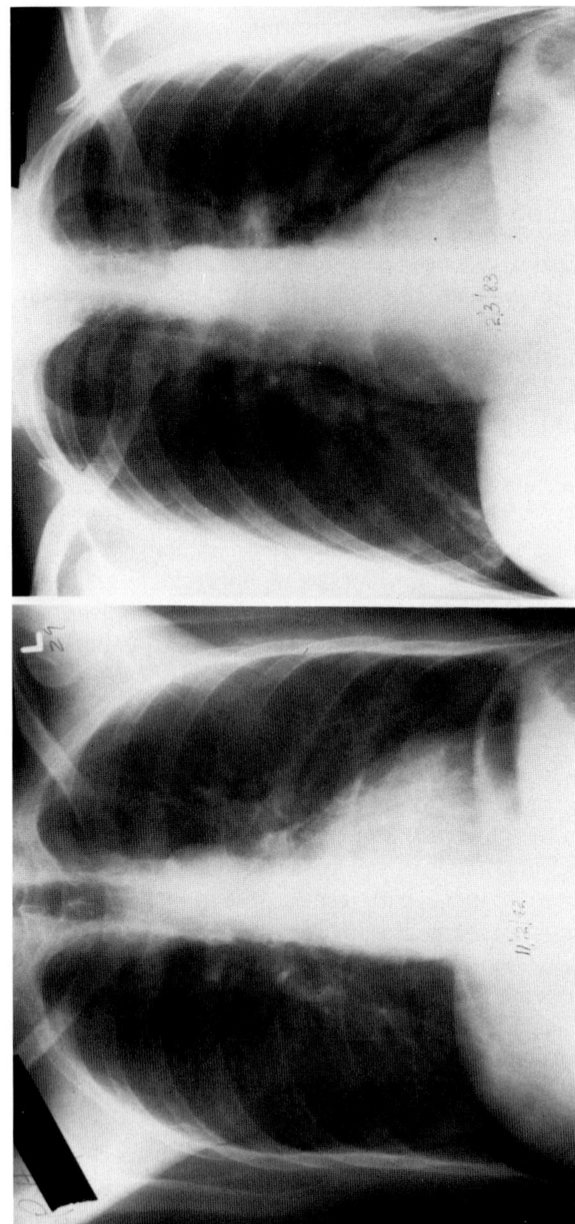

Figure 4 Chest roentgenogram in patient with asymptomatic *P. carinii* pneumonia showing minimal diffuse hazy infiltrate (*left*) which cleared after treatment (*right*).

increased air flow rates and a decreased diffusing capacity argues strongly for the presence of *P. carinii* pneumonia. For example, a homosexual patient with absolutely no symptoms of pneumonia had a minimally abnormal routine chest roentgenogram (Figure 4) which prompted spirometry revealing an increased $FEV_1/FVC\%$. Subsequently, a formal pulmonary function test confirmed the high flow rates (as reflected by an FEV_1/FVC of 89%) associated with a decreased diffusing capacity 19 ml/min × mmHg, 69% of predicted). Because he lacked pulmonary symptoms, the patient and his primary physician were reluctant to accept a bronchoscopic evaluation. The patient consented to a gallium lung scan which was diffusely positive grade 4 (Figure 5). On this basis, the patient agreed to bronchoscopy which was positive for *P. carinii* pneumonia. Three weeks after treatment with trimethoprim-sulfamethoxazole, repeat bronchoscopy showed resolution of *P. carinii* pneumonia. Similarly, a repeat gallium lung scan was negative (Figure 5). At that time, the pulmonary function showed resolution of his decreased diffusing capacity for carbon monoxide (38 mg/min × mmHg, 104% of predicted) as well as a decrease toward normal of his flow rates (FEV_1/FVC of 82%).

I. Diagnosis

Before the AIDS epidemic, the diagnosis of *P. carinii* pneumonia had traditionally required lung biopsy although other diagnostic techniques had been employed with variable success: transthoracic needle aspiration of the lung

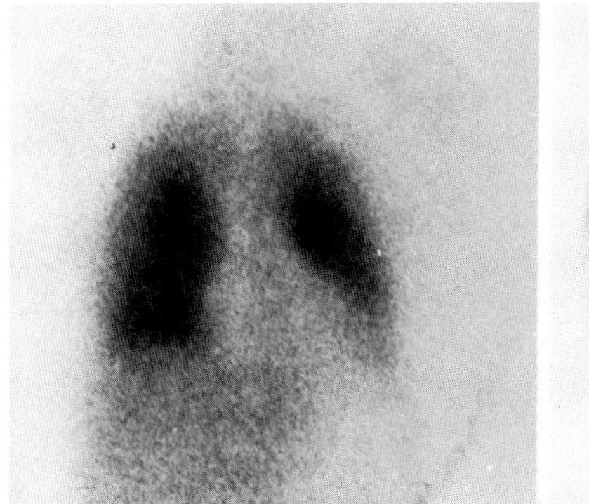

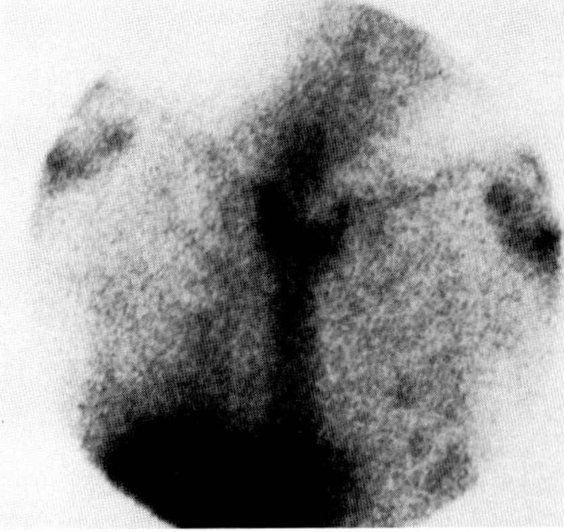

Figure 5 Gallium lung scan in patient with asymptomatic *P. carinii* pneumonia showing (*left*) diffuse grade 4 uptake which resolved (*right*) after therapy.

(62-64), cuffed catheter lavage (65), translaryngeal aspiration (66), and the collection of hypopharyngeal material or expectorated sputum (67-69). Recently, fiberoptic bronchoscopy with transbronchial biopsy has replaced open lung biopsy (6). In our initial reports in patients with AIDS, bronchoscopic procedures including transbronchial biopsy had a diagnostic yield for *P. carinii* pneumonia of over 90% (6,70). In our most recent comparative report, lavage was diagnostic of *P. carinii* pneumonia in 89% of instances while transbronchial biopsy was diagnostic in 93%; both transbronchial biopsy and lavage together had a yield of 100% for *P. carinii* pneumonia (71).

Interest in bronchoalveolar lavage employing the fiberoptic bronchoscope was stimulated by the complications and expense associated with transbronchial biopsy. Transbronchial biopsy through the fiberoptic bronchoscope is usually performed with fluoroscopic localization but still results in a 5% incidence of pneumothorax (72). Substantial hemorrhage (more than 50 ml of blood) also occurs (73,74). Even before the present epidemic, experience with lavage had already suggested its potential utility (65,75,76). The results of lavage in patients with AIDS has been similarly impressive (77-82). In 40 consecutive AIDS patients at risk for *P. carinii* pneumonia, lavage was diagnostic in 34 of 35 patients (83).

The effectiveness of lavage in detecting *P. carinii* is consistent with the pathology of *P. carinii* pneumonia and the alveolar sampling afforded by lavage. In *P. carinii* pneumonia the alveolar air spaces become filled with cysts and trophozoites (Figure 1) (29). An average lavage samples an estimated one million alveoli and cellular constituents from lavage samples are similar to cell extracts made from lung parenchyma obtained by open lung biopsy (84). In experimental *P. carinii* pneumonia induced in rats by administration of steroids, lavage could detect *P. carinii* as early as sections of lung tissue (75).

Finally, sputum induction for the diagnosis of *P. carinii* pneumonia was advocated even before the AIDs epidemic (67-69). In the context of AIDS, Bigby reported that induced sputum had a diagnostic accuracy for *P. carinii* pneumonia of 61% (85). However, in this report, the negative predictive value of sputum evaluation was only 44%. Further, sputum evaluation was not evaluated in patients with mild *P. carinii* pneumonia associated with normal chest x-ray. Also, it is possible that other infectious agents may be missed by sputum evaluation that would be detected by lavage. Finally, the expertise required for evaluation of sputum for *P. carinii* may only be available in large institutions where AIDS is a frequent problem.

J. Serological Diagnosis

There is no serological test for the presence of *P. carinii* pneumonia (7). Various workers have developed complement fixation and indirect immunofluorescence methods for detection of antibody against *P. carinii*; counter-immunoelectrophoresis for *P. carinii* antigen detection has also been described (7,14,86).

Complement fixation studies have detected antibody to *P. carinii* in 75-90% of infants with endemic infantile *P. carinii* pneumonia; however, serial conversion occurred two to three weeks after the onset of clinical *P. carinii* pneumonia. Further, the test is insensitive among immunosuppressed patients inasmuch as they may be unable to respond by antibody production as evidenced by only half of the patients with established *P. carinii* pneumonia having antibody detected and changes in titer were not diagnostically helpful either (87). Further, a positive test may be nonspecific vis-à-vis disease as over two-thirds of normal subjects develop this antibody due to prior subclinical infection (9,14).

Circulating *P. carinii antigen* can be detected in 79% (19,36) of bone marrow transplant patients with established *P. carinii* pneumonia; half of these patients had antigenemia detected prior to or within 72 h of diagnosis, making the test potentially useful diagnostically (86,87). However, detecting the presence of antigen also appears to be nondiagnostic in that 15% of cancer patients without pneumonia were positive, 35 of 52 bone marrow transplant patients with viral or idiopathic pneumonia were positive, and 11 of 25 bone marrow transplant patients without any pneumonia were positive for *P. carinii* antigen. It may be that lung injury is the common denominator for the development of a positive antigen among these patients because none of 120 normal children had antigen detected and only one of 50 normal bone marrow donors had detectable antigen (88).

K. Present Approach to the Diagnosis of *P. carinii* Pneumonia

It should be stressed that empiric therapy for *P. carinii* pneumonia should be discouraged because the clinical and chest x-ray findings of *P. carinii* pneumonia are nonspecific (89); 228 of 441 patients with AIDS (48%) had other opportunistic infections besides *P. carinii* pneumonia (5). Moreover, side effects of therapy for *P. carinii* pneumonia are surprisingly high and merit a precise diagnosis.

Presently any patient with an appropriate exposure history and an undiagnosed penumonia should have sputum induction or lavage (Figure 6). If these studies are negative, repeat bronchoscopy should be undertaken for lavage and transbronchial biopsy. Using this approach, we have not had to resort to an open lung biopsy in the context of AIDS. If sputum evaluation and bedside or outpatient lavage continue to be high yield modalities, then expensive and time consuming screening procedures such as pulmonary function assessment, exercise arterial blood gas analysis, or gallium lung scanning can be obviated even among patients with mild presentations associated with

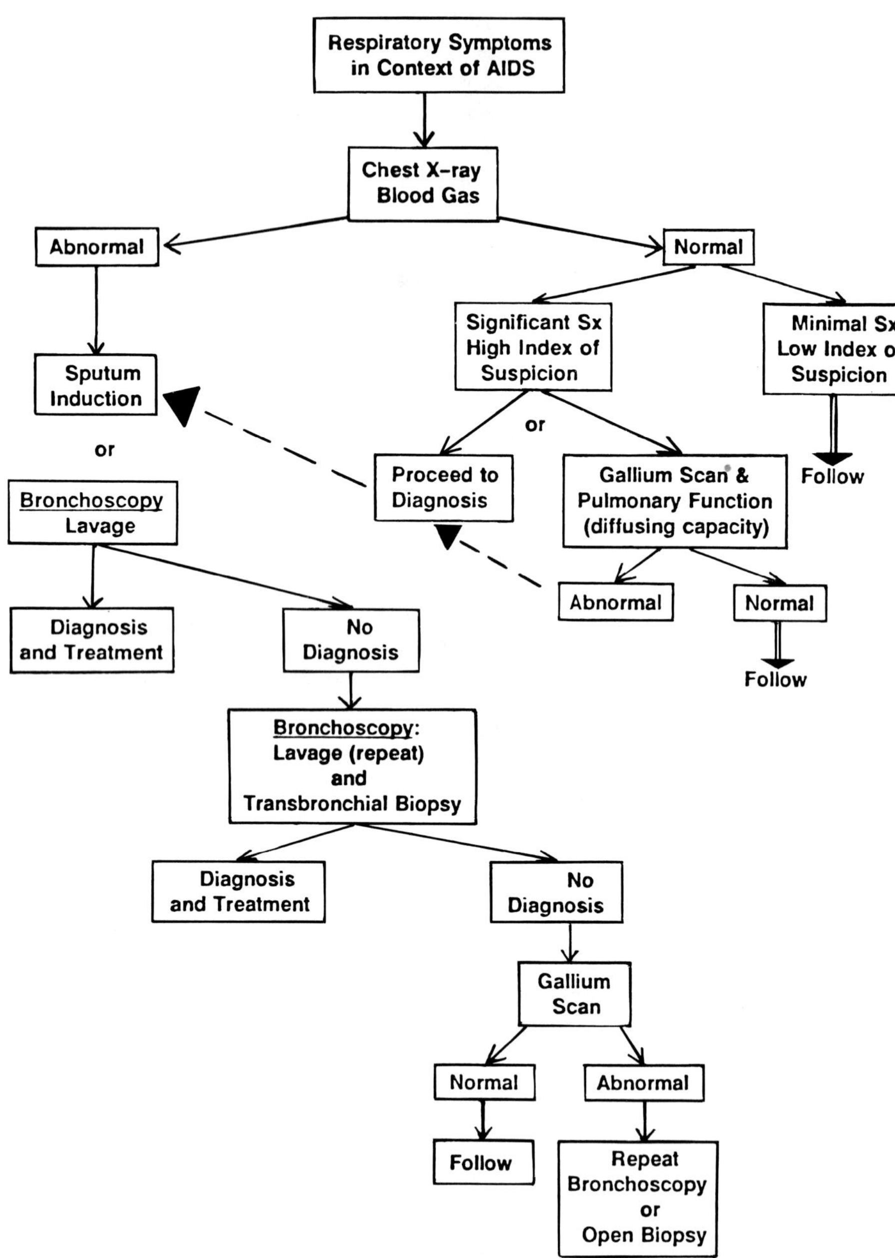

Figure 6 Diagnostic algorithm for the pulmonary complications of AIDS.

normal arterial blood gases and/or normal chest roentgenograms. Given the benign nature of sputum induction and lavage, it is likely that patients and their physicians will consider diagnostic evaluation earlier in the presence of even mild symptoms that are now recognized as being consistent with *P. carinii* pneumonia. At this time patients are less hypoxic and more likely to respond to therapy (4).

L. Treatment of *P. carinii* Pneumonia Prior to the AIDS Epidemic

Without therapy, *P. carinii* pneumonia in the immunosuppressed host is virtually 100% fatal, and among malnourished or premature infants, *P. carinii* pneumonia is 50% fatal (90). In 1958, Ivady and Paldy first used pentamidine isethionate for *P. carinii* pneumonia and reduced the mortality of *P. carinii* pneumonia among malnourished and/or premature infants to 2%. Since 1967 pentamidine has been available only through the CDC. A report from the CDC involving 163 confirmed *P. carinii* pneumonia cases prior to the AIDS epidemic revealed a therapeutic response rate to pentamidine of 63% among patients who received at least nine days of therapy (91). However, 47% of patients had pentamidine-related side effects: azotemia, liver function abnormalities, intramuscular injection site sterile abscesses, hypoglycemia, hypotension, rash, and hypocalcemia (91,92).

In 1974, Hughes et al. showed the combination of trimethoprim-sulfamethoxazole (TMP-SMX) was effective in the prevention and treatment of *P. carinii* pneumonia in cortisone-treated rats (93). Subsequently, TMP-SMX was found to be effective in treating children and adults with *P. carinii* pneumonia (90,94,95). Side effects, primarily rash and nausea, occurred in 13% of patients (90).

In 1978, prior to the AIDS epidemic, Hughes et al. compared the effectiveness of pentamidine and TMP-SMX among children with *P. carinii* pneumonia. The drugs were found to be equally effective (about 75%) (96). However, given the 47% incidence of toxicity with pentamidine compared with 13% incidence of adverse events related to TMP-SMX, TMP-SMX became the drug of choice.

M. Treatment of *P. carinii* Pneumonia in AIDS Patients

The treatment of *P. carinii* pneumonia should be undertaken with the knowledge that, at the present time, AIDS-related immune suppression is untreatable and the relapse rate for *P. carinii* pneumonia in AIDS patients is between 30% and 50%. Even after successful therapy of *P. carinii* pneumonia, the mean survival of AIDS patients is 7.7 months; few patients with prior

P. carinii pneumonia in the context of AIDS have lived more than two years (3,5,35). It should be stressed that quality of life must be balanced with diagnostic and therapeutic manipulations (97).

Retrospective and prospective studies of *P. carinii* pneumonia among AIDS patients have shown pentamidine and TMP-SMX to be similarly effective (4,38,41,48,98,99). However, in contrast to the pre-AIDS experience in which a 13% toxicity rate was found, the incidence of adverse reactions to therapy with TMP-SMX is at least 50% (96,100,101).

Dose, Route, and Duration of Therapy

Trimethoprim-Sulfamethoxazole: The usual dose of TMP-SMX is 15-20 mg/kg of the trimethoprim and 75-100 mg/kg of sulfamethoxazole daily in four divided doses intravenously for 21 days. In pre-AIDS *P. carinii* pneumonia studies with TMP-SMX, oral therapy was as effective as intravenous therapy except in patients with gastrointestinal diseases. Low blood levels of TMP-SMX in these cases reflected poor absorption and was predictive of ineffective therapy (95). Similarly, among complaint AIDS patients without gastrointestinal problems, oral TMP-SMX can be used effectively (38). If the presence of an intact gastrointestinal system is unclear, it has been recommended that patients on oral therapy have a blood level one and a half hours after a dose to insure absorption (90). The blood level of trimethoprim should be above 5 μg/ml and the sulfamethoxazole level should be at least 100 μg/ml.

The common TMP-SMX-related side reactions among AIDs patients include rash, leukopenia, thrombocytopenia, and nausea. Rash and/or leukopenia usually begin at about days 8-10 of TMP-SMX therapy. Several anecdotal reports described anaphylaxis at the time of retreatment with TMP-SMX among AIDS patients who have had a prior TMP-SMX adverse reaction, especially rash (5).

The role of folinic acid therapy in treating or preventing hematological problems due to TMP-SMX has not been defined. Although rare among patients treated with TMP-SMX without AIDS, there is a 30% incidence of significant cytopenia with TMP-SMX among AIDS patients. Trimethoprim inhibits dihydrofolate reductase in bacteria and presumably *P. carinii* and thereby decreases the conversion of dihydrofolate to tetrahydrofolate (90). In vitro studies also suggest that trimethoprim can inhibit erythroid and granulocyte hematopoiesis in man which can be reversed with folinic acid (102-104). However, in our experience and that of others, folate supplementation has not reversed the cytopenia that developed in AIDS patients during therapy with TMP-SMX (4,101). The mechanism of TMP-SMX induced cytopenia among AIDS patients is not clear and one study suggests an immune mechanism rather than folate deficiency (105).

Pentamidine: Presently there are two forms of pentamidine available. The dose of pentamidine isethionate is 4 mg/kg given once per day. The dose of the pentamidine methanesulfonate salt is expressed as the weight of pentamidine base only (2.3 mg of pentamidine base/kg once per day) (48). Classically, therapy with pentamidine is intramuscular, but injection site aseptic abscesses can develop. Therefore, pentamidine has been used intravenously in 250 ml of 5% dextrose in water infused slowly over 2-3 h to avoid hypotension (5,106).

Pentamidien toxicity has always been a major problem. In the context of AIDS, pentamidine adverse reactions occur in as many as 78% of patients (99). Serious early adverse reactions include hypotension and hypoglycemia; other reactions include neutropenia, rash, fever, hepatitis, decreased renal function, hematuria (107), pancreatitis (108), as well as intramuscular abscess formation. Recently, preliminary studies suggest that the aerosolized route of pentamidine delivery may be helpful. Animal experiments showed that aerosolized pentamidine resulted in a "comparatively high concentration of pentamidine in the lungs" with less pentamidine delivered to the liver and kidney relative to intramuscular therapy (109,110). Further, immunosuppressed rats with *P. carinii* penumonia can be successfully treated with aerosolized pentamidine (110a). Most recently we have shown that inhaled pentamidine in AIDS patients with *P. carinii* pneumonia is an effective treatment (110b-110d). Inhaled pentamidine did not result in significant toxicity relative to the intravenous route of administration. The lack of toxicity is probably due to the lack of systemic drug absorption following inhaled therapy. Also, in terms of therapeutic effectiveness, the level of pentamidine in bronchoalveolar lavage fluid was 10 times higher after inhaled pentamidine than following intravenous drug administration.

Monitoring Therapeutic Effectiveness

Patients must be monitored closely for therapeutic effectiveness as well as adverse drug reaction. In general, compared with patients without AIDS, AIDS patients with *P. carinii* pneumonia present with a more insidious onset of symptoms associated with less hypoxia; as noted above, this condition contrasts with the more fulminant course of respiratory dysfunction associated with *P. carinii* pneumonia in immunosuppressed patients without AIDS (38,49,111). The AIDS patients with the more insidious presentation and less respiratory failure at the time of diagnosis are more likely to survive with therapy relative to patients who present with severe respiratory failure (4). Recent studies suggest that therapeutic effectiveness is as high as 90% with earlier diagnosis of the disease (112). Patients presenting with respiratory failure requiring intubation and mechanical ventilation have, at best, a 14% chance of surviving (5).

Among patients who respond to therapy, the fever usually decreases by five to eight days, the PaO_2 increases by at least 10 mmHg by day 8 to 10, and the chest x-ray shows improvement by day 12 to 13 (5). Of note, 50% of the patients who subsequently responded to therapy had an initial worsening of their chest x-ray (49). In general, by day 4 or 5 if the patient is clinically worse, it is recommended that therapy be changed. It should be stressed that switching patients to pentamidine due to failure of initial therapy with SMX-TMP is associated with a 90% mortality from that episode of *P. carinii* pneumonia. In contrast, changing to pentamidine because of TMP-SMX-related side effects in patients responding to initial therapy with SMX-TMP usually results in continued therapeutic response (6).

Duration of Therapy

The duration of therapy for *P. carinii* pneumonia in AIDS patients is not clear because cure has not been defined (48). Just as AIDS patients often present with prolonged mild symptoms, they tend to respond to therapy slowly and, as noted, there is a striking 30-50% relapse rate of *P. carinii* pneumonia (48). Repeat lung biopsy after successful therapeutic response frequently reveals persistent organisms (99,111,113,114).

Persistence of *P. carinii* pneumonia after conventional therapy may be an important factor in the recurrence of this infection in AIDS patients; alternatively, these persistent organisms may be nonviable (39). It is not clear if prolonging therapy would decrease the striking incidence of persistent organisms and/or recurrent *P. carinii* pneumonia in AIDS patients (48,115). In patients with prior *P. carinii* pneumonia who subsequently develop new onset temperature elevation and respiratory symptoms, interpretation of bronchoscopic findings is often complicated by the known persistence of *P. carinii* pneumonia among AIDS patients (113).

Other Drugs

In view of the therapeutic inadequacy of conventional therapy, especially in terms of adverse reactions, and the epidemic nature of AIDS, new therapeutic modalities are being investigated. Using both TMP-SMX and pentamidine together has not been effective, in part, because of drug toxicity (116).

Benefit from use of steroid therapy in certain cases of *P. carinii* pneumonia failing conventional therapy has been reported (39,117). Even before the AIDS epidemic it had been noted that *P. carinii* pneumonia was suppressed with steroid therapy (118,119). However, steroid therapy for asthma or dermatitis in patients at risk for AIDS has been associated with subsequent fulminate *P. carinii* pneumonia (120). Obviously the benefit versus risk associated with the use of steroids in patients presenting with severe *P. carinii* pneumonia needs to be studied.

Other possibly effective compounds are presently undergoing evaluation. Difluoromethylornithine (DFMO), an inhibitor of polyamine synthesis, was found effective in six patients in whom conventional therapy had either failed or had been associated with unacceptable adverse reactions (121). When used as initial therapy for *P. carinii* pneumonia, DFMO resulted in some clinical, radiological, and gas exchange improvement in six of eight patients; this change was not sustained consistent with the concept that this drug is static against *P. carinii* and should not be used as initial exclusive therapy for this infection. Alternatively, benefit from DFMO in patients failing prior therapy may have resulted from improved lung healing possibly afforded by DFMO (122).

Hughes has shown that dapsone (diaminodiphenylsulfone) can be effective therapy for murine *P. carinii* pneumonia. The drug was synergistic with trimethoprim in successfully treating *P. carinii* pneumonia in this animal model (123). In two preliminary reports, dapsone 100 mg/d and trimethoprim at a dose of 20 mg/kg per day in four divided doses, was effective in at least 8 or 11 patients. The majority of patients however developed significant adverse reactions including nausea, vomiting, rash, pancytopenia, and hemolytic anemia (124-126). However, recent studies suggest that dapsone alone is not effective in the treatment of *P. carinii* pneumonia in AIDS patients (127).

N. Prophylaxis Against *P. carinii* Pneumonia

The attack rate of *P. carinii* pneumonia among AIDS patients is at least 30% per year, relative to an attack rate of 0.1-1.1% among non-AIDS immunosuppressed patients. Moreover, the tendency for *P. carinii* pneumonia to recur among AIDS patients has stimulated tremendous interest in prophylactic therapy for *P. carinii* pneumonia. Hughes first showed the dramatic benefit of the prophylactic use of TMP-SMX (at a dose of trimethoprim 5 mg/kg per d and sulfamethoxazole 25/mg/kg per d) in 160 children with immune suppression who were at risk for *P. carinii* pneumonia. Over a two-year period none of 80 treated patients acquired *P. carinii* pneumonia while 17 of 80 patients on placebo developed *P. carinii* pneumonia (128). However, studies in animals and patients with AIDS showed that prophylaxis with TMP-SMX or pentamidine does not eradicate *P. carinii* organisms, and that patients are only protected while they are actively taking prophylactic therapy (95,129). It has been advocated that patients continue prophylactic therapy with TMP-SMX after successful therapy for *P. carinii* pneumonia. However, the adverse reactions to this compound in AIDS patients is limiting (129).

The utility of Fansidar (pyrimethamine and sulfadoxine) is presently being evaluated for *P. carinii* pneumonia prophylaxis (2,129). Before the AIDS epidemic Fansidar was found to be as effective as pentamidine in therapy of *P. carinii* pneumonia among experimental animals, but only limited human studies had been undertaken. (130-132) Severe life-threatening reactions have been reported in otherwise healthy patients using the drug for malaria prophylaxis (48,133).

We recently showed that inhaled pentamidine significantly decreased the occurrence of *P. carinii* pneumonia among patients with AIDS. Further, in those patients on monthly inhaled pentamidine prophylaxis who did develop *P. carinii* pneumonia, the illness was very mild.

III. Cytomegalovirus

Disease caused by cytomegalovirus (CMV) infection of immunosuppressed patients often involves many organs probably reflecting hematogenous spread: lung, central nervous system (134, 135), gastrointestinal tract (136, 137), eye (138,139), liver, bone marrow, etc. Adrenal involvement has recently been emphasized as a cause of a hypoadrenal status in AIDS patients (140-142). Although reported, pneumonia in otherwise healthy patients with CMV mononucleosis is uncommon (143). The precise relative contributions of host and viral factors in the development of CMV pneumonia are unknown. Some studies suggest that host factors, including peripheral and lung CMV specific cytotoxic T lymphocytes, natural killer cells, and alveolar macrophages are involved in protecting the host from disease due to this ubiquitous organism (144-147).

Clinically, CMV pneumonia is associated with cough, dyspnea, fever, hypoxia, and liver function test abnormalities with chest x-ray evidence of bilateral patchy or interstitial basilar infiltrates (143). Pathological findings include monouclear cells with distinctive intranuclear inclusions (148).

There is a debate as to what constitutes CMV disease versus infection in patients with AIDS (149). The specific diagnosis of CMV pneumonia ultimately depends on finding cells with intranuclear inclusions on histological evaluation. However, it should be emphasized that new research techniques such as detection of viral DNA by *in situ* hybridization or detection of viral antigen by direct immunofluroescence have greatly improved the sensitivity for detecting CMV (150-152).

Bronchoscopy is effective in diagnosing the presence of CMV in the lungs of AIDS patients; 95 of 221 (43%) bronchoscopic evaluations detected the virus by characteristic histology and/or culture of bronchoscopically derived secretions and lung tissue (71). Lavage had twice the yield for CMV as transbronchial biopsy (71, 81). In one study, CMV was never isolated from lavage, either by culture or typical cytology, without histological evidence of pneumonitis (153). However, the significance of recovering CMV from culture of bronchoscopically derived lung tissue or secretions in patients with AIDS without histological or clinical pneumonia is not clear (143,150). Because AIDS patients are often viremic with CMV (154), a transbronchial biopsy sample which grows CMV without histological evidence of inclusions may simply be an artifact of hemorrhagic transbronchial biopsy.

Another related debate is the clinical significance of diagnosing CMV infection and/or disease in AIDS patients. In our first 20 AIDS patients presenting with *P. carinii* pneumonia, 17 had pulmonary coinfection with CMV. All but three of these patients responded to therapy for *P. carinii* pneumonia. This therapeutic response to *P. carinii* pneumonia makes less likely a pathological role for CMV in terms of disease (149). Similarly, in the study of Brodie et al.of 69 AIDS patients with *P. carinii* pneumonia undergoing their first bronchoscopy, CMV was also isolated in 31 patients (155). Their median life expectancy from the time of bronchoscopy was the same as the patients with *P. carinii* pneumonia alone. Even stratifying the patients with CMV by degree of virus burden did not imply an important pathogenic role for CMV. Further, the presence of viral inclusion bodies did not affect survival. Therefore the recovery of CMV in the lungs of patients with AIDS had no effect on mortality in this study (155). However, other centers have shown pulmonary CMV to have an important effect on survival. In Stover's experience, patients with *P. carinii* pneumonia without CMV had a 14% mortality, while patients with *P. carinii* pneumonia and CMV had a 92% mortality (49). Similarly, in an autopsy series of 15 patients dying of AIDS, CMV was found to be the principal cause of death in 47% of these patients and the leading cause of respiratory insufficiency—in seven of nine (78%). Of note, 14 of these 15 patients (93%) at autopsy had evidence of widely disseminated CMV infection. Antemortem, 14 of these 15 patients had positive CMV blood cultures initially requiring two to three weeks to grow, but subsequently the cultures became positive at progressively shorter intervals, suggesting increased viral burden in their blood (154,156).

The apparent difference in clinical significance of CMV pulmonary infection between centers may relate to patient selection and specifically whether patients are early or late in their course with AIDS. As Kovaks et al (4) point out, at the time of lung biopsy in patients relatively early in their course, histopathological evidence of CMV infection was seen in 10% of cases but CMV inclusion cells were sparse in number and clinical outcome depended on successful therapy of *P. carinii* pneumonia. In an autopsy series CMV inclusion cells were more common. This finding suggested that CMV may not be an important factor contributing to pulmonary dysfunction when patients initially present with *P. carinii* pneumonia. However, later in the course of AIDS progressive CMV disease associated with an increased viral burden is more likely to contribute to morbidity and mortality (4).

For treatment, an acyclovir derivative, dihydroxypropoxymethylguanine (DHPG, Syntex), and an apparently identical compound B759μ (Burroughs Wellcome) are presently undergoing clinical trials. Some therapeutic benefit has been reported but not confirmed by other studies (150, 157).

Other viruses beside CMV have been isolated from the lungs of AIDS patients. In our study involving 104 bronchoscopic procedures, six (6%) were positive for adenovirus by cell culture and direct fluorescence (158).

IV. Bacterial Pulmonary infections in AIDS

A. Atypical *Mycobacterium avium-intracellulare* or *Mycobacterium avium* Complex (MAC)

This bacterial complex is a frequent environmental contaminant found in soil and water as well as in a variety of birds and mammals (159-161). The portal of entry in humans is probably the respiratory tract, although ingestion, as documented in chickens may be another route of entry (112, 162).

Prior to 1982 there had been fewer than 100 patients reported with disseminated atypical mycobacterial infection, the most common species was MAI, and the most common associated immunosupressive disease was hairy cell leukemia (163). In AIDS patients there is a dramatic incidence of disseminated MAC noted on autopsy. All five of the first AIDS patients presenting at University of California, Los Angeles died with disseminated MAI and another center reported autopsy evidence of widely disseminated MAI in 55% (30/55) of patients dying with AIDS (164). Sites of dissemination include lung, blood, lymph node, bone marrow, liver, spleen, adrenal gland, eye, brain, pancreas, prostate, testes, thyroid, thymus, heart, and gastrointestinal tract; disseminated MAC has been associated with bowel lesion simulating Whipple's disease (165). Pulmonary infection in 441 AIDS patients involved MAC in 17% of cases (5), either alone or associated with other AIDS-related lung infections. In that multicenter study, the bronchoscopic yield for pulmonary MAC was high, 78%, but the bronchoscopic diagnosis was often delayed pending culture results (5,6). Smears and cultures of bronchial lavage positive for MAC do not necessarily imply the presence of invasive pulmonary disease (112, 150). Moreover, AIDS patients often do not make well-formed granulomas, so biopsy material should be stained and cultured for acid fast bacteria, even in the absence of granulomas (166-169).

The clinical presentation of MAC in AIDS patients is difficult to determine because of frequent coinfection with other agents. In general, AIDS patients with MAC have a prolonged, downhill course associated with fever and weight loss, poor response to therapy, and usually a fatal outcome. The clinical presentation of non-AIDS patients with MAC also reveals a prolonged, five-month interval between onset of symptoms, especially fever and weight loss, prior to diagnosis (162). Of note, in 30 non-AIDS patients with MAC, pulmonary symptoms occurred in only 27% but chest x-ray evidence of pulmonary MAC involvement was present in 67%. In contrast to AIDS patients, these patients with MAC, even in the setting of immunosuppression, still made granulomas in over 80% of cases. In further contrast to patients with AIDS, 60% of these patients with MAC, but without AIDS, had a sustained therapeutic response, and the patients who failed therapy had tremendous tissue burdens of MAC organisms (162).

Diagnosis of Atypical *Mycobacterium avium-intracellulare*

Even before the AIDS epidemic it had been noted that finding MAC in sputum did not constitute a diagnosis of disease. However, finding MAC in multiple organ sites usually denotes disease; in AIDS patients it has been reported that positive blood cultures for MAC have always been associated with widespread organ dissemination (164). Nevertheless, because of the presence of other infections in AIDS patients, it is not clear what role MAC has in this syndrome or its course (170).

In view of the disseminated nature of the infection noted at autopsy, it is not surprising that organisms can be detected in many body fluids and tissues (159). New blood culture techniques for MAC involving lysing of leukocytes and erythrocytes have shown a tremendous and sustained quantitative MAC bacteremia burden associated with an even greater tissue burden of organisms (163,164,171). This high grade MAC infection has been likened to lepromatous leprosy (171).

This large number of organisms probably makes MAC difficult to treat (162,171). Even before the AIDS epidemic the overall success rate for treatment of localized pulmonary MAC even in patients without apparent immune suppression was only between 45% and 65% (5). Lack of success is largely due to multiple drug resistance, perhaps because the organism appears to have a permeability barrier to therapeutic agents (172). Recently MAC has been shown to have some sensitivity for ansamycin, a rifampin derivative, as well as to clofazamine (164). The CDC released ansamycin for 318 AIDS patients with MAC. About one-third of these patients had some response to therapy but eradication of MAC infection was uncommon; clofazamine did not improve survival (173).

Mycobacterium Tuberculosis

An increased incidence of *Mycobacterium* tuberculosis has also been observed in AIDS patients (112,169). This finding reflects reactivation of latent disease as it is most likely to occur among AIDS patients from regions with a high incidence of tuberculosis, such as Haiti (174). Similarly, AIDS patients who are intravenous drug abusers from American localities with high rates of tuberculosis in the general population also are at risk for tuberculosis (169).

Clinically, tuberculosis in AIDS patients involves a continuum from lymphadenitis to disseminated tuberculosis with meningitis; positive blood cultures have been reported (174). Haitian AIDS patients are more likely to have extrapulmonary tuberculosis than American-born AIDS patients. Similarly, in their respective non-AIDS general populations, Haitians are more likely to have extrapulmonary tuberculosis than that found in the general American population with tuberculosis. Haitian AIDS patients have the same incidence of atypical MAC as American-born AIDS patients. This observation reflects similar rates of this infection in these two populations (174).

The chest roentgenogram in one series of AIDS patients with tuberculosis resembled progressive primary tuberculosis (169). Lower lobe infiltration with hilar adenopathy was more common than apical changes. In addition to the atypical radiographic pattern, the diagnosis was not made by skin test or sputum evaluation and generally required an invasive diagnostic approach (169). It should be noted that tuberculosis preceded AIDS per se by a mean of six months (range, 1-17 months). Finally, even in AIDS patients with severe and disseminated tuberculosis, therapy has been generally effective (169,174).

B. Other Bacterial Infections

In addition to mycobacterial infections, other bacterial infections have been well documented in AIDS patients (112). In the setting of T-cell immune dysfunction, infection by *Legionella* species is not surprising (112). *Legionella* infections among AIDS patients have been severe and have included unusual presentations such as sinus involvement (175). Similarly, *Nocardia asteroides* pleural-pericardial infection has been described (112).

Although AIDS is associated with a profound T-cell deficiency, B-cell dysfunction has also been documented (176,177). In the series of Stover et al., 7% of AIDS patients had bacterial pneumonia (49). Patients with AIDS have a well-documented inability to respond with antibody production to pneumococcal antigen (177-179). *Streptococcus pneumoniae* occurs with increased frequency among AIDS patients (112). Although this organism usually causes a lobar infiltrate, the chest roentgenogram in the setting of this infection in AIDS patients has been described as patchy. Similarly, *Haemophilus influenzae* results in a diffuse pneumonia resembling *P. carinii* pneumonia. Finally, the occurrence of nosocomial bacterial pneumonia such as due to *Pseudomonas aerugenosa* among severely ill, hospitalized AIDS patients is not surprising. In formulating empiric therapy, coverage for bacterial processes should be considered (112). In one series of bacterial pneumonias in AIDS patients, 88% had a curative response with specific antibacterial therapy (180).

V. Fungal Pulmonary Infections

Despite the known frequent occurrence of *Candida* oropharyngeal infection, pulmonary infection with fungus occurs in only a few percent of patients with AIDS, and in some large series not at all (5). The nonspecific radiographic manifestations of fungal infections include diffuse interstitial infiltrates with a reticular nodular pattern, as well as masslike appearances. Bronchoscopy has been effective in identifying the presence of pulmonary fungal infection (181). In the NHLBI study of 441 AIDS patients with pulmonary disease, nine had *Cryptococcus* and nine had other fungal pulmonary diseases (5). Cryptococcal antigen titers in both serum and cerebrospinal fluid were extremely high in AIDS patients with this infection. In one autopsy series, cryptococcal meningitis was a presenting clinical manifestation of AIDS in 3 of 10 patients; all three patients died due to cryptococcal meningitis despite aggressive therapy. This fungal infection in AIDS patients often recurs after apparent successful therapy. It has been suggested that weekly amplotericin B should be continued "indefinitely" (112). Pulmonary involvement in AIDS secondary to disseminated histoplasmosis, and, less commonly, due to coccidioidomycosis has also been reported (181,182). These infections have occurred outside their usual endemic settings.

VI. Respiratory Cryptosporidiosis

Cryptosporidiosis caused by the coccidial protozoan *Cryptosporidium* has been associated with severe diarrhea in AIDS patients. Pulmonary involvement by this organism has now been documented in AIDS (183,184). Oocysts of *Cryptosporidium* as seen on Giemsa and acid-fast stains of respiratory secretions should be differentiated from *Toxoplasma* and *P. carinii* organisms. One report described the utility of the modified cold Kinyoun stain to distinguish *Cryptosporidium* from these other microbes (183). Patients presented with copious sputum associated in some cases with bilateral interstitial infiltrates on chest x-ray. Although respiratory involvement by this organism occurs in fowl (183) and was recently described in an infant with severe combined immune deficiency (185), the role of this organism in producing pulmonary impairment and symptoms is not clear.

VII. Kaposi's Sarcoma of the Lung

Although not an infectious pulmonary complication of AIDS, Kaposi's sarcoma (KS), even before the AIDS epidemic, had been considered an opportunistic tumor occurring in the presence of immunosuppressive diseases and/or therapy (186). Pulmonary KS by itself can result in respiratory failure (187). Given the lack of sufficient autopsy data in AIDS patients, the precise incidence of pulmonary involvement by KS is unknown. Generally, one-third to one-half of AIDS patients have KS and the incidence of pulmonary KS in AIDS patients with pulmonary dysfunction has been reported between 8% and 13% (6,49,187). In one study, 19 of 32 KS patients (60%) had pulmonary involvement by this tumor (188). In autopsy series of AIDS patients, pulmonary KS was reported in over 25% of patients (170,187,189).

The presence of pulmonary KS must be in the differential of AIDS-related pulmonary dysfunction. In the lung, KS can involve proximal major airways, including the larynx, lung parenchyma, and/or the pleura (186, 187,190). Further, the development of pulmonary KS has no relation to the time course or extent of clinically apparent disease and can occur even in the presence of tumor regression (187). Finally, although mucocutaneous KS is usually evident, the tumor can first present in the lung in a mild form or associated with rapidly progressive respiratory failure (191,192).

Clinically, the presentation of pulmonary KS cannot be distinguished from pulmonary opportunistic infection. Cough and dyspnea with or without fever are common complaints (190). Because KS lesions are hemorrhagic and involve major airways as well as the pleura, the complaint of wheezing and/or stridor, hemoptysis, or pleuritic pain with hemorrhagic exudative pleural effusion may suggest the diagnosis. Similarly, the chest x-ray associated with pulmonary KS may reveal diffuse parenchymal infiltrates indistinguishable from opportunistic infections. In contrast to *P. carinii* pneumonia, however, diffuse KS of the lung on chest radiograph tends to be nodular and commonly associated with hilar and mediastinal adenopathy and/or pleural effusion (193-196). Further, KS can result in diffuse lung infiltration on chest radiograph due to diffuse alveolar or interstitial hemorrhage as well as pulmonary edema secondary to lymphatic obstruction (194).

Although usually unnecessary, the histological diagnosis of pulmonary KS requires an open lung biopsy (187). Transbronchial biopsy has on occasion been diagnostic of pulmonary KS but it is usually nondiagnostic and carries a risk of hemorrhage (6,187,191,193). Moreover, crush artifact, hemorrhage, granulation tissue, and fibrosis may all mimic histological features of KS on a small, transbronchial biopsy lung sample. Finally, open lung biopsy, which gives a larger sample size is usually unnecessary since the bronchoscope can be useful for simply visualizing the characteristic flat, bright red to violacious KS lesions lining the airway mucosa, even when these lesions are negative on bronchoscopic biopsy (188).

Other AIDS-related tumors and/or proliferative processes may involve the thorax. Non-Hodgkin's lymphoma in AIDS patients is extremely aggressive and is almost always associated with extranodal spread (197,198). In one large series, 8% of AIDS patients with non-Hodgkin's lymphoma had pulmonary involvement including hilar and mediastinal adenopathy and parenchymal nodules or masses.

VIII. Lymphocytic Interstitial Pneumonia

In general, the pulmonary manifestations of AIDS are similar in pediatric and adult patients (199,200). However, in contrast to adults, lymphocytic interstitial pneumonia (LIP) has been a prominent feature of pediatric AIDS (46,199,201-203). As initially defined by Liebow and Carrington in 1966, LIP refers to diffuse infiltration of alveolar walls by mature lymphocytes, plasma cells, and reticuloendothelial cells (204). Although initially described as a distinct pathological entity, other authors consider LIP a nonspecific pathological pattern: LIP is associated with various immune deficiencies and auto-immune diseases, especially Sjogren's, and has a variable natural history including the transformation into lymphoma (201,204-207). Prior to the AIDS epidemic, LIP was very rarely described in pediatric patients (206, 208,209).

In AIDS, up to half the pediatric patients in some series have LIP (46, 199,201-203). Some adult AIDS patients have now also been identified with this pulmonary disease (210,211). The histology of LIP in AIDS patients is distinct from the classic description (212). The pulmonary infiltrate is composed of atypical lymphocytes that invade bronchioles, rather than mature monocytes that simply surround bronchioles and vessels. Also, the air spaces in some patients are filled with numerous mononuclear cells resembling desquamative interstitial pneumonia (199,212).

Another important difference between LIP in patients with and without AIDS relates to the T-cell subset that comprises the infiltrate. The interstitial lymphocytes in both patients with and without AIDS are comprised primarily of T cells (208,210,212). However, in patients without AIDS these lymphocytes are of the helper-inducer subset, while in AIDS patients these T cells are primarily cytotoxic-suppressor cells (208,212).

The etiology of LIP in AIDS patients is unclear. The occurrence of LIP is usually described without concomitant opportunistic pulmonary infections ascribed to AIDS (213,214). However, we, and others (214), have recovered the AIDS retrovirus in lung lymphocytes obtained by lavage from patients with opportunistic infections as well as with LIP. The AIDS retrovirus has also been isolated from lymph nodes with similar cytotoxic-suppressor lymphocytosis (214). Indeed, LIP may represent a pulmonary expression of reactive lymphoplasmacytosis involving lymph nodes and other organs (46, 199,202,211,214). Alternatively, the retrovirus itself could cause the lymphocytosis noted in various organs in AIDS patients, including the lung (214).

The clinical presentation of LIP is constant but very nonspecific (206). Patients have dyspnea and a nonproductive cough with or without fever. There is an increased respiratory rate but rales are usually absent. The chest x-ray reveals a diffuse miliary pattern that has been mistaken for tuberculosis. With time the radiograph may reveal confluent infiltrates with air bronchograms (201,213). The physiological pattern is similar to that of *P. carinii* pneumonia: restrictive lung volumes with decreased diffusing capacity associated with hypoxia and a respiratory alkalosis (205,213). The diagnosis requires an open lung biopsy in that transbronchial biopsy usually produces too small a sample (199).

The natural history and response to therapy is unclear. Prior to the AIDS epidemic LIP was associated with an inconsistent response to therapy with steroids and/or alkylating agents (205). Pediatric AIDS patients with LIP may be a subgroup with a better prognosis than patients presenting with opportunistic pulmonary infections (199). The pediatric AIDS patients have been noted to spontaneously clear their LIP with stable followup for over two years (202,204). Steroid therapy has been effective in selected AIDS patients with severe LIP over a four-year period (212). However, other patients with initial prompt steroid response have abruptly died of infectious complications (202).

References

1. Centers for Disease Control. Acquired immunodeficiency syndrome (AIDS) update—United States. MMWR 1983; 32:309-11.
2. Hardy D, Wolfe PR, Gottlieb MS, Knight S, Mitsuyasu R, Young LS. Fansidar prophylaxis for *Pneumocystis carinii* pneumonia (PCP). In: The International Conference on the Acquired immunodeficiency Syndrome. Abstracts. Philadelphia: American College of Physicians, 1985.
3. Fauci AS, moderator. Acquired immunodeficiency syndrome: epidemiologic, clinical, immunologic, and therapeutic considerations. Ann Intern Med 1984; 100:92-106.
4. Kovacs JA, Hiemenz MD, Macher AM, et al. *Pneumocystis carinii* pneumonia: a comparison between patients with the acquired immunodeficiency syndrome and patients with other immunodeficiencies. Ann Intern Med 1984; 100:663-71.
5. Murray JF, Felton CP, Garay SM, et al. Pulmonary complications of the acquired immunodeficiency syndrome. N Engl J Med 1984; 310:1682-8.
6. Hopewell PC, Luce JM. Pulmonary involvement in the acquired immunodeficiency syndrome. Chest 1985; 1:104-12.
7. Hughes WT. Pneumocystis carinii. In: Mandell GL, Douglous RG, Bennett JE, eds. Principles and practice of infectious diseases. New York: John Wiley & Sons, 1979:2137-42.
8. Campbell WG Jr. Ultrastructure of *Pneumocystis* in human lung. Arch Pathol 1972; 93:312-24.
9. Hughes WT. *Pneumocystis carinii* pneumonia. N Engl J Med 1977; 297:1381-3.
10. Pifer LL, Hughes WT, Murphy MJ Jr. Propagation of *Pneumocystis carinii in vitro*. Pediatr Res 1977; 11:305-16.
11. Cushion MT, Ruffolo JJ, Linke MJ, Walzer PD. *Pneumocystis carinii*: growth variables and estimates in the A549 and WI-38 VA13 human cell lines. Exp Parasitol 1985; 60:43-54.
12. Masur H, Jones TC. The interactiion in vitro of *Pneumocystis carinii* with macrophages and L-cells. J Exp Med 1978; 147:157-70.

13. Henshaw NG, Carson JL, Collier AM. Ultrastructural observations of *Pneumocystis carinii* attachment to rat lung. J Infect Dis 1985; 151:181-6.
14. Pifer LL, Hughes WT, Stagno S, Woods D. *Pneumocystis carinii* infection: evidence for high prevalence in normal and immunosuppressed children. Pediatrics 1978; 61:35-41.
15. Walzer P, Rutledge ME. Comparison of rat, mouse, and human *Pneumocystis carinii* by immunofluorescence. J Infect Dis 1980; 142:449.
16. Perera DR, Western KA, Johnson HD, Johnson WW, Schultz MG, Akers PV. *Pneumocystis carinii* pneumonia in a hospital for children. JAMA 1970; 214: 1074-8.
17. Watanabe JM, Chinchinian H, Weitz C, McIlvanie SK. *Pneumocystis carinii* pneumonia in a family. JAMA 1965; 193:119-20.
18. Lyons HA, Vinijchaikul K, Hennigar GR. *Pneumocystis carinii* pneumonia unassociated with other disease. Arch Intern Med 1961; 108:173-80.
19. Frenkel JK, Good JT, Schultz JA. Latent Pneumocystis infection of rats, relapse, and chemotherapy. Lab Invest 1966; 15:1559-77.
20. Walzer PD, Schnelle V, Armstrong D, Rosen PP. Nude mouse: a new experimental model for *Pneumocystis carinii* infection. Science 1977; 197:177-9.
21. Hughes WT. Natural mode of acquisition for de novo infection with *Pneumocystis carinii*. J Infect Dis 1982; 145:842-48.
22. Singer C, Armstrong D, Rosen PP, Schottenfeld D. *Pneumocystis carinii* pneumonia: a cluster of eleven cases. Ann Intern Med 1975; 82:772-7.
23. Gentry LO, Remington JS. *Pneumocystis carinii* pneumonia in siblings. J Pediatr 1970; 76:769-71.
24. Giron JA, Martinez S, Walzer PD. Should inpatients with *Pneumocystis carinii* be isolated? Lancet 1982; 2:46.
25. Walzer PD, LaBine M, Redington J, Cushion MT. Lymphocyte changes during chronic administration of and withdrawal from corticosteroids: relation to *Pneumocystis carinii* pneumonia. J Immunol 1984; 133:2502-08.
26. Herrod HG, Valenski WR, Woods DR, Pifer LL. The *in vitro* response of human lymphocytes to *Pneumocystis carinii* antigen. J Immunol 1981; 126:59-61.
27. Furata T, Euda K, Kyuua S, Fujiwara K. Effect of T-cell transfer or *Pneumocystis* infection in nude mice. Jpn J Exp Med 1984; 54:59-64.
28. Furuta T, Ueda K, Fujiwara K, Yamanouchi K. Cellular and humoral immune responses of mice subclinically infected with *Pneumocystis carinii*. Infect Immun 1985; 47:544-8.
29. Price RA, Hughes WT. Histopathology of *Pneumocystis carinii* infestation and infection in malignant disease in childhood. Hum Pathol 1974; 5:737-52.
30. Woodward SC, Sheldon WH. Subclinical *Pneumocystis carinii* pneumonitis in adults. Bull Johns Hopkins Hosp 1961; 109:148-59.
31. Hamlin WB. *Pneumocystis carinii*. JAMA 1968; 204:171-72.
32. Esterly JA. *Pneumocystis carinii* in lungs of adults at autopsy. Am Rev Respir Dis 1968; 97:935-7.
33. Sueishi K, Hisano S, Sumiyoshi A, Tanaka K. Scanning and transmission electron microscopic study of human pulmonary pneumocytosis. Chest 1977; 72: 213-6.

34. Price RA, Hughts WT. Histopathology of *Pneumocystis carinii* infestation and infection in malignant disease in childhood. Hum Pathol 1974; 5:737-52.
35. Barnett RN, Hull JG, Vortel V, Schwarz J. *Pneumocystis carinii* in lymph nodes and spleen. Arch Pathol 1969; 88:175-80.
36. Awen CF, Baltzan MA. Systemic dissemination of *Pneumocystis carinii* pneumonia. CMA J 1971; 10]4:809-12.
37. Rahimi SA. Disseminated *Pneumocystis carinii* in thymic alymphoplasia. Arch Pathol 1974; 97:162-5.
38. Haverkos HW. Assessment of therapy for *Pneumocystis carinii* pneumonia. Am J Med 1984; 76:501-8.
39. Engelberg LA, Lerner CW, Tapper ML. Clinical features of *Pneumocystis* pneumonia in the acquired immune deficiency syndrome. Am Rev Respir Dis 1984; 130:689-94.
40. Golden JA, Opportunistic pulmonary infection in AIDS: modalities of diagnosis and follow-up. Symposium on Acquired Immunodeficiency Syndrome, American Thoracic Society, 1983, Kansas City.
41. Garay SM, Belenko M, Schwiep F, Kamelhar D, Greene J. *Pneumocystis carinii* pneumonia in the acquired immunodeficiency syndrome. In: The International Conference on the Acquired Immunodeficiency Syndrome: Abstracts. Philadelphia: American College of Physicians, 1985.
42. Stern RG, Gamsu G, Golden JA, Hirji M, Webb WR, Abrams DI. Intrathoracic Adenopathy: differential feature of AIDS and diffuse lymphadenopathy syndrome. AJR 1984; 142:689-92.
43. Milligan SA, Stulbarg MS, Gamsu G, Golden J. *Pneumocystis carinii* pneumonia radiographically simulating tuberculosis. Am Rev Respir Dis 1985; 132:1124-6.
44. Brown RKJ, Huberman RP, Vanley G. Pulmonary features of Kaposi sarcoma. AJR 1982; 139:659-60.
45. Kornfeld H, Axelrod JL. Pulmonary presentation of Kaposi's sarcoma in a homosexual patient. Am Rev Respir Dis 1983; 127:248-9.
46. Silverman BA, Rubinstein A. Serum lactate dehydrogenase levels in adults and children with acquired immunodeficiency syndrome (AIDS) and AIDS-related complex: possible indicator of B cell lymphoproliferation and disease activity. Am J Med 1985; 78:728-36.
47. Sanyal SK, Mariencheck WC, Hughes WT, Parvey LS, Tsiatis AA, Mackert PW. Course of pulmonary dysfunction in children surviving *Pneumocystis carinii* pneumonitis. Am Rev Respir Dis 1981; 124:161-6.
48. Catterall JR, Potasman I, Remington JS. *Pneumocystis carinii* pneumonia in the patient with AIDS. Chest 1985; 88:758-62.
49. Stover DE, White DA, Romano PA, Gellene RA, Robeson WA. Spectrum of pulmonary diseases associated with the acquired immunodeficiency syndrome. Am J Med 1985; 78:429-37.
50. Gibson GJ, Pride NB. Lung distensibility: the static pressure-volume curve of the lungs and its use in clinical assessment. Br J Dis Chest 1976; 7:143-84.
51. Weitzman RH, Wilson AF. Diffusing capacity and overall ventilation: perfusion on asthma. Am J Med 1974; 57:767-74.
52. Zapletal A, Motoyana EK, Gibson CE, Bouhuys A. Pulmonary mechanics on asthma and cystic fibrosis. Pediatrics 1971; 48:64-72.

53. Overland ES, Nolan AJ, Hopewell PC. Alteration of pulmonary function on intravenous drug abusers: prevalence, severity, and characterization of gas exchange abnormalities. Am J Med 1980; 68:231-7.
54. Dodek PM, Coleman DL, Golden JA, Luce JM, Murray JF, Gold WM. *Pneumocystis* pneumonia in patients with acquired immunodeficiency syndrome: correlation between pulmonary function testing and fiberoptic bronchoscopy, abstract. Am Rev Respir Dis 1983; 127:81.
54a. Tsan M. Mechanism of gallium-67 accumulation in inflammatory lesions. J Nuc Med 1985; 26:88-92.
54b. Montgomery AB, Lipavsky A, Turner J, Murray JF. Pulmonary extravascular protein accumulation is not affected by continuous positive airway pressure (CPAP). Amer Rev Respir Dis 1987; 135:A168 (Abstract).
55. Coleman DL, Hattner RS, Luce JM, Dodek PM, Golden JA, Murray JF. Correlation between gallium lung scans and fiberoptic bronchoscopy in patients with suspected *Pneumocystis carinii* pneumonia and the acquired immune deficiency syndrome. Am Rev Respir Dis 1984; 130:1166-9.
56. Siemsen JK, Grebe SF, Waxman AD. The use of gallium-67 in pulmonary disorders. Semin Nucl Med 1978; 8:245-9.
57. Liebman R, Ryo UY, Bekerman C, Pinsky SM. Ga-67 scan of a homosexual man with *Pneumocystis carinii* pneumonia. Clin Nuc Med 1982; 10:480-1.
58. Parthasarathy KL, Bakshi S, Bender MA. Radiogallium scan in *P. carinii* pneumonia. Clin Nuc Med 1982; 7:71-4.
59. Levin M, McLeod R, Young Q, Abrahams C, Chambliss M, Walzer P, Kabins SA. *Pneumocystis* pneumonia: importance of Gallium scan for early diagnosis and description of a new immunoperoxidase technique to demonstrate *Pneumocystis carinii*. Am Rev Respir Dis 1983; 128:182-5.
60. Turbiner EH, Yeh SDJ, Rosen PP, Bains MS, Benua RS. Abnormal gallium scintigraphy in *Pneumocystis carinii* pneumonia with a normal chest radiograph. Radiology 1978; 127:437-8.
61. Levenson SM, Warren RD, Richman SD, Johnston GS, Chabner BA. Abnormal pulmonary Gallium accumulation in *P. carinii* pneumonia. Radiology 1978; 127:437-8.
62. Kim H-K, Hughes WT. Comparison of methods for identification of *Pneumocystis carinii* in pulmonary aspirates. Am J Clin Pathol 1973; 60:462-6.
63. Jacobs JB, Vogel C, Powell RD, DeVita VT. Needle biopsy in *Pneumocystis carinii* pneumonia. Radiology 1969; 93:525-30.
64. Johnson HD, Johnson WW. *Pneumocystis carinii* pneumonia in children with cancer. Diagnosis and treatment. JAMA 1970; 214:1067-73.
65. Drew WL, Finley TN, Mintz L, Klein HZ. Diagnosis of *Pneumocystis carinii* pneumonia by bronchopulmonary lavage. JAMA 1974; 230: 713-5.
66. Rifkind D, Faris TD, Hill RB. *Pneumocystis carinii*. Studies on diagnosis and treatment. Ann Intern Med 1966; 65:943-56.
67. Erchul JW, Williams LP, Meighan PP. *Pneumocystis carinii* in hypopharyngeal material. N Engl J Med 1962; 267:926-7.
68. Fortuny IE, Tempero KF, Amsden TW. *Pneumocystis carinii* pneumonia diagnosed from sputum and successfully treated with pentamidine isethionate. Cancer 1970; 26:911-3.

69. Tan-Vihn L, Cochard A-M, Vu-Trieu-Dong, Solonar W. Diagnostic in vivo de la pneumonie a "Pneumocystis." Arch Fr Pediatr 1963; 20:773-92.
70. Coleman Dl, Dodek PM, Luce JM, Golden JA, Gold WM, Murray JF. Diagnostic utility of fiberoptic bronchoscopy in patients with *Pneumocystis carinii* pneumonia and the acquired immune deficiency syndrome. Am Rev Respir Dis 1983; 128:795-99.
71. Broaddus C, Dake MD, Stulbarg MS, et al. Bronchoalveolar lavage and transbronchial biopsy for the diagnosis of pulmonary infections in the Acquired Immunodeficiency Syndrome. Ann Intern Med 1985; 102:747-52.
72. Fulkerson, WJ. Current concepts: fiberoptic bronchoscopy. N Engl J Med 1984; 311:511-15.
73. Zavala D. Pulmonary hemorrhage in fiberoptic transbronchial biopsy. Chest 1976; 70:584-8.
74. Flick G, Barbers R, Gong J. Bedside fiberoptic bronchoscopy and bronchoalveolar lavage for the diagnosis of *Pneumocystis carinii* pneumonia in patients with the Acquired Immunodeficiency Syndrome. Am Rev Respir Dis 1985; 131:A221.
75. Kelley J, Landis JN, Davis GS, Trainer TD, Jakab GJ, Green GM. Diagnosis of pneumonia due to pneumocystis by subsegmental pulmonary lavage via the fiberoptic bronshoscope. Chest 1978; 74:24-8.
76. Stover DE, Zaman MB, Hajdu DI, Lange M, Gold J, Armstrong D. Bronchoalveolar lavage in the diagnosis of diffuse pulmonary infiltrates in the immunosuppressed host. Ann Intern Med 1984; 101:1-7.
77. Stover DE, White DA, Romano PA, Gellene RA. Diagnosis of pulmonary disease in Acquired Immune Deficiency Syndrome (AIDS). Am Rev Respir Dis 1984; 130:659-62.
78. Broaddus C, Dake M, Stulbarg M, Golden J, Hopewell P. Bronchoalveolar lavage in the diagnosis of opportunistic infections in patients with the Acquired Immune Deficiency Syndrome (abstract). Am Rev Respir Dis 1984; 129:A35.
79. Ognibene FP, Shelhamer J, Bill V, et al. The diagnosis of *Pneumocystis carinii* pneumonia in patients with the Acquired Immunodeficiency Syndrome, using subsegmented bronchoalveolar lavage. Am Rev Respir Dis 1984; 129:929-32.
80. Orenstein M, Webber CA. Pulmonary infections in Acquired Immunodeficiency Syndrome diagnostic yield utilizing fiberoptic bronchoscopy and bronchoalveolar lavage (abstract). Am Rev Respir Dis 1984; 129:A188.
81. Dake M, Broaddus C, Stulbarg M, Golden J, Hopewell P. The spectrum of opportunistic *Pneumocystis carinii* pneumonia in patients with Acquired Immune Deficiency Syndrome. Am Rev Respir Dis 1984; 129:A188.
82. Caughey H, Wong H, Gamsu G, Golden JA. Nonbronchoscopic bronchoalveolar lavage for the diagnosis of *Pneumocystis carinii* pneumonia in the Acquired Immunodeficiency Syndrome. Chest 1985; 88:659-62.
84. Keogh Ba, Crystal RG. Alveolitis: The key to the interstitial lung disorders. Thorax 1982; 37:1-10.
85. Bigby T, Margolskee D, Curtis J, et al. The usefulness of induced sputum in the diagnosis of *Pneumocystis carinii* pneymonia in patients with Acquired Immunodeficiency Syndrome. Am Rev Respir Dis 1985; 131:A222.

86. Meyers JD, Pifer LL,, Sale GE, Thomas ED. The value of *Pneumocystis carinii* pneumonia after marrow transplantation. Am Rev Resp Dis 1979; 120:1283-7.
87. Maddison SE, Hayes GV, Slemenda SB, Norman LG, Ivey MH. Detection of specific antibody by enzyme-linked immunosorbent assay and antigenemia by counterimmunoelectrophoresis in humans infected with *Pneumocystis carinii*. J Clin Microbiol 1982; 15:1036-43.
88. Pifer LL. Serodiagnosis of *Pneumocystis carinii*. Chest 1985; 87:698-9.
89. Naharian JS, Ascher NL. Pulmonary complications of AIDS. N Engl J Med 1984; 311:1182-3.
90. Winston DJ, Lau WK, Gale RP, Young LS. Trimethoprim-sulfamethoxazole for treatment of *Pneumocystis carinii* pneumonia. Ann Intern Med 1980; 92:762-9.
91. Walzer PD, Perl DP, Krogslad DJ, Rawson PG, Schultz MG. *Pneumocystis carinii* pneumonia in the United States: epidemiologic, diagnostic, and clinical features. Ann Intern Med 1974; 80:83-9.
92. Western KA, Perera DR, Schultz MG. Pentamidine isethionate in the treatment of *Pneumocystis carinii* pneumonia. Ann Intern Med 1970; 73:695-702.
93. Hughes WT, McNabb PC, Macues TD, Feldman S. Efficacy of trimethoprim and sulfamethoxazole in the prevention and treatment of *Pneumocystis carinii* pneumonitis agents. Antimicrob Agents Chemother 1974; 5:289-93.
94. Hughes WT, Feldman S, Sanyal SK. Treatment of *Pneumocystis carinii* pneumonitis with trimethoprim-sulfamethoxazole. Can Med Assoc J 1975; 112 (suppl): 47S-50S.
95. Lau WK, Young LS. Trimethopeim-Sulfamethoxazole treatment of *Pneumocystis carinii* pneumonia in adults. N Engl J Med 1976; 295:716-8.
96. Hughes WT, Feldman S, Chaudhary SC, Ossi MJ, Cox F, Sanyal SK. Comparison of pentamidine isethionate and trimethoprim-sulfamethoxazole in the treatment of *Pneumocystis carinii* pneumonia. J Pediatr 1978; 92:285-91.
97. Steinbrook R, Lo B, Moulton J, Saika G, Hollander H, Volberding PA. Preferences of homosexual men with AIDS for life-sustaining treatment. N Eng J Med 1986; 314:457-60.
98. Wharton JM, Coleman DL, Wofsy CB, Luce JM, Blumenfeld W, Hadley WK, et al. Trimethoprim-sulfamethoxazole or pentamidine for *Pneumocystis carinii* pneumonia in the acquired immunodeficiency syndrome. Ann Intern Med 1986; 105:37-44.
99. Wharton M, Coleman DL, Fitz G, et al. Prospective randomized trial of trimethoprim-sulfamethoxazole versus pentamidine for *Pneumocystis carinii* pneumonia on the Acquired Immunodeficiency Syndrome (abstract). Am Rev Respir Dis 1984; 129:188A.
100. Gordin FM, Simon GL, Wofsy CB, Mills J. Adverse reactions to trimethoprim-sulfamethoxazole in patients with the acquired immunodeficiency syndrome. Ann Intern Med 1984; 100:495-99.
101. Jaffe HS, Abrams DI, Ammann AJ, Lewis BJ, Golden TA. Complications of Co-trimoxazole treatment oi AIDS-associated *Pneumocystis carinii* pneumonia on homosexual men. Lancet 1983; 11:1109-11.

102. Golde DW, Bersch N, Quan SG. Trimethoprim and sulphamethoxa-zole inhibition of hematopoiesis *in vitro*. Br J Haematol 1978; 40:363-7.
103. Small CB, Garris CA, Friedland GH, Klein RS. The treatment of *Pneumocystis carinii* pneumonia in the acquired immunodeficiency syndrome (abstract). Am Rev Respir Dis 1984; 129:188A.
104. Kinzie BJ, Taylor JW. Trimethoprim and folinic acid. Ann Intern Med 1984; 101:565.
105. Outwater E, McCutchan JA. Neutrophil-associated antibodies and granulocytopenia in the sulfonamide reaction in AIDS. In: The International Conference on the Acquired Immunodeficiency Syndrome. Abstracts. Philadelphia: American College of Physicians, 1985.
106. Sklarek HM, Mantovani RP, Erens E, Heisler D, Niederman MS, Fein AM. AIDS in a bodybuilder using anabolic steroids. N Engl J Med 1984; 311:1701.
107. Suster M, Dunn M. Pentamidine and hematuria. Ann Intern Med 1986; 105:146.
108. Salmeron S, Petitpretz P, Katlama C, Herve P, Brivet F, Simonneau G, et al. Pentamidine and pancreatitis. Ann Intern Med 1986; 105:140-1.
109. Waldman RH, Pearce DE, Martin RA. Pentamidine isothionate levels in lungs, livers, and kidneys of rats after aerosol or intramuscular administration. Am Rev Resp Dis 1973; 108:1004-6.
110. Bernard EM, Donnelly HJ, Koo HP, Armstrong D. Aerosol administration improves delivery of pentamidine to the lungs (abstract). In: Program and Abstracts of the 25th Interscience Conference on Antimicrobial Agents and Chemotherapy, 1985, No. 552, p. 193.
110a. Debs RJ, Blumenfeld W, Brunette EN, et al. Successful treatment with aerosolized pentamidine of Pneumocystis carinii pneumonia in rats. Antimicrobe Agents Chemother 1987; 31:37-41.
110b. Golden JA, Hollander H, Conte JE. Inhaled pentamidine or low-dose intravenous pentamidine as novel therapy for Pneumocystis carinii pneumonia in the acquired immunodeficiency syndrome. Amer Rev Respir Dis 1987; 135:A168 (Abstract)
110c. Conte JE, Hollander H, Golden JA. Inhaled or redduced intravenous pentamidine for Pneumocystis carinii pneumonia: a pilot study. Ann Int Med 1987; 107:495-8.
110d. Montgomery AB, Luce JM, Turner J, Lin ET, Debs RJ, Corkery KJ, et al. Aerosolized pentamidine as sole therapy for Pneumocystis carinii pneumonia in patients with acquired immunodeficiency syndrome. Lancet 1987; 2:480.
111. Sterling RP, Bradley BB, Khalil KG, Kerman RH, Conklin RH. Comparison of biopsy-proven *Pneumocystis carinii* pneumonia in acquired immune deficiency syndrome patients and renal allograft recipients. Ann Thorac Surg 1985; 38:494-8.
112. Armstrong D, Gold JWM, Dryjanski J, et al. Treatment of infections in patients with the Acquired Immunodeficiency Syndrome. Ann Intern Med 1985; 103:738-43.
113. Delorenzo LJ, Maguire GP, Wormser GP, Davidian M, Stone DJ. Persistence of *Pneumocystis carinii* pneumonia in the Acquired Immunodeficiency Syn-

drome. In: The International Conference on the Acquired Immunodeficiency Syndrome. Abstracts. Philadelphia: American College of Physicians, 1985.

114. Shelhamer JH, Ognibene GP, Macher AM, et al. Persistence of *Pneumocystis carinii* in lung tissue of acquired immunodeficiency syndrome patients treated for *Pneumocystis* pneumonia. Am Rev Respir Dis 1984; 130:1161-5.

115. Michael P, Brodie H, Wharton M, Bryan C, Wofsy C, Hopewell P. Significance of persistence of *P. carinii* after completion of treatment. In: The International Conference on the Acquired Immunodeficiency Syndrome: Abstracts. Philadelphia: American College of Physicians, 1985.

116. Kluge RM, Spaulding CM, Spain AJ. Combination of pentamidine and trimethoprim-sulfamethoxazole in the therapy of *Pneumocystis carinii* pneumonia on rats. Antimicrob Agents Chemother 1978; 13:975-8.

117. Foltzer MA, Hannan SE, Kozak AJ. *Pneumocystis* pneumonia: respone to corticosteroids. JAMA 1985; 253:979.

118. Rifkind D, Starzl TE, Marchioro TL, Waddell WR, Rowlands DT, Hill RB. Transplantation pneumonia. JAMA 1964; 189:114-8.

119. Slapak M, Lee HM, Hume DM. Transplat lung—a new syndrome. B Med J 1968; 1:80-4.

120. Shafer RW, Offit K, Mecris NT, Horbar GM, Ancona L, Hoffman IR. Possible risk of steroid administration in patients at risk for AIDS. Lancet 1985; 1:934-5.

121. Golden JA, Sjoerdsma A, Santi DV. *Pneumocystis carinii* pneumonia treated with difluoromethylornithine—a prospective study among patients with the acquired immunodeficiency syndrome. West J Med 1984; 141:613-23.

122. Giri SN, Hyde DM, Schwartz LW, Younker WR. The effect of a difluoromethylornithine on the development of bleomycin-induced pulmonary fribosis in hamsters. Am J Pathol 1982; 109:115-22.

123. Hughes, WT. Developmental therapeutics for *Pneumocystis carinii* pneumonia (PCP). In: The International Conference on the Acquired Immunodeficiency Syndrome. Abstracts. Philadelphia: American College of Physicians, 1985.

124. Richardson S, Fanning M, Bruton J, Salit I, Read S, Shepherd F. Diaminodiphenylsulfone (Dapsone) as treatment for *Pneumocystis carinii* pneumonia in AIDS patients in combination with trimethoprim. In: The International Conference on the Acquired Immunodeficiency Syndrome. Abstracts. Philadelphia: American College of Physicians, 1985.

125. Leoung Gs, Mills J, Hughes W, Hopewell P, Wofsy C. Treatment of first Episode *Pneumocystis carinii* pneumonia (PCP) in AIDS patients with dapsone and trimethoprim (DS/TMP). In: The International Conference on the Acquired Immunodeficiency Syndrome. Abstracts. Philadelphia: American College of Physicians, 1985.

126. Leoung GS, Mills J, Hopewell PC, Hughes W, Wofsy C. Dapsone-trimethoprim for *Pneumocystis carinii* pneumonia in the acquired immunodeficiency syndrome. Ann Intern Med 1986; 105:45-8.

127. Mills J, Leoung G, Medina I, Hughes W, Hopewell P, Wofsy C. Dapsone is less effective than standard therapy for Pneumocystis pneumonia in AIDS patients. (abstract). Am Rev Respir Dis 1986; 133:A184.

128. Hughes WT, Kuhn S, Chaudhary S, et al. Successful chemoprophylaxis for *Pneumocystis carinii* pneumonitis. N Engl J Med 1977; 297:1419-25.
129. Gottlieb MS, Knight S, Mitsuyasu R, Weisman J, Roth M, Young LS. prophylaxis of *Pneumocystis carinii* infection in AIDS with pyrimethamine-sulfadoxine. Lancet, 1984; 2:398-99.
130. Kirby HB, Kenamore B, Guckian JC. *Pneumocystis carinii* pneumonia treated with pyrimethamine and sulfadiazine. Ann Intern Med 1971; 75:505-9.
131. Post C, Fakouhi T, Dutz W, Bandarizadeh B, Kohout EE. Prophylaxis of epidemic infantile pneumocystis with a 20:1 sulfadoxine + pyrimethamine combination. Curr Ther Research 1971; 13:273-9.
132. Navin TR, Miller KD, Satriale RF, Lobel HO. Adverse reactions associated with pyrimethamine-sulfadoxine prophylaxis for *Pneumocystis carinii* infections in AIDS. Lancet, 1985; 1:1332.
133. Lazar HP, Murphy RL, Phair JP. Fansidar and hepatic granulomas. Ann Intern Med 1985; 102:722.
134. Vital C, Vital A, Vignoly B, et al. Cytomegalovirus encephalitis in a patient with acquired immunodeficiency syndrome. Arch Pathol Lab Med 1985; 109:105-6.
135. Edwards RH, Messing R, McKendall RR. Cytomegalovirus meningoencephalitis in a homosexual man with Kaposi's sarcoma: Isolation of CMV from CSF cells. Neurology 1985; 35:560-2.
136. Pass HI, Potter DA, Macher AM, et al. Thoracic ma ifestations of the acquired immune deficiency syndrome. J Thorac Cardiovasc Surg 1984; 88:654-8.
137. Blackman E, Vimadalal S, Nash G. Significance of gastrointestinal cytomegalovirus infection in homosexual males. Am J Gastoenterol 1984; 79:935-40.
138. Friedman AH, Freeman WR, Orellana j, Kraushar MF, Starr MB, Luntz MH. Cytomegalovirus retinitis and immunodeficiency in homosexual males. Lancet 1982; 1:958.
139. Jampol LM. ocular findings of acute cytomegalovirus infection. N Eng J Med 1982; 307:1584.
140. Guenthner EE, Rabinowe SL, Van Niel A, naftilan A, Dluhy RG. Primary Addison's disease in a patient with the acquired immunodeficiency syndrome. Ann Intern Med 1984; 100:847.
141. Tapper ML, Rotterdam HZ, Lerner CW, Al'Khafaji K, Seitzman PA. Adrenal necrosis in the acquired immunodeficiency syndrome. Ann Intern Med 1984; 100:239.
142. Greene LW, Cole W, Greene JB, et al. Adrenal insufficiency as a complication of the Acquired Immunodeficiency Syndrome. Ann Intern Med 1984; 101:494-8.
143. Cohen JI, Corey GR. Cytomegalovirus infection in the normal host. Medicine 1985; 64:100-13.
144. Reddehase MJ, Weiland F, Munch K, Jonjic S, Luske A, Koszinowski UH. Interstitial murine cytomegalovirus pneumonia after irradiation: characterization of cells that limit viral replication during established infection of the lungs. J Virol 1985; 55:264-73.
145. Quinnan GV, Kirmani N, Rook AH, et al. Cytotoxic T cells in cytomegalovirus infection. N Engl J Med 1982; 307:7-13.

146. Shanley JD, Ballas ZK. Alteration of bronchoalveolar cells during murine cytomegalovirus interstitial pneumonitis. Am Rev Respir Dis 1985; 132:77-81.
147. Miller SA, Bia FJ, Coleman DL, Lucia HL, Young KR, Root RK. Pulmonary macrophage function during experimental cytomegalovirus interstitial pneumonia. Infect Immun 1985; 47:211-6.
148. Craighead JE. Pulmonary cytomegalovirus in the adult. Am J Pathol 1971; 3:487-99.
149. Golden JA. Cytomegalovirus infection or disease. Ann Intern Med 1984; 101:882.
150. Levy JA, Hopewell PC, Wofsy C, Mills J. Acquired immune deficiency syndrome. Am Rev Respir Dis 1985; 132:1337-8.
151. Myerson D, Hackman RC, Meyers JD. Diagnosis of cytomegaloviral pneumonia by in situ hybridization. J Infect Dis 1984; 150:272-7.
152. Myerson D, Hackman RC, Nelson JA, Ward DC, McDougall JK. Widespread presence of histologically occult cytomegalovirus. Hum Pathol 1984; 15:430-9.
153. Stover DE, White DA, Romano PA, Gellene RA. Diagnosis of pulmonary disease in acquired immune deficiency syndrome (AIDS); role of bronchoscopy and bronchoalveolar lavage. Am Rev Respir Dis 1984; 130:659-62.
154. Macher AM, Reichert CM, Straus SE, et al. Death in the AIDS patient: role of cytomegalovirus. N Engl J Med 1983; 309-1454.
155. Brodie HR, Broaddus C, Blumenfeld W, Hopewell PC, Moss A, Mills J. Is cytomegalovirus (CMV) a cause of lung disease in patients with AIDS? In: The International Conference on the Acquired Immunodeficiency Syndrome. Abstracts. Philadelphia; American College of Physicians, 1985.
156. Reichert CM, O'Leary TJ, Levens DL, Simrell CR, Macher AM. Autopsy pathology in the acquired immune deficiency syndromw. Am J Pathol 1983; 112:357-82.
157. Masur H, Lane HC, Palestine A, et al. Effect of 9-(1,3-dihydroxy-2-propoxymethyl) quanine on serious cytomegalovirus desease in eight immunosuppressed homosexual men. Ann Intern Med 1986; 104:41-4.
158. Brodie HR, Drew WL, Hopewell PC, Weinberg P, Golden JA, Wilber J. Adenovirus pneumonis in homosexual males. Am Rev Respir Dis 1984; 129:A188.
159. Macher AM, Kovacs JA, Gill V, et al. Baceremia due to *Mycobacterium avium-intracellulare* in the acquired immunodeficiency syndrome. Ann Intern Med 1983; 99:782-5.
160. Parker BC, Ford MA, Gruft H, Falkinham JO. Epidemiology of infection by nontuberculous mycobacteria. IV. Preferential aerosolization of *Mycobacterium Intracellulare* from natural waters. Am Rev Respir Dis 1983; 128:652-6.
161. Berlin OGW, Zakowski P, Bruckner DA, Clancy MN, Johnson BL. *Mycobacterium avium:* a pathogen of patients with acquired immunodeficiency syndrome. Diagn Microbiol Infect Dis 1984; 2:213-8.
162. Horsburgh CR, Mason UG, Farhi DC, Iseman MD. Disseminated infection with *Mycobacterium avium-intracellulare*. Medicine 1985; 64:36-48.
163. Winter SM, Bernard EM, Gold JWM, Armstrong D. Humoral response to dissimented infection by *Mycobacterium avium-Mycobacterium intracellulare* in acquired immunodeficiency syndrome and hairy cell leukemia. J Infect Dis 1985; 151:523-27.

164. Kiehn TE, Edwards FF, Brannon P, et al. Infections caused by *Mycobacterium avium* complex in immunocompromised patients: diagnosis by blood culture and fecal examination, antimicrobial susceptibility tests, and morphological and seroagglutination characteristics. J Clin Microbiol 1985; 21:168-73.
165. Strom RL, Gruninger RP. AIDS with *Mycobacterium avium-intracellulare* lesions resembling those of Whipple's disease. N Engl J Med 1983; 309:1323-4.
166. Giron JA, Mandel LJ, Wollschlager C, et al. Mycobacterial culture in acquired immunodeficiency syndrome. Ann Intern Med 1983; 98:1028-9.
167. Cohen RJ, Samoszuk MK, Busch D, Lagios M. occult infections with *M. intracellulare* in bone-marrow biopsy specimens from patients with AIDS. N Engl J Med 1983; 308:1475-6.
168. Greene JB, Sidhu GS, Lewin S, et al. *Mycobacterium avium-intracellulare*: a cause of disseminated life-threatening infection in homosexuals and drug abusers. Ann Intern Med 1982; 97:539-46.
169. Sunderam G, McDonald RJ, Maniatis T, Oleske J, Kapila R, Reichman LB. Tuberculosis as a manifestation of the acquired immunodeficiency syndrome (AIDS). JAMA 1986; 256:362-6.
170. Nash G, Fligiel S. pathologic features of the lung in the acquired immune deficiency syndrome (AIDS): an autopsy study of seventeen homosexual males. Am J Clin Pathol 1984; 81:6-12.
171. Wong B, Edwards FF, Kiehn TE, et al. Continuous high-grade *Mycobacterium avium-intracellulare* bacteremia in patients with the acquired immune deficiency syndrome. Am J Med 1985; 78:35-40.
172. Mizuguchi Y, Udou T, Yamada T. Mechanism of antibiotic resistance in *Mycobacterium intracellulare*. Microbiol Immunol 1983; 27:425-31.
173. Mess TP, Hadley WK, Wofsy CB. Bacteremia due to *Mycobacterium* tuberculosis (MTS) and *Mycobacterium avium intracellulare* (MAI) in homosexual males. In: The International Conference on the Acquired Immunodeficiency Syndrome. Abstracts. Philadelphia: American College of Physicians, 1985.
174. Pitchenik AE, Cole C, Russell BW, Fischl MA, Spira TJ, Snider DE. Tuberculosis, atypical mycobacteriosis, and the acquired immunodeficiency syndrome among Haitian and non-Haitian patients in South Florida. Ann Intern Med 1984; 101:641-5.
175. Schlanger G, Lutwick LI, Kurzman M, Hoch B, Chandler FW. Sinusitis caused by *Legionella pneumophila* in a patient with the acquired immune deficiency syndrome. Am J Med 1984; 77:957-60.
176. Lane HC, Masur H, Edgar LC, et al. Abnormalities of B-cell activation and immunoregulation in patients with the acquired immunodeficiency syndrome. N Engl J Med 1983; 309:453-8.
177. Ammann AJ, Schiffman G, Abrams D, Volberding P, Ziegler J, Conant M. B-cell immunodeficiency in acquired immune deficiency syndrome. JAMA 1983; 251:1447-9.
178. Garbowit DL, Alsip SG, Griffin FM. *Hemophilus influenzae* bacteremia in a patient with immunodeficiency caused by HTLV-III. N Engl j Med 1986; 314:56.
179. Simberkoff MS, El Sadr W, Schiffman G, Rahall JJ. *Streptococcus pneumoniae* infections and bacteremia in patients with acquired immune deficiency syndrome,

with report of a pneumococcal vaccine failure. Am Rev Respir Dis 1984; 130: 1174-6.

180. Kolsky B, Gold JWM, Whimbey E, et al. Bacterial pneumonia in patients with the acquired immunodeficiency syndrome. Ann Intern Med 1986; 104:38-41.
181. Bonner JR, Alexander WJ, Dismukes WE, et al. Disseminated histoplasmosis in patients with the acquired immune deficiency syndrome. Arch Intern Med 1984; 144:2178-81.
182. Abrams DI, Robia M, Blumenfeld W, Simonson J, Cohen MB, Hadley WK. Disseminated coccidioidomycosis in AIDS. N Engl J Med 1984; 310:986-7.
183. Ma P, Villanueva TG, Kaufman D, Gillooley JF. Respiratory cryptosporidiosis in the acquired immune deficiency syndrome; use of modified cold kinyoun and hemacolor stains for rapid diagnoses. JAMA 1984; 252:1298-301.
184. Forgacs P, Tarshis A, Ma P, et al. Intestinal and bronchial cryptosporidiosis in an immunodeficient homosexual man. Ann Intern Med 1983; 99:793-4.
185. Kocoshis SA, Cibull ML, Davis TE, et al. Intestinal and pulmonary cryptosporidiosis in an infant with severe combined immune deficiency. J Pediatr Gastroenterol Nutr 1984; 3:149-59.
186. Misra DP, Sunderrajan EV, Hurst DJ, Maltby JD. Kaposi's sarcoma of the lung: radiography and pathology. Thorax 1982; 37:155-6.
187. Ognibene FP, Steis RG, Macher AM, et al. Kaposi's sarcoma causing pulmonary infiltrates and respiratory failure in the acquired immunodeficiency syndrome. Ann Intern Med 1985; 102:471-5.
188. Garay SM, Belenko M, Fazzini E, Schinella R. Pulmonary Kaposi's sarcoma in the Acquired Immunodeficiency Syndrome. In: The International Conference on the Acquired Immuno-deficiency Syndrome. Abstracts. Philadelphia: American College of Physicians, 1985.
189. Welch K, Finkbeiner W, Alpers CE, et al. Autopsy findings in the acquired immune deficiency syndrome. JAMA 1984; 252:1152-9.
190. Pitchenik AE, Fischl MA, Saldana MJ. Kaposi's sarcoma of the tracheobronchial tree: clinical, bronchoscopic and pathologic features. Chest 1985; 87:122-4.
191. Nash G, Fligiel S. Kaposi's sarcoma presenting as pulmonary disease in the acquired immunodeficiency syndrome: diagnosis by lung biopsy. Hum Pathol 1984; 15:999-1001.
192. Rucker L, Meador J. Kaposi's sarcoma presenting as homogeneous pulmonary infiltrates in a patient with acquired immunodeficiency syndrome. West J Med 1985; 142:831-3.
193. Ciment LM, Rotbart A, Blaustein A, Galbut RN, Grieder D. Asthma, Kaposi's sarcoma, and nodular pulmonary infiltrates. Ches 1983; 84:281-2.
194. Touboul JL, Mayayd CM, Fouret P, Akoun GM. Pulmonary lesions of Kaposi's sarcoma, intra-alveolar hemorrhage, and pleural effusion. Ann Intern Med 1985; 103:808.
195. McCauley DI, Naidich DP, Leitman BS, Reede DL, Laubenstein L. Radiographic patterns of opportunistic lung infections and Kaposi sarcoma in homosexual men. AJR 1982; 139:653-8.
196. Hill CA, Harle TS, Mansell PWA. The prodrome, Kaposi sarcoma, and infections associated with acquired immunodeficiency syndrome: radiologic findings in 39 patients. Radiology 1983; 149:393-9.

197. Schoeppel SL, Hoppe RT, Dorfman RF, et al. Hodgkin's disease in homosexual men with generalized lymphadenopathy. Ann Intern Med 1985; 102:68-70.
198. Ziegler JL, Beckstead JA, Volberding PA, et al. Non-Hodgkin's lymphoma in 90 homosexual men: relation to generalized lymphadenopathy and the acquired immunodeficiency syndrome. N Eng J Med 1984; 311:565-70.
199. Joshi VV, Oleske JM, Minnefor AB, Saad S, Klein KM, Singh R, et al. Pathologic pulmonary findings in children with the acquired immunodeficiency syndrome. Hum Pathol 1985; 16:241-6.
200. Scott GB, Buck BE, Leterman JG, Bloom FL, Parks WP. Acquired immunodeficiency syndrome in infants. N Engl J Med 1984; 310:76-81.
201. Saldana MJ, Mones JM, Scott GB, Fischl MA. Lymphoid interstitial pneumonia in the acquired immunodeficiency syndrome. In: The International Conference on the Acquired Immunodeficiency Syndrome. Abstracts. Philadelphia: American College of Physicians, 1985.
202. Solal-Celigny P, Couderc LJ, Herman D, Herve P, Schaffar-Deshayes L, Brun-Vezinet F. Lymphoid interstitial pneumonitis in acquired immunodeficiency syndrome-related complex. Am Rev Respir Dis 1985; 131:956-60.
203. Oleske J, Minnefor A, Cooper R, Thomas K, delaa Cruz A, Ahdieh H, et al. Immune deficiency syndrome in children. JAMA 1983; 249:2345-9.
204. Grieco MH, Chinoy-Acharya P. Lymphocytic interstitial pneumonia associated with the acquired immune deficiency syndrome. Am Rev Respir Dis 1985; 131:952-5.
205. Strimlan CV, Rosenow EC, Weiland LH, Brown LR. Lymphocytic interstitial pneumonia. Ann Intern Med 1978; 88:616-21.
206. Church JA, Isaacs H, Saxon A, Keens TG, Richards W. Lymphoid interstitial pneumoitis and hypogammaglubulinemia in children. Am Rev Respir Dis 1981; 124:491-6.
207. O'Brodovich HM, Moser MM, Lu L. Familial lymphoid interstitial pneumonia: a long-term follow-up. Pediatrics 1980; 65:523-8.
208. Church JA, Nye CA, Isaacs H. Lymphocyte subsets in lymphoid interstitial pneumonitis. Arch Pathol Lab Med 1984; 108:861-50.
209. Lovell D, Lindsley C, Langston C. Lymphoid interstitial pneumonia in juvenile rheumatoid arthritis. J Pediat 1984; 105:947-50.
210. Couderc LJ, Materon S, Solal-Celigny PH, Caubarrere I, Saimot AG, Clauvel JP, et al. Lymphoid interstitial pneumonitis (LIP) in Haitians and Africans: an AIDS-linked entity? In: The International Conference on the Acquired Immunodeficiency Syndrome. Abstracts. Philadelphia: American College of Physicians, 1985.
211. Saldana MJ, Mones J, Buck BE. Lymphoid interstitial pneumonia in Haitian residents of Florida. Chest 1984; 84:347.
212. Kornstien MJ, Pietra GG, Hoxie JA, Conley ME. Pathology and treatment of interstitial pneumonitis in two infants with AIDS. Am Rev Respir Dis 1986; 133:1196-8.
213. Scully RE, Mark EJ, McNeely BU. Case records of the Massachusetts General Hospital. N Engl J Med 1986; 314:629-40.

214. Ziza JM, Brun-Vezinet F, Venet A, Rouzioux CH, Traversat J, Israel-Biet B, et al. Lymphadenopathy-associated virus isolated from bronchoalveolar lavage fluid in AIDS-related complex with lymphoid interstitial pneumonitis. N Engl J Med 1985; 313:183.

17

Hairy Leukoplakia and Other Oral Features of HIV Infection

John S. Greenspan
School of Dentistry
and School of Medicine
University of California
San Francisco, California

Deborah Greenspan
School of Dentistry
University of California
San Francisco, California

I. Introduction

The oral cavity may be the location of the first signs and symptoms of many diseases. This fact is particularly true in the case of human immunodeficiency virus (HIV) infection. Among the earliest descriptions of acquired immunodeficiency syndrome (AIDS) was included the mention of oral lesions of Kaposi's sarcoma (KS), oral candidiasis, and chronic herpes simplex (1). This observation should not be surprising, because the oral cavity and its surrounding structures are well known to be particularly prone to the effects of opportunistic infections and neoplasia. For example, these diseases are common in individuals with leukemia, kidney transplant and bone marrow recipients, and other patients receiving chemotherapy (2). Many physicians have not had the opportunity to become familiar with oral soft tissue examination. Furthermore, neither they nor most dentists see the full range of oral manifestations of disease with any frequency. This unfamiliarity with oral lesions, which are the subject of this chapter, can lead to their underdiagnosis or misdiagnosis. Therefore, we wish to emphasize that a thorough oral examination by a clinician familiar with oral soft tissue disease is an important part of the workup of any patient suspected of having HIV infection. The oral examination should include careful assessment of all mucosal surfaces with an adequate light source, a mouth mirror, examination gloves, and the use of guaze squares to hold and extend the tongue. The clinician should assess the color, contour, and consistency of the mucosa and the presence of abnormalities including lesions and also dryness (xerostomia). The gingiva and periodontium should be included. Any oral lesions discovered should be investigated using smears, culture, or biopsy where indicated.

Oral lesions may fall into several of the Centers for Disease Control (CDC) groups of manifestations of HIV infection (3). Oral ulceration may be part of group 1: acute infection associated with seroconversion. Group 4, subgroup C, category C 2, includes oral hairy leukoplakia and oral candidiasis, while subgroup D includes oral KS and oral lesions of AIDS-associated lymphoma.

Oral lesions of HIV infection have been classified as fungal, bacterial, viral, neoplastic, and of unknown etiology (4). These have been described in detail elsewhere (5-9). In this chapter we will concentrate on those lesions that can reflect the course of HIV infection.

II. Oral Hairy Leukoplakia

Oral hairy leukoplakia (HL) is a white lesion that was first seen in San Francisco in 1981 in a group of homosexual men (10). Over 300 cases have now been observed in San Francisco and HL has been seen in different parts of the United States and in many areas of the world including Europe, South America, and Africa (11-14).

A. Clinical Appearance

Hairy leukoplakia appears on the lateral margin of the tongue and sometimes on the buccal or labial mucosa and floor of the mouth [Figs. 1, 2 (Plates III, IV, facing page 357), and 3]. It is white and does not rub off. The surface may be smooth, corrugated, or markedly prolific with projections giving a "hairy" appearance. The corrugations tend to run vertically along the lateral margin of the tongue. The lesion may appear on the lateral margins of the tongue either unilaterally or bilaterally, in one or more small areas, or in a

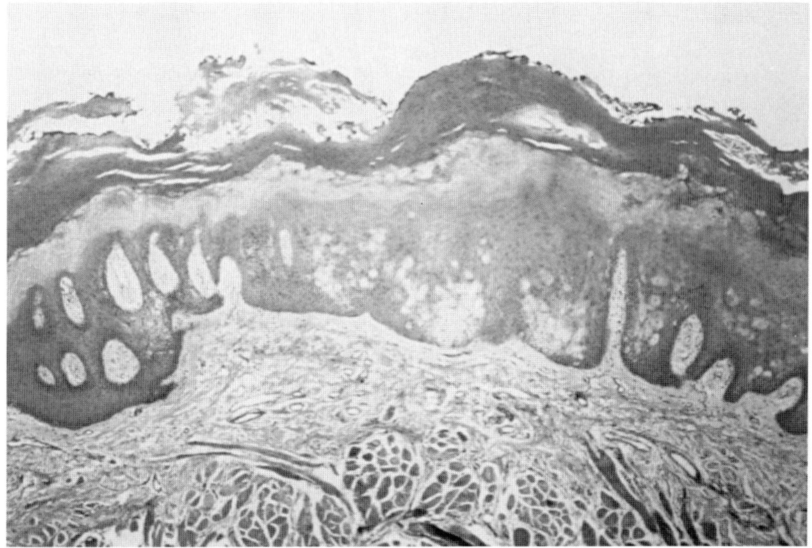

Figure 3 Histopathology of hairy leukoplakia showing surface corrugations, acanthosis, and koilocytosis. No round cell infiltrate is present. Original magnification multi X16.

single, extensive area. It may extend onto the ventral suface of the tongue, where it may appear flat, and also onto the dorsal surface of the tongue, where it appears "hairy."

B. *Candida* and Hairy Leukoplakia

At first, the lesion was thought to be a form of candidiasis, and indeed it may have been included in several reports of oral lesions in AIDS and AIDS-related complex (ARC). *Candida albicans* was found in a smear and culture in 71 of 140 patients studied (15). All the smears and cultures became negative after antifungal therapy, but the lesions did not disappear.

C. Histopathology

Biopsy (Figure 4) reveals a characteristic appearance with folds or "hairs," hyperparakeratosis, acanthosis, vacuolation of bands or clumps of prickle cells, and little, if any, subepithelial inflammation (10,11). Further studies have revealed some immunocytochemical and ultrastructural appearances suggestive of a papillomavirus (Figure 5), although we have not yet identified human papillomavirus (HPV) DNA in Southern blot on in situ hybridization

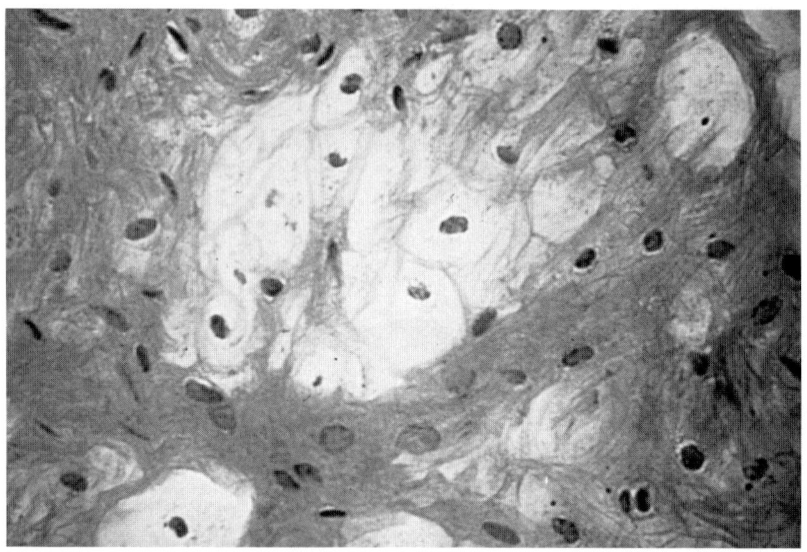

Figure 4 Histopathology of hairy leukoplakia showing details of koilocytes. Original magnification X40.

(Greenspan J., et al., unpublished data). The presence of Epstein-Barr virus (EBV) has been established using multiple techniques (15) (see below).

D. Electron Microscopy

Electron microscopic examination of specimens from 25 patients, which involved the viewing of at least 150 epithelial cells, revealed (in each specimen) some prickle cells with individual structures whose appearance resembled that of individual papillomavirus particles in genital condylomata, reported in some studies (16,17). These structures were polygonal particles, approximately 46-52 nm in diameter, with a poorly defined internal structure. They were observed only within nuclei. Arrays resembling those of typical papillomavirus particles (18) were seen in a few specimens. Twenty-three of the 25 specimens showed numerous particles of the herpes-type virus described previously (10). These were 100-nm naked capsids within the prickle-cell nuclei, accompanied in nine cases by numerous arrays of ill-defined particles (65-75 nm in diameter) (Figure 5). Enveloped virions (150-200 nm in diameter) were seen in the cytoplasm and in the intercellular spaces. Both herpes-type virus particles and papillomavirus-like particles were seen in the same epithelial cells in three specimens (Figure 5).

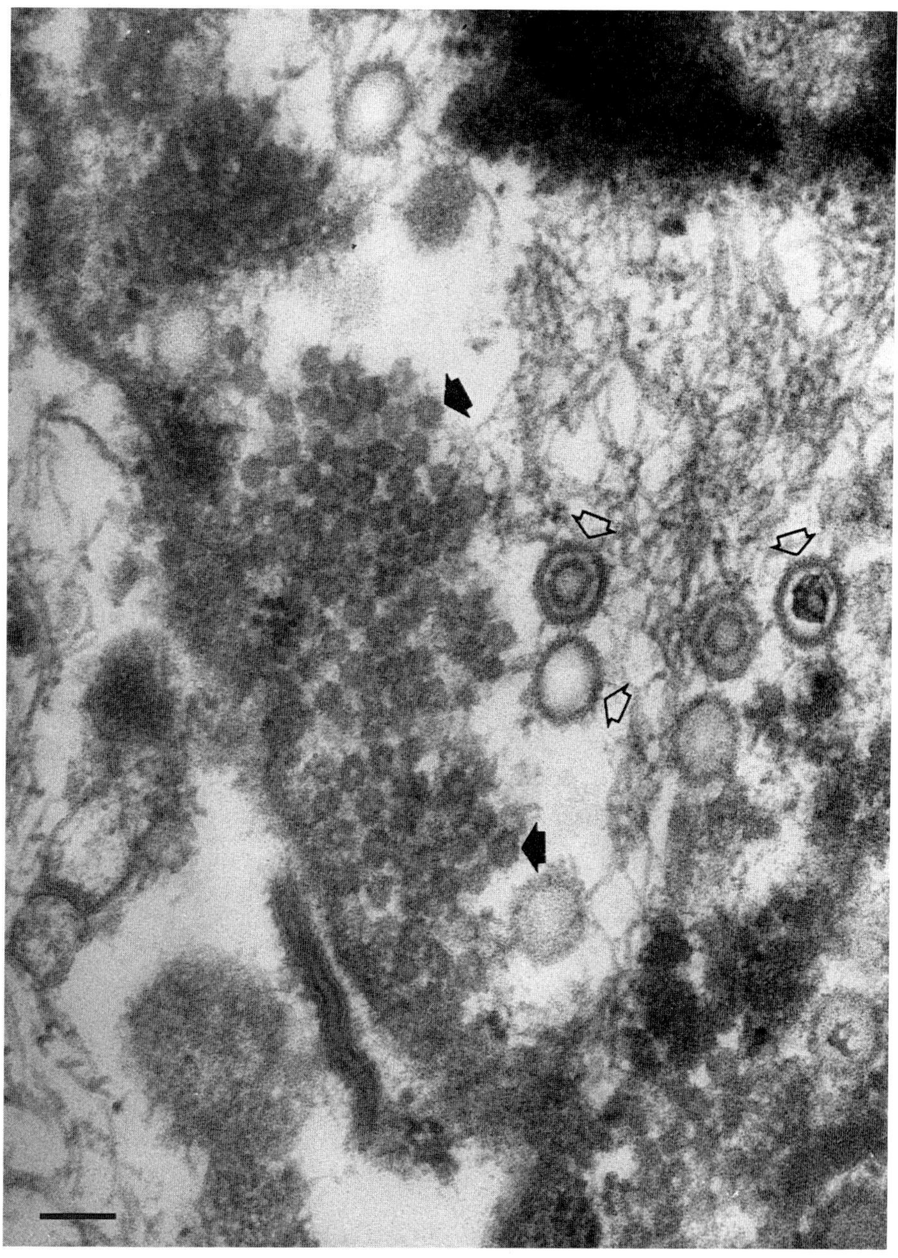

Figure 5 Intranuclear EBV particles (*hollow arrows*) and particles resembling papillomavirus (*solid arrows*). Original magnification X123,000. Bar, 0.1 μ.

E. Virology

Using culture and a number of immunohistochemical techniques, no evidence has been found of herpes simplex, varicella zoster, or cytomegalovirus, but EBV has been detected (15). Anticomplement immunofluorescence with human reference sera containing antibodies to EBV capsid antigen produced distinctive nuclear staining in 10 of 21 specimens tested. Negative controls included nonlesional mucosa from the same cases as well as biopsies of other oral diseases. Southern blot hybridization with probes for EBV revealed the typical EBV-specific pattern (Figure 6). Reconstruction hybridization indicated that more than 200 viral DNA copies per cellular genome were present in many cases. Nonlesional biopsies from the same patients were negative. High-complexity probes generated from the DNA of each lesional specimen hybridization at many positions. These findings suggested that the entire EBV genome was present (Figure 4).

F. Epstein-Barr Virus Serology

The results of the EBV serological tests (Figure 7) revealed a fivefold difference between the geometric means of the igG antibody titers to the viral capsid antigen of heterosexual subjects (geometric mean 367) and those of apparently healthy homosexual men (geometric mean 1778). The patients with HL appeared to be a subgroup of the homosexual group, since their antibody titers to the viral capsid antigen (geometric mean 2198) were noticeably higher than those of either of the other groups. There were no biologically important differences among the three groups in the titers of antibodies to the early-antigen diffuse and restricted components or to the EBV-associated nuclear antigens (see Chapter 19).

G. Langerhans' cells

Intraepithelial Langerhans' cells are reduced or absent in the HL lesion, and this decrease correlates with the presence of viral antigens (19).

H. Human Immunodeficiency Virus Status

Most individuals with HL have antibodies to HIV. Of 101 people tested, 100 were positive for antibodies to HIV. Over 75% of the individuals examined had infectious HIV recovered from their peripheral blood cells. Moreover, in close to 60% of these virus-positive individuals, high titers of virus were observed in cultures of their peripheral blood cells (20). These results on virus isolation are unusual for HIV-infected people and have been observed only in clinically healthy individuals or in individuals with late symptoms of HIV infection. When the immune response of patients with hairy leukoplakia

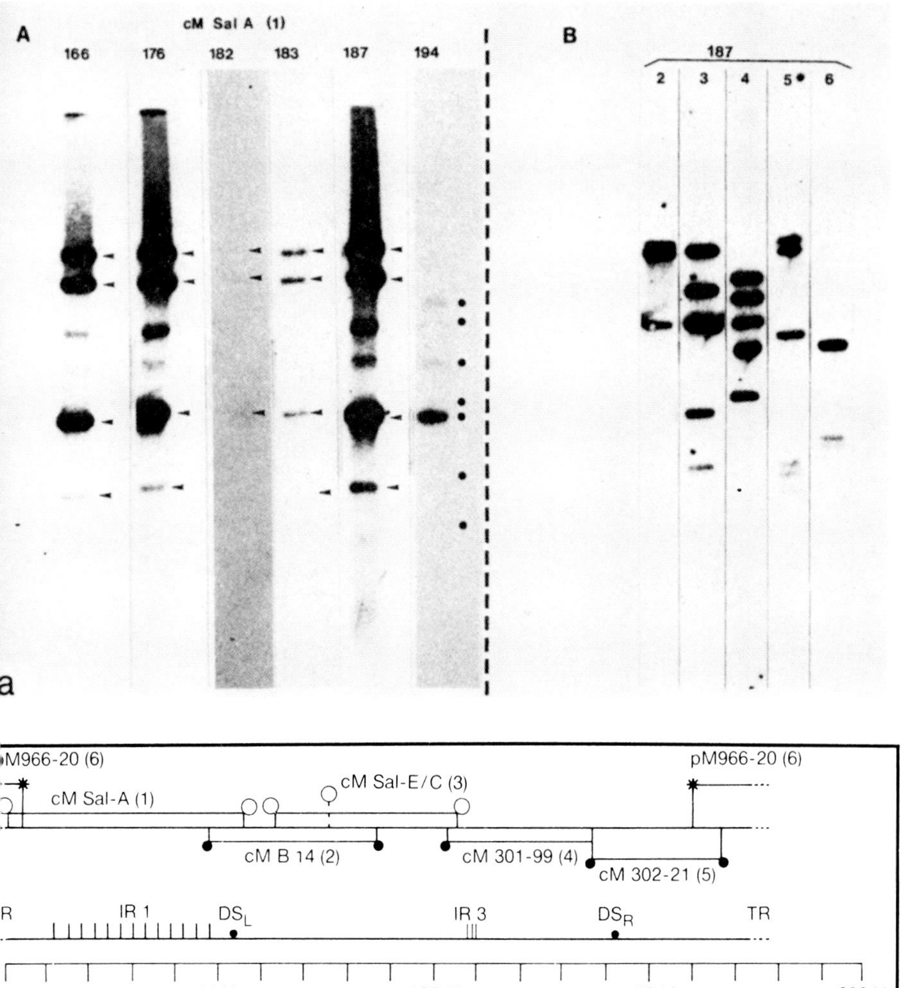

Figure 6 Detection of the whole genome of EBV in hairy leukoplakia tissue by southern blot hybridization. (*A*) High-complexity probe hybridization of ^{32}P-labeled DNA from six specimens of hairy leukoplakia (166-194, top) with restriction-enzyme-digested plasmid cM Sal-A (1) recombinant DNA (0.05 pmol). A *Sal*/I/*Bg*/II digest of the same clone was used for specimen 194. The map region of the EBV genome that is represented within this clone is shown in *b*. (*B*) High-complexity probe hybridization of ^{32}P-labeled DNA from hairy leukoplakia specimen 187 with DNA (0.05 pmol) from each of the following: a *Sal*/I digest of cMB14 (2), an *Eco*RI digest of cM Sal-E/C (3), a *Bam*HI digest of cM301-99 (4), a *Hind*III digest of cM302-21 (5), and a *Sal*I, *Bg*II, *Hind*III triple degest of pM966-20. (From Ref. 15.)

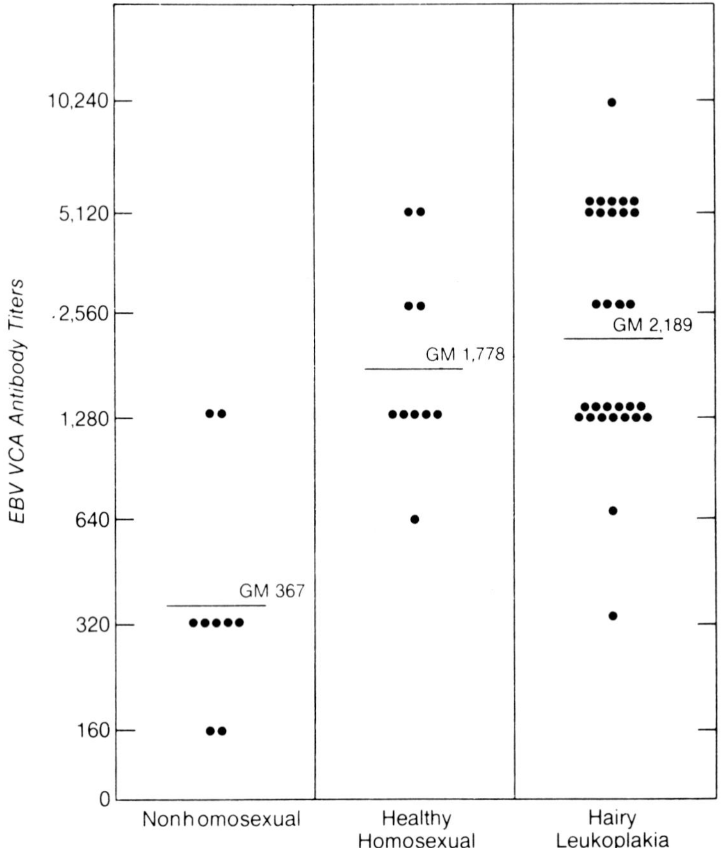

Figure 7 Titers of serum IgG antibodies to Epstein-Barr virus viral capsid antigen (EBV VCA) in patients with hairy leukoplakia and nonhomosexual and healthy homosexual control subjects. GM geometric mean. (From Ref. 15.)

is examined by immunoblot procedures, it is noteworthy that these individuals show strong reactions against the precursor envelope protein gp160 and *gag* protein p55. Moreover, substantial response is noted to the envelope gp120 and gp41, polymerase p65 and p31, and *gag* p25. This profile of serological response in HL is surprising since this group has a high frequency of development of AIDS within a short period of time (see below). Generally, antibodies to p25 are low in the severely ill individuals. The results suggest that other factors besides the immunological profile need to be examined in terms of predicting outcome in individuals who first present with HL.

I. Hairy Leukoplakia and AIDS

The incidence of development of AIDS in those patients with HL who did not have the full syndrome when first seen was investigated in a prospective study (20). The study population consisted of the 143 homosexual or bisexual male patients with HL but without AIDS seen between October 1981 and October 1985. The "Life-Test" procedure of the Statistical Analysis System (SAS, version 5) was used to calculate the product-limit estimate of the survival curve for the development of AIDS. Of the 143 patients who did not have AIDS at the time of diagnosis of HL, 43 developed AIDS from 1 to 31 months after the diagnosis of HL. Since only 33 patients were followed for more than a year before developing AIDS, the confidence intervals are wide at longer lengths of followup. The probability of the development of AIDS was 48% (34-63%) by 16 months, and by 31 months the point estimate was that 83% of patients develop AIDS with a 95% confidence limit of 57.5-100%.

Of the 43 patients who developed AIDS, 32 (74%) presented with *Pneumocystis carinii* pneumonia (PCP), 7 (16%) with KS, and 4 with other opportunistic infections. This distribution is significantly different from that of the other 1488 AIDS patients diagnosed in San Francisco at that time, where only 55% of patients developed PCP and 36% developed KS. This rate of the development of AIDS is very high and comfirms that HL is an important predictor of the eventual development of the full-blown syndrome. It is not known why PCP and other opportunistic infections predominate so dramatically among the HL patients who develop AIDS. However, it is speculated that something in the pathogenesis of HL may reflect biological events which predispose to more serious life-threatening opportunistic infections such as PCP.

J. Hairy Leukoplakia in Other Risk Groups

Until recently HL has been reported only in homosexual men. Recently, HL has been described in four patients, seropositive for HIV antibodies, from other risk groups (21). Three patients were seen in San Francisco and one in New York. The first patient was a 53-year-old man whose only risk factor was a blood transfusion four years previously. He developed HL on the lateral margins of the tongue and two months later was diagnosed with PCP. The second patient was a 29-year-old hemophiliac in whom HL developed in early 1986. He developed PCP four months later. The third patient was a 43-year-old woman who was the partner of a HIV-infected man. HL appeared on the lateral margin of the tongue. She developed toxoplasmosis within two months of diagnosis of HL. She denied IV drug use and there was no history of blood transfusions. The fourth patient seen in New York was a 56-year-old woman who was the partner of a seropositive IV drug user. The diagnosis of HL was confirmed by biopsy, except in the case of the hemophiliac, where in situ hybridization for EBV was performed on cytospin preparations of epithelial cells obtained by scraping the surface of the lesion (22). It had been suggested that HL might be associated with some aspect of the homosexual lifestyle because all of the first reports were in male homosexuals. However, the occurrence of the lesion in a transfusion recipient, two women, and a hemophiliac, all of whom were HIV-seropositive, suggests that the lesion is not restricted to homosexual men. In male homosexuals HL is an important predictor for the subsequent development of AIDS. The occurrence of opportunistic infections, characteristic of AIDS, in three of our patients within several months of the diagnosis of HL suggests prognostic implications similar to those seen in homosexual men. It is reasonable to assume that this clinically obvious and readily diagnosable oral mucosal lesion will be an important sign of HIV infection in other risk groups.

K. Hairy Leukoplakia at Other Sites

Hairy leukoplakia is associated with EBV and possibly with papillomavirus. Because EBV is found in other mucosal surfaces and because papillomaviruses can be passed sexually, it seemed appropriate to investigate whether HL occurs on mucous membranes other than those of the mouth.

The study (23) involved 19 consecutive homosexual or bisexual men; 14 had biopsy confirming HL and 5 had a presumptive diagnosis based on clinical criteria. Full anoscopic examination without bowel preparation was done as part of the initial evaluation. Eleven patients had entirely normal findings, six had internal or external hemorrhoids, and four had perianal condyloma accuminata. No patient had anal canal or rectal lesions suggestive of HL. The unique location of HL in the oral cavity is unexplained.

L. Differential Diagnosis and Diagnostic Criteria

Hairy leukoplakia may be confused with white sponge nevus, leukoplakia due to other causes, and oral candidiasis. Current diagnostic criteria are clinical appearance and histopathology. Where biopsy is not possible, failure to respond to antifungal therapy is an appropriate consideration. Noninvasive techniques including demonstration of EBV in surface epithelial cells are under development, but are not currently widely available.

M. Pathogenesis

Hairy leukoplakia appears to be an epithelial hyperplasia of the oral mucosa associated with EBV and possibly a second virus. No examples of malignant transformation of HL have been described. Absence of Langerhans' cells (LC) and coexistent systemic immunosuppression caused by HIV appear to be involved. It is not clear in what order and to what extent these factors contribute to the pathogenesis of HL. One possible schema is as follows:

1. HIV causes T_4 lymphocyte depletion.
2. T_4 lymphocyte reduction results in failure of lymphokine production, upon which LC depend directly or indirectly (via macrophages).
3. Loss of LC function in LC-deficient areas of the tongue allows expression of latent EBV and a possible second virus or else infection by those viruses.
4. EBV (and perhaps the second virus) causes epithelial hyperplasia. Moreover, HIV may be found to infect Langerhans' cells and thus be directly involved in the progression to HL.

N. Treatment

The lesion is usually asymptomatic and treatment may not be indicated. However, patients with HL are often concerned about the appearance of the lesion and soreness that can be associated with coexisting *Candida* infection. While antifungal therapy may, by eliminating *Candida*, reduce the symptoms, no drug is known to eliminate the lesion permanently. A preliminary observation with acyclovir being used at high doses for the treatment of herpes zoster showed temporary reduction in the clinical extent of the lesion (24).

O. Significance

Hairy leukoplakia is a specifically HIV-associated lesion found in several of the adult AIDS risk groups and is highly predictive of the development of AIDS (20). It is HIV-associated, never has been described before the AIDS epidemic, and has not been seen outside the AIDS risk groups. It is the first form of oral leukoplakia that shows consistent evidence for the presence of a virus, although human papillomavirus may be found in some cases of the common forms of leukoplakia. Also, HL is the first lesion in which EBV is consistently found in fully expressed virion form, although EBV-DNA and some EBV antigens are found in Burkitt's lymphoma, nasopharyngeal carcinoma, and some other carcinomas. The lesion also shows that persistent productive EBV infection can occur in oral epithelial cells. Until the issue of the nature of the second virus in HL is settled, the possibility exists of simultaneous infection by two viruses.

III. Oral Candidiasis

Candidiasis is a common oral fungal disease. *Candida albicans* is the species most often involved, although *C. stellatoides* and *C. tropicalis* are occasionally seen. *C. albicans* can be found as a commensal in the mouth in the absence of overt mucosal lesion. Publications on AIDS often inadequately describe oral candidiasis. Candidiasis of the esophagus is one of the opportunistic infections seen in AIDS. Oral candidiasis is a very common feature of HIV infection (1,5-7,25), occurring in about 75% of both ARC and AIDS patients (26). Indeed, oral candidiasis among risk groups may be of predictive value for the subsequent development of AIDS (25,27,28). Little is known of the pathogenesis of HIV-associated oral candidiasis. In other populations, the development of oral candidiasis can be related to a number of predisposing factors including antibiotic therapy, diabetes, xerostomia, and defects in cell-mediated immunity. The destruction of T-helper cells by HIV cytopathic effects and the subsequent profound immunodeficiency are presumably steps in the pathway that leads to oral candidiasis. However, the exact mechanism whereby these systemic abnormalities are expressed as local mucosal changes, which permit colonization and even invasion by candidal hyphae, are unknown.

Oral candidiasis associated with HIV infection has several different clinical presentations (29). These include pseudomembranous [Figure 8 (Plate IV, facing page 357)] and atrophic candidiasis [Figure 9 (Plate IV, facing page 357)] as well as angular cheilitis. Pseudomembranous candidiasis, sometimes called thrush, has a characteristic appearance. White curdy plaques are scattered upon bright red oral mucosa. These white plaques can be removed readily, often revealing a bleeding surface. Any part of the oral cavity may be involved. The atrophic form of candidiasis appears clinically as a red lesion and the most common locations are the palate and dorsum of the tongue. When candidiasis affects the dorsal surface of the tongue, patchy depapillated areas appear. Angular cheilitis may be present either alone or in conjunction with either of the other forms.

In association with HIV infection, oral candidiasis may persist for months if untreated. Diagnosis or oral candidiasis can be made from examination of a Gram stain or potassium hydroxide suspension of smears, showing the presence of hyphae and blastospores. Culture is used to determine the species involved and the number of colonies. A high colony count suggests colonization and active infection rather than the commensal state.

Oral candidiasis is a major and often the first expression of HIV infection. Accurate and early diagnosis of this lesion is an essential component of the physical examination of people in the AIDS risk groups. Treatment involves the use of systemic or topical antifungal medication.

IV. Gingivitis and Periodontal Disease

Even in good health, the gingival crevice contains a rich and varied microflora. Among HIV-infected individuals, many show a tendency to develop severe gingival inflammation and progressive destructive periodontal disease (30, 31). The gingivitis resembles acute necrotizing ulcerative gingivitis (ANUG) but is of prolonged duration and is severe. The gingiva appear bright red and swollen with ulcers at the tips of the interdental papillae. pain and halitosis are marked. In HIV-associated periodontitis [Figure 10 (Plate IV, facing page 357)], the sign is rapid and progressive destruction of the supporting tissues, periodontal ligament, and alveolar bone, with loosening and even exfoliation of teeth. A mixed flora is present and has yet to be studied in detail. The pathogenesis of these lesions is also poorly understood. In particular, no information is yet available on the contribution to the tissue damage made by microbial pathogens and by the host response, notably polymorphonuclear leukocytes, macrophages, lymphocytes, and humoral factors.

Treatment

Treatment consists of local debridement, irrigation with povidine-iodine (Betadine) 10%, and followup for prophylaxis and management. This procedure may require referral to a periodontist. Penicillin is not effective in management; ANUG in association with HIV infection behaves differently and may not respond to the use of antibiotics. Chlorhexidine is of use in controlling painful exacerbations.

V. Other Microbial Pathogens

Case reports have described HIV-associated oral lesions due to *Mycobacterium avium intracellulare* (32), histoplasmosis (33), *Klevsiella pneumoniae,* and *Enterobacteria cloacae* (34).

VI. Oral Viral Lesions

Just as potentially pathogenic fungi are able to take advantage of the immune paralysis induced by HIV infection, several viruses become able to colonize or become reactivated in the mouth, producing lesions. These include herpes group viruses and papillomaviruses. Hairy leukoplakia may also represent opportunistic viral infection.

Human papillomaviruses cause warts, including oral papillomas, condylomata, and focal epithelial hyperplasia (35). Immunosuppressed individuals show an increased tendency to develop skin warts, while anogenital warts occur as a sexually transmitted disease in male homosexuals, and in promiscuous heterosexual individuals of both sexes (36). We have seen many cases of oral warts in HIV-infected individuals.

Herpes simplex can frequently produce recurrent painful episodes of ulceration, most commonly appearing on the palate. The patient may report small vesicles which erupt to form ulcers. Diagnosis can be made from culture or from cytological smears showing characteristic viral giant cells (37). Recently, more accurate confirmation has become available using monoclonal antibodies. Herpes zoster causes by varicella zoster virus also can produce oral ulceration.

VII. Oral Neoplasia

The neoplastic diseases associated with AIDS may be analogous to the opportunistic infections seen in the same group of individuals. Carcinogens and oncogenic viruses are probably rendered more effective by failure of some part of the immune system such as the tumor surveillance mechanism. These diseases include Kaposi's sarcoma, non-Hodgkin's lymphoma, and perhaps oral squamous cell carcinoma. Kaposi's sarcoma is a multicentric neoplasm that may occur intraorally either alone or in association with skin, visceral, and lymph node lesions. The first lesions of KS are often seen in the mouth (8, 38, 39). Additionally KS can appear as a red, blue or purple lesion which may be flat or raised, solitary or multiple (Figures 8 and 9) (see Chapter 13). The most common oral site reported is the hard palate, although the lesion may be found on any part of the oral mucosa, including the gingiva, soft palate, and buccal mucosa.

The etiology and histology of KS are discussed in Chapter 13.

VIII. Conclusion

The AIDS epidemic has focused renewed attention on oral soft tissue diseases. A plethora of oral lesions are involved at every stage of HIV infection, and may herald the transition to the very serious and even fatal phases. Some oral lesions in HIV infection are new diseases, such as HL and perhaps the gingival and periodontal lesions. These entities raise fundamental questions about the pathogenesis of oral mucosal hyperplasia and infections and inflammatory disease. Other oral lesions seen in HIV infection are also seen in the general population. Studies of their etiology and pathogenesis are facilitated by investigations of their HIV-associated manifestations.

References

1. Gottlieb MS, Schroff R, Schanker HM, Weisman JD, Fan PT, Wolf RA, Saxon A. *Pneumocystis carinii* pneumonia and mucosal candidiasis in previously healthy homosexual men: evidence of a new acquired cellular immunodeficiency. N Engl J Med 1981; 305:1425-31.

2. Peterson DE, Sonis ST, eds. Oral complications of cancer chemotherapy. The Hague: Martinus Nijhoff, 1983.
3. Centers for Disease Control. Classification system for human T-lymphotropic virus type III/lymphadenopathy-associated virus infections. MMWR 1986; 35:334-9.
4. Greenspan D, Greenspan JS, Pindborg JJ, Schiødt M. In: AIDS and the dental team. Copenhagen: Munksgaard, 1986.
5. Silberman S, Migliorati CA, Lozada-Nur R, Greenspan D, Conant M. Oral findings in people with or at high risk for AIDS: a study of 375 homosexual males. J Am Dent Assoc 1986; 112:187-92.
6. Reichardt P, Pohle H-D, Gelderblom H, Strunz V. AIDS—orale manifestationen. Dtsch Zahnärztl 1986; 41:374-6.
7. Safai B, Johnson KG, Myskowski PL. The natural history of Kaposi's sarcoma in the acquired immunodeficiency syndrome. Ann Intern Med 1985; 103:744-50.
8. Lozada F, Silverman S Jr, Migliorati CA, Conant MA, Volberding PA. Oral manifestations of tumor and opportunistic infections in the acquired immunodeficiency syndrome (AIDS): findings in 53 homosexual men with Kaposi's sarcoma. Oral Surg 1983; 56:491-4.
9. Greenspan D, Silverman Jr S. Oral lesions of human immunodeficiency virus infection. Calif Dent Assoc J 1987; 15:28-33.
10. Greenspan D, Greenspan JS, Conant M, Petersen V, Silverman S Jr, de Souza Y. Oral "hairy"leukoplakia in male homosexuals: evidence of association with both papillomavirus and a herpes-group virus. Lancet 1984; 2:831-4.
11. Eversole LR, Jacobsen P, Stone CE, Freckleton V. Oral condyloma planus (hairy leukoplakia) among homosexual men: a clinicopathologic study of thirty-six cases. Oral Surg 1986; 61:249-55.
12. Centers for Disease Control. Oral viral lesion (hairy leukoplakia) associated with acquired immunodeficiency syndrome. MMWR 1985; 34:549-50.
13. Greenspan JS, Greenspan D, Lennette ET, Abrams DI, Conant MA, Petersen VH. Oral viral leukoplakia—a new AIDS-associated condition. Adv Exp Med Biol 1985; 187:123-8.
14. De Maubeuge J, Ledoux M, Feremans W, Zissis G, Goens J, Andre J, Gourdain JM, Menu R, De Wit S, Cran S, Clumeck N, Achten G. Oral "hairy" leucoplakia in an African AIDS patient. J Cutan Pathol 1986; 13:235-41.
15. Greenspan JS, Greenspan D, Lennette ET, Abrams DI, Conant MA, Petersen V, Freese UK. Replication of Epstein-Barr virus within the epithelial cells of oral "hairy" leukoplakia, an AIDS-associated lesion. N Engl J Med 1986; 313:1564-71.
16. Dunn AEG, Ogilvie MM. Intranuclear virus particles in human genital wart tissue: observations on the ultrastructure of the epidermal layer. J Untrastruct Res 1986; 22:282-95.
17. Oriel JD, Almeida JD. Demonstration of virus particles in human genital warts. Br J Vener Dis 1970; 46:37-42.
18. Williams MG, Howatson AF, Almeida JD. Morphological characterization of the virus of the human common wart (*Verruca vulgaris*). Nature 1961; 189:895-7.
19. Daniels TE, Greenspan D, Greenspan JS, Lennette E, Petersen V, de Souza Y. Langerhans' cell absence correlates with viral antigen presence in hairy leukoplakia. J Dent Res 1986; 65:766.

20. Greenspan D, Greenspan JS, Hearst NG, Pan L-Z, Conant MA, Abrams DI, Hollander H, Levy JA. Oral hairy leukoplakia: human immunodeficiency virus status and risk for development of AIDS. J Infect Dis 1987; 155:475-81.
21. Greenspan D, Hollander H, Friedman-Kien A, Freese UK, Greenspan JS. Oral hairy leucoplakia in two women, a haemophiliac and a transfusion recipient. Lancet 1986; 2:978-9.
22. de Souza YG, Greenspan D, Hammer M, Hartzog GA, Felton JR, Greenspan JS. Demonstration of Epstein-Barr virus DNA in the epithelial cells of oral hairy leuloplakia. J Dent Res 1986; 65:765
23. Hollander H, Schiødt M, Greenspan D, Stringari S, Greenspan J. Hairy leukoplak ia and the acquired immunodeficiency syndrome. Ann Intern Med 1986; 104:892.
24. Friedman-Kien AE. Viral origin of hairy leukoplakia. Lancet 1986; 2:694.
25. Klein RS, Harris CA, Small CB, Moll B, Lesser M, Friedland GH. Oral candidiasis in high-risk patients as the initial manifestation of the acquired immunodeficiency syndrome. N Engl J Med 1984; 311:354-8.
26. Pindborg JJ, Rindum J, Schiodt M, Hansen HJ. Suggestion for a classification of oral candidiasis in patients with AIDS, ARC, and serum antibodies for LAV/HTLV-III. J Dent Res 1986; 65:765.
27. Chandrasekar PH, Molinari JA. Oral candidiasis: forerunner of acquired immunodeficiency syndrome (AIDS)? oral Surg 1985; 60:532-4.
28. Murray HW, Hillman JK, Rubin BY, Kelly CD, Jacobs JL, Tyler LW, Donelly DM, Carriero SM, Godbold JH, Roberts RB. Patients at risk for AIDS-related opportunistic infections. N Engl J Med 1985: 313:1504-10.
29. Greenspan D, Greenspan JS, Pindborg JJ, Schiødt M. AIDS and the dental team. Copenhagen: Munksgaard, 1986:36.
30. Winkler JR, Murray PA, Greenspan D, Greenspan JS. AIDS virus associated periodontal disease. J Dent Res 1986; 65:741.
31. Winkler JR, Murray PA. Periodontal disease as related to HIV infection. Calif Dent Assoc J 1987; 15:20-4.
32. Volpe F, Schwimmer A, Barr C. Oral manifestations of disseminated mycobacteruim avium intracellulare in a patient with AIDS. Oral Surg 1985; 60:567-70.
33. Fowler CB, Nelson JF, Smith BR. A case of acquired immunodeficiency syndrome presenting as a palatal perforation: report of a case and review of the literature. Presented at 40th Meeting of American Academy of Oral Pathology, Toronto, May 1986.
34. Greenspan D, Greenspan JS, Pindborg JJ, Schiodt M. AIDS and the Dental Team. Copenhagen: Munksgaard, 1986:p. 45.
35. Scully C, Prime S, Maitland N. Papillomaviruses: their possible role in oral disease. Oral Surg 1985; 60:166-74.
36. Owen WF. Sexually transmitted disease and traumatic problems in homosexual men. Ann Intern Med 1980; 92:805-11.
37. Fung JC, Shanley J, Tilton RC. Comparison of herpes simplex virus-specific DNA probes and monoclonal antibodies. J Clin Microbiol 1985; 22:748-53.

38. Green TL, Beckstead JH, Lozada-Nur F, Silverman S Jr, Hansen LS. Histopathologic spectrum of oral Kaposi's sarcoma. Oral Surg 1984; 58:306-14.
39. Eversole LR, Leider AS, Jacobsen PL, Shaber EP. Oral Kaposi's sarcoma associated with acquired immunodeficiency syndrome among homosexual males. J Am Dent Assoc 1983: 107:248-53.

18

Other Infections Associated with AIDS

Stephen E. Follansbee
School of Medicine
University of California
San Francisco, California

I. Introduction

Unlike the complications of AIDS discussed in earlier chapters, there are a number of infections that are present either in a disseminated form or, while presenting with focal findings, are indeed disseminated at the onset. In addition, there are some infections discussed elsewhere in this book that present outside the expected foci. These include extrapulmonary legionellosis and focal cryptococcal abscesses outside the central nervous system. This chapter will discuss some of these other infections complicating AIDS. The pathogens involved, their sites of infection, approaches for their detection, and treatment are summarized in Table 1.

The spectrum of infectious agents causing disease in persons with human immunodeficiency virus (HIV) infection spans the microbiological kingdom. The cell-mediated immune deficiency associated with HIV infection predisposes to a variety of viral, parasitic, and fungal infections. The B-cell dysregulation also associated with AIDS predisposes to infections due to

Table 1 Summary of Other Infections in AIDS

Infectious Agent	Sites	Method of Detection	Treatment
Bacterial	Various, including sepsis, pneumonia, gastrointestinal, skin, pericardium, central nervous system, sinusitis esophagitis	Direct stain Gram's Dieterle (*Legionella*) Acid-fast (*Nocardia*) IFA (*Legionella*) Culture CYE (*Legionella*) Serology (syphilis)	Antibiotics available for all established infection. Treatment may be more prolonged and recurrences common. Gammaglobulin for recurrent infections due to encapsulated bacteria.
Fungal			
Candida	Central nervous system, esophageal and other gastrointestinal, fungemia	Direct stain Culture	Amphotericin B intravenously for invasive disease, with possible renal, metabolic, and bone marrow toxicity. Ketoconazole for suppression or prolonged therapy of invasive disease, with possible hepatitis and adrenal suppression. Topical imidazoles for mucocutaneous disease.
Coccidioides immitis	Progresive pulmonary or disseminated to one or more organs; "sepsis"	Direct stain Culture, with attention of mycology personnel to possible contagion.	Amphotericin B for life-threatening invasive disease, including renal and central nervous system. Ketoconazole for progressive pulmonary and maintenance.

Histoplasma capsulatum	Progressive pulmonary; disseminated; sepsis; lower gastrointestinal mass.	Direct stain of biopsied material, blood (Giemsa methenamine silver) Culture Radioimmunoassay for fungal antigen (not generally available).	As for *Coccidioides*.
Cryptococcus	Sepsis; pulmonary; meningitis; focal abscesses; peritonitis; disseminated.	Stain (India Ink) Cryptococcal antigen (serum; cerobrospinal fluid) Culture, will grow on routine blood agar.	Amphotericin B 5-flucytosine, with attention to possible marrow toxicity. Ketoconazole for suppression of extra-central nervous system disease (preliminary observations).
Protozoal			
Coccidia: Cryptosporidia and *Isospora*	Gastrointestinal with diarrhea, abdominal pain, malabsorption; biliary tract; bronchial tract.	Stain, modified Ziehl-Neelsen; Giemsa.	No standard effective therapy, with suggested benefit from Spiramycin, α-difluoromethyl-ornithine, furazolidone. Trimethoprim-sulfamethoxazole sometimes effective for *Isospora*.
Toxoplasma gondii	Central nervous system; pulmonary; testicular.	Peroxidase-antiperoxidase stain.	Often initiated in appropriate clinical situation for ''empiric'' trial. Pyrimethamine-sulfadiazine with attention to bone marrow and allergic reactions. Clindamycin (up to 2.7 g/d) in the sulfadiazine intolerant patient. Chronic suppression mandatory.

Table 1 (*continued*)

Infectious Agent	Sites	Method of Detection	Treatment
Strongyloides stercoralis	Intestinal; hyperinfection with pulmonary migration.	Wet prep of sputum; Enterotest® ; Stool ova and parasite examination.	Thiabendazole
Mycobacterial *M. avium* complex and *M. tuberculosis*; other atypicals.	Disseminated; skin; lymphadenitis; focal or diffuse pulmonary; gastrointestinal.	Acid-fast stain of secretions, drainage, stool, or biopsy material.	Standard regimens for suspected *M. tuberculosis* (see Table 2). Controversial for *M. avium*. Multidrug therapy indicated. Fever control using nonsteroidal anti-inflammatory agents.

IFA, immunofluorescent antibody; CYE, charcoal yeast extract.

other pathogens including the encapsulated bacteria. These include the pneumococcus, *Haemophilus*, and meningococcus. Moreover, many of the conditions associated with AIDS lead to other factors which predispose to additional infections. These factors include the frequent reliance on intravascular devices, disruption of the integrity of skin and mucous membranes by Kaposi's sarcoma (1) or superficial infections, prolonged hospitalization, and neutropenia associated with chemotherapeutic regimens. Rarely, primary neutropenia has also been associated with AIDS (2).

It is not possible to rank these other infections with respect to frequency. Their incidence in AIDS varies with the risk group demographics (3). There are problems associated with a passive surveillance system in collecting accurate statistics. An additional problem is that at times multiple pathogens may be isolated concurrently. It may be difficult to assess which is primarily involved in the disease manifestations necessitating therapy against all treatable pathogens in some instances.

Evaluation for other opportunistic infections in the setting of AIDS is an often repeated and sometimes exhaustive process. It is difficult to dictate in an algorithmic approach the evaluation of fever, night sweats, chills, or any of the other initial manifestations of a new opportunistic infection. Clearly, such pathogens as *Cryptosporidium* should be quickly demonstrated in a patient with diarrhea. In contrast, other pathogens may present in a nonspecific manner with few focal findings, with or without fever. If a thorough history and physical examination do not reveal any etiology, it may be helpful for more specific evaluation to search for evidence of mycobacterial infection, *Cryptococcus* or other fungal infection, cytomegalovirus disease, or such bacterial pathogens as *Salmonella.* A gallium scan may be helpful to locate pulmonary or lymph node disease not otherwise appreciated clinically. Cultures of blood for fungi, bacteria, and viruses may also reveal an otherwise unsuspected pathogen. Isolates from normally sterile sites should not be dismissed as "contaminants" in an expanding array of clinical situations. An example is the occurrence of prolonged bacteremia associated with lung abscesses secondary to *Rhodococcus equi* (*Corynebacterium equi*) in persons with AIDS (4-6). Even when the diagnosis seems clinically evident, blood cultures during febrile episodes often reveal additional unexpected pathogens. Two-thirds of septicemia, both inpatient and outpatient acquired, have been reported due to organisms not considered opportunists in T-cell deficiency states (7). Therefore, empirical therapy must often anticipate a broad spectrum of potential pathogens. The purpose of this chapter is to describe some of these other pathogens and the spectrum of illness seen in the setting of AIDS.

II. Bacterial Infections

A. *Streptococcus pneumoniae* (pneumococcus) and *Haemophilus influenzae*

Epidemiology

Children and adults with AIDS are at increased risk for bacterial infection. The streptococci and *Haemophilus* species are ubiquitous and infections occur in both adults (8) and children (9). Moreover, the relative risk is estimated to be as high as 5.7 cases of pneumococcal bacteremia/100 patients per year (10). As many as 70% of the nonmycobacterial bacteremias in persons with AIDS are associated with organisms such as these that are not usually associated with defective T-cell lymphocyte function (11). One study following 46 children documented serious bacterial infections in 26 children, including 27 episodes of sepsis in 21 of them (9). Likewise, a high recurrence rate of bacterial infections has been reported in adult AIDS patients (12).

Disease Manifestations

The spectrum of diseases includes sinusitis, bronchitis, cellulitis, and lower respiratory infections (13). The cough is usually productive of purulent sputum, but may be minimally productive, mimicking *Pneumocystis carinii* pneumonia (see Chapter 16). Patients often present with multilobar involvement. Although chest roentgenograms may show classic alveolar consolidation, both pneumococcal and *Haemophilus* pneumonia have been associated with a diffuse interstitial pattern, again easily confused with that of pneumocystis pneumonia. Bacteremia is seen in 20-60% of cases of pneumonia. Recurrence of pneumonia has been observed in some patients as well (13). Recently *Haemophilus parainfluenzae* prostatitis has been described in a young man with evidence of HIV infection but not defined AIDS (14).

Diagnosis

As mentioned above, blood cultures are frequently positive for these bacteria. Sputum may be difficult to obtain, but Gram stain of sputum or bronchial washing may help guide initial therapy. In patients with sudden onset of pulmonary complaints, such as pleuritic chest pain or rigor, it may be warranted to obtain blood and routine sputum cultures along with the chest roentgenogram and to initiate antibacterial therapy first, before looking for other opportunistic pulmonary pathogens. Although these pathogens are most often associated with sinusitis, the spectrum of organisms that can cause clinically similar symptoms includes the coliform bacteria, *Cryptococcus* and other fungi, and even *Acanthamoeba* (15). Therefore, it is useful to obtain sinus cultures before empirical therapy, or at least obtain cultures if the clinical response is suboptimal in five to seven days.

Treatment

A high index of suspicion will often dictate initial therapy prior to the results of cultures. Penicillin G remains the treatment of choice for pneumococcal disease. For *Haemophilus influenzae* infections, treatment is dictated by the β-lactamase test. Longer-acting parenteral second- or third-generation cephalosporins, such as cefuroxime, cefonicid, or ceftriaxone, are useful pending the results of this test. These drugs can be conveniently administered on an outpatient basis for patients allergic to penicillin, ampicillin, or trimethoprim-sulfamethoxazole and suffering from serious pulmonary or other infections.

Prevention

Despite reports suggesting a subnormal antibody response (16), the pneumococcal vaccine may offer some protection and is recommended to patients with AIDS. An apparent vaccine failure has been reported (10). In addition, the use of intravenous gammaglobulin in adults with recurrent pneumococcal or hemophilus infections may be useful. Such preparations have been widely accepted in pediatric AIDS patients (16) and suggested in adult patients (17). Lastly, the high fatality rate reported in nosocomial bacterial infection associated with AIDS (12) underscores the need for a high index of suspicion and early recognition and empirical therapy in the hospitalized patient with new onset fever or shock.

B. *Staphylococcus aureus*

Epidemiology

This organism is ubiquitous and the incidence of colonization in patients with AIDS seems increased. As in other persons with frequent hospitalizations, undergoing frequent invasive procedures, and needing intravascular devices, this organism is a frequent pathogen in persons with AIDS. In patients with Kaposi's sarcoma, the cancer may break the integrity of the pulmonary barriers and predispose the tissue to staphylococcal or other bacterial pneumonia.

Diseases

The spectrum of disease includes folliculitis, impetigo, and cellulitis, superficial or deep abscesses, life-threatening toxic-shock syndrome, and pneumonia. More invasive illness such as sinusitis and staphylococcal subcutaneous abscesses are common. Patients with chronic indwelling intravascular lines are at risk for staphylococcus bacteremia and bacterial endocarditis.

A small number of patients, with no apparent risk factors other than AIDS, present with overwhelming *Staphylococcus* bacteremia. Recently bacterial esophagitis has been described in persons with other immunosuppresive disorders and may be seen in patients with AIDS (18).

Treatment

The use of appropriate antibiotics and removal of intravascular lines is standard in the bacteremic patient. Initial identification of staphylococcal species may be delayed but often treatment must be initiated before the isolate is identified. Vancomycin intravenously in this situation is the drug of choice pending sensitivity reporting. Although on occasion indwelling intravascular line-related infection may be treated *in situ,* most often the line will need to be removed unless there is another focus of bacteremia evident.

Prevention

Because of the high frequency of skin colonization and risk for serious infection from the patient's own endogenous flora, chlorhexidine or other antimicrobial-containing soaps are recommended for routine skin care. In addition, frequent assessment and meticulous care of intravascular lines, as well as the avoidance of unnecessary venipuncture or other invasive devices should lower the risk for serious staphylococcal disease. Finally, unnecessary hospitalizations will reduce the chance of nosocomial infection.

C. *Salmonella* and *Shigella* Infections

Epidemiology

Enterocolitis due to *Salmonella enteritidis* and *Shigella* species has been noted prior to the AIDS epidemic in individuals at risk for AIDS (e.g., homosexual men). *Shigella, Salmonella,* as well as other enteric pathogens such as *Campylobacter,* may act as sexually transmitted pathogens through fecal-oral spread. These agents, though not strictly meeting the early Centers for Disease Control criteria for the diagnosis of AIDS, often cause life-threatening and recurrent disease (11). As in other conditions such as organ transplantation, sarcoidosis or hemolytic anemias, the incidence of serious disease from *Salmonella* is increased. The prevalence of this infection is estimated to be as high as 20 times that in healthy populations (19); it is as high as 1867 per 100,000 cases in the San Francisco experience (20).

Diseases

With respect to *Salmonella enteritidis* infection, septic enterocolitis appears to be the most frequent presentation. However, there is not a typical set of signs or symptoms characteristic of this syndrome (20a). The incidence of bacteremia approaches 75-80% (21). In addition, relapses of bacteremia are common; 62.5% of cases recurred in one report (22). Four of five patients have documented gastrointestinal infections from at least one other organism. This finding suggests that this coinfection may increase the risk for bacteremia (23). However, bacteremia may occur in patients without gastrointestinal symptoms (24). Because of this observation, the febrile patient with AIDS without diarrhea must still be evaluated for *Salmonella* sepsis. Other sites of infection, such as endocarditis, pyelonephritis, and cholecystitis, should also be considered.

Shigella bacteremia has been reported in persons with AIDS (11). It has occurred concurrently with colitis due to cytomegalovirus and often leads to prolonged diarrhea, recurrent disease, and a slower response to appropriate therapy.

Treatment

The antibiotic used depends on the pathogen isolated and antimicrobial sensitivities. Unfortunately, many isolates of *Salmonella* and *Shigella* are resistant to ampicillin. There has been a tendency to avoid chloramphenicol because of preexisting leukopenia in many instances. As discussed elsewhere (see Chapter 16), many patients are already manifesting allergic reaction to trimethoprim and/or sulfamethoxazole, or develop allergic reactions during the course of therapy. In addition, this combination may further suppress the bone marrow. Occasionally, certain of the third-generation cephalosporins have been reported to be effective in these instances (24). Quinolone antimicrobials (norfloxacin, ciprofloxacin, and others) can be effective both orally and parenterally (25). As with other antimicrobial regimens, relapses with the quinolones have been seen.

Prevention

These pathogens are transmitted sexually, as well as through other routes of fecal/oral contamination. Guidelines to minimize the risk for sexual transmission of HIV are appropriate for minimizing the risk for acquiring these enteric pathogens. In addition, patients should be advised of appropriate precautions if travelling to areas of the world where enteric pathogens are endemic. The most common source in the United States of nonsexually acquired salmonellosis is poultry and poultry products (26). Precautions regarding cleaning and storage of eggs and fresh and cooked chicken should be advised. Other factors, such as decreased gastric acidity and prior use of antibiotics (27), may be difficult to control. Invasive *Salmonella dublin* infections have been associated with drinking raw milk (28) and have been seen in patients with AIDS. Metastatic infection developed in 33% of patients reported and can be difficult to eradicate. Therefore, recommendations against drinking unpasteurized milk are appropriate.

The role of chronic antimicrobial suppression is unclear, especially in light of the multiple drug intolerances often seen in this patient population. In addition, there is a risk for developing antibiotic resistance and superinfection. However, as in certain other conditions such as chronic granulomatous disease (29) and renal transplantation (30). chronic therapy after relapse of salmonella infection may be indicated.

D. *Listeria monocytogenes*

Epidemiology

This small, aerobic, motile Gram-positive bacillus is well described as a pathogen in other settings, including the extremes of age, chronic steroid use, and other immunosuppressed conditions. It is nearly ubiquitous in nature. The portal of entry in most instances has been the gastrointestinal tract. The fact that it has been seen, although infrequently, in persons with AIDS has been discussed (31).

Diseases

Infection with this organism has presented as meningitis (32, 33) or bacteremia (34). In humans the bacterium has also caused amniotitis and endophthalmitis. It has also been associated with maternal death in the setting of AIDS.

Treatment

The treatment involves ampicillin, chloramphenicol, or trimethoprim-sulfamethoxazole (34a). Cephalosporins are unreliable. The new quinolones may have a role in the penicillin and trimethoprim-sulfamethoxazole-allergic patient.

Prevention

Most cases of listeriosis are sporadic. Although outbreaks of listeriosis have been associated with contaminated milk products (35) and other foodstuffs, no means of prevention is well defined (35a).

E. *Campylobacter* Species

Epidemiology

This short, motile, comma- or "seagull"-shaped Gram-negative rod has been well recognized as a cause of enterocolitis (36). *Campylobacter fetus* ssp. *jejuni* is a more frequent cause of diarrhea than *Salmonella* or *Shigella* in the United States. Chronic or recurrent diarrhea due to campylobacter has been associated with hypogammaglobulinemia. *C. fetus* ssp. *jejuni* has been found in the stool specimens of 6.3% of homosexual men with and 2.7% of homosexual men without intestinal symptoms (37). In addition, *C. fetus* ssp. *fetus* has been described to cause disease in this population. Typically, those persons infected with this latter organism include elderly people with underlying illnesses, including alcoholism, malignancy, immunodeficiency, malnutrition, diabetes mellitus, chronic renal failure, and cardiovascular disease. Less often associated with symptomatic intestinal disease, clinical manifestations of *C. fetus* ssp. *fetus* include sepsis, endocarditis, pericarditis, mycotic aneurysms, thrombophlebitis, pneumonia, empyema, abscesses, septic arthritis, and spontaneous peritonitis, as well as infections of the urinary and biliary tracts (38). A case of recurrent bacteremia and gangrenous cholecystitis in a person with AIDS has been reported (39). It is notable that despite the high incidence of carriage in homosexual men, profound *Campylobacter* enteritis in persons with AIDS has been an infrequent problem.

Diseases

Patients with AIDS present with diarrhea, which may be bloody, and associated with severe abdominal cramps and tenesmus. Correlating stool carriage with symptoms revealed that 23% of AIDS patients carrying the organism had diarrhea, compared with only 4.5% of healthy male homosexuals (11). Although apparently rare, more serious disease should be expected and any of the foci listed above, including endovascular sites and the central nervous system, should be considered. In addition to the report of a person with gangrenous cholecystitis mentioned above, there has been another report of bacteremia in two homosexual men (40). Neither of these men had gastrointestinal symptoms. In the presence of fever without an apparent source, it may be valuable to take a stool specimen for *Campylobacter* culture and alert the clinical microbiology laboratory to the possibility of campylobacteremia.

Treatment

Erythromycin (500 mg four times daily) is the treatment of choice for gastrointestinal disease. Doxycycline or tetracycline may be effective in the erythromycin intolerant patient. Parenteral therapy, in combination with an aminoglycoside, or chloramphenicol may be necessary in invasive disease, particularly in central nervous system infection. Rifampin has also been used in serious infection as an adjunct to other antibiotics. Because of emerging resistance patterns, in special situations of frequent relapse, it may be necessary to ask for special antibiotic sensitivities of the isolate (41).

Prevention

Recommendation for behavior patterns to decrease acquisition of other enteric pathogens are appropriate for *Campylobacter* as well. Outbreaks of *Campylobacter* associated with raw milk ingestion have been reported (40, 42, 43).

F. *Legionella* Infections

Epidemiology

Legionella species, including *L. pneumophila*, are small, fastidious, Gram-negative organisms. They appear to be ubiquitous and are particularly associated with comtaminated water supplies. Difficulty in identifying this pathogen in early epidemics was due to the fastidious growth requirements of the legionella species. Person-to-person spread has not been documented.

Diseases

The role of *Legionella* in both outpatient and nosocomial pulmonary infections has been well described. Extrapulmonary infections have been noted, including the pericardium (44,45), myocardium (46), prosthetic heart valves (47), and blood (48). A patient with AIDS has been described with *Legionella* sinusitis (49). An AIDS patient with pericarditis, necrotizing myositis, and probable cellulitis secondary to overwhelming legionellosis (*Legionella longbeachiae*) has been observed (personal observation).

Diagnosis

Extrapulmonary disease may be difficult to document unless one has a high index of suspicion. Routine culture media, including blood culture systems, will not support the growth of this fastidious organism. The organism can be seen on Gram stain as weakly Gram-negative (50, 51), although the Dieterle silver impregnation stain, or direct fluorescent antibody staining is more specific (52). Most isolates will grow on charcoal yeast extract agar within three to five days.

Treatment

Erythromycin in doses up to 1 g every 6 h, either orally or parenterally, is the treatment of choice. Rifampin has been added in resistant infections.

Prevention

Awareness of this organism as a nosocomial pathogen is key to preventing subsequent cases. No other means of prevention exist.

G. *Nocardia asteroides* and Other *Actinomycetales* Organisms

Epidemiology

Nocardia is a Gram-positive, filamentous rod capable of causing serious disease in immunocompromised individuals. The organism is an ubiquitous soil-borne aerobic bacterium of the order *Actinomycetales. Nocardia* infection has been observed in the setting of AIDS (53). That report also described another case of cervical lymphadenitis due to a streptomyces species, related to *Nocardia.* An association with prior nocardiosis and the subsequent development of nontuberculous mycobacteriosis in cardiac allograft recipients has been described (54). Recently, a report of cervicofacial actinomycosis in a man with generalized lymphadenopathy and evidence of HIV infection has appeared (55).

Diseases

Nocardia is most often acquired through the respiratory tract and presents as a pulmonary infection. Rarely, infection of skeleton, central nervous system, lymph nodes, and other organs has been encountered. In the setting of AIDS, direct extension from a pulmonary focus may lead to regional lymphadenitis and pericarditis. *Actinomyces* species are found commonly in the oral cavity and most infections have been localized to this area.

Diagnosis

The organism is not visualized in hematoxylin-eosin or periodic acid-Schiff (PAS) preparations. *Nocardia* may be seen as weakly Gram-positive. Diagnosis is confirmed with appropriate special stains, including a modified acid-fast stain. *Nocardia* are weakly acid-fast, although *Actinomyces* are not. Unfortunately, organisms may not be seen on expectorated sputum or in transbronchial lung biopsy specimens in cases of pulmonary disease. Reasons include predominence of other organisms in expectorated specimens, or sampling error due to patchy foci of pulmonary involvement (56). Bronchoalveolar lavage fluid may be more helpful in diagnosis. Growth will occur on blood agar or Sabouraud's dextrose agar, but longer incubation may be required, up to twenty-one days. In addition, coexistence with other pathogens, including *Salmonella* and mycobacteria, must be suspected in the setting of AIDS (53). In extrapulmonary disease, biopsy and culture are necessary.

Treatment

Unfortunately, in vitro sensitivity testing of *Nocardia* is difficult to perform, not standardized, and difficult to extend to clinical situations. The sulfonamide drugs, including trimethoprim-sulfamethoxazole, have been recommended and treatment may be prolonged. Because of allergic reactions to the sulfa-containing medications, alternative antibiotic therapy may be necessary. Recommendations include minocycline, cycloserine, some of the newer β-lactam drugs, and aminoglycosides, particularly amikacin (57). When possible, surgical debridement will help shorten the course of antibiotic therapy. Likewise, *Actinomyces* infections require long-term therapy. However, these are most often sensitive to pencillin, which is the drug of choice for invasive disease.

H. Syphilis

Epidemiology

Many of the people at risk for HIV infection have been at risk for syphilis as well as other sexually and congenitally transmitted diseases (57a). Although the incidence of syphilis among homosexually active men in the United States has been falling, its incidence among heterosexually active individuals has not (57b).

Disease Manifestations

The manifestations of *Treponema pallidum* infection will not be reviewed in detail. The clinical signs and symptoms of secondary syphilis are protean and may involve the skin, mucous membranes, genitalia, central nervous system (including the ocular and auditory systems), kidney, liver, and intestinal wall, as well as joints and periosteum. In general, *Treponema pallidum* has not been an opportunist in the setting of HIV infection. The possibility has been discussed (57c) in response to reports of several cases of apparently aggressive neurosyphilis in four individuals with HIV infection (57d).

Diagnosis

Darkfield examination of material from chancres of primary lesions establishes early diagnosis. Most have relied on serodiagnosis for later stages, including latent infection (57e). A recent report suggests that seroconversion may be delayed in some HIV-infected individuals who acquire syphilis (57f). A high index of suspicion in the setting of unusual skin eruptions and central nervous system disease is necessary to rule out this pathogen. Negative serology should not discourage further evaluation for syphilis, such as silver-stain or the more cumbersome Warthin-Starry stain for spirochetes in appropriately obtained material. Repeat serology in 14-21 days may also establish the diagnosis.

Treatment

The standard treatment regimens using penicillin G are well outlined (57g). Various reports have suggested that the single injection of benzathine penicillin for early syphilis may not be sufficient and relapses occur (57h). Clearly the spinal fluid results should prompt aggressive therapy with intravenous penicillin G (24 mU per day in six divided doses) for 10 to 14 days if they support the diagnosis of neurosyphilis in one of its many forms. At present there are not enough data to modify the recommendations for 2.4 mU of benzathine Penicillin G intramuscularly at weekly intervals for three doses for uncomplicated latent syphilis.

Prevention

Serological screening is mandatory in the setting of possible HIV infection if sequelae of untreated spirochetal infection are to be prevented. Safer sex guidelines will diminish the incidence of new acquisition of this pathogen.

III. Fungi

Mycoses complicate the clinical course of every patient with AIDS. These run the spectrum from superficial and easily treated dermatitis or mucositis to life-threatening disseminated infections. Some of these infections have been reviewed recently (58). The major pathogens in the setting of HIV infection are discussed. Miscellaneous syndromes include disseminated cutaneous *Sporotrichosis schenckii* infection reported in an immunodeficient, HIV-infected female factor VIII recipient (59). Rare cases of invasive aspergillosis have appeared (60,61).

A. *Candida albicans* and Non-albicans Species

Epidemiology

Candida species are found all over the environment. *Candida* infections are very common in the immunosuppressed, and are familiar infections to most patients with AIDS and to those with less serious manifestations of HIV infection.

Diseases

The organism presents with a broad spectrum of manifestations. Patients with AIDS are familiar with the white exudative plaque of oral candidiasis coating the oropharynx. Often, other mucous and cutaneous sites may be infected, including the perineal area. The pathogen may be more invasive. *Candida* esophagitis may lead to severe symptoms of dysphagia and odynophagia, the more common symptom. Fungemia associated with indwelling intravenous lines is unfortunately all too common and on occasion associated with deep-seated abscesses.

Diagnosis

Diagnosis may require only simple visualization of the characteristic lesions of the oropharynx, or may require histological and culture evidence of invasive or disseminated disease. A recent report suggested that oral candidiasis is a marker for esophageal involvement in patients with AIDS (62). These authors suggest that upper endoscopy is not necessary before initiating therapy in patients with esophageal symptoms and oral candidiasis. However, endoscopy may be necessary in patients whose symptoms persist despite appropriate antifungal therapy. The funduscopic examination may aid in the diagnosis of systemic disease. Suspicion for invasive disease should be raised in patients who are febrile, leukopenic, and have mucocutaneous colonization and/or deep intravascular lines.

Treatment

The treatment depends on the site and severity of involvement. There is often individually expressed preferences for one or the other of the topical agents available. Oral ketoconazole may be necessary in patients with *Candida* esophagitis, but treatment failures have been reported (63). Ketoconazole may also be useful in more extensive mucocutaneous disease. This drug is often well tolerated. However, this drug should be used cautiously in this patient population already at high risk for hepatitis, both from viruses and other medications, as well as at risk for adrenal insufficiency for a variety of reasons, including cytomegalovirus and mycobacterial infection. Systemic disease requires removal of any intravascular lines that may be implicated, as well as the use of intravenous amphotericin B. Unlike many of the other disseminated fungal infections which necessitate long term therapy, a short course of amphotericin B, in a cumulative dosage of 500 mg, may be curative.

Prevention

Decreasing the intensity of skin and mucous membrane colonization should help lessen the risk for serious disseminated infection. Avoiding prolonged courses of antibacterial medications should also help in this regard.

B. *Coccidioides immitis*

Epidemiology

Coccidioides immitis is endemic to the southwestern and far western United States. The most common illness is self-limited respiratory infection in immunocompetent individuals. There is a well-described difference in risk for dissemination based on racial background. Sites of dissemination include the skin, lymphnodes, urinary tract, and central nervous system. Reactivation of *Coccidioides* infection has been seen in renal transplant patients (64).

Disease

In the immunodeficient individual, this fungal pathogen may readily disseminate or lead to progressive pulmonary disease. Several cases of disseminated disease have been described in patients with AIDS (65). The disease often takes a more aggressive course with higher rate of fungemia and multiple organ disease (66).

Diagnosis

Unfortunately, diagnosis may require invasive procedures. The diagnosis should be entertained in the setting of development of diffuse bilateral reticulonodular or nodular infiltrates on chest roentgenogram. Skin test anergy is common even in the immunocompetent with disseminated or extrapulmonary coccidioidomycosis. However, in persons with AIDS, the serologic tests may also be unremarkable. One person had no reaction to either coccidioidin 1:100 or spherulin 1:100, and over a two-month interval showed no antibody production as determined by precipitin (IgM), complement fixation (IgG), counter immunoelectrophoresis (IgG), and immunodiffusion (both IgM and IgG) (65). However, a more recent report found verification of coccidioidal infection in initial serologic testing in five of seven patients using tests for tube-precipitating antigen, complement-fixing antibodies for coccidioidan, or both (66).

Treatment

Amphotericin B is the drug of choice. Some isolates may be sensitive to the imidazoles. However, currently available imidazoles do not penetrate the central nervous system or the urinary tract well. Therapy may need to be indefinite, as is occasionally the case in otherwise immunocompetent individuals with disseminated disease.

Prevention

Although there is a vaccine undergoing clinical trial, it is not widely available. Coccidioidomycosis will remain a problem for the immunodeficient patient in endemic areas, especially since most disease in patients with AIDS represents reactivation of latent foci from prior infection. Of note, ketoconazole therapy up to 400 mg/d did not prevent the development of disseminated disease in some reported patients (66). Microbiology laboratory personnel should be alert to the possibility of *Coccidioides* infection in high-risk patients to reduce the risk of laboratory acquired infection.

C. *Histoplasma capsulatum*

Epidemiology

Like *Coccidioides*, *Histoplasma* is an environmental (soil) organism. In the United States it is seen most commonly in the region of the Ohio River Valley. However, individuals from the Caribbean or South America should also be considered at risk for disseminated histoplasmosis (67). *Histoplasma* most often causes a self-limited or inapparent pulmonary infection in the immunocompetent person, with up to 500,000 new cases per year. As many as 80% of the population in endemic areas are skin test reagin positive. *Histoplasma* is a dimorphic fungus that exists in the soil in the mycelial phase. The smaller spores (microconidia) can be inhaled and reach the smaller bronchioles and alveoli where infection is established.

Disease

Like *Coccidioides immitis*, *Histoplasma* can cause focal pulmonary infection, or a variety of disseminated syndromes (68). It has been well described in persons with AIDS (69,70), including those who have left the endemic area years before presentation. Disease most often follows reactivation of an old focus of infection, and procedes to unchecked dissemination. Infection may present with a septic shocklike picture (71,72), disseminated disease with a normal chest roentgenogram, or progressive pulmonary disease (69). Cultures have been positive from the blood in five of seven cases (69), as well as bone marrow, brain, liver, sputum, and lymph node (70). In addition, a variety of skin lesions have been described (73), including pustular, follicular, erythematous plaquelike, and ulcerated perianal lesions in a single patient (74). Furthermore, a case of gastrointestinal histoplasmosis has been reported in a person at risk for AIDS presenting with a large cecal mass (75).

Diagnosis

The cultures and smears of involved tissue, including blood (76), are reported to be positive. The lysis-centrifugation blood culture technique appears to offer more rapid recovery over conventional methods (77). In addition, *Histoplasma* serological tests have been found positive in all patients reported in one series (68). However, some cases required that immunodiffusion as well as complement fixation be done for both the yeast and mycelial phases, since the complement fixation titer to mycelial antigen may not be positive in all patients tested (67). In the absence of positive culture or histology, these serological tests do not distinguish between past and active infection. A recent study reporting on the results of a radioimmunoassay for *H. capsulatum* antigen appears promising in the context of disseminated histoplasmosis (78). Some of the patients in this series with antigenemia and antigenuria had AIDS as the predisposing condition to disseminated disease. Until antigen detection tests for histoplasma become standardized, the diagnosis is most reliably established by isolating the organism. *H. capsulatum* does not stain well with hematoxylin-eosin but does appear well with either the Giemsa's stain or methenamine silver stain. *Histoplasma* grows well on either potato yeast extract or Sabouraud's agar.

Treatment

Although *Histoplasma* is generally more sensitive than coccidioides to the imidazole antibiotics, the treatment of choice for disseminated disease is still amphotericin B. Relapses after 35 mg/kg of amphotericin B have been reported, and prolonged suppression may be necessary. Ketoconazole in doses of 400-600 mg/d may be necessary for continued suppression of disease.

Prevention

None known. Person-to-person transmission is not reported.

D. *Cryptococcus neoformans*

Epidemiology

Like many of the other pathogens associated with opportunistic infections in persons with AIDS, the *Cryptococcus* is ubiquitous. Most clinical disease is associated with encapsulated *C. neoformans.* However, poorly encapsulated and non-neoformans species have been identified as well (79).

Disease

Although on occasion the cause of clinical illness in the immunocompetent individual (80) (less than 300 cases per year), cryptococcus is a pathogen in the immunosuppressed individual. The central nervous system presentations are known (see Chapter 15), and represent the most common site of infection, 66-84% of cases (81). However, many of these cases are also disseminated, with other foci of infection identified, including the prostate (82). Cryptococcal disease may present without central nervous system involvement in persons with AIDS, and as the initial manifestation of AIDS (83).

Patients may have a fever with no obvious source, and have few focal complaints. They may present septicemic, with or without concurrent meningitis. Skin lesions appearing like those of molluscum contagiosum have been reported (73). Disease of the lungs (81), myocardium (84), bone marrow, kidney, liver, and even joint space (85) has been reported. A case of cellulitis with necrotizing vasculitis in the setting of immunosuppressive therapy for a cadaveric renal allograph has been recently described (86). It is not uncommon to obtain a growth of *C. neoformans* from culture material submitted from a transbronchial biopsy in a patient with *Pneumocystis carinii* pneumonia a week or more after completion of successful therapy for the pneumocystis. In addition, numerous cases have been reported to present simultaneously with central nervous system toxoplasmosis (87).

Diagnosis

As part of a fever assessment, the serum cryptococcal antigen may be the most sensitive initial test for this pathogen (88). Serum titers as high as 1:2,000,000 have been reported (89). However, there have been instances where the soluble serum antigen is not detected in invasive disease (90). In situations where patients present with extra-central nervous system complaints suggesting either focal or systemic disease due to *Cryptococcus*, a spinal tap is mandatory. The serum and cerebral spinal fluid cryptococcal antigen, India ink preparation of spinal fluid, and appropriate cultures may help determine the duration of therapy.

Treatment

Cryptococcal meningitis and the other disseminated forms require prolonged and often indefinite therapy with amphotericin B (90). 5-flucytosine is often used in combination with amphotericin B. However, this oral antifungal agent is often associated with hematological toxicity, limiting its usefulness in chronic treatment. Many patients require chronic suppressive therapy with up to 1 mg/kg amphotericin B, once or twice weekly to prevent relapse of disease (91). Some patients with disease limited to the lung, with no evidence for systemic or central nervous system infection, have been treated with shorter courses of amphotericin B, i.e., 500-1000 mg, and followed carefully. If the serum cryptococcal antigen is negative, these patients can be followed at monthly intervals with repeat serum antigen determination, without suppressive therapy. In addition, high doses of ketoconazole (1000 mg/d) have been used in some patients after six to eight weeks of amphotericin therapy with successful suppression of recurrence (92). Investigational imidazoles such as fluconazole may prove more useful. Some investigators have recommended the use of an Ommaya reservoir for treating patients with slowly responsive or unresponsive central nervous system disease and AIDS. However, recent anecdotes have suggested that Ommaya reservoirs may not always be useful (93).

Prevention

Unfortunately, there is no prevention for this ubiquitous environmental organism. Development of disseminated cryptococcal disease has been seen in patients on lower doses of ketoconazole for other conditions (up to 400 mg/d) (94).

IV. Protozoa

As a group, the protozoa remain some of the most common and devastating opportunistic pathogens in AIDS patients (95). Pneumocystosis and central nervous system toxoplasmosis are discussed in Chapters 16 and 15, respectively. Management of infections due to *Giardia lamblia*, *Entamoeba histolytica*, and other common intestinal protozoa have not proven to be particularly complex in the setting of AIDS and will not be discussed.

A. Cryptosporidiosis and Infection Due to *Isospora belli*

Epidemiology

Cryptosporidia and *Isospora* have been identified in several mammals, birds and reptiles, apparently lacking much host specificity (96). These intestinal protozoa are increasingly recognized as a cause of self-limited diarrheal syndromes in a number of situations. A waterborne outbreak of cryptosporidiosis attributed to a common source of fecally contaminated water has been described (97). It is a frequent finding in patients with diarrhea (98) and in children in day care centers (99). The organism has been acquired as a human zoonosis, and person-to-person transmission is well described, both sexually and nonsexually, through fecal to oral contamination. In the setting of AIDS, it is seen most commonly in homosexual men and children (100). The incubation period is usually 4-12 days and the mean duration of symptoms is usually 10-14 days. In immunosuppressed patients, cryptosporidiosis can be devastating and life-threatening (101).

Diseases

The microbiology and pathogenesis of cryptosporidiosis has been recently reviewed (102). In summary, *Cryptosporidia* infect the microvillus border of the small intestine and can be seen diffusely along other mucosal surfaces, from the esophagus (103) to the rectum and bronchi. Although considered intracellular parasites, they are "extracytoplasmic." The pathogenesis of disease is still unclear, but appears to involve enterotoxic mechanisms leading to the histopathological picture of epithelial cell loss, villous atrophy and fusion, crypt elongation, and minimal inflammatory cell response.

Both pathogens can present with indistinguishable syndromes in the immunosuppressed patient. The pattern of secretory diarrhea without inflammatory cells or red blood cells can result in crampy abdominal pain and voluminous watery diarrhea. In one series *Cryptosporidium* was the most common cause of abdominal pain in patients with AIDS (104). Quantities of up to 20 liters of stool per day have been reported. Usually the patients are not febrile or have only low grade temperature elevation, unless there is concurrent infection with other intestinal pathogens, such as *Salmonella*, *Shigella*, cytomegalovirus, or *Mycobacterium avium-intracellulare*. In addition, patients may present with cholecystitis (11,105) and bronchial disease (101).

Diagnosis

A variety of methods for staining the macrogametes, microgametes, and oocysts are available. Stool specimens may yield the oocysts on either a modified Ziehl-Neelsen stain (106) or modified Sheather's sugar flotation method. Esophageal, gastric, intestinal, or bronchial biopsies reveal the organism on Giemsa stain. The oocysts of *Isospora belli* are much larger and oval rather than round, as seen in *Cryptosporidia.* In addition, they have two sporoblasts, whereas the oocyst of *Cryptosporidium* species release four sporozoites. The number of negative specimens necessary to confirm the absence of this pathogen has not been established. In immunocompetent individuals the organism can be shed asymptomatically, but a majority of specimens of infected symptomatic individuals are positive (78/90 or 86.7% in one series [107]).

Treatment

There is no established therapy for cryptosporidiosis (108). A variety of antimicrobials have been tried and occasionally appear successful (109). Spiramycin (Rovamycin), up to 3 g/d orally (110), α-difluoromethyl-ornithine (111), and furazolidone have received some attention and have been used with occasional success (11). Although symptoms may improve in some, parasitic cure is unusual with these agents. A preliminary report describing improvement of diarrhea in five of eight patients after treatment with oral bovine transfer factor is encouraging (112). Trimethoprim-sulfamethoxazole has been used in isospora infections, but recurrence appears to be high (113). Other reports suggest trimethoprim-sulfamethoxazole may not always be useful in *Isospora* infections (114). Therefore, treatment is mostly symptomatic with one or more antiparastaltic agents as tolerated and fluid replacement. Occasionally nonsteroidal antiinflammatory drugs have led to symptomatic improvement, possibly by blocking cyclic AMP production.

Prevention

Since the organism is transmitted by the fecal-oral route, earlier recommendations for avoiding other enteric pathogens are appropriate.

B. *Strongyloides stercoralis*

Epidemiology

Strongyloides is found in the southern United States, as well as in other warm, moist climates. The pathogen is usually acquired through penetration of intact skin by infective larvae residing in moist soil. It has been described as a venereal pathogen as well (114a). Usually asymptomatic carriage is not a problem, unless the patient is immunosuppressed. A hyperinfection syndrome often heralded by Gram-negative rod sepsis has been described in other immunosuppressed patients (115). Serious infection has only recently been described in the setting of AIDS (115a). Extraintestinal disease is omitted in some case definitions of AIDS (116).

Diseases

The pathogenesis of this disease involves chronic reinfection via the intestinal tract and portal system, with subsequent migration of the infective filariform larva to the liver and then lungs. Pulmonary infiltrates, cough, and sputum production are associated with eosinophilia. Patients may present with enteric bacteremia.

Diagnosis

A high index of suspicion is the mainstay of diagnosis. Diagnosis is most often established by examination of intestinal contents. The stool may reveal the rhabditiform larva. The string test (Enterotest) is often positive. Occasionally, the diagnosis is established by examination of sputum or tracheal-bronchial secretions. A direct wet smear or cytologic examination of sputum may yield the filariform larva.

Treatment

Thiabendazole (Vermox) may be curative. The standard dosage regimen is 25 mg/kg b.i.d. for two days. Unfortunately, often the patients are very ill and prolonged therapy seems indicated. Mortality rate is high, due to continued sepsis or other complicating infections.

Prevention

Acquisition can be avoided by wearing shoes out of doors. Unfortunately, stool examination in high-risk patients does not seem to predict later development of the hyperinfection syndrome.

C. *Toxoplasma gondii*

Epidemiology

This protozoan is covered extensively elsewhere (Chapter 15). A brief mention is made because it may be disseminated in patients with AIDS.

Diseases

Other organs are often infected by *T. gondii* concurrent with central nervous system manifestations. The pulmonary form most often occurs with other pulmonary pathogens, and the contribution of this protozoan to the clinical symptoms is unclear (117). Pulmonary disease attributed to toxoplasma appears to mimic *Pneumocystis carinii* pneumonia, with diffuse infiltrates and a scant, often nonproductive cough. The heart is the other organ most commonly infected in persons with AIDS and disseminated disease at autopsy. Two cases of testicular toxoplasmosis have been reported in patients dying with known central nervous disease (118) and a patient presenting with weakness, hypothermia, headache, nausea, and hypotension secondary to toxoplasma hypothalamic infection (119) has been reported. Despite the frequency of retinal disease in persons with AIDS and the high incidence of toxoplasmosis, toxoplasmic retinochoroiditis appears to be fairly uncommon (120), but can be seen, often in the absence of identified cortical brain lesions. The differential diagnosis includes cytomegalovirus and syphilis (121).

Diagnosis

Unlike central nervous system disease, that may be treated empirically based on a compatible presentation and multiple lesions visualized on either a computed axial tomography (CAT) or magnetic resonance image (MRI) scan of the head, disease elsewhere requires visualization of the organism in tissue. This has been aided with a peroxidase-antiperoxidase stain.

Treatment

Treatment consists of a combination of pyrimethamine and sulfadiazine, 25-50 mg/day and 1-2 g q.i.d., respectively. Since this combination of folate antagonists can interfere with mammalian folic acid and therefore nucleic acid biosynthesis, it is occasionally necessary to supplement with folinic acid, either as Brewer's yeast, or occasionally leukovorin. Because of the frequency of allergic reactions and bone marrow toxicity, clindamycin, up to 2.7 g/d parenterally followed by 1200-2400 mg/d orally, has been substituted for the sulfadiazine with some success in central nervous system disease (122). Spiramycin has generally not been successful (123). Relapses occur often once therapy is discontinued. Therefore, long-term maintenance therapy is indicated (123a). It is usually established by the minimum dose of medication necessary to maintain asymptomatic central nervous system disease after radiographic resolution of lesions.

Prevention

Since the organism is ubiquitous, most patients present with reactivation of old disease and not new acquisition. It is recommended to check all patients serologically for presence of past infection at the time of diagnosis of AIDS. This procedure may help heighten one's index of suspicion for recurrent disease should central nervous system or other compatible organ system complaints appear. Unfortunately, trimethoprim-sulfamethoxazole prophylaxis against recurrent *Pneumocystis carinii* pneumonia does not seem to prevent development of central nervous system toxoplasmosis. Patients are advised not to eat raw meat and to avoid contact with dry cat feces to prevent new acquisition of this pathogen.

V. *Mycobacterium* Infections

Mycobacterium infections are the most common bacteremic illness complicating AIDS (124). Discussion will be divided into the *M. avium* complex (MAC) infections and *M. tuberculosis hominis* infections. However, other mycobacteria have been reported in association with AIDS. *Myocbacterium haemophilum* infection has been reported to cause tenosynovitis and multiple subcutaneous abscesses in persons with AIDS (125). Although smears for acid-fast bacilli of lesion aspirates may be markedly positive, growth will only occur in hemin-supplemented medium. Other atypical isolates reported include *M. simiae* (126), *M. xenopi*, *M. fortuitum*, *M. gordonae*, *M. kansasii* (127), *M. malmoense*, and *M. scrofulacium*. Standard drugs used as antimycobacterial agents are described in Table 2.

A. *Mycobacterium avium* Complex Infections

Epidemiology

The complex is found ubiquitously in the environment, including soil, water, and house dust, and MAC has been noted to cause disease in other mammal and bird species. It is found during life in 10-20% and at autopsy in up to 50% of persons with AIDS (128). Unlike the situation with *Mycobacterium tuberculosis*, there appears to be no difference in occurence based on AIDS risk group. Person-to-person transmission is not documented. Many believe the organism is acquired through the gastrointestinal tract. The role of MAC as a possible cofactor in the development of AIDS has been suggested (129).

Diseases

Prior to AIDS, MAC was most often described as a pulmonary opportunist, in patients with underlying severe lung disease (130). It has often been implicated as a common cause of scrofula in children. Its most common presentation in persons with AIDS is that of a disseminated infection. Patients present most often with fever as high as 104 to 105 degrees, chills, night sweats, malaise, weight loss, and fatigue. There may be a mild cough and dyspnea. Patients also may have a variety of gastrointestinal syndromes, including chronic abdominal pain with diarrhea, chronic malabsorption with Whipple's disease-like histology, and extrabiliary obstruction with or without jaundice and abdominal pain secondary to regional lymphadenopathy (11). MAC can be a major cause of malabsorption and weight loss (131) as well as skin lesions (73) and oral ulcerative lesions (132).

Table 2 Antituberculous Agents

Drug	Supplied	Dosage	Comments
Isoniazid	Tabs: 300 mg 100 mg	300 mg p.o.	Role as adjunct therapy in MAC infection unclear. May cause hepatitis, peripheral neuritis.
Rifampin	Caps: 300 mg	600 mg p.o.	May be replaced by Rifabutin. May cause hepatitis, allergic skin or febrile reaction.
Rifabutin	Caps: 150 mg	300-450 mg p.o.	Investigational and optimal dosage not known. Side effects as with Rifampin.
Ethambutol	Tabs: 400 mg 100 mg	15-25 mg/kg per d p.o.	Optic neuritis in high dosage. Must be adjusted for renal failure. May cause skin rash, gastrointestinal upset.
Clofazimine	Caps: 100 mg	100-200 mg p.o.	Skin discoloration (red-brown), ocular pigmentation, abdominal pain, diarrhea are dose-related.
Amikacin sulfate	Vials for injection	Up to 10 mg/kg i.v. or i.m.	May cause worsening nephro- or ototoxicity. Role suggested for initial therapy of symptomatic MAC infection.
Ciprofloxacin	Caps: 500 mg 750 mg	Up to 1.5 g p.o.	Investigational but good in vitro activity against MAC.
Pyrazinamide	Tabs: 500 mg	25 mg/kg up to 2 g p.o.	Hepatic toxicity; hyperuricemia.
Cycloserine	Caps: 250 mg	15 mg/kg up to 1 g p.o.	Not well tolerated in AIDS because of CNS (personality) changes, but sometimes good MAC activity.
Ethionamide	Caps: 250 mg	15 mg/kg up to 1 g p.o.	Not well tolerated because of gastrointestinal intolerance, but sometimes good MAC activity.

MAC, *Mycobacterium avium* complex.

Diagnosis

The diagnosis is most often established by isolation or visualization of the organism from one or more specimens (133). High-grade mycobacteremia is well described (134). A variety of systems have been used to document bacteremia (135). A lysis-centrifugation system will often confirm the diagnosis in 7-14 days of incubation from blood specimens. More immediate diagnosis can be obtained by direct visualization in body fluids, such as stool, or tissue such as lymphnode, liver biopsy, gastrointestinal biopsy (136), skin biopsy (137), and on occasion bone marrow (138). In only 4 of 10 bone marrow specimens which subsequently yielded MAC on culture were granulomas visualized (139). Three of the 10 positive cultures were obtained from specimens showing both granuloma and a positive acid-fast stain, whereas four of the positive cultures occurred in specimens that revealed neither granuloma nor acid-fast bacilli. *Mycobacterium kansasii* dissemination to the bowel in patients with AIDS appears to be distinguished from MAC infection by the absence of foamy macrophages in the former infection despite the presence of diffuse inflammation and positive acid-fast smears of intestinal biopsy specimens (127).

Treatment

Treatment is controversial. Most isolates are resistant to the conventional antituberculosis medications, including isoniazid, ethambutol, and rifampin by the standard agar colony reduction techniques. Of note, a recent report suggested that bacteriocidal activity of ethambutol against MAC can be demonstrated in broth (140). Differences in in vitro susceptibility test patterns between isolates of *M. avium* from patients with AIDS and patients with respiratory disease but no AIDS have been reported (141). Susceptibility to cycloserine and ethionamide for those isolates from AIDS patients with disseminated disease has been noted. Occasionally isolates are sensitive to streptomycin. Two additional antimicrobial agents, ansamycin (Rifabutin) and clofazamine (Lamprene), have been used. In vitro culture systems and liquid media suggest a variety of other potentially effective antimicrobials, including some quinolone antibiotics and some of the third-generation cephalosporins.

Most clinicians agree that this condition is not curable (142), and patients remain mycobacteriologically infected. However, antituberculosis therapy may improve some of the symptoms, although the literature documenting this impression in the setting of AIDS is unclear (143). This finding contrasts to pulmonary *M. avium* infection in the non-AIDS setting where correlation between in vitro sensitivity testing and response to therapy has recently been suggested (144). In AIDS patients, conversion to culture negativity often does not correlate with clinical improvement. Symptoms of fever, chills, night sweats may be intermittent in some and make assessment of response to any single chemotherapeutic regimen difficult.

Initiation of therapy is usually reserved for those individuals with a compatible clinical illness, prolonged symptoms of fever, chills, and night sweats, and an organism identified on either smear or culture from a normally sterile site, in the absence of other identified treatable pathogens. It is unclear whether initiating therapy for individuals documented to be infected in the absence of symptoms offers any advantage. Many clinicians use standard doses of isoniazid (300 mg/d) and ethambutol (15 to 25 mg/kg per d) as basis for therapy. Rifabutin can be obtained from the Parasitic Drug Section, Centers for Disease Control. Clofazimine in doses of 100-200 mg/d has been used. It has recently been released in the United States for the treatment of leprosy. In the short course, parenteral aminoglycosides and cephalosporins have been used for very ill patients. However, the chronicity of infection makes long term administration of these generally impractical. Studies to date have failed to affirm the superiority of any single proposed drug regimen (142). Ongoing research using in vitro culture systems and a beige mouse model of disseminated MAC infection should define more efficacious therapeutic regimens (124).

Prevention

This organism is not known to be transmissible person-to-person. No preventive measures are established.

B. *Mycobacterium tuberculosis hominis*

Epidemiology

With respect to AIDS, *M. tuberculosis* is most often isolated from those individuals who would be expected to be at risk for prior acquisition of the pathogen, such as intravenous drug users, emigrants from developing countries, and individuals with a history of extensive travel to or residence in highly endemic areas, such as Africa. However, a recent report suggests that this is not always the case and that all AIDS risk groups should be considered to be at risk for tuberculosis (145,146). An increase in cases of *M. tuberculosis* has occurred in those areas where an increased incidence in AIDS has also been seen, i.e., southern Florida, New York City, New Jersey, and San Francisco. Given that there are estimated to be about 10 million people with latent tuberculosis infection in the United States, and as many as 1.5 million people with HIV infection, it is expected that overlap in these two populations may result in an increased number of clinically evident cases of tuberculosis. In half of cases or more, tuberculous disease precedes the diagnosis of AIDS, by as much as five years (147).

Diseases

Tuberculosis is more likely to present in a disseminated (55% of patients) or extrapulmonary (72% of patients) form in the presence of HIV infection. Bone marrow, lymph node, liver, central nervous system (148), peritoneum (149), choroidal (150), and renal infections have been described. The symptoms include fever, chills, and night sweats, but granulomatous response may be impaired. The radiographic findings have been noted to include hilar and or mediastinal adenopathy (59%) and localized or diffuse pulmonary infiltrates (65%) (151). A miliary pattern and cavitation are rarely seen, but normal chest roentgenograms are common (12%).

Diagnosis

Given the unusual presentations listed above, an aggressive and invasive approach to diagnosis may be necessary. Tuberculin skin test reactivity is often impaired. Of 31 patients with both culture-proven *Mycobacterium tuberculosis* infection and AIDS reported to the San Francisco Department of Public Health between 1981 and 1985, only 10 (32%) had a skin test (Purified Protein Derivative) reaction of greater than or equal to 10 mm (152). Acid-fast bacilli seen in well-formed granulomatous lesions on biopsy of involved organs favors *M. tuberculosis* infection rather than MAC infection. However, this pathogen has been isolated in the absence of any documented inflammatory response (149). Appropriate specimens to establish a culture-confirmed diagnosis of tuberculosis include respiratory secretions, urine, blood (153), lymph node, bone marrow, liver, or other tissue or body fluid that is indicated clinically (154).

Treatment

Most of the reported isolates are sensitive to a variety of antituberculous medications. In general, treatment should include at least three drugs initially. Definitive treatment, with the ultimate drug choice determined by the antimicrobial sensitivity of the isolate, may need to be more prolonged than standard, but response appears to be good (145,155). Fatal cases appear to occur more often in the most deep-seated infections, including those in the pericardium and central nervous system (147). After completion of therapy, patients should be watched carefully for recurrence of disease (154).

Prevention

It is recommended that persons testing positive for HIV infection should have a PPD skin test early in the course of the identification of HIV infection (156,157). Persons in high-risk groups for AIDS and HIV infection who have a positive PPD reaction should receive isoniazid chemoprophylaxis regardless of age (154). In addition, visualization of acid-fast bacilli in pulmonary secretions should prompt appropriate respiratory precautions, pending identification of the isolate, to prevent the potential spread of tuberculosis to others.

References

1. Glaser JB, Landesman SH. *Streptococcus bovis* bacteremia and acquired immunodeficiency syndrome (letter). Ann Intern Med 1983; 99:878.
2. Spivak JL, Bender BS, Quinn TC. Hematologic abnormalities in the acquired immune deficiency syndrome. Am J Med 1984; 77:224-8.
3. Blaser MJ, Cohn DL. Opportunistic infections in patients with AIDS: clues to the epidemiology of AIDS and the relative virulence of pathogens. Rev Infect Dis 1986; 8:21-30.
4. Sane DC, Durack DT. Infection with *Rhodococcus equi* in AIDS (letter). N Engl J Med 1986; 314:64.
5. Samies JH, Hathaway BN, Echols RM, Veazey JM Jr, Pilon VA. Lung abscess due to *Corynebacterium equi*: report of the first case in a patient with acquired immune deficiency syndrome. Am J Med 1986; 80:685-8.
6. Wang HH, Tollerud D, Danar D, Hanff P, Gottesdiener K, Rosen S. Another Whipple-like disease in AIDS? N Engl J Med 1986; 314:1577-8.
7. Whimbey E, Gold JWM, Polsky B, Dryjanski J, Hawkins C, Blevins A, Brannon P, Kiehn TE, Brown AE, Armstrong D. Bacteremia and fungemia in patients with the acquired immunodeficiency syndrome. Ann Intern Med 1986; 104:511-4.
8. White S, Tsou E, Waldhorn RE, Katz P. Life-threatening bacterial pneumonia in male homosexuals with laboratory features of the acquired immunodeficiency syndrome. Chest 1986; 87:486-8.
9. Bernstein LJ, Krieger BZ, Novick B, Sicklick MJ, Rubinstein A. Bacterial infection in the acquired immunodeficiency syndrome of children. Pediatr Infect Dis 1985; 4:472-5.
10. Simberkoff MS, El Sadr W, Schiffman G, Rahal JJ Jr. *Streptococcus pneumoniae* infections and bacteremia in patients with acquired immune deficiency syndrome, with report of a pneumococcal vaccine failure. Am Rev Respir Dis 1984; 130:1174-6.
11. Grant IE, Armstrong D. Management of infectious complications in acquired immunodeficiency syndrome. Am J Med 1986; 81 (Suppl 1A):59-72.
12. Witt DJ, Craven DE, McCabe WR. Bacterial infections in adult patients with the acquired immune deficiency syndrome (AIDS) and AIDS-related complex. Am J Med 1987; 82:900-6.
13. Polsky B, Gold JWM, Whimbey E, Dryjanski J, Brown AE, Schiffman G, Armstrong D. Bacterial pneumonia in patients with acquired immunodeficiency syndrome. Ann Intern Med 1986; 104:38-41.
14. Clairmont GJ, Zon LI, Groopman JE. *Hemophilus parainfluenzae* prostatitis in a homosexual man with chronic lymphadenopathy syndrome and HTLV-III infection. Am J Med 1987; 82:175-7.
15. Fischl MA, Dickinson GM. Sinus disease associated with the acquired immunodeficiency syndrome. Second International Conference on AIDS (1986), Paris, France. Poster 517.

16. Ammann AJ, Schiffman G, Abrams D, Volberding P, Ziegler J, Conant M. B-cell immunodeficiency in acquired immune deficiency syndrome. JAMA 1984; 251:1447-9.
17. Sanders N, Dietrich S, Robinson K, Bowlen A, Ewing N, Friedman A. Intravenous immune gamma globulin (IVGG) in hemophilia patients with AIDS or AIDS-related complex (ARC). Second International Conference on AIDS (1986), Paris, France. Poster 553.
18. Walsh TJ, Belitsos NJ, Hamilton SR. Bacterial esophagitis in immunocompromised patients. Arch Intern Med 1986; 146:1345-8.
19. Smith PD, Macher AM, Bookman MA, Boccia RV, Steis RG, Gill V, Manischewitz J, Gelmann E. *Salmonella typhimurium* enteritis and bacteremia in the acquired immunodeficiency syndrome. Ann Intern Med 1985; 102:207-9.
20. Celum CL, Chaisson RE, Echenberg DF, Barnhart JL, Rendon C, Rutherford GW. The epidemiology of salmonellosis in patients with acquired immune deficiency syndrome in San Francisco. Second International Conference on AIDS (1986), Paris, France. Poster 516.
20a. Sperber SJ, Schleupner CJ. Salmonellosis during infection with human immunodeficiency virus. Rev Infect Dis 1987; 9:925-34.
21. Fischl MA, Dickinson GM, Sinave C, Pitchenik AE. *Salmonella* bacteremia as manifestation of acquired immunodeficiency syndrome. Arch Intern Med 1986; 146:113-5.
22. Glaser JB, Morton-Kute L, Berger SR, Weber J, Siegal FP, Lipez C, Robbins W, Landesman SH. Recurrent *Salmonella typhimurium* bacteremia associated with the acquired immunodeficiency syndrome. Ann Intern Med 1985; 102: 189-93.
23. Jacobs JL, Gold JWM, Murray HW, Roberts RB, Armstrong D. *Salmonella* infections in patients with the acquired immunodeficiency syndrome. Ann Intern Med 1985; 102:186-8.
24. Nadelman RB, Mathur-Wagh U, Yancovitz SR, Mildvan D. Salmonella bacteremia associated with the acquired immunodeficiency syndrome (AIDS). Arch Intern Med 1985; 145:1968-71.
25. Bryan JP, Rocha H, Scheld WM. Problems in salmonellosis: rationale for clinical trials with newer beta-lactam agents and quinolones. Rev Infect Dis 1986; 8:189-207.
26. Aserkoff B, Schroeder SA, Brachman PS. Salmonellosis in the United States—a five-year review. Am J Epidemiol 1970; 92:13-24.
27. Profeta S, Forrester C, Eng RHK, Liu R, Johnson E, Palinkas R, Smith SM. *Salmonella* infections in patients with acquired immunodeficiency syndrome. Arch Intern Med 1985; 145:670-2.
28. Fierer J. Invasive *Salmonella dublin* infections associated with drinking raw milk. West J Med 1983; 138:665-9.
29. Burniat W, Toppet M, De Mol P. Acute and recurrent salmonella infections in three children with chronic granulomatous disease. J Infect 1980; 2:263-8.
30. Dupuis F, Vereerstraeten P, van Geertruyden J, Kinnaert P, Schoutens E, Toussant C. *Salmonella typhimurium* urinary infection after kidney transplantation. Report of seven cases. Clin Nephrol 1974; 2:131-5.

31. Jacobs JL, Murray HW. Why is *Listeria monocytogenes* not a pathogen in the acquired immunodeficiency syndrome (editorial)? Arch Intern Med 1986; 146: 1299-300.
32. Koziol K, Rielly KS, Bonin RA, Salcedo JR. *Listeria monocytogenes* meningitis in AIDS. Can Med Assoc J 1986; 135:43-4.
33. Gould IA, Belok LC, Handwerger S. *Listeria monocytogenes*: a rare cause of opportunistic infection in the acquired immunodeficiency syndrome (AIDS) and a new cause of meningitis in AIDS. A case report. AIDS Res 1986; 2: 231-4.
34. Real FX, Gold JWM, Krown SE, Armstrong D. *Listeria monocytogenes* bacteremia in the acquired immune deficiency syndrome (letter). Ann Intern Med 1984; 101:883-4.
34a. Spitzer PG, Hammer SM, Karchmer AW. Treatment of *Listeria monocytogenes* infection with trimethoprim/sulfamethoxazole: Case report and review of the literature. Rev Infect Dis 1986; 8:427-30.
35. Centers for Disease Control. Listeriosis outbreak associated with Mexican style cheese. MMWR 1985; 34:357-9.
35a. Mascola L, Lieb L, Chiu J, Fannin SL, Linnan MJ. Listeriosis: An uncommon opportunstic infection in patients with acquired immunodeficiency syndrome. Am J Med 1988; 84:162-4.
36. Blaser MJ, Wells JG, Feldman RA, Pollard RA, Allen JR, Collaborative Diarrheal Disease Study Group. *Campylobacter* enteritis in the United States: a multicenter study. Ann Intern Med 1983; 98:360-5.
37. Quinn TC, Goodell SE, Fennell CL, Wang SP, Schuffler MD, Holmes KK, Stamm WE. Infections with *Campylobacter jejuni* and *Campylobacter*-like organisms in homosexual men. Ann Intern Med 1984; 101:187-92.
38. Mendleson MH, Nicholas P, Malowany M, Lewis S. Subdural empyema caused by *Campylobacter fetus* ssp. *fetus* (letter). J Infect Dis 1986; 153:1183-4.
39. Costel EE, Wheeler AP, Gregg CR. *Campylobacter fetus* ssp *fetus* cholecystitis and relapsing bacteremia in a patient with acquired immunodeficiency syndrome. South Med J 1984; 77:927-8.
40. Pasternak J, Bolivar R, Hopfer RL, Fainstein V, Mills K, Rios A, Bodey GP, Fennell CL, Totten PA, Stamm WE. Bacteremia caused by *Campylobacter*-like organisms in two male homosexuals. Ann Intern Med 1984; 101:339-41.
41. Dworkin B, Wormser GP, Abdoo RA, Cabello F, Aguero ME, Sivak SL. Persistence of multiply antibiotic-resistant *Campylobacter jejuni* in a patient with the acquired immune deficiency syndrome. Am J Med 1986; 80:965-70.
42. Blaser MJ, Sazie E, Williams LP Jr. The influence of immunity on raw milk-associated *Campylobacter* infection. JAMA 1987; 257:43-6.
43. Centers for Disease Control. *Campylobacter* outbreak associated with raw milk provided on a dairy tour—California. MMWR 1986; 35:311-2.
44. Mayock R, Skale B, Kohler RB. *Legionella pneumophila* pericarditis proved by culture of pericardial fluid. Am J Med 1983; 75:534-6.
45. Friedland L, Snydman DR, Weingarden AS, Hedges TR, Brown R, Busky M. Ocular and pericardial involvement in Legionnaires' disease. Am J Med 1984; 7:1105-7.

46. Nelson DP, Rensimer ER, Burke CM, Raffin TA. Cardiac legionellosis (editorial). Chest 1984; 86:807-8.
47. McCabe RE, Baldwin JC, McGregor CA, Miller DC, Vosti KL. Prosthetic valve endocarditis caused by *Legionella pneumophila.* Ann Intern Med 1984; 100:525-7.
48. Martin RS, Marrie TJ, Best L, Sumarah RK, Peppard R. Isolation of *Legionella pneumophila* from the blood of a patient with Legionnaires' disease. Can Med Assoc J 1984; 131:1085-7.
49. Schlanger G, Lutwick LI, Kurzman M, Hoch B, Chandler FW. Sinusitis caused by *Legionella pneumophila* in a patient with the acquired immune deficiency syndrome. Am J Med 1984; 77:957-60.
50. Liu F, Wright DN. Gram stain in Legionnaires' disease. Am J Med 1984; 77:549-50.
51. Baptiste-Desruisseaux D, Duperval R, Marcoux JA. Legionnaires' disease in the immunocompromised host: usefulness of the Gram's stain. Can Med Assoc J 1985; 133:117-8.
52. Edelstein PH, Meyer RD, Finegold SM. Laboratory diagnosis of Legionnaires' disease. Am Rev Respir Dis 1980; 121:317-27.
53. Holtz HA, Lavery DP, Kapila R. Actinomycetales infection in the acquired immunodeficiency syndrome. Ann Intern Med 1985; 102:203-5.
54. Simpson GL, Raffin TA, Remington JS. Association of prior nocardiosis and subsequent occurrence of nontuberculous mycobacteriosis in a defined, immunosuppressed population. J Infect Dis 1982; 146:211-9.
55. Yeager BA, Hoxie J, Weisman RA, Greenberg MS, Bilaniuk LT. Actinomycosis in the acquired immunodeficiency syndrome-related complex. Arch Otolaryngol Head Neck Surg 1986; 112:1293-5.
56. Rodriguez JL, Barrio JL, Pitchenik AE. Pulmonary nocardiosis in the acquired immunodeficiency syndrome: diagnosis with bronchoalveolar lavage and treatment with non-sulfur containing drugs. Chest 1986; 90:912-4.
57. Wallace RJ, Jr., Wiss K, Curvey R, Vance PH, Steadham J. Differences among *Nocardia* spp. in susceptibility to aminoglycosides and beta-lactam antibiotics and their potential use in taxonomy. Antimicrob Agents Chemother 1983; 23:19-21.
57a. Moss AR, Osmond D, Bacchetti P, Chermann JC, Barre-Sinoussi F, Carlson J. Risk factors for AIDS and HIV seropositivity in homosexual men. Am J Epidemiol 1987; 125:1035-47.
57b. Centers for Disease Control. Increases in primary and secondary syphilis—United States. MMWR 1987; 36:393-7.
57c. Jordon KG. Neurosyphilis and HIV infection (letter). N Engl J Med 1987; 317:1473-4.
57d. Johns DR, Tierney M, Felsenstein D. Alteration in the natural history of neurosyphilis by concurrent infection with the human immunodeficiency virus. N Engl J Med 1987; 316:1569-72.
57e. Hart G. Syphilis tests in diagnostic and therapeutic decision making. Ann Intern Med 1986; 104:368-76.

57f. Hicks CB, Benson PM, Lupton GP, Tramont EC. Seronegative secondary syphilis in a patient infected with the human immunodeficiency virus (HIV) with Kaposi sarcoma. Ann Intern Med 1987; 107:492-6.
57g. Centers for Disease Control. 1985 STD treatment Guidelines. MMWR 1985; 34:94S-9S.
57h. Berry CS, Hooton TM, Collier AC, Lukehart SA. Neurologic relapse after benzathine penicillin therapy for secondary syphilis in a patient with HIV infection. N Engl J Med 1986; 316:1587-601.
58. Holmberg K, Meyer RD. Fungal infections in patients with AIDS and AIDS-related complex. Scand J Infect Dis 1986; 18:179-92.
59. Bibler MR, Luber JH, Glueck HI, Estes SA. Disseminated sporotrichosis in a patient with HIV infection after treatment for acquired Factor VIII inhibitor. JAMA 1986; 256:3125-6.
60. Henochowicz S, Mustafa M, Lawrinson WE, Pistole M, Lindsay J Jr. Cardiac aspergillosis in acquired immune deficiency syndrome. Am J Cardiol 1985; 55: 1239-40.
61. Jones PG, Cohen RL, Batts DH, Silva J Jr. Disseminated histoplasmosis, invasive pulmonary aspergillosis, and other opportunistic infections in a homosexual patient with the acquired immunodeficiency syndrome. Sex Transm Dis 1983; 10:202-4.
62. Tavitian A, Raufman JP, Rosenthal LE. Oral candidiasis as a marker for esophageal candidiasis in the acquired immunodeficiency syndrome. Ann Intern Med 1986; 104:54-5.
63. Tavitian A, Raufman JP, Rosenthal LE, Weber J, Webber CA, Dincsoy HP. Ketoconazole-resistant candida esophagitis in patients with acquired immunodeficiency syndrome. Gastroenterology 1986; 90:443-5.
64. Seltzer J, Broaddus VC, Jacobs R, Golden JA. Reactivation of coccidioides infection. West J Med 1986; 145:96-8.
65. Roberts CJ. Coccidioidomycosis in acquired immune deficiency syndrome; depressed humoral as well as cellular immunity. Am J Med 1984; 76:734-6.
66. Bronnimann DA, Adam RD, Galgiani JN, Habib MP, Petersen EA, Porter B, Bloom JW. Coccidioidomycosis in the acquired immunodeficiency syndrome. Ann Intern Med 1987; 106:372-9.
67. Mandell W, Goldberg DM, Neu HC. Histoplasmosis in patients with the acquired immune deficiency syndrome. Am J Med 1986; 81:974-8.
68. Goodwin RA, Jr., Shapiro JL, Thurman GH, Thurman SS, Des Prez RM. Disseminated histoplasmosis: clinical and pathologic correlations. Medicine 1980; 59:1-33.
69. Wheat LJ, Slama TG, Zeckel ML. Histoplasmosis in the acquired immune deficiency syndrome. Am J Med 1985; 78:203-10.
70. Bonner JR, Alexander WJ, Dismukes WE, App W, Griffin FM, Little R, Shin MS. Disseminated histoplasmosis in patients with the acquired immune deficiency syndrome. Arch Intern Med 1984; 144:2178-81.
71. Dietrich PY, Pugin P, Regamey C, Bille J. Disseminated histoplasmosis and AIDS in Switzerland (letter). Lancet 1986; 2:752.

72. Brivet F, Roulot D, Naveau S, Delfraissy JF, Goujard C, Tertian G, Cartier I, Brouhet E, Dupont B. The acquired immunodeficiency syndrome. Histoplasmosis (letter). Ann Intern Med 1986; 104:447.
73. Penneys NS, Hicks B. Unusual cutaneous lesions associated with acquired immunodeficiency syndrome. J Am Acad Dermatol 1985; 13:845-52.
74. Hazelhurst JA, Vismer HF. Histoplasmosis presenting with unusual skin lesions in acquired immunodeficiency syndrome (AIDS). Br J Dermatol 1985; 113: 345-8.
75. Haggerty CM, Britton MC, Dorman JM, Marzoni FA Jr. Gastrointestinal histoplasmosis in suspected acquired immunodeficiency syndrome. West J Med 1985; 143:244-6.
76. Henochowicz S, Sahovic E, Pistole M, Rodrigues M, Macher A. Histoplasmosis diagnosed on peripheral blood smear from a patient with AIDS. JAMA 1985; 253:3148.
77. Paya CV, Roberts GD, Cockerill FR, III. Laboratory methods for the diagnosis of disseminated histoplasmosis: clinical importance of the lysis-centrifugation blood culture technique. Mayo Clin Proc 1987; 62:480-5.
78. Wheat LJ, Kohler RB, Tewari RP. Diagnosis of disseminated histoplasmosis by detection of *Histoplasma capsulatum* antigen in serum and urine specimens. N Engl J Med 1986; 314:83-8.
79. Bottone EJ, Johansson BE, Szporn A, Toma M, Poon M, Wormser GP. Poorly encapsulated *Cryptococcus neoformans* from AIDS patients: morphologic, cultural, and pathogenic correlates. First International Conference on Acquired Immunodeficiency Syndrome (AIDS), 1985, Atlanta, Georgia. Poster W-20.
80. Shah B, Taylor HC, Pillay I, Chung-Park M, Dobrinich R. Adrenal insufficiency due to cryptococcosis. JAMA 1986; 256:3247-9.
81. Gal AA, Koss MN, Hawkins J, Evans S, Einstein H. The pathology of pulmonary cryptococcal infections in the acquired immunodeficiency syndrome. Arch Pathol Lab Med 1986; 110:502-7.
82. Lief M, Sarfarazi F. Prostatic cryptococcosis in acquired immune deficiency syndrome. Urology 1986; 28:318-9.
83. Witt D, McKay D, Schwam L, Goldstein D, Gold J. Acquired immune deficiency syndrome presenting as bone marrow and mediastinal cryptococcosis. Am J Med 1987; 82:149-50.
84. Lewis W, Lipsick J, Cammarosano C. Cryptococcal myocarditis in acquired immune deficiency syndrome. Am J Card 1985; 55:1240.
85. Ricciardi DD, Sepkowitz DV, Berkowitz LB, Bienenstock H, Maslow M. Cryptococcal arthritis in a patient with acquired immune deficiency syndrome. Case report and review of the literature. J Rheumatol 1986; 13:455-8.
86. Shrader SK, Watts JC, Dancik JA, Band JD. Disseminated cryptococcosis presenting as cellulitis with necrotizing vasculitis. J Clin Microbiol 1986; 24:860-2.
87. Bahls F, Sumi SM. Cryptococcal meningitis and cerebral toxoplasmosis in a patient with acquired immune deficiency syndrome. J Neuro Neurosurg Psychiatry 1986; 49:328-30.
88. Roux P, Touboul JL, Feuilhade de Chauvin M, Delacour T, Revuz J, Basset D, Mayaud C, Lancastre F. Disseminated cyrptococcus diagnosis in AIDS patient by screening for soluble serum antigens (letter). Lancet 1986; 1:1154.

89. Eng RHK, Bishburg E, Smith SM, Kapila R. Cryptococcal infections in patients with acquired immune deficiency syndrome. Am J Med 1986; 81:19-23.
90. Zuger A, Louie E, Holzman RS, Simberkoff MS, Rahal JJ. Cryptococcal disease in patients with the acquired immunodeficiency syndrome: diagnostic features and outcome of treatment. Ann Intern Med 1986; 104:234-40.
91. Kovacs JA, Kovacs AA, Polis M, Wright C, Gill VJ, Tuazon CU, Gelmann EP, Lane C, Longfield R, Ovirturt G, Macher AM, Fauci AS, Carrillo JE, Bennett JE, Masur H. Cryptococcosis in the acquired immunodeficiency syndrome. Ann Intern Med 1985; 103:533-8.
92. Mess TP, Hadley WK, Wofsy CB. Use of high dose oral ketoconazole in AIDS patients for prevention of relapse in cryptococcal infections. Second International Conference on AIDS, 1986, Paris, France. Poster 544.
93. DeVita VT Jr, Broder S, Fauci AS, Kovacs JA, Chabner BA. Developmental therapeutics and the acquired immunodeficiency syndrome. Ann Intern Med 1987; 106:568-81.
94. Follansbee SE, Busch DF. Cryptococcal meningitis (CM) complicating AIDS: analysis of 22 cases. First International Conference on Acquired Immunodeficiency Syndrome (AIDS), 1985, Atlanta, Georgia. Poster W-17.
95. Wong B. Parasitic diseases in immunocompromised hosts. Am J Med 1984; 76:479-86.
96. Tzipori S. Cryptosporidiosis in animals and humans. Microbiol Rev 1983; 47: 84-96.
97. D'Antonio RG, Winn RE, Taylor JP, Gustafson TL, Current WL, Rhodes MM, Gary W, Jr., Zajac RA. A waterborne outbreak of cryptosporidiosis in normal hosts. Ann Intern Med 1985; 103:886-8.
98. Jokipii L, Pohjola S, Jokipii AMM. Cryptosporidium: a frequent finding in patients with gastrointestinal symptoms. Lancet 1983; 2:358-60.
99. Taylor JP, Perdue JN, Dingley D, Gustafson TL, Patterson M, Reed LA. Cryptosporidiosis outbreak in a day care center. Am J Dis Child 1985; 139: 1023-25.
100. Navin TR, Hardy AM. Cryptosporidiosis in patients with AIDS (letter). J Infect Dis 1987; 155:150.
101. Forgacs P, Tarshis A, Ma P, Federman M, Mele L, Silverman ML, Shea JA. Intestinal and bronchial cryptosporidiosis in an immunodeficient homosexual man. Ann Intern Med 1983; 99:793-4.
102. Navin TR, Juraneu DP. Cryptosporidiosis: clinical, epidemiologic, and parasitologic review. Rev Infect Dis 1984; 6:313-27.
103. Kazlow PG, Shah K, Benkov KJ, Dische R, LeLeiko NS. Esophageal cryptosporidiosis in a child with acquired immune deficiency syndrome. Gastroenterology 1986; 91:1301-3.
104. Barone JE, Gingold BS, Nealon TF, Jr., Arvanitis ML. Abdominal pain in patients with acquired immune deficiency syndrome. Ann Surg 1986; 204: 619-23.
105. Margulis SJ, Honig CL, Soave R, Govoni R, Mouradian JA, Jacobson IM. Biliary tract obstruction in the acquired immunodeficiency syndrome. Ann Intern Med 1986; 105:207-10.

106. Ng E, Markell EK, Fleming RL, Fried M. Demonstration of *Isospora belli* by acid-fast stain in a patient with acquired immune deficiency syndrome. J Clin Microbiol 1984; 20:384-6.
107. Jokipii L, Jokipii ANN. Timing of symptoms and oocyst excretion in human cryptosporidiosis. N Engl J Med 1986; 315:1643-7.
108. Centers for Disease Control. Update: treatment of cryptosporidiosis in patients with acquired immunodeficiency syndrome (AIDS). MMWR 1984; 33: 117-9.
109. Centers for Disease Control. Cryptosporidiosis: assessment of chemotherapy of males with acquired immune deficiency syndrome (AIDS). MMWR 1982; 31:589-92.
110. Spicehandler D, Agins B, El-Sadr W, Simberkoff MS, Rahal JJ. Evaluation of efficacy of Spiramycin in intestinal cryptosporidiosis. First International Conference on AIDS, 1985, Atlanta, Georgia. Poster W-32.
111. Rolston KVI, Hoy J, Mansell PWA. Diarrhea caused by "nonpathogenic amoebae" in patients with AIDS (letter). N Engl J Med 1986; 315:192.
112. Louie E, Borkowsky W, Klesius PH, Haynes TD, Gordon S, Lawrence HS. Treatment of cryptosporidiosis with oral bovine transfer factor. Second International Conference on AIDS, 1986, Paris, France. Poster 548.
113. DeHovitz JA, Pape JW, Boncy M, Johnson WD Jr. Clinical manifestations and therapy of *Isospora belli* infections in patients with the acquired immunodeficiency syndrome. N Engl J Med 1986; 315:87-90.
114. Tietze KJ, Gaska JA, Cosgrove EM. Treatment of *Isospora belli* enteritis in patients with AIDS (letter). Clin Pharm 1986; 5:191.
114a. Phillips SC, Mildvan D, Williams DC, Gelb AM, White MC. Sexual transmission of enteric protozoa and helminths in a venereal-disease-clinic population. N Engl J Med 1981; 305:603-6.
115. Purtilo DT, Meyers WM, Connor DH. Fatal strongyloidiasis in immunosuppressed patients. Am J Med 1974; 56:488-93.
115a. Maayan S, Wormser GP, Widerhorn J, Sy ER, Kim YH, Ernst JA. *Strongyloides stercoralis* hyperinfection in a patient with the acquired immune deficiency syndrome. Am J Med 1987; 83:945-8.
116. Pettithory JC, Perouin F. AIDS and strongyloidiasis in Africa (letter). Lancet 1987; 1:921.
117. Catterall JR, Hofflin JM, Remington JS. Pulmonary perspective: pulmonary toxoplasmosis. Am Rev Respir Dis 1986; 133:704-5.
118. Nistal M, Santana A, Paniaqua R, Palacios J. Testicular toxoplasmosis in two men with the acquired immunodeficiency syndrome (AIDS). Arch Pathol Lab Med 1986; 110:744-6.
119. Milligan SA, Katz MS, Craven PC, Strandberg DA, Russel IJ, Becker RA. Toxoplasmosis presenting as panhypopituitarism in a patient with the acquired immune deficiency syndrome. Am J Med 1984; 77:760-4.
120. Parke DW, II, Font RL. Diffuse toxoplasmic retinochoroiditis in a patient with AIDS. Arch Ophthalmol 1986; 104:571-5.
121. Stoumbos VD, Klein ML. Syphilitic retinitis in a patient with acquired immunodeficiency syndrome-related complex (letter). Am J Ophthalmol 1987; 103:103-4.

122. Rolston KVI, Hoy J. Role of clindamycin in the treatment of central nervous system toxoplasmosis. Am J Med 1987; 83:551-4.

123. Leport C, Volde JL, Katlama C, Regnier B, Matheron S, Saimot AG. Failure of spiramycin to prevent neurotoxoplasmosis in immunosuppressed patients (letter). JAMA 1986; 255:2290.

123a. Leport C, Raffi F, Matheron S, Katlama C, Regnier B, Saimot AG, Marche C, Vedrenne C, Vilde JL. Treatment of central nervous system toxoplasmosis with pyrimethamine/sulfadiazine combination in 35 patients with the acquired immunodeficiency syndrome. Am J Med 1988; 84:94-100.

124. Young LS, Inderlied CB, Berling OG, Gottlieb MS. Mycobacterium infections in AIDS patients, with an emphasis on the *Mycobacterium avium* complex. Rev Infect Dis 1986; 8:1024-33.

125. Males BM, West TE, Bartholomew WR. *Mycobacterium haemophilum* infection in a patient with acquired immune deficiency syndrome. J Clin Microbiol 1987; 25:186-90.

126. Levy-Frebault V, Pangon B, Bure A, Katlama C, Marche C, David HL. *Mycobacterium simiae* and *Mycobacterium avium-M. intracellulare* mixed infection in acquired immune deficiency syndrome. J Clin Microbiol 1987; 25: 154-7.

127. Sherer R, Sable R, Sonnenberg M, Cooper S, Spencer P, Schwimmer S, Kocka F, Muthuswamy P, Kallick C. Disseminated infection with *Mycobacterium kansasii* in the acquired immunodeficiency syndrome. Ann Intern Med 1986; 105:710-2.

128. Marinelli DL, Albelda SM, Williams TM, Kern JA, Iozzo RV, Miller WT. Nontuberculous mycobacterial infection in AIDS: clinical, pathologic and radiographic features. Radiology 1986; 160:77-82.

129. Collins FM. *Mycobacterium avium*-complex infections and development of the acquired immunodeficiency syndrome: casual opportunist or causal cofactor? Int J Leprosy 1986; 54:458-74.

130. Bass JB Jr. *Mycobacterium avium-intracellulare*—rational therapy of chronic pulmonary infection (editorial)? Am Rev Respir Dis 1986; 134:431-2.

131. Gillin JS, Shike M, Alcock N, Urmacher C, Krown S, Kurtz RC, Lightdale CJ, Winawer SJ. Malabsorption and mucosal abnormalities of the small intestine in the acquired immunodeficiency syndrome. Ann Intern Med 1985; 102:619-22.

132. Volpe F, Schwimmer A, Baer C. Oral manifestations of disseminated *Mycobacterium avium intracellulare* in a patient with AIDS. Oral Surg Oral Med Oral Pathol 1985; 60:567-70.

133. Kiehn TE, Cammerata R. Laboratory diagnosis of mycobacterial infections in patients with acquired immunodeficiency syndrome. J Clin Microbiol 1986; 24:708-11.

134. Wong B, Edward FF, Kiehn TE, Whimbey E, Donnelly H, Bernard EM, Gold JWM, Armstrong D. Continuous high-grade *Mycobacterium avium-intracellulare* bacteremia in patients with the acquired immune deficiency syndrome. Am J Med 1985; 78:35-40.

135. Macher AM, Kovacs JA, Gill V, Roberts GP, Ames J, Park CH, Straus S, Lane HC, Parrillo JE, Fauci AS, Masur H. Bacteremia due to *Mycobacterium avium-intracellulare* in the acquired immunodeficiency syndrome. Ann Intern Med 1983; 99:782-5.
136. Roth RI, Owen RL, Keren DF, Volberding PA. Intestinal infection with *Mycobacterium avium* in acquired immune deficiency syndrome (AIDS): histologic and clinical comparison with Whipple's disease. Dig Dis Sci 1985; 30: 497-504.
137. Kwan TH, Kaufman HW. Acid-fast bacilli with cytomegalovirus and herpesvirus inclusions in the skin of an AIDS patient. Am J Clin Pathol 1986; 85: 236-8.
138. Bishburg E, Eng RHK, Smith SM, Kapila R. Yield of bone marrow culture in the diagnosis of infectious diseases in patients with acquired immunodeficiency syndrome. J Clin Microbiol 1986; 24:312-4.
139. Castella A, Croxson TS, Mildvan D, Witt DH, Zalusky R. The bone marrow in AIDS: A histologic, hematologic, and microbiologic study. Am J Clin Pathol 1985; 84:425-32.
140. Heifets LB, Iseman MD, Lindholm-Levy PJ. Ethambutol MICs and MBCs for *Mycobacterium avium* complex and *Mycobacterium tuberculosis*. Antimicrob Agents Chemother 1986; 30:927-32.
141. Horsburg CR Jr, Cohn DL, Roberts RB, Masur H, Miller RA, Tsang AY, Iseman MD. *Mycobacterium avium-Mycobacterium intracellulare* isolates from patients with or without acquired immunodeficiency syndrome. Antimicrob Agents Chemother 1986; 30:955-7.
142. Hawkins CC, Gold JWM, Whimbey E, Kiehn TE, Brannon P, Cammarata R, Brown AE, Armstrong D. *Mycobacterium avium* complex infections in patients with the acquired immunodeficiency syndrome. Ann Intern Med 1986; 105:184-8.
143. Masur H, Tuazon C, Gill V, Grimes G, Baird B, Fauci AS, Lane HC. Effect of combined Clofazimine and Ansamycin therapy on *Mycobacterium avium-Mycobacterium intracellulare* bacteremia in patients with AIDS. J Infect Dis 1987; 155:127-9.
144. Horsburgh CR, Jr., Mason UG, III, Heifets LB, Southwick K, Labrecque J, Iseman MD. Response to therapy of pulmonary *Mycobacterium avium-intracellulare* infection correlates with results of *in vitro* susceptibility testing. Am Rev Respir Dis 1987; 135:418-21.
145. Louie E, Rice LB, Holzman RS. Tuberculosis in non-Haitian patients with acquired immunodeficiency syndrome. Chest 1986; 90:542-5.
146. Guarner J, del Rio C, Slade B. Tuberculosis as a manifestation of the acquired immunodeficiency syndrome (letter). JAMA 1986; 256:3092.
147. Sunderam G, McDonald RJ, Maniatis T, Oleske J, Kapila R, Reichman LB. Tuberculosis as a manifestation of the acquired immunodeficiency syndrome (AIDS). JAMA 1986; 256:362-6.
148. Bishburg E, Sunderam G, Reichman LB, Kapila R. Central nervous system tuberculosis with the acquired immunodeficiency syndrome and its related complex. Ann Intern Med 1986; 105:210-3.

149. Barnes P, Leedom JM, Radin DR, Chandrasoma P. An unusual case of tuberculosis peritonitis in a man with AIDS. West J Med 1984; 144:467-9.
150. Croxatto JO, Mestre C, Puente S, Gonzalez G. Nonreactive tuberculosis in a patient with acquired immune deficiency syndrome (letter). Am J Ophthalmol 1986; 102:659-60.
151. Pitchenik AE, Rubinson HA. The radiographic appearance of tuberculosis in patients with the acquired immune deficiency syndrome (AIDS) and Pre-AIDS. Am Rev Respir Dis 1985; 131:393-6.
152. Tuberculosis and acquired immunodeficiency syndrome, San Francisco, 1981-1985. San Francisco Epidemiologic Bulletin, June, 1986; 2, No. 6.
153. Saltzman BR, Motyl MR, Friedland GH, McKitrick JC, Klein RS. *Mycobacterium tuberculosis* bacteremia in the acquired immunodeficiency syndrome. JAMA 1986; 256:390-1.
154. Centers for Disease Control. Diagnosis and management of mycobacterial infection and disease in persons with human T-lymphotropic virus type III/lymphadenopathy-associated virus infection. MMWR 1986; 35:448-51.
155. Pitchenik AE, Cole C, Russell BW, Fischl MA, Spire TJ, Snider DE Jr. Tuberculosis, atypical mycobacteriosis, and the acquired immunodeficiency syndrome among Haitian and non-Haitian patients in south Florida. Ann Intern Med 1984; 101:641-5.
156. Centers for Disease Control. Tuberculosis and the acquired immunodeficiency syndrome—Florida. MMWR 1986; 35:587-90.
157. Rieder HL, Snider DE Jr. Tuberculosis and the acquired immunodeficiency syndrome (editorial). Chest 1986; 90:469-70.

19

Other Virus Infections in AIDS

I. Cytomegalovirus

W. Lawrence Drew *Mount Zion Hospital and Medical Center, San Francisco, California*

A. Introduction

Cytomegalovirus (CMV) is a member of the herpesvirus (*Herpetoviridae*) family, which also includes herpes simplex, varicella-zoster, and Epstein-Barr viruses. These DNA viruses, which are approximately 150 to 200 nm in diameter, are composed of an inner core, a capsid, and an envelope. CMV is quite labile and is destroyed rapidly by heat, low pH, and cycles of freezing and thawing, but loses titer only slowly if held at 4 °C. If it is necessary to freeze a specimen containing this virus, 50-70% sorbitol provides stabilization. Strain differences are identified by restriction endonuclease techniques (1), which indicate that most human strains differ from one another.

B. Epidemiology of CMV Infection

In less developed countries, nearly 100% of the population is infected with CMV during infancy or childhood. In contrast, only about 20% of individuals in the United States and Europe are infected by age 20 (Figure 1), and most of these are infected perinatally (2). Nearly 1% of all babies born in the United States are congenitally infected with this virus (3,4). Another 5-10% of babies become infected by CMV during birth as a result of exposure to the virus in the maternal cervix (5). This mode of acquisition is similar to

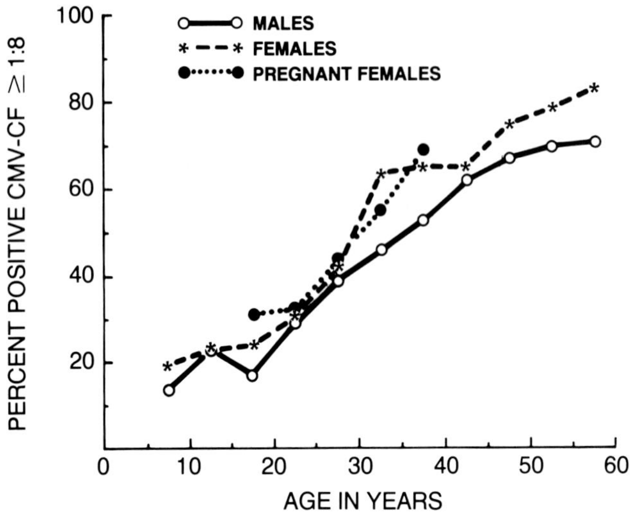

Figure 1 Prevalence of complement-fixing antibody to cytomegalovirus (CMV) by age and sex. (From Ref. 2.)

that of neonatal infection with chlamydia, group B streptococci, *Neisseria gonorrhoeae*, and herpes simplex virus. Breast milk may also be an important vehicle of transmission to neonates (6,7). By adulthood, when approximately 20% of the population has been infected by CMV (8,2), the rate of new infections averages 1-2% per year. For many adults, sexual transmission appears to be an important means of spread (see below). CMV can also be transmitted by blood transfusion (9) and organ transplantation (10). It has been estimated that approximately 3% of units of blood may transmit CMV.

Evidence for Sexual Transmission of CMV

The evidence for sexual transmission of CMV may be summarized as follows:

1. The virus does not spread readily among adults by ordinary, nonsexual, person-to-person contact (11), even during prolonged exposure to individuals known to be excreting the virus (12,13).
2. The prevalence of CMV antibody more than doubles during the sexually active ages of 15 to 35 years (8,2).
3. CMV has been isolated from the cervix of 13% (14) to 23% (15) of women attending clinics for suspected venereal disease.
4. CMV has been isolated from semen (16).

5. Active CMV infection (virus recovered from the cervix and a positive CMV IgM antibody titer) was described in the female sexual partner of a man whose semen had been virus-positive for 5 months (16). In addition, Chretien et al. (17) reported CMV mononucleosis in two men after sexual contact with a woman whose cervix and urine were CMV-positive. Evidence of recent CMV infection was also found in another female sexual contact of one of the two male patients. In contrast, roommates of these patients who were not their sexual partners had negative CMV complement fixation (CF) antibody titers.
6. High rates of CMV infection are found in homosexual men (see below).

Cytomegalovirus Infection in Homosexual Men

We observed urinary excretion of CMV in 14 (7.4%) of 190 homosexual men, but in none of 101 heterosexual men attending the same sexually-transmitted-disease clinic ($p < 0.005$) (18). Similarly, antibody to CMV was detected in 130 (93.5%) of 139 homosexual men, but in only 38 (54.3%) of 70 heterosexual men ($p < 0.005$).

In a subsequent prospective study of 237 homosexual men participating in the Western Study Group Hepatitis Vaccine Trial at the San Francisco City

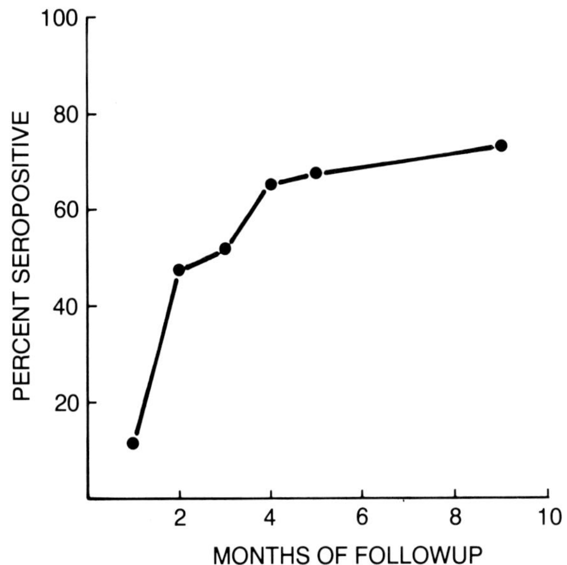

Figure 2 Acquisition of CMV antibody in a cohort of 31 CMV-seronegative homosexual men in San Francisco, 1981.

Clinic, we again noted a high prevalence of CMV IgG serum antibody—206 of 237, or 86.9% (19). Of the 31 men lacking CMV antibody on initial testing, 22 experienced seroconversion within 9 months of follow-up, for an attack rate of 71% during this time period (Figure 2).

During a mean follow-up period of 14.3 months (range, 2-20 months), 66 (32%) of the 206 initially seropositive men excreted CMV in their urine on one or more occasions. Both a urine and a semen specimen were obtained during a single visit from 52 of the homosexual men. CMV was recovered from 18 of the semen specimens, but from only three of the 18 corresponding urine samples. Specimens from a single individual grew CMV from the urine but not from the semen. Semen would therefore appear to be nearly five times as sensitive as urine in detecting the presence of CMV. Clearly, the widespread occurrence of CMV viruria and "virusemenia" in this sexually active population makes exposure to the virus all but inevitable and accounts for the extraordinarily high attack rate of CMV infections among previously seronegative homosexual men.

Data on the prevalence of CMV IgM antibody suggest that homosexuals may experience repeated episodes of CMV infection. (The conventional course of antibody response during acute CMV infection is shown in Figure 3.) CMV IgM antibody was detected on one or more occasions in the sera of

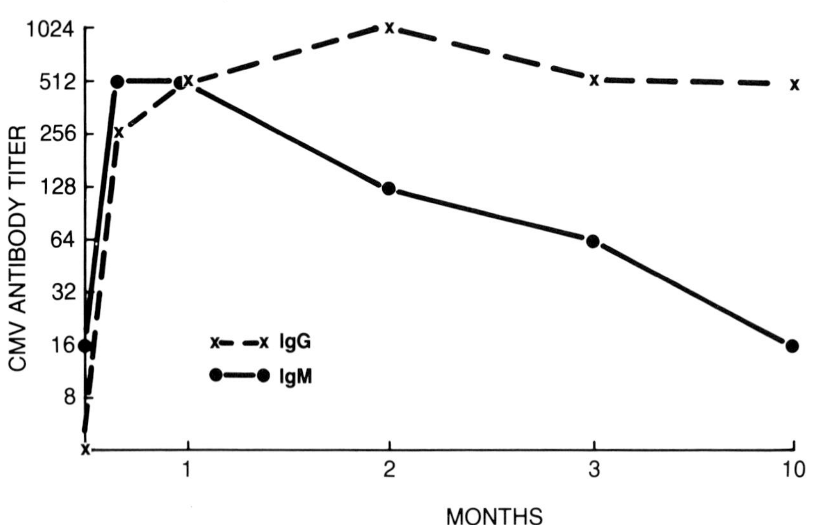

Figure 3 Time course for the development of CMV IgM and IgG antibody during acute primary CMV infection.

Table 1 Presence of CMV IgM Antibody in Prospectively Studied Homosexual Men

Group	Subjects no. positive/no. tested (%)	Serum Samples no. positive/no. tested (%)
Seronegatives	0/9 (0)	0/54 (0)
Seropositives	196/206 (95)	165/1136 (67)
Seroconverters	20/22 (91)	46/86 (53)[a]

[a]Samples obtained after seroconversion.
Source: Ref. 19.

more than 90% of the homosexual men and tended to appear, disappear, and then reappear over the course of time (19). In contrast, IgM antibody to CMV was detected in only 2.8% of 103 serum specimens randomly collected from volunteer male blood donors. Among the homosexual men there was no temporal correlation between the presence of CMV viruria and serum IgM antibody titers. CMV IgM antibody was detected in a significantly ($p < 0.05$) higher proportion of serum samples from the 206 initially seropositive men (67% of 1135 samples) than in the postconversion samples obtained from the 22 seroconverters (53% of 86 samples). These data are summarized in Table 1. The higher prevalence of CMV IgM antibody in longstanding seropositive men than in recent seroconverters suggests that the former group is continually being re-exposed to (and possibly reinfected with) exogenous strains of the virus. We, and others, have recently determined that patients with acquired immunodeficiency syndrome (AIDS) may be infected with more than one strain of CMV (1). Using restriction enzyme techniques to distinguish different isolates, we found that four of four AIDS patients had at least two different isolates from their autopsy organ cultures (1).

In a study by our laboratory, questionnaires concerning demographic data, clinical histories, and sexual practices were completed by 78 subjects. Fifty-four of these individuals were initially seropositive and 24 seronegative, including 17 of the 22 seroconverters and seven of the nine who remained persistently seronegative. Among the men who were seropositive on initial testing, those who excreted CMV during the study period were significantly younger (mean age, 26.6) than those who did not (mean age, 32.7) ($p < 0.05$). This finding confirms our earlier observation that CMV excretion by healthy homosexual men rarely occurs beyond age 30 (18) and suggests that viruria tends to decrease with time.

Information was also obtained regarding the frequency of participation in the following sexual practices: kissing, oral-genital contact, and anal-genital contact (19) (Table 2). Only passive (receptive) anal intercourse correlated with the initial presence of anti-CMV antibody or with seroconversion

Table 2 Prevalence of Cytomegalovirus Among 78 Homosexual Men According to Sexual Practice

Sexual practice	No. of men	No. antibody-positive (%)
Kissing		
yes	77	70 (91)
no	1	1 (100)
Oral-genital contact (active)		
yes	78	71 (91)
no	0	—
Oral-genital contact (passive)		
yes	71	64 (90)
no	7	7 (100)
Anal-genital contact (active)		
yes	74	67 (91)
no	4	4 (100)
Anal-genital contact (passive)[a]		
yes	59	57 (97)
no	19	14 (74)
Oral-anal contact (active)		
yes	47	44 (94)
no	31	27 (87)
Oral-anal contact (passive)		
yes	66	61 (92)
no	12	10 (83)

[a]$p = 0.008$ by Fisher's exact test (correlation of six other sexual practices with cytomegalovirus infection not significant).
Source: Ref. 19.

Table 3 Prevalence of CMV Antibody Among Homosexual Men

	No. of men	No. positive (%)
1. Homosexual men: passive anal intercourse	59	57 (96.6)
2. Homosexual men: no passive anal intercourse	19	14 (73.7)
3. Heterosexual men	70	38 (54.3)

1 vs. 2: $p < 0.01$.
1 vs. 3: $p < 0.001$.
2 vs. 3: not statistically significant.
Source: Ref. 19.

to this virus during the course of the study. Of 59 men who engaged in passive anal intercourse, CMV antibody was present in 96.6%; of the 19 men who did not engage in this practice, antibody was present in only 73.7% ($p < 0.01$) (Table 3). The latter figure does not differ significantly from the prevalence of CMV antibody among heterosexual men attending a venereal disease clinic. These data suggest that exposure of the anorectal mucosa to CMV-infected semen constitutes a major route of acquisition of CMV infection by homosexual men. The same conclusion has been made for transmission of the AIDS virus by the anal-genital route (see Chapter ??).

C. Clinical Conditions Associated with CMV

Infection with CMV in AIDS can result in several clinical syndromes, including chorioretinitis, pneumonia, encephalitis, adrenalitis, colitis, and hepatitis (20). Not all patients with blood, urine, or tissue cultures positive for CMV have clinical illness related to the infection, and a diagnosis of disease caused by CMV should be made by tissue biopsy with histological evidence of virus-mediated damage.

Chorioretinitis

Ocular disease due to CMV occurs only in patients with severe immunodeficiency and is common in patients with AIDS. Blurring of vision or visual loss is a frequent complaint, and ophthalmological examination reveals large, yellowish-white granular areas with perivascular exudates and flame-shaped hemorrhages. Histologically, coagulation necrosis and microvascular abnormalities are present (21,22).

It is important to distinguish between CMV retinitis and cotton-wool spots due to AIDS per se. Cotton-wool spots are common in AIDS patients, but they are asymptomatic, regress spontaneously, and have an excellent prognosis. On ophthalmological examination, cotton-wool spots appear as fluffy white lesions with indistinct margins and are not associated with exudates or hemorrhages (21,22).

A high index of suspicion is essential in the diagnosis of CMV chorioretinitis in AIDS. All patients should have a thorough ophthalmological examination, with pupillary dilation, at regular intervals. AIDS patients with new visual complaints should be evaluated as soon as possible, and patients with suspected or confirmed CMV chorioretinitis should be considered for treatment with 9-(1,3-dihydroxy-2-propoxymethyl)guanine (DHPG).

Pneumonia

Isolation of CMV from pulmonary secretions or lung tissue in AIDS patients with pneumonia undergoing bronchoscopy is common, but a true pathogenic role of the virus in the disease process is not always apparent. Many patients with pulmonary disease and CMV isolation have infection with other pathogens, especially *Pneumocystis carinii* (see Chapter 16). Many of the patients respond to therapy directed at *Pneumocystis carinii* pneumonia (PCP) alone, raising the question of whether CMV is a true pulmonary pathogen. Some patients with CMV infection and pulmonary disease who have no other pathogens present on diagnostic bronchoscopy, however, probably do have invasive CMV pneumonia. Diagnosis, therefore, should be made on the basis of a combination of factors, including positive CMV culture from lung tissue or pulmonary secretions, the presence of pathognomonic cells with intranuclear or intracytoplasmic inclusion bodies, and the absence of other pathogenic organisms.

When CMV causes pulmonary disease in AIDS, the presenting syndrome is that of an interstitial pneumonia. Patients complain of gradually increasing shortness of breath, dyspnea on exertion, and a dry, nonproductive cough. The heart and respiratory rates are elevated, and auscultation of the lungs often reveals minimal findings with no evidence of consolidation. Chest x-ray shows diffuse interstitial infiltrates similar to those present in PCP. Hypoxemia is invariably present.

Central Nervous System Infection

Subacute encephalitis caused by CMV probably occurs in AIDS, but recent evidence suggests that many instances of encephalitis in AIDS result from infection by the human immunodeficiency virus (HIV) (see Chapter 15). It is not uncommon to find both pathogens in the brains of AIDS patients. CMV is not considered a neurotropic virus, but occasional reports of the isolation or identification of CMV from brain tissue or cerebrospinal fluid support the hypothesis that CMV can, on occasion, produce central nervous system infection (23-25).

The presentation of CMV encephalitis in AIDS is similar to that of "subacute" encephalitis due to other etiologies. Personality changes, difficulty in concentrating, headaches, and somnolence are frequent findings. Diagnosis can be confirmed only by brain biopsy, with evidence of perventricular necrosis, giant cells, intranuclear and intracytoplasmic inclusions, and isolation or identification of the virus (23).

Gastrointestinal Infection

Histological and culture evidence of CMV enterocolitis has been reported. Colonic ulceration, lower-gastrointestinal (GI) bleeding, and mucosal vasculitis have been described in the presence of positive CMV cultures and histopathology suggestive of CMV enterocolitis (26-28).

Patients with CMV colitis present with diarrhea, weight loss, anorexia, and fever. The differential diagnosis includes other GI pathogens, including cryptosporidium, *Giardia*, *Entamoepae*, *Shigella*, *Camphylobacter*, and HIV (see Chapter 18). Sigmoidoscopy reveals diffuse submucosal hemorrhages and diffuse mucosal ulcerations. Biopsy specimens often reveal vasculitis with neutrophilic infiltration, CMV-infected endothelial cells, and nonspecific inflammation.

Adrenalitis

An unexpected finding in patients with AIDS has been the frequent occurrence of CMV infection of the adrenal gland with adrenal gland necrosis and Addison's disease. In one study, eight of 10 patients with AIDS had CMV adrenalitis documented at autopsy by the demonstration of inclusion bodies in adrenal cells with inflammatory cells (29). Adrenal necrosis was present in all patients with histological evidence of CMV adrenal gland infection. Other autopsy studies have confirmed the frequent occurrence of CMV adrenalitis in AIDS patients with CMV infection, and have noted that many AIDS patients had clinical evidence of adrenal dysfunction (hyponatremia, hypotension) prior to death (30,31). Subsequent reports have also cited the frequent development of adrenal gland dysfunction in patients with AIDS and have suggested routine testing of adrenal gland function in patients with AIDS who have clinical evidence of hypoadrenalism (32-34).

Patients with primary or secondary hypoadrenalism present with nonspecific symptoms (weight loss, weakness, hypotension) and electrolyte abnormalities (hyponatremia, hyperkalemia). AIDS patients with clinical findings consistent with adrenal gland dysfunction and evidence of CMV infection should undergo evaluation of adrenal gland function. Adrenal function can be assessed by determining baseline cortical levels and the cortisol response to ACTH administration. Normal adrenal function allows for an increase of more than 50% in the plasma cortisol level 30 to 60 minutes after the IM or IV administration of 25 units ACTH. AIDS patients with CMV adrenalitis do not develop an increase in cortisol levels after administration of ACTH and should be maintained on replacement glucosteroid therapy.

D. Diagnosis of CMV Infection

General Considerations

The diagnosis of CMV *infection* is substantiated by a positive culture from any site or by seroconversion. The diagnosis of CMV *disease* is a much more difficult problem. Patients may excrete virus in urine, semen, or the cervix for years after acquiring the virus. Thus, a positive culture from these sites does not by itself prove that CMV is causing the patient's symptom complex. Recovery of the virus from blood is suggestive of active disease due to CMV, but patients may be asymptomatic even when viremic. Recovery of the virus from a lung culture supports a diagnosis of CMV pneumonitis, especially if characteristic viral inclusions are seen in the tissue. In the absence of inclusions, a positive lung culture may be only the equivalent of a positive blood culture and not explain a pneumonia. If CMV is recovered from lung, and no other pathogen or pathological process is identified, CMV may be the cause of the pneumonia even when inclusions are absent. Sorting out a contributing role for CMV in pneumonia is frequently complicated by the identification of coexisting pathogens such as *Pneumocystis carinii* (see Chapter 16). Indeed, these two particular agents are found together so frequently that a synergistic relationship between them is suspected (see below).

Similar interpretive problems pertain to recovery of CMV from intestinal and esophageal biopsies. Again, if no other pathogen is identified, CMV may explain a colitis/esophagitis, especially when viral inclusions are present. When CMV is recovered from other organs, such as the brain, the liver, and the adrenal glands, it is likely that the virus is responsible for disease in these sites, especially when inclusions are also seen. Viral inclusions are not a sine qua non for proving disease because they are quite rare and can be missed due to sampling error.

Virus Isolation

With standard tissue culture procedures, CMV may require 4 weeks or more to develop recognizable cytopathic effects (CPE) in human diploid fibroblast cultures. Investigators at the Mayo Clinic and elsewhere have reported excellent correlation of an overnight tissue-culture method with the standard procedure (35). In the rapid method, specimens are inoculated by centrifuging a shell vial containing a coverslip seeded with human diploid fibroblast cells. After overnight culture, the coverslip cells are stained with a specific monoclonal CMV antibody. This procedure—or subsequent modifications—offers a practical method for rapid identification of CMV in urine. Further studies will be needed to determine if it is equally effective for cultures from other sites.

Other Methods of Viral Detection

Detection of CMV antigen in clinical specimens: During the past 5 years, a number of laboratories have reported their experiences with direct detection of CMV antigen in clinical specimens. Urine samples were among the first to be evaluated, but in general they have been subject to high background levels of enzymatic activity or autofluorescence and poor sensitivity (36). The emphasis in recent research has been the detection of CMV antigen in respiratory specimens such as lung lavage or lung biopsy (37,38). Hackman et al. (39) reported their experience with lung biopsy using a single monoclonal antibody directed at a late antigen. Immunofluorescence (IF) was positive in

27 lung biopsies of patients with bone marrow transplants complicated by interstitial pneumonia; in seven of these, histologic findings were not indicative of CMV pneumonitis but culture was positive in five of seven. Overall, culture and IF were of equivalent sensitivity and any differences were probably due to sampling variation. Both procedures were, however, more sensitive than histology for detecting CMV infection, but it is unclear whether cases lacking histologic confirmation are true instances of CMV pneumonia (see earlier discussion).

Bronchoalveolar lavage (BAL) specimens have also been used to detect CMV antigen and diagnose CMV pneumonitis. Emanuel et al. (38) found that BAL stained with monoclonal antibodies was 100% sensitive; i.e., nine of nine patients with CMV pneumonitis meeting the combination of clinical, radiologic, virologic, and pathological criteria were positive by BAL. All these patients had >0.5% of BAL cells positive for CMV antigen by IF. Three additional patients were positive by IF, but less than 0.1% of cells exhibited antigen. These patients were thought to have other etiologies for their pneumonitis, although mild, concurrent, nonfatal CMV pneumonitis could not be completely excluded. One of the patients had a *Pneumocystis carinii* pneumonia, a second had herpes simplex pneumonitis, and the third appeared to have bacterial pneumonia. The antibody used in these studies was initially a human monoclonal, but because of high background fluorescence a pool of six mouse monoclonal antibodies, directed against both early and late CMV antigens, was employed in the later phase of the study. Cordonnier et al. (40) reported essentially similar results comparing IF with culture and cytology on BAL specimens. Martin and Smith (41), however, found that direct IF was only 33.6% as sensitive as an overnight shell viral culture procedure and 27% as sensitive as conventional tube cultures. They ascribed this poor sensitivity of BAL direct IF to poor preservation of cellular morphology by the cytocentrifuge, but the use of a monoclonal antibody directed only at an immediate early antigen may have been partly responsible. For optimal detection of CMV antigen(s) in clinical specimens, it is probably best to use a pool of monoclonal antibodies directed against both early and late antigens.

Nucleic acid hybridization: DNA-DNA hybridization to detect CMV in clinical samples directly was first described by Chou and Merigan (42) and by Myerson et al. (43). The former ultracentrifuged urine, immobilized the sample on nitrocellulose filters, and hybridized with a 32p-labeled cloned probe prepared by Eco R1 digestion of CMV, strain AD-169. Although the test could be performed in 24 hours it was somewhat insensitive. Fourteen (29%) of 48 culture-positive samples were negative. Virtually all samples with titers <500 cfu/ml were negative. No false positives were encountered.

Other laboratories have reported improved sensitivity on urine (92%) but occasional false positives (3% to 12%) (44,45). False positives in comparison to culture were especially common with buffy coat cultures. On the basis of additional clinical and laboratory data, the authors suggest that the cultures of their patients were false negative rather than that the hybridization assay was false positive (45). Further studies are necessary to resolve this issue. Myerson and co-workers used three different biotinylated CMV probes on formalin-fixed, paraffin-embedded lung tissue to detect CMV in situ. Five of eight culture-positive lung specimens were positive for in situ CMV (43).

Serology

Development of CMV antibody in a patient previously seronegative indicates primary CMV infection. Titers of CMV antibody may wax and wane during life, so fourfold or other low-level increases of antibody should not be interpreted as being diagnostic of active viral infection. Over a prolonged period of observation, complement fixing (CF) antibody titers may even decrease below detectable levels so that presumed seroconversions may occur if CF is the procedure used for detection of antibody.

CMV-specific IgM antibody may be helpful in indicating recent or active infection, especially if seroconversion has already occurred by the time the first blood specimen is obtained. In primary CMV infection, IgM antibody generally will develop and then disappear over a period of 6-9 months (Figure 3). Theoretically, CMV-specific IgM antibody develops only during primary infection, but in fact it may reappear during reactivation of CMV. IgM antibody is common in the sera of homosexual men (18,19), presumably as a result of reactivation of CMV, although repeated exposure to differing strains of the virus may account for its presence in some individuals (1). Theoretically, CMV-specific IgM antibody should be useful in identifying infants with congenital CMV infection. Unfortunately, this test has low sensitivity and specificity in infants (46) and is not as helpful as a urine culture obtained at birth or within the first 2 to 3 weeks of life.

E. CMV as a Cofactor in AIDS

CMV and Immune Suppression

Data from a number of studies suggest a possible cofactor role for CMV infection in AIDS. As noted above, CMV infection is highly prevalent both among patients with AIDS and among homosexual men in general. Of 164 AIDS patients (including homosexual men, intravenous drug users, and hemophiliacs) tested by the Centers for Disease Control for CMV antibody, 162 were positive (47). The two with negative results may have been end-stage AIDS patients, who, in our experience, are often unable to maintain antibody responses.

CMV is known to cause T-cell dysfunction during the syndrome of acute CMV mononucleosis. T-helper lymphocytes and mitogen responses are suppressed and then revert to normal after convalescence (48,49). There is also an increase of T-suppressor cells, which persists for several months. A review of the immunological consequences of acute CMV mononucleosis has been published (50).

Since CMV infects T lymphocytes, it may therefore interact with the AIDS retrovirus in infected lymphocytes. Rice et al. (51) reported in vitro infection of human peripheral blood T and B lymphocytes, natural killer cells, and monocytes by low-passage CMV isolated from patients with various clinical syndromes. Virus expression was limited to the synthesis of immediate-early CMV polypeptides; viral replication did not occur. "Wild" virus strains were more infectious than laboratory adapted viruses, suggesting that the latter are highly adapted to fibroblasts, whereas in "nature" CMV may be more lymphotropic. Immunocompetent mononuclear cells infected by CMV had diminished mitogenic and antigenic responses. These results correlate with previous observations of decreased lymphocyte proliferative responses to mitogens and antigens in patients with acute CMV infection (52-54). The latter also show a transient defect in cytotoxic lymphocyte responses to allogeneic cells.

We have investigated the relationship between CMV serologic status and T-cell imbalance in homosexual men (55). Normal T-helper/T-suppressor (H/S) ratios (>1.0) were found in 40 of 42 homosexual men without antibodies to CMV versus only 34 (51%) of 67 homosexual men with antibodies to the virus ($p < 0.001$). In order to determine whether asymptomatic primary CMV infection in homosexual men induces immunological abnormalities, 34 of the 42 CMV-seronegative men were enrolled in a prospective study to document the time of seroconversion and relate it to H/S ratio results. During an average follow-up period of 13.6 months, 12 (35%) seroconverted, 10 of whom were asymptomatic. All 12 had H/S ratios ⩾1.0 in the month prior to seroconversion, and these ratios all dropped below 1.0 within 1 to 3 months following seroconversion (average nadir, 0.62) (Table 4). H/S ratios remained ⩽1.0 for an average of 9.6 months. Of the seven seroconverters who have been followed for at least 12 months, three remain <1.0. The degree of abnormality of H/S ratio did not differ in the asymptomatic versus the symptomatic patients. Of 20 seronegative men whose initial H/S ratio was >1.0 and who have remained seronegative, only one developed an H/S ratio that has been consistently below 1.0. Three of the 12 CMV seroconverters have developed antibodies to HIV. Our results suggest that cytomegalovirus is responsible for at least some of the immunological abnormalities occurring in homosexual men. Even asymptomatic CMV infection induces profound disturbances in the ratio of helper to suppressor T lymphocytes, and these may persist for prolonged periods of time. These abnor-

Table 4 Relation of Helper:Suppressor T-Cell Ratios to Primary Cytomegalovirus Infectio

Patient	Ratio before seroconversion	Ratio at seroconversion	Duration of ratio of ⩽1.0 mo.	Duration of follow-up (mo.)	Current HIV antibod status
1	1.9	0.47	9	42	+[a]
2	1.8	0.69	15	21	−
3	1.6	0.7	3	16	−
4	1.3	0.4	18	18	+[b]
5	3.6	0.2	2	8	−
6	1.38	0.96	5	8	−
7	1.4	0.9	2	6	−
8	1.0	0.1	12	12	−
9	2.9	0.65	1	1	−
10	NA	0.23	43	43	+[c]
11	NA	0.96	23	24	−
12	NA	0.7	10	18	−
Average	1.87	0.58	11.91	18.08	

[a]HIV antibody acquired prior to or simultaneously with CMV.
[b]HIV and CMV infection acquired simultaneously.
[c]HIV antibody acquired after CMV infection.
Data measured monthly throughout the study.
NA = not available.
Source: Ref. 56.

malities appear to occur prior to, and independently of, infection by HIV. In summary, we suspect that CMV infection may be an important cofactor in the acquisition of HIV infection and that in many cases CMV infection may be a necessary cofactor for the full expression of infection by HIV (56).

CMV as a Cofactor in Kaposi's Sarcoma

There is increasing evidence that in a suitably predisposed (i.e., immunocompromised) host, CMV may be a cofactor in the pathogenesis of KS. This conclusion is based on the following lines of evidence (see also Table 5).

1. CMV has been considered a possible human oncogenic virus by virtue of its ability to stimulate synthesis of DNA and RNA in host cells (57) and its ability to transform human embryo fibroblasts (58). The transformed cells can grow as sarcomatous tumors when transplanted into immunosuppressed mice (58). Several investigators have now identified a transforming segment of the CMV genome through studies in vitro (59).

2. The prevalence of CMV antibody detected in 46 elderly European and American patients with KS was significantly higher than it was in two age-matched control groups without KS. This serologic difference was not seen

Table 5 Evidence Suggesting that Cytomegalovirus (CMV) Is Associated with Kaposi's Sarcoma (KS)

A. Oncogenic potential of CMV
   1. Stimulates DNA and RNA synthesis in host cells (57).
   2. Transforms human embryo fibroblasts that grow as sarcomas in mice (58).
   3. Transforming segment of the genome identified (59).

B. CMV genome or proteins in Kaposi's sarcoma tissue
   1. CMV DNA in 6 of 12 African biopsies by reassociation kinetics (60), 0 of 6 by Southern blot analysis (63).
   2. CMV DNA in 8 of 12 epidemic KS biopsies by in situ hybridization (62).
   3. CMV RNA detected in 8 of 14 (57%) KS biopsies (60,61).
   4. CMV antigen, especially IFA, found in 23 of 37 (62%) KS biopsies, but late antigens are not detected (60,61,64).

C. Epidemiological studies
   1. All patients with KS are seropositive to CMV (60,62).
   2. Specific serologic association with CMV but not with HSV-1, HSV-2, or EBV (60).
   3. The virus can be isolated from urine, semen, liver, lung tissue of KS patients (62); on rare occasions, CMV recovered from tumor biopsy in tissue culture (61).
   4. Occurrence of KS in seropositive renal transplant recipients (65).
   5. Relative paucity of KS cases in IV drug users who as a group are not universally CMV seropositive (67,72).
   6. Decreasing prevalence of KS in homosexual men correlates with decreasing acquisition of CMV.

with antibodies to EBV, herpes simplex (HSV), and varicella-zoster viruses (64).

3. CMV nucleic acids have been demonstrated in some KS tumor biopsies. Boldogh et al. (60), for example, detected CMV DNA in six of 12 and CMV RNA in three of nine biopsies from African patients with KS. EBV and HSV type 2 sequences were not detected. We reported the presence of CMV RNA by hybridization in situ in two of three KS biopsies from homosexual men whose tumor cultures were negative for replicating CMV (61). More recently, Spector and co-workers (62) used the technique of hybridization in situ to detect CMV DNA specifically within tumor cells of KS tissue specimens. They used as probes, instead of whole virus genome, subgenomic fragments of CMV DNA, which had previously been shown not to cross-hybridize with host-cell human DNA. With this technique, they were able to detect CMV genetic sequences in tumor cells from six of 10 evaluable KS specimens but

not in sections of uninvolved skin (62). Other investigators have not been able to detect CMV DNA or RNA in KS tissues. For example, Rüger and colleagues (63), using a Southern blot procedure, were not able to detect CMV DNA in six AIDS-related KS tissues. In biopsies from eight African KS patients, they detected marginal hybridization in only two. In summary, it appears that CMV genome or subgenomic fragments may be found in some but not all KS tissues.

4. CMV antigens have been detected in KS tissue. Boldogh and associates (60) and Ciraldo and colleagues (64) reported the presence of CMV early antigens in tumor tissues from patients with classic and endemic forms of KS. We detected CMV early antigens by a similar procedure in six of nine KS biopsy specimens from homosexual men with AIDS (61), and more recently have found this antigen in an additional nine of 18 cases examined. Biopsies of normal skin from 21 of 22 of our patients were negative for CMV antigens, and all KS biopsies were also negative for CMV by culture. The presence of CMV early antigens, coupled with the apparent absence of CMV late antigens or whole virus in KS biopsies (60,61), suggests that CMV genome may be present in a nonreplicative, and hence more likely oncogenic, state. The observation rules out the possibility that viral presence results simply from disseminated CMV infection or from a tropism of the virus for dermal or tumor tissue.

5. KS is prevalent in two groups of individuals who share the dual features of immunosuppression and extremely high rates of active CMV infection: renal transplant patients and homosexual men with AIDS. There have been at least 36 reports of KS in renal transplant patients (65); it has been estimated that KS accounts for more than 3% of all malignancies occurring in organ transplant recipients (65). Although CMV studies have not been specifically reported in these studies, renal transplant recipients as a group are subject to extremely high rates of primary or reactivated CMV infection (66), and all these patients are, of course, immunosuppressed during the posttransplantation period. KS appears an average of 16 to 36 months after transplantation, suggesting an approximate incubation period for the development of the tumor in immunocompromised patients.

6. High rates of CMV infection in homosexual men with AIDS have been amply documented. To date, we have studied 57 homosexual men with KS for CMV antibody, and all are positive. Of 39 KS patients who have had appropriate secretion cultures, 24 (62%) have been positive.

7. There is a marked discrepancy in the incidence of KS cases among homosexual versus heterosexual AIDS patients. In New York City, KS occurs in 46% of AIDS cases among homosexual men, but in only 3.8% of AIDS

cases among heterosexual men (67). This striking discrepancy suggests that a cofactor may be present in homosexual men that is not present in heterosexuals. This cofactor may be CMV infection, since IV drug users, most of whom are heterosexual, do not have high rates of CMV infection. Of 143 IV drug users in San Francisco and New York City, only 92 (46%) were seropositive; this rate is similar to that observed in the general population (68) and vastly different from that observed in homosexual men (93.5%) (18). Such antibody prevalence rates underestimate the *magnitude* of CMV exposures in a group such as homosexual men, since there may be multiple, repetitive exposures to—and infection by—the virus, yet antibody only measures a single exposure (70). Indeed, an estimate of the extent of CMV exposure among gay men can be inferred from the finding that, even on a single sample, the semen of 25% of homosexual men is CMV culture-positive (71).

A further epidemiological clue to a cofactor in KS may be the recent decline in KS as the presenting manifestation of AIDS in homosexual men, as reported by Rutherford et al. (72) (Table 6) and Des Jarlais and his colleagues (67). Might this change be paralleled by a decrease in CMV transmission among homosexual men? To investigate this question, homosexual men were recruited from clinics for sexually transmitted diseases and from epidemiological studies in San Francisco. CMV antibody was measured by immunofluorescence (74) and seroconversion was defined as the develop-

Table 6 Decline in Rates of KS and in CMV Seroconversion in Homosexual Men (%)

Year	Prevalence of KS as presenting manifestation of AIDS in homosexual men (72)	Seroconversion of CMV antibody in cohorts of initially CMV seronegative homosexual men
1981	63	71
1982	54	57
1983	46	25
1984	35	10
1985	24	4

ment of a CMV antibody titre of 8 or more in a previously seronegative man. CMV antibody was sought on entry into the study and every 2-6 months, irrespective of clinical symptoms or signs. Data on the rate of KS as the initial manifestation of AIDS were provided by the San Francisco AIDS surveillance unit.

The rate of new primary CMV infections among seronegative homosexual men fell from 71% in 9 months in 1980-1981 to 4% in the 12 months of 1985. This decline parallels a fall in KS as the presenting manifestation of AIDS in homosexual men (Table 6).

The decline in KS may reflect diminished exposure to any one of several sexually transmitted disease, other than CMV, and to other putative cofactors such as amyl nitrite. Thus, the correlation of decreased KS with decreased CMV infection may be fortuitous. However, in view of the many threads of evidence implicating CMV in KS (73), we suggest that the declining incidence of KS may reflect diminishing exposure to CMV.

The development of Kaposi's sarcoma in homosexual men is clearly a complication of their immunocompromised state. Indeed, whether or not CMV is a cofactor in the pathogenesis of AIDS, we feel that the evidence is suggestive that the virus makes a contribution to the development of Kaposi's sarcoma. Definitive proof of an etiological role for CMV in the genesis of KS requires further studies and possibly the demonstration of protection by a vaccine.

CMV as a Cofactor in *P. carinii* Pneumonia

We have reported evidence for CMV infection in 10 homosexual patients with *P. carinii* pneumonia (56). In all 10 patients, evidence was found for either past or present infection with CMV. All patients had CMV-specific IgG antibody, and nine had CMV-specific IgM antibody. The virus was recovered from lung tissue in seven of the eight cases in which viral culture was attempted. In several instances we can infer that the virus was present in extremely high titer. Recovery of CMV from lung tissue in 88% of homosexual men with *P. carinii* pneumonia suggests an association between these two infectious agents. Coexistent CMV and *P. carinii* pneumonia have been described previously. If CMV infection predisposes persons to *P. carinii* infection, what is the mechanism? The alveolar macrophages of both man (75) and mouse (76) can be infected by CMV; in the mouse model, CMV has been shown to impair phagocytosis of bacteria (76). Histological studies suggest that the macrophage is an important component of the host response to *P. carinii*. It may be that CMV infection of alveolar macrophages impairs their ability to interact with *P. carinii* by impairing cell-mediated immune responses, as mentioned above.

F. Treatment

During the past several years the following drugs have been investigated for possible anti-CMV effect.

Idoxuridine

Because of its in vitro activity, idoxuridine (IDU) was studied in patients with CMV infection as early as 1968 (77). IDU is an analog of thymidine, which is incorporated into viral DNA, causing inhibition of DNA synthesis. This drug has potential activity against all DNA viruses, including herpes simplex, varicella-zoster, Epstein-Barr, and cytomegalovirus. Barton and Tobin (78) used IDU to treat neonatal CMV infection. All of the treated infants experienced a reduction in CMV titer in their urine, but there was no clinical improvement, and severe toxicity was noted. IDU is presently considered too toxic and insufficiently effective for systemic administration.

Cytosine Arabinoside

Cytosine arabinoside (Ara-C) inhibits the synthesis of the DNA precursor deoxycytidine. The treatment of congenital CMV infection with Ara-C was studied in three trials. A moderate decrease in the titer of urinary CMV was found in one study of four infants (79), but this finding was accompanied by both hematological and hepatic toxicity, and no clinical improvement was noted in any of the patients. Plotkin and Statler (80) used Ara-C to treat three infants, all of whom showed clinical improvement, but severe thrombocytopenia limited the use of the drug. A third study of two infants by Kraybill et al. (81) showed variable antiviral effects, but again there was substantial toxicity in the forms of vomiting, neutropenia, and thrombocytopenia.

Adenine Arabinoside

Adenine arabinoside (Ara-A) was synthesized in the early 1960s as an anticancer drug. It is converted to the triphosphate intracellularly and acts by inhibiting DNA-polymerase (82). After demonstrating efficacy for treatment of herpetic keratitis and encephalitis as well as herpes zoster infection, Ara-A (vidarabine) was studied in patients with CMV infection. Pollard et al. treated seven organ-transplant recipients who had CMV retinitis (83). Five of the seven vidarabine-treated patients had a favorable clinical response, but this result was not significantly different from the improvement noted in three of six placebo recipients. In an open study of treatment of various CMV syndromes in both normal and immunosuppressed patients, Ch'ien and colleagues (84) found that vidarabine was well tolerated but that there was only a transient antiviral effect in the normal hosts; immunosuppressed patients showed only a slight reduction in urine virus titers, and viremia persisted.

Interferon

Human leukocyte (alpha) interferon is part of the natural response to a variety of viral infections (85). Administration of exogenous alpha interferon has been shown to be effective for the prevention and treatment of a variety of viral infections. A double-blind, placebo-controlled trial of interferon for prevention of CMV infections was performed in renal transplant patients receiving standard immunosuppressive therapy with or without antithymocyte globulin (86). There was substantially less CMV viremia in the group receiving interferon, but this finding was limited to those patients who did not receive antithymocyte globulin. Alpha-interferon therapy was also studied in four patients with CMV retinitis (87). Three of these patients suffered from AIDS and the fourth had Hodgkin's disease. The urine viral titers increased in two patients and decreased in the other two. All three patients with AIDS experienced progression of the CMV retinitis; the retinal lesions stabilized in the subject with Hodgkin's disease. Bone-marrow-transplant patients with CMV pneumonia showed no clinical improvement when treated with interferon (88) or combined vidarabine and interferon (89).

CMV Immune Globulin

CMV immune globulin (derived from plasma with a high titer of CMV antibody) was reported to have limited efficacy in preventing CMV infection

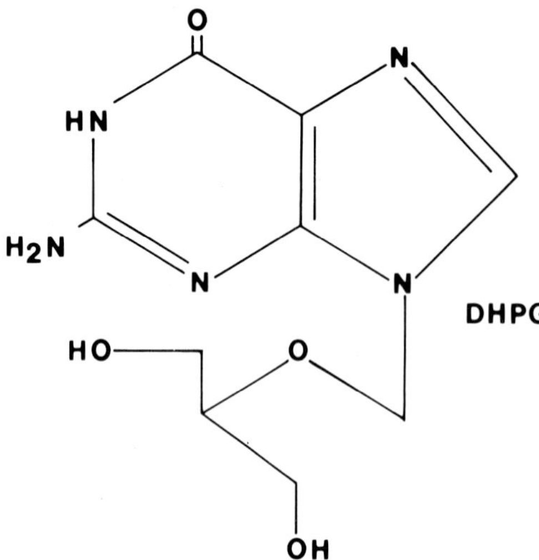

Figure 4 Structure of DHPG.

in seronegative patients undergoing bone-marrow transplants, but a more recent trial did not demonstrate any benefit (90). Others have reported success with CMV immune globulin or high-dose human gamma globulin in treating patients with CMV infection, but these trials were uncontrolled (91, 92).

9-(1,3-Dihydroxy-2-Propoxymethyl) Guanine*

9-(1,3-Dihydroxy-2-Propoxymethyl) guanine (DHPG) is a guanosine analog, differing from acyclovir (ACV) by only one hydroxyl side chain (Figure 4). With this structural change, the drug is approximately 50-fold more active than ACV against CMV. In cytomegalovirus-infected cells, DHPG is phosphorylated to DHPG-monophosphate by a cellular deoxyguanosine kinase (T. R. Matthews, personal communication), then further phosphorylated to the triphosphate form by other cellular enzymes. DHPG appears to be phosphorylated about 10-fold more in virus-infected cells, and this provides some selectivity to the compound. DHPG-triphosphate competitively inhibits binding of deoxyguanosine triphosphate to DNA polymerase, preventing DNA synthesis and terminating DNA elongation. The drug has been used to treat serious CMV infections in patients with AIDS (93). In most patients in whom CMV infection was virologically confirmed, clinical status improved or stabilized, although in a few the status of some affected organs did not improve or deteriorated. Fourteen of 18 patients with adequate viral-culture data had clearing of CMV from all cultured sites. Patients with CMV pneumonia often responded poorly; four of seven died before completing 14 days of DHPG therapy. The condition of 11 of 13 patients with CMV retinitis and five of eight with gastrointestinal disease stabilized or improved. However, clinical and virological relapses occurred in 11 (79%) of 14 patients when DHPG was discontinued. As a result, it is now clear that many patients responding to an initial course of DHPG treatment must continue on maintenance DHPG as long as there is evidence of CMV infection and immunocompromise. Neutropenia is the most frequent adverse reaction, occurring in approximately 20% of recipients.

Given the toxicity of DHPG, patients who are candidates for treatment with this drug must be carefully selected (Table 7). Immunocompromised patients with retinitis usually pursue a relentless course of deteriorating vision, eventuating in blindness. In addition, these patients may experience systemic infection with CMV with multiple organ involvement. We therefore suggest that patients with retinitis, as well as those with other end organ disease such as pneumonitis, colitis, esophagitis, hepatitis, and the generalized

---

*Ganciclovir.

Table 7 CMV Infections Warranting Consideration of DHPG Treatment

1. Immunocompromised patients with CMV end-organ disease, e.g.:
   Retinitis
   Pneumonitis
   Enteritis
   Encephalitis
   "Wasting" syndrome
2. Infants with severe congenital or acquired disease
3. Nonimmunocompromised patients with acute severe primary CMV infection

"wasting" syndrome, are candidates for therapy with this potentially toxic agent.

DHPG has been shown to have a salutary effect on CMV chorioretinitis in approximately 80% of AIDS patients, although lesions tend to recur if therapy is discontinued (94,95). Approximately 50% of AIDS patients with CMV pneumonia have responded to treatment with DHPG. Therapy with DHPG should be considered when a patient has documented CMV pulmonary infection as the only pathogen and a progressive deteriorating clinical course (96).

No effective treatment is known for confirmed CMV encephalitis. Administration of DHPG could be considered, but no data on its efficacy is available. The majority of AIDS patients with CMV colitis respond to a course of DHPG treatment and, in many, remission of this syndrome is sustained.

Similarly, neonates with severe congenital disease and those infants who have life-threatening acquired disease (97,98) should also be considered for treatment with DHPG.

References

1. Drew WL, Mocarski ES, Sweet E, Miner RC. Multiple infections with CMV in AIDS patients: Documentation by Southern blot hybridization. J Infect Dis 1984; 150:952.
2. Wentworth BB, Alexander ER. Seroepidemiology of infections due to members of the herpesvirus group. Am J Epidemiol 1971; 94:496-507.
3. Birnbaum G, Lynch JI, Margileth AM, Lonergan WM, Sever JL. Cytomegalovirus infections in newborn infants. J Pediatr 1969; 789-95.
4. Starr JG, Bart RD, Gold E. Inapparent congenital cytomegalovirus infection: clinical and epidemiologic characteristics in early infancy. N Engl J Med 1970; 282:1075-8.
5. Reynolds DW, Stagno S, Hosty TS, Tiller M, Alford CA Jr. Maternal cytomegalovirus excretion and perinatal infection. N Engl J Med 1973; 289:1-5.

6. Leinikki P, Heinonen K, Pettay O. Incidence of cytomegalovirus infections in early childhood. Scand J Infect Dis 1972; 4:1-5.
7. Stagno S, Reynolds DW, Pass RF, Alford CA. Breast milk and the risk of cytomegalovirus infection. N Engl J Med 1980; 302:1073-6.
8. Stern H, Elek SD. The incidence of infection with cytomegalovirus in a normal population: a serological study in Greater London. J Hyg Camb 1965; 63:79-87.
9. Kaariainen L, Klemola E, Plaoheimo J. Rise of cytomegalovirus antibodies in infectious-mononucleosis-like syndrome after transfusion. Br Med J 1966; 1: 270-2.
10. Betts RF, Freeman RB, Douglas Jr RG, Talley TE, Rundell B. Transmission of cytomegalovirus infection with renal allograft. Kidney Int 1975; 8:387-94.
11. Wenzel RP, McCormick DP, Davies JA, Berling C, Beam WE. Cytomegalovirus infection: a seroepidemiologic study of a recruit population. Am J Epidemiol 1973; 97:410-4.
12. Betts RF, Cestero RVM, Freeman RB, Douglas RG. Epidemiology of cytomegalovirus infection in end stage renal disease. J Med Virol 1979; 4:89-96.
13. Tolkoff-Rubin NE, Rubin RH, Keller EE, Baker GP, Stewart JA, Hirsch MS. Cytomegalovirus infection in dialysis patients and personnel. Ann Intern Med 1978; 89:625-8.
14. Jordan MC, Rousseau WE, Noble GR, Stewart JA, Chin TDY. Association of cervical cytomegalovirus with venereal disease. N Engl J Med 1973; 288:932-4.
15. Wentworth BB, Bonin P, Holmes KK, Butman L, Wiesner P, Alexander ER. Isolation of viruses, bacteria and other organisms from venereal disease clinic patients: methodology and problems associated with multiple isolations. Health Lab Sci 1973; 10:75-81.
16. Lang DJ, Kummer JF, Hartley DP. Cytomegalovirus in semen: persistence and demonstration in extracellular fluids. N Engl J Med 1974; 291:121-3.
17. Chretien JH, McGinnis CG, Muller A. Venereal causes of cytomegalovirus mononucleosis. JAMA 1977; 238:1644-5.
18. Drew WL, Mintz L, Miner RC, Sands M, Ketterer B. Prevalence of cytomegalovirus infection in homosexual men. J Infect Dis 1981; 143:188-92.
19. Mintz L, Drew WL, Miner RC, Braff EH. Cytomegalovirus infections in homosexual men: An epidemiological study. Ann Intern Med 1983; 99:326-9.
20. Armstrong D, Gold JWM, Dryjanski J, et al. Treatment of infections in patients with the acquired immunodeficiency syndrome. Ann Intern Med 1985; 103:738-43.
21. Teich S, Orellana J. Retinal lesions in cytomegalovirus infection. Ann Intern Med 1986; 104:132.
22. Akula SK, Mansell PWA, Ruiz R. Complications of the acquired immunodeficiency syndrome. Ann Intern Med 1986; 104:726-7.
23. Hawley DA, Schaefer JF, Schulz DM, Muller J. Cytomegalovirus encephalitis in acquired immunodeficiency syndrome. Am J Clin Pathol 1983; 80:874-7.
24. Dix RD, Bredesen DE, Erlich KS, Mills J. Recovery of herpesviruses from cerebrospinal fluid of immunodeficient homosexual men. Ann Neurol 1985; 18: 611-4.
25. Dix RD, Bredesen DE, Davis RL, Mills J. Herpesvirus neurological diseases associated with AIDS: Recovery of viruses from central nervous system (CNS)

tissues, peripheral nerve, and cerebrospinal fluid (CSF) (abstract). Atlanta: International Conference on AIDS, 1985:43.

26. Meiselman MS, Cello JP, Margaretten W. Cytomegalovirus colitis: Report of the clinical, endoscopic, and pathologic findings in two patients with the acquired immune deficiency syndrome. Gastroenterology 1985; 88:171-5.
27. Knapp AB, Horst DA, Eliopoulos G, Gamm HF, Gaber LW, Falchuk KR, Falchuk M, Trey C. Widespread cytomegalovirus gastroenterocolitis in a patient with acquired immunodeficiency syndrome. Gastroenterology 1983; 85:1399-402.
28. Gertler SL, Pressman J, Price P, Brozinsky S, Miyai K. Gastrointestinal cytomegalovirus infection in a homosexual man with severe acquired immunodeficiency syndrome. Gastroenterology 1983; 85:1403-6.
29. Tapper ML, Rotterdam HZ, Lerner CW, Al'Khafaji K, Seitzman PA. Adrenal necrosis in the acquired immunodeficiency syndrome. Ann Intern Med 1984; 100:239-41.
30. Glasgow BJ, Steinsapir KD, Anders K, Layfield LJ. Adrenal pathology in the acquired immunodeficiency syndrome. Am J Clin Pathol 1985; 84:594-7.
31. Weiss CD. The human immunodeficiency virus and the adrenal medulla (letter). Ann Intern Med 1986; 105:300.
32. Klein RS, Mann DN, Friedlan GH, Surks MI. Adrenocorticol function in the acquired immunodeficiency syndrome (letter). Ann Intern Med 1983; 99:566.
33. Greene LW, Cole W, Green JB, Levy B, Louie E, Raphael B, Waitkevicz J, Blum M. Adrenal insufficiency as a complication of the acquired immunodeficiency syndrome. Ann Intern Med 1984; 101:497-8.
34. Guenther EE, Rabinowe SL, Van Niel A, Naftilan A, Dluthy RG. Primary Addison's disease in a patient with the acquired immunodeficiency syndrome. Ann Intern Med 1984; 100:847-8.
35. Gleaves CA, Smith TF, Shuster EA, Pearson GR. Rapid detection of cytomegalovirus in MRC-5 cells inoculated with urine specimens by using low-speed centrifugation and monoclonal antibody to an early antigen. J Clin Microbiol 1984; 19:917-9.
36. McKeating JA, Stagno S, Stirk PR, Griffiths PD. Detection of cytomegalovirus in urine samples by enzyme-linked immunosorbent assay. J Med Virol 1985; 16: 367-73.
37. Antonio V, Whitley RJ, Ceballos R, Stagno S. Rapid diagnosis of pneumonia due to cytomegalovirus with specific monoclonal antibodies. J Infect Dis 1983; 147:1119-20.
38. Emanuel D, Peppard J, Stover D, Gold J, Armstrong D, Hammerling U. Rapid immunodiagnosis of cytomegalovirus pneumonia by bronchoalveolar lavage using human and murine monoclonal antibodies. Ann Intern Med 1986; 104:476-81.
39. Hackman RC, Myerson D, Meyers JD, Shulman HM, Sale LC, Goldstein LC, Rastetter M, Flournoy N, Thomas ED. Rapid diagnosis of cytomegaloviral pneumonia by tissue immunofluorescence with a murine monoclonal antibody. J Infect Dis 1985; 151:325-9.
40. Cordonnier C, Escudier E, Nicolas J, Fleury J, Deforges L, Ingrand D, Bricout F, Bernaudin J. Evaluation of three assays on alviolar lavage fluid in the diag-

nosis of cytomegalovirus pneumonitis after bone marrow transplantation. J Infect Dis 1987; 155:495-500.

41. Martin WJ, Smith TF. Rapid detection of cytomegalovirus in bronchoalveolar lavage specimens by a monoclonal antibody method. J Clin Micro 1986; 23: 1006-8.
42. Chou S, Merigan TC. Rapid detection and quantitation of human cytomegalovirus in urine through DNA hybridization. N Engl J Med 1983; 308:921-5.
43. Myerson D, Hackman RC, Nelson JA, Ward DC, McDougall JK. Widespread presence of histologically occult cytomegalovirus. Hum Pathol 1984; 15:430-8.
44. Buffone GJ, Schimbor CM, Demmler GJ, Wilson DR, Darlington GJ. Detection of cytomegalovirus in urine by nonisotopic DNA hybridization. J Infect Dis 1986; 154:163-6.
45. Spector SA, Rua JA, Spector DH, McMillan R. Detection of human cytomegalovirus in clinical specimens by DNA-DNA hybridization. J Infect Dis 1984; 150:121-6.
46. Stagno S, Pass RF, Reynolds DW, Moore MA, Nahmins AJ, Alford CA. Comparative study of diagnostic procedures for congenital cytomegalovirus infection. Pediatrics 1980; 65:251-7.
47. Centers for Disease Control. Preliminary results reported at NIH Conference on AIDS. Bethesda, MD: May 1983.
48. Rinaldo CR, Carney WP, Richter BS, Black PH, Hirsch MS. Mechanisms of immunosuppression in cytomegaloviral mononucleosis. J Infect Dis 1980; 141: 488-95.
49. Carney WP, Rubin RH, Hoffman RA, Hansen WP, Healey K, Hirsch MS. Analysis of T lymphocyte subsets in cytomegalovirus mononucleosis. J Immunol 1981; 126:2114-6.
50. Hirsch MS, Felsenstein D. Cytomegalovirus-induced immunosuppression. In Selikoff IJ, Teirstein AS, Hirschman SZ, eds. Acquired Immune Deficiency Syndrome. New York. Ann NY Acad Sci 1984; 437:8-15.
51. Rice GPA, Schrier RD, Oldstone MBA. Cytomegalovirus infects human lymphocytes and monocytes: Virus expression is restricted to immediate early gene products. Proc Natl Acad Sci USA 1984; 61:6134-8.
52. Rinaldo CR, Black PH, Hirsch MS. Virus-leukocyte interactions in cytomegalovirus mononucleosis. J Infect Dis 1977; 136:667-8.
53. Levin MJ, Rinaldo CR, Leary PL, Zaia JA, Hirsch MS. Immune response to herpes virus antigens in adults with acute cytomegalovirus mononucleosis. J Infect Dis 1979; 140:851-7.
54. Carney WP, Iacoviello V, Hirsch MS. Functional properties of T lymphocytes and their subsets in cytomegalovirus mononucleosis. J Immunol 1983; 130:390-3.
55. Drew WL, Mills, J, Levy JA, Dylewski J, Casavant C, Ammann A, Brodie H, Merigan TC. Cytomegalovirus infection and abnormal T lymphocyte subset ratios in homosexual men. Ann Intern Med 1985; 103:61-3.
56. Follansbee SE, Busch DF, Wofsy CB, et al. An outbreak of *Pneumocytis carinii* pneumonia in homosexual men. Ann Intern Med 1982; 96:705-13.

57. St Jeor SC, Albrecht TB, Frank FD, Rapp R. Stimulation of cellular DNA synthesis with human cytomegalovirus. J Virol 1974; 13:353-62.
58. Geder L, Lausch R, O'Neill F, Rapp F. Oncogenic transformation of human embryo lung cells by human cytomegalovirus. Science 1976; 192:1134-7.
59. Nelson J, Fleckenstein B, Galloway DA, McDougall JK. Transformation of NIH 3T3 cells with cloned fragments of human cytomegalovirus AD-169. J Virol 1982; 43:83-91.
60. Boldogh I, Beth E, Huang E-S, Kyalwazi SK, Giraldo G. Kaposi's sarcoma. IV. Detection of CMV DNA, CMV RNA, and CMNA in tumour biopsies. Int J Cancer 1981; 28:469-74.
61. Drew WL, Miner RC, Ziegler JL, Gullett JH, Abrams DI, Conant MA, Huang ES, Groundwater JR, Volberding P, Mintz L. Cytomegalovirus and Kaposi's sarcoma in young homosexual men. Lancet 1982; 2:125-7.
62. Spector DH, Shaw SB, Hock LJ, Abrams D, Mitsuyasu RT, Gottlieb MS. Association of human cytomegalovirus with Kaposi's sarcoma. In Gottlieb MS, Groopman JE, eds. Acquired Immune Deficiency Syndrome. New York: Alan R. Liss, 1984:109-26.
63. Ruger R, Colimon R, Fleckenstein B. Search for DNA sequences of human cytomegalovirus in Kaposi's sarcoma tissues with cloned probes. In Giraldo G, Beth E, eds. Epidemic of Acquired Immune Deficiency Syndrome (AIDS) and Kaposi's Sarcoma: Antibiotics and Chemotherapy. Vol. 32. New York: Karger, 1983:43-7.
64. Giraldo G, Beth E, Henle W, Henie G, Mike V, Safar B, Huraux JM, McHardy J. Antibody patterns to herpesviruses in Kaposi's sarcoma. II. Serological association of American Kaposi's sarcoma with cytomegalovirus. Int J Cancer 1978; 22:126-31.
65. Penn I. Kaposi's sarcoma in organ transplant recipients. Transplantation 1979; 27:8-11.
66. Fiala M, Payne JE, Berne TV, Moore TC, Henle W, Montogomerie JZ, Chatterjee SN, Guze LB. Epidemiology of cytomegalovirus infection after transplantation and immunosuppression. J Infect Dis 1975; 132:421-32.
67. De Jarlais DC, Marmor M, Thomas P, Chamberland M, Zolla-Pazner S, Sencer DJ. Kaposi's sarcoma among four different AIDS risk groups. N Engl J Med 1984; 310:1119.
68. Brodie HR, Drew WL, Maayan S. Prevalence of Kaposi's sarcoma in AIDS patients reflects differences in rates of cytomegalovirus infection in high risk groups. AIDS Memorandum 1984; 1(7):12.
69. Marmor M, Des Jarlais DC, Spira T, et al. AIDS and cytomegalovirus exposure in New York City drug abusers (poster). International Conference on AIDS. Atlanta, GA, April 1985:52.
70. Drew WL, Mocarski ES, Sweet E, Miner RC. Multiple infections with CMV in AIDS patients: Documentation by southern blot hybridization. J Infect Dis 1984; 150:952.
71. Mintz L, Drew WL, Miner RC, Braff EH. Cytomegalovirus infections in homosexual men: An epidemiological study. Ann Intern Med 1983; 99:326-9.
72. Rutherford GW, Echenberg DF, Rauch KJ, Piland TH, Barnhart JL, Warner WL, Wu AC. The epidemiology of AIDS-related Kaposi's sarcoma in San Francisco:

evidence for decreasing incidence (poster). 2nd International Conference on AIDS. Paris, France, June 25, 1986 (abstract 680).
73. Mintz L, Miner RC, Yeager AS. Anti-complement immunofluorescence test that uses isolated fibroblast nuclei for detection of antibodies to human cytomegalovirus. J Clin Microbiol 1980; 12:562-6.
74. Giraldo G, Beth E, Bounaguro FM. Kaposi's sarcoma: a natural model of interrelationships between viruses, immunologic responses, genetics, and oncogenesis. Antibiot Chemother 1984; 32:1-11.
75. Drew WL, Mintz L, Hoo R, Finley TN. Growth of herpes simplex and cytomegalovirus in cultured human alveolar macrophages. Am Rev Respir Dis 1979; 119:287-91.
76. Shanley JD, Pesanti EL. Replication of murine cytomegalovirus in lung macrophages: Effect on phagocytosis of bacteria. Infect Immun 1980; 29:1152-9.
77. Conchie AF, Barton BW, Tobin JO. Congenital cytomegalovirus infection treated with idoxuridine. Br Med J 1968; 4:162-3.
78. Barton BW, Tobin J. The effect of idoxuridine on the excretion of cytomegalovirus in congenital infection. Ann NY Acad Sci 1970; 173:90-5.
79. McCracken GJ Jr, Luby JP. Cytosine arabinoside in the treatment of congenital cytomegalic inclusion disease. J Pediatr 1972; 80:488-95.
80. Plotkin SA, Stetler H. Treatment of congenital cytomegalic inclusion disease with antiviral agents. Antimicrob Agents Chemother 1969; 9:372-7.
81. Kraybill EN, Sever JL, Avery GB, Movassaghi N. Experimental use of cytosine arabinoside in congenital cytomegalovirus infection. J Pediatr 1972; 80:485-7.
82. Whitley R, Alford C, Hess F. Vidarabine: a preliminary review of its pharmacological properties and therapeutic use. Drugs 1980; 20:267-82.
83. Polland RB, Egbert P, Gallagher J, Merigan TC. Cytomegalovirus retinitis in immunosuppressed hosts. I. Natural history and effects of treatment with adenine arabinoside. Ann Intern Med 1980; 93:655-4.
84. Ch'ien LT, Cannon N, Whitley R. Effect of adenine arabinoside on cytomegalovirus infections. J Infect Dis 1974; 130:32-9.
85. Finter NB, ed. Interferons and Interferon Inducers. New York: Elsevier, 1973: 363-390.
86. Cheeseman SH, Rubin R, Stewart J. Controlled clinical trial of prophylactic human-leukocyte interferon in renal transplantation. N Engl J Med 1979; 300: 1345-49.
87. Chou SW, Dylewski JS, Gaynon MW, Egbert PR, Merigan TC. Alpha-interferon administration in cytomegalovirus retinitis. Antimicrob Agents Chemother 1984; 25:25-8.
88. Meyers JD, McGuffin R, Neiman P, Singer J, Thomas E. Toxicity and efficacy of human leukocyte interferon for the treatment of cytomegalovirus pneumonia after marrow transplantation. J Infect Dis 1980; 141:555-62.
89. Meyers JD, McGuffin R, Bryson Y, Cantell K, Thomas E. Treatment of cytomegalovirus pneumonia after marrow transplant with combined vidarabine and human leukocyte interferon. J Infect Dis 1982; 146:80-4.
90. Condie RM, Hall BL, Howard RJ, Fryd D, Simmons RL, Najarian JS. Treatment of life-threatening infections in renal transplant recipients with high-dose intravenous human IgG. Transplantation Proc 1979; 11:66-8.

91. Meyers JD, Leszczynski J, Zaia JA, Flournoy N, Newton B, Snydman DR, Wright GG, Levin MJ, Thomas ED. Prevention of cytomegalovirus infection by cytomegalovirus immune globulin after marrow transplantation. Ann Intern Med 1983; 98:442-6.
92. Nicholls AJ, Brown CB, Edward N, Cuthbertson B, Yap PL, McClelland DBL. Hyperimmune immunoglobulin for cytomegalovirus infections. Lancet 1983; 1: 532-3.
93. Collaborative DHPG Treatment Study Group. Treatment of serious CMV infection using DHPG in patients with AIDS and other immunodeficiencies. N Engl J Med 1986; 314:801-5.
94. Felsenstein D, D'Amico DJ, Hirsch MS, Neumeyer DA, Cederberg DM, de Miranda P, Schooley RT. Treatment of cytomegalovirus retinitis with 9-[2-hydroxy-1-(hydroxymethyl)ethoxymethyl] guanine. Ann Intern Med 1985; 103: 377-80.
95. Bach MC, Bagwell SP, Knapp NP, Davis KM, Hedstrom PS. 9-(1,3-dihydroxy-2-propoxymethy) guanine for cytomegalovirus infections in patients with the acquired immunodeficiency syndrome. Ann Intern Med 1985; 103:381-2.
96. Shepp DH, Dandliker PS, de Miranda P, Burnette TC, Cederberg DM, Kirk LE, Meyers JD. Activity of 9-[2-hydroxy-1-(hydroxymethyl)ethoxymethyl] guanine in the treatment of cytomegalovirus pneumonia. Ann Intern Med 1985; 103: 368-73.
97. Arvin AM, Yeager AS, Merigan TC. Effect of leukocyte interferon on urinary excretion of cytomegalovirus in infants. J Infect Dis 1976; 133:A205-10.
98. Ballard RA, Drew WL, Hufnagle KG, Riedel PA. Acquired cytomegalovirus infection in preterm infants. Am J Dis Child 1979; 133:482-5.

II. Herpes Simplex Virus

Kim S. Erlich and John Mills *School of Medicine, University of California, San Francisco, California*

A. Overview

Herpes simplex virus (HSV) infections have been occurring in humans throughout most of recorded history. Early references to HSV orolabial eruptions appear in recordings of Herodotus in 100 A.D.; genital HSV infections were not described until the 1700s but were probably occurring much earlier (1). In recent years, both orolabial and genital HSV infections have continued to plague populations throughout the world, and AIDS patients appear to be infected at an equal or greater frequency than the general population (2). Often only an uncomfortable and mildly debilitating infection in the immunocompetent host, HSV infection in the AIDS patients can be extensive and locally destructive, and may result in disseminated lesions that can become life-threatening (3). Unlike other virus infections, there is no evidence that HSV acts as a cofactor in the pathogenesis of AIDS.

Management of HSV infections in AIDS patients can be difficult. Recurrence rates and the severity of eruptions can increase as the immune status of the AIDS patient deteriorates. The occasional atypical clinical presentation can lead to a delay in diagnosis and hence in the initiation of proper therapy. Recent advances in the development of effective antiviral agents allow for safe and effective therapy of HSV infections. Two intravenous agents in particular, vidarabine and acyclovir, have been demonstrated to be superior to placebo in the treatment of severe HSV infections in both immunocompetent and immunosuppressed individuals. The current availability of acyclovir capsules also enables successful management of HSV infections in the outpatient setting.

B. Epidemology

The prevalence of HSV infection in the general population is high. Reported prevalence rates depend on the HSV type studied and on the social and demographic characteristics of the population (4). Precise data on the prevalence rates of HSV infections in the AIDS population are not available, but evidence suggests that the rate of infection parallels or exceeds that in the general population. Of 50 homosexual AIDS patients extensively evaluated in 1983, serum antibodies to HSV were present in all 50 patients as well as in 95% of their non-sexual-contact friends (5). The virus requires a moist environment for survival, and there is no known animal vector; human-to-human spread appears to be the only important mode of transmission. In classic teachings, HSV type 1 (HSV-1) and HSV type 2 (HSV-2) have been associated with infection of the orolabial and genital areas, respectively; this association is not absolute, and infection with either virus may occur at any anatomical site.

HSV-1 Infection

Serologic studies indicate that HSV-1 exposure commonly occurs during childhood between the ages of 6 months and 5 years (4). Prevalence rates for orolabial HSV-1 in the general population vary widely. The risk of HSV-1 infection is higher in low socioeconomic classes in crowded living conditions, where prevalence rates can approach 80 to 100%. High prevalence rates in lower-class, urban populations are probably related to the close person-to-person contact necessary for virus transmission. A study of 254 healthy homosexual men in New York City revealed a 95% infection rate for HSV-1 (5). The prevalence rates of HSV in other AIDS subpopulations and in more affluent groups are probably lower. Many seropositive individuals have no recollection of a clinical outbreak, while other apparently immunocompetent people suffer from frequently recurring symptomatic eruptions. Recurrences can be triggered by several well-described external events, such as sunlight, febrile illnesses, menstruation, and stress. Although the variability individual recurrence rates is poorly understood, subtle alterations in host immune status or the presence of unrecognized external triggering events may explain this difference.

Seropositive individuals undergoing immunosuppression have an increased likelihood of developing recurrences of herpes. This phenomenon has been demonstrated in bone-marrow-transplant recipients and in individuals with other underlying states of deficient cell-mediated immunity (6,7). As most patients with AIDS have serologic evidence of previous exposure to HSV-1, it would be expected that the immunosuppressive state induced by HIV would lead to an increased incidence of clinical herpetic recurrences. Although not universal, many AIDS patients do report frequent and severe orolabial HSV recurrences during their illness that may become more severe as immunosuppression becomes more profound (3). In a study of 34 patients with AIDS, eight had clinical or virological evidence of active HSV recurrences at the time of screening (8).

HSV-2 Infection

Infection with HSV-2 follows a different pattern from that of HSV-1. Although neonates can be infected at birth, infection with HSV-2 generally occurs at adolescence with the onset of sexual activity (4). Transmission is usually by sexual contact and, as with other sexually transmitted diseases, the risk of infection increases with the number of sexual partners. Prevalence rates for HSV-2 vary between 10 and 70%, depending on the level of sexual activity and socioeconomic level of the population studied (4). Promiscuous homosexual men are at an especially high risk of becoming infected with HSV-2, with prevalence rates exceeding 90% in some studies (5), while other groups at risk of developing AIDS may have prevalence rates similar to those of the general population. As with HSV-1, recurrence rates for HSV-2 are variable and may increase with immunosuppression. Most genitally infected normal individuals who are symptomatic during their primary infection develop symptomatic recurrences thereafter (9).

Anorectal infections with HSV-2 are frequently seen in homosexual men with proctitis; a recent study evaluating 102 men with proctitis attributed the illness to HSV-2 in 23 patients. A small number of patients in the same study had subclinical recurrences of HSV-2 proctitis; three of 75 asymptomatic homosexual men had evidence of active HSV-2 rectal infection on examination (10,11).

C. Pathogenesis

The structure and mode of replication of HSV are similar to those of other herpes viruses. A double-stranded DNA nucleoprotein core surrounded by an icosahedral protein capsid is in turn surrounded by a lipid and glycoprotein outer membrane. Transmission of the virus occurs by direct inoculation of infected droplets to a susceptible mucosal surface or by entry through a break in the normally protective skin surface. After resolution of the acute mucocutaneous infection, HSV develops latency in neural tissues; usually in the trigeminal or sacral ganglia (12). Evidence suggests that early in the course of infection viral particles travel from the site of inoculation along sensory nerves to the correponding nerve root ganglia. At the level of the ganglia, a poorly understood interaction between the virus and the host cells occurs. Viral DNA can be demonstrated in the ganglion cells at this time by in situ hybridization techniques, but viral antigens and complete virions are not produced (12,12a). Once viral latency is established, the virus may "reactivate" at any time by mechanisms that are incompletely understood. Viral replication occurs at the level of the sensory ganglia, and viral particles travel peripherally along sensory nerves to cause active infection at mucosal or epithelial surfaces (7). Infection with one HSV type induces cell-mediated immunity and the production of type-specific antibodies that are partially cross-reactive with the other HSV type. Although these immune mechanisms do not affect the underlying state of viral latency, they probably play a key role in regulating the number of clinical recurrences and in minimizing viral replication at epithelial surfaces. Antibodies elicited by previous HSV-1 infection do not afford complete protection against subsequent infection with HSV-2, but do result in a milder clinical course than that which occurs in a completely seronegative individual (9).

D. Clinical Presentation

The clinical presentation of both initial and recurrent HSV infections in AIDS is variable and often differs significantly from that in the normal host. The severity of the outbreak depends on several factors, including the degree of immunosuppression, the site of initial viral infection, and whether preexisting, cross-reacting anti-HSV antibodies are present at the time of initial infection (13).

Orolabial Infection

After an incubation period of 2 to 12 days, orolabial infection with HSV often results in a gingivostomatitis. This infection, while usually caused by HSV-1, may also be due to HSV-2. Symptoms can be mild enough to go unnoticed, but when present take the form of a painful vesicular eruption on the lips, tongue, or buccal mucosa (14). As many as 20 distinct vesicles can appear, which rapidly coalesce and rupture to form shallow ulcers covered with a whitish-yellow necrotic material. Fever and cervical lymphadenopathy may be present if the pharynx and tonsils are involved (15).

In the normal host, primary herpetic lesions heal over a 7- to 10-day period by re-epithelialization without scarring. In AIDS patients, and in other immunocompromised individuals, the clinical course can be more protracted, with lesions persisting for several weeks and showing minimal evidence of tissue repair. Continued viral replication, local progresion of cutaneous lesions, extensive tissue destruction, and occasional viral dissemination to distant sites during primary infection can occur (3,16).

Orolabial HSV-1 recurrences may develop spontaneously or in association with various poorly understood external triggering events (e.g., sunlight, febrile illnesses, stress, or menstruation). States of relative immunosuppression may also increase the risk of developing clinical recurrences, and AIDS patients may develop clinical recurrences of orolabial disease in association with other external stimuli, such as an unrelated opportunistic infection or the administration of systemic chemotherapy. Recurrent eruptions are often preceded by a 1- to 2-day prodrome consisting of paresthesias at the area of impending eruption, and tend to occur in the same general area as the initial primary infection. In the normal host, orolabial recurrences are associated with a clinical course milder than that of the primary infection (14).

Recurrent HSV-1 infection in AIDS patients can be identical to that seen in the immunocompetent host, but can also be highly atypical in manifestation. The infection may be mild and indolent with minimal inflammation, or severe and persistent with large ulcerative lesions and extensive tissue destruction (3). Viral dissemination to distant sites during recurrences of HSV infection has not been clearly documented in AIDS patients.

Genital Infection

Many individuals who acquire HSV-2 through sexual contact have circulating polyclonal cross-reactive anti-HSV antibodies from previous HSV-1 orolabial infection. This "nonprimary" infection is somewhat less severe than the "primary" infection seen in patients who have no previous exposure to either herpes type (13). Both HSV types are capable of causing genital infection, although 65 to 95% of genital isolates from patients with primary infections are HSV-2 (9), and most rectal infections are also caused by HSV-2 (10).

After an incubation period of 2 to 12 days, initial primary genital infection in the normal host causes local symptoms in 95% of men and 99% of women (Table 8). Small papules develop, which rapidly evolve to form painful

Table 8 Signs and Symptoms Present During Primary Genital HSV Infection in the Normal Host

Clinical findings	Frequency (%) Men (63 pts.)	Women (26 pts.)
Local pain	95	99
Tender inguinal lymphadenopathy	80	81
Dysuria	44	83
Urethral or vaginal discharge	27	85
Systemic symptoms (fever, headache, myalgias, malaise)	39	68
Meningitis	11	36

Source: Modified from Ref. 13.

vesicles. The vesicles typically rest on an erythematous base and are tender to palpation. They can appear as closely situated clusters or widely spaced, distinct lesions. The vesicles ulcerate rapidly and heal by crusting and re-epithelialization. In the normal host, healing of primary infection averages 16.5 days in men and 19.7 days in women. Some patients will take longer to heal completely; signs and symptoms can occasionally last as long as 4 to 6 weeks. Systemic symptoms, consisting of fever, headache, myalgias, and malaise, occur in about a third of men and more than two-thirds of women with primary genital herpes. These symptoms are usually resolved by the end of the first week of illness (13). Genital or orolabial infection with HSV in homosexual men usually occurs before the development of AIDS; hence, true "primary" genital HSV infection in this group of patients is unusual (2,5). A primary HSV infection in an AIDS patient would be likely to parallel the presentation seen in other immunocompromised individuals, with more severe local infection, a prolonged healing time, an increased risk of viral dissemination, and more severe systemic symptoms during the illness (16). In contrast to "primary" infection, recurrent genital eruptions in AIDS patients develop frequently during the course of their illness and can be a major source of morbidity (3). Genital HSV is more likely to recur if the initial infection was due to HSV-2 rather than HSV-1 (9). As in orolabial infection, many patients report prodromal symptoms, such as paresthesias, itching, or tingling, at the area of impending eruption. These symptoms may begin up to 48 hours prior to the development of visible lesions. Occasionally, patients will have "false prodromes," with prodromal symptoms but no subsequent clinical outbreak (13).

In the normal host, the number of vesicles, the degree of discomfort, and the duration of viral shedding during HSV recurrences are less than during the initial infection. In some AIDS patients, however, recurrences of genital HSV can become more frequent and more severe as HIV-induced immunosuppression persists. Progressive genital ulcerations accompanied by severe local pain and prolonged viral shedding occur frequently (3), and secondary infection of macerated genital ulcers with bacterial or fungal pathogens can occur. However, recurrent HSV infections of some AIDS patients are clinically mild and indolent. Small, shallow ulcerations can be the only evidence of a clinical recurrence, but viral shedding may continue for days to weeks.

Anorectal Infection

Severe, chronic ulcerative HSV lesions of the perianal area were reported as one of the first opportunistic infections in AIDS (17). Since that time, HSV has been recognized to be the most frequent cause of nongonococcal proctitis in sexually active homosexual men (10). Most clinically apparent episodes of true HSV proctitis are probably due to initial infection with HSV-2, although HSV-1 infection and subacute HSV recurrences can occur (10,11). Anorectal pain, perianal ulcerations, constipation, and tenesmus are prominent symptoms of HSV proctitis. Other symptoms that frequently present include fever, inguinal adenopathy, rectal discharge, hematochezia, sacral paresthesias, and difficulty in initiating urination. Neurological symptoms in the distribution of the sacral plexus aids in differentiating proctitis due to HSV from proctitus 'due to other causes (Table 9).

Table 9 Signs and Symptoms in Patients with HSV Proctitis and Proctitis due to Other Causes

	Frequency (%)	
Clinical findings	HSV proctitis (23 pts.)	Non-HSV proctitis (79 pts.)
Anorectal pain[a]	100	77
Tenesmus[a]	100	77
Anal discharge	91	82
Constipation[a]	78	41
Perianal lesions[a]	70	8
Inguinal lymphadenopathy	57	11
Fever[a]	48	16
Neurological symptoms[a]	52	13
Hematochezia	61	41
Abdominal pain	9	22

[a]Significant difference ($p < 0.01$) by Fisher's exact test.
Source: Modified from Ref. 11.

Anorectal and sigmoidoscopic examination usually reveals a friable mucosa with vesicular or pustular lesions and diffuse mucosal ulceration. Recurrent HSV eruptions at the perianal area are common in AIDS patients who have been previously infected. Local pain and itching, and pain on defecation, are prominent symptoms, and shallow ulcerative lesions are typically present on external examination. In many AIDS patients, an indolent fissurelike ulceration of the gluteal crease is particularly common and may not be accompanied by perianal lesions. Viral shedding may be prolonged in AIDS patients during recurrences, and healing may occur slowly without treatment (11).

E. Diagnosis of HSV Infection

Clinical Diagnosis

Genital HSV infection is usually suspected from the characteristic appearance of the visible, external lesions. Multiple tender, bilaterally distributed, ulcerative lesions are typical of first-episode infections, while only a few small lesions in a single area may be present in recurrent infections (13, 18). In individuals with predisposing risk factors, the presence of cutaneous herpes lesions for several weeks without healing suggests a diagnosis of AIDS (19). Proctitis due to HSV often presents similar to proctitis due to other causes, but the presence of anorectal pain, perianal ulcerations, difficulty in urinating, and sacral neurological findings help to identify HSV as the etiological agent (11). Diagnosis is usually suspected in a sexually active homosexual man on clinical grounds, but should always be confirmed virologically. Findings on sigmoidoscopy include diffuse, shallow, ulcerative lesions with occasional intact vesicles and a friable mucosa (11). In very slender or cachectic patients, nonhealing fissurelike HSV ulcers in the gluteal crease or perirectal area are often misdiagnosed as sacral decubitus. A high index of suspicion must be maintained with regard to any genital or perirectal lesion in the AIDS patient to assure rapid diagnosis of HSV and early initiation of therapy.

Encephalitis due to HSV is usually caused by reactivation of previously latent type 1 infection, although HSV-2 encephalitis in AIDS patients has been reported (21,22). Diagnosis of HSV encephalitis on clinical grounds is difficult since AIDS patients may present with atypical findings (21,22). Lumbar puncture findings are nonspecific; cerebrospinal fluid usually reveals elevated protein, a lymphocytic pleocytosis, occasional erythrocytes, and negative viral cultures. Computed axial tomography (CAT) scanning or electroencephalographic studies are abnormal in the majority of cases and are helpful in locating areas of involvement for diagnostic biopsy (20). Definitive diagnosis is made only by brain biopsy, where the virus or viral antigen is identified in cerebral tissue. The typical histopathology seen in normal hosts with HSV encephalitis, that of hemorrhagic cortical necrosis and lymphocyte infiltration, may not be present in the AIDS patient (21,22). Diagnostic brain biopsy should be considered early in the AIDS patient with suspected HSV encephalitis since effective treatment is available and early institution of therapy is associated with a more favorable outcome.

Laboratory Procedures

Virus culture: There are many methods for laboratory diagnosis of HSV infection, but direct culture of suspected lesions remains the method of choice. Viral culture is more sensitive and more specific than either demonstration of multinucleated giant cells or inclusion bodies by the Tzanck smear, direct staining by immunofluorescence or immunoperoxidase, or detection of viral particles by electron microscopy (23-25). Specimens for viral culture from an external lesion are obtained by scraping the erythematous base gently with a Dacron or cotton-tipped applicator. Alternatively, intact vesicles can be unroofed or carefully aspirated with a small-bore needle. Specimens from the rectal mucosae for culture should be obtained directly during proctoscopy. Care should be taken to avoid introducing stool, blood, alcohol, soap, or detergent into the material to be cultured, since these substances can inactivate the virus and result in a false-negative culture. Moreover, as drying destroys the virus, specimens should be kept moist during transport. Commercially available viral transport media, such as Hank's Balanced Saline with 1% fetal calf serum, Leibovitz-Emory medium, and Stuart's medium, will maintain the virus without serious loss of infectivity for up to 72 hours if refrigerated at 4°C (26).

Material to be cultured is usually inoculated into one or more of several available continuous tissue culture cell lines. Typical changes in the cell morphology—cytopathic effects (CPE)—are usually observed within 24 to 48 hours, and progress rapidly as virus is released into the media from cell lysis. Both HSV-1 and HSV-2 produce similar CPEs in most infected cell cultures and cannot be reliably differentiated by culture alone.

HSV typing: Since relapse rates for HSV-1 and HSV-2 vary for different anatomical sites, differentiation between the two HSV types may have prognostic implications (9). Typing is usually performed with commercially available fluorescein conjugated monoclonal antibodies. More sophisticated techniques, such as restriction endonuclease fingerprinting of the virus DNA, can identify differences in strains within the same HSV types, or confirm that two isolates are identical strains. In rare clinical settings, this technique can be used to confirm case-to-case transmissions (27). For practical purposes, however, strain typing has little utility in the clinical management of herpes infections in AIDS patients.

Serologic studies: Serologic studies are rarely useful in the clinical setting, since prevalence rates for HSV antibodies in AIDS patients are high and the readily available techniques cannot reliably differentiate between antibodies to HSV-1 and those to HSV-2 (2,28). Newer investigational techniques using monoclonal-antibody-purified glycoprotein antigens are more accurate in differentiating between antibody types, but these methods are not yet commercially available. Antibody studies can be useful, however, after a suspected initial infection when both acute and convalescent sera are available (23). A fourfold or greater increase in measured antibody titer over a period of several weeks is indicative of a "first-episode" infection. The presence of detectable antibody in the acute sample, with a subsequent fourfold or greater increase in titer, implies that the infection is "nonprimary," i.e., that the patient has been previously infected with the other HSV type. Recurrent HSV eruptions are only rarely associated with a rise in antibody titer.

F. Complications and Sequelae

Encephalitis caused by HSV occurs infrequently, but it is the most severe and life-threatening complication of HSV infection. Encephalitis either occurs as a result of primary HSV infection or develops secondarily from reactivation of previously latent orolabial disease. The virus preferentially infects the orbitofrontal and temporal lobes, possibly as the result of ascending spread along nerve fibers from the trigeminal ganglia to the anterior and middle fossae (29). Both HSV-1 and HSV-2 have been described as causing encephalitis in AIDS patients, and other patients have had dual infection of the central nervous system with both HSV and cytomegalovirus (CMV) (21, 22).

The most common clinical presentation of HSV brain involvement in normal hosts is that of an acute encephalitis. Nonspecific findings (fever, headache, nausea, confusion, and maningismus), along with temporal lobe findings (focal seizures, aphasia, or olfactory hallucinations), are characteristic. Localizing neurological signs, such as transient hemiparesis and cranial nerve defects, are also frequently present. If left untreated, the illness progresses rapidly, resulting in obtundation, generalized seizures, coma, and death. Lumbar puncture reveals an increased intracranial pressure, elevated cerebrospinal fluid (CSF) protein, a lymphocytic pleocytosis, and the occasional presence of erythrocytes. Viral cultures of CSF are usually negative, and diagnosis must be confirmed by brain biopsy (30).

HSV encephalitis in AIDS patients can be atypical, with many patients developing subtle neurological abnormalities during their illness, suggesting a "subacute" form of encephalitis (31). Diagnosis based on clinical criteria can be extremely difficult, as encephalopathy due to human immunodeficiency virus (HIV) or other opportunistic pathogens may mimic that due to HSV. Noninvasive methods can suggest the diagnosis of HSV encephalitis, but an uncertain diagnosis should be confirmed by brain biopsy (20). The electroencephalogram is frequently abnormal early in the course of the illness, showing spikes and slow wave abnormalities localized to the area of cerebral involvement. CAT scans are frequently normal early in the illness but may later reveal localized edema, low-density focal lesions, mass effect, contrast enhancement, and hemorrhage (32).

Aseptic meningitis is a frequent complication of primary genital and rectal infection in immunocompetent hosts and occurs in up to one-third of infected patients (13). Headache, photophobia, and meningismus are frequent complaints, but most nonimmunocompromised patients are not ill enough to require hospitalization. CSF examination reveals a slightly elevated opening pressure, elevated protein, normal or slightly low glucose level, a lymphocytic pleocytosis, and negative viral cultures (33).

HSV can occasionally be isolated from the CSF of AIDS patients with meningitis (31,34). Both HSV-1 and HSV-2 have been recovered from CSF and may be associated with either a primary or recurrent genital or anorectal eruption.

Autonomic nervous system dysfunction occurs commonly in association with genital or anorectal infection; neurogenic bladder, constipation, impotence, and sacral anesthesia probably occur as the result of sacral nerve root involvement (11,13). Ascending myelitis and Mollaret's meningitis have also been reported (35,36).

Extragenital lesions are often found during initial infection and may be secondary to neural spread (zosteriform herpes), bloodborne dissemination, or autoinoculation. Extensive dissemination can cause a presentation similar to that of chickenpox or shingles, and differentiation by laboratory means may be necessary for definitive diagnosis.

G. Treatment

Early institution of therapy for HSV infections in AIDS patients helps to minimize the morbidity and mortality associated with the illness. Treatment regimens should be chosen for each patient on an individual basis, and should take into account the location and severity of the infection, the immune status of the host, whether the infection is a first episode or a recurrence, and whether the patient is ill enough to require hospitalization (Table 10).

Antiviral Chemotherapy: Acyclovir

Specific antiviral chemotherapy is effective in the management of HSV infections in the compromised host (16,37-44). Acyclovir (9-[(2-hydroxyethoxy)methyl]guanine), an acyclic nucleoside analog of guanosine, is the drug

Table 10 Treatment Regimens for Herpes Simplex Virus Infections in Patients with AIDS

Clinical presentation	Setting	Antiviral therapy	Duration of treatment
Genital or rectal (first episode)	Outpatient	Acyclovir 200 mg PO 5 times daily	Until lesions are crusted
	Hospitalized	Acyclovir 5 mg/kg IV q8 hours[a]	Until lesions are crusted
Genital or rectal (recurrence)	Outpatient	Acyclovir 200 mg PO 5 times daily	Until lesions are crusted
Genital or rectal (prophylaxis for frequent recurrences)	Outpatient	Acyclovir 200 mg PO 3 times daily	Daily up to 2 years
Encephalitis	Hospitalized	Acyclovir 10 mg/kg IV q8 hours[a]	Minimum of 10 days
Disseminated infection	Hospitalized	Acyclovir 10 mg/kg IV q8 hours[a]	Minimum of 10 days

[a]Vidarabine 15 mg/kg/day IV can be used as an alternative antiviral in patients with life-threatening HSV infections who are unable to tolerate acyclovir.

Table 11 Dosage Adjustment of Intravenous Acyclovir in Patients with Renal Dysfunction

Creatinine clearance (ml/min/1.73 m^2)	% of standard dose[a]	Dosing interval (hr)
>50	100	8
25 to 50	100	12
10 to 25	100	24
0 to 10	50	24

[a]Usually 5 mg/kg; 10 mg/kg employed for HSV central nervous system infections.

of choice for treatment of HSV infections in AIDS. The activity of acyclovir against HSV-infected cells results from the drug's selective monophosphorylation by the viral enzyme thymidine kinase. Acyclovir monophosphate is subsequently converted to the triphosphate form by host cellular kinases. Acyclovir triphosphate, the active antiviral, is a selective inhibitor of viral DNA polymerase and is slightly more active against HSV-1 than HSV-2. Acyclovir is distributed into all tissues, including the brain and CSF, and is cleared from the bloodstream by the kidney. The serum half-life in patients with normal renal function is 2-3 hours, and the intravenous dose should be adjusted for patients with renal impairment (Table 11). Acyclovir is available in intravenous, oral, and topical forms. The serum levels of the drug and the clinical response to therapy are dependent on the route of administration, the amount of drug administered, and the duration of therapy.

Intravenous acyclovir: Acyclovir administered by IV infusion shortens the clinical illness in immunocompetent or immunosuppressed patients with primary or recurrent HSV infection (16,37-39,45). In normal patients with severe first-episode genital herpes treated with IV acyclovir 15 mg/kg per day for 5 days, there was a marked reduction in viral shedding, duration of symptoms, numbers of new lesions, more rapid healing of all external lesions (45).

Immunosuppressed patients with chronic mucocutaneous HSV infections also respond well to IV acyclovir (16,37,38). In a study evaluating 34 bone-marrow-transplant patients with severe HSV infections, administration of acyclovir 750 mg/m^2 per day for 7 days significantly decreased symptoms, viral shedding, and the time for healing of lesions when compared to placebo (37). After completion of therapy, however, patients receiving acyclovir had a shorter interval of time until their next HSV outbreak, and these outbreaks were more severe than those in the placebo group. This effect has been observed in other studies as well, suggesting that immune mechanisms responsible for the control of HSV recurrences may require the presence of replicating virus as antigenic stimulation.

Acyclovir is effective in the treatment of HSV encephalitis, and has been shown to be superior to the previously standard treatment of intravenous vidarabine. Recent multicenter studies concluded that patients receiving acyclovir 30 mg/kg per day for 10 days had a lower mortality rate (28% versus 54%) and a lower incidence of severe sequelae (63% versus 85%) than patients treated with vidarabine 15 mg/kg per day for the same length of time (46,47).

Intravenous acyclovir is also useful for prophylaxis of HSV recurrences in immunosuppressed patients with latent HSV infection (40,41). Bone-marrow-transplant recipients with serologic evidence of HSV infection who received acyclovir 750 mg/m^2 per day for 21 days at the time of marrow transplantation had a lower incidence of HSV recurrence while receiving therapy than did patients receiving placebo (40). Many of the acyclovir-treated patients subsequently developed HSV recurrences, however, upon discontinuation of the drug.

Oral acyclovir: In immunocompetent patients with primary genital HSV infection, oral acyclovir (200 mg five times daily for 10 days) reduces the duration of viral shedding, the subjective discomfort, and the number of new lesions when compared to placebo-treated controls (48). Acyclovir also has a similar beneficial effect in patients with recurrent genital HSV infection, although the effects are less dramatic (49). Oral acyclovir is also effective for treatment of acute recurrent HSV infections in immunosuppressed patients; the clinical response does not appear to be as dramatic as with IV acyclovir, but no comparative studies have been done (16,39).

Continuous administration of oral acyclovir prevents HIV recurrences in immunocompetent and immunocompromised patients with frequently recurring HSV infections (42-44,50,51). Recurrences that develop while on chronic suppressive therapy are shorter and milder as compared with those in placebo-treated controls. Patients have been maintained on chronic administration of acyclovir for up to 24 months with no observed increase in side effects or toxicity. One disadvantage of this suppressive therapy is that once the drug is discontinued, patients often develop an initial HSV recurrence more severe than those previously experienced.

Topical acyclovir: Acyclovir ointment, a 5% solution in polyethylene glycol, has a modest beneficial effect when administered to immunocompetent patients with primary genital HSV or to immunosuppressed patients with chronic mucocutaneous lesions (52,53). Subjective symptoms and shedding of virus are slightly reduced by the topical drug, but there is no effect on healing of lesions or on new lesion formation. Topical acyclovir appears to have no effect on healing of recurrent herpes in immunocompetent patients.

Vidarabine

Adenine arabinoside (vidarabine), an analog of the nucleoside adenine deoxyribose, has in vitro activity against many viruses, including HSV. Its mechanism of action is incompletely understood, but vidarabine undergoes intracellular phosphorylation to a triphosphate form and is a potent inhibitor of viral DNA polymerase. Vidarabine is not absorbed when given orally, is poorly soluble, and requires a large amount of intravenous fluid for administration. It is excreted by the kidney and has a half-life of 3.5 hours. Side effects are common, including gastrointestinal, neurological, and hematological toxicity.

Vidarabine was the first antiviral agent shown to be safe and effective in the treatment of serious HSV infections. Treatment with vidarabine 15 mg/kg per day for 10 days in HSV encephalitis reduced the mortality from 70% to 30% (54). Additional studies demonstrated the effectiveness of vidarabine in the treatment of herpes neonatorum (55). A multicenter study evaluating vidarabine in the treatment of immunocompromised patients with mucocutaneous HSV infection revealed a modest beneficial effect in patients over 40 years old on fever, pain control, and virus shedding when compared to placebo (56).

As noted previously, a multicenter trial comparing vidarabine and acyclovir in the treatment of HSV encephalitis concluded that acyclovir is a superior agent, as mortality and long-term sequelae were lower in the acylovir-treated group (46).

In view of the superiority of acyclovir in treatment of HSV and the difficulties associated with vidarabine administration, the latter drug should be used only if a patient with serious HSV infection develops an adverse reaction to acyclovir or is infected with an acyclovir-resistant strain.

Resistance to acyclovir occurs infrequently in individuals receiving the drug for severe HSV infection (57,58), but can be easily produced by growth of virus in subinhibitory concentrations of acyclovir or by infection of animals receiving low doses of the drug (59,60). Acyclovir resistance can occur by at least three mechanisms, including loss of thymidine kinase activity, alteration in the substrate specificity for thymidine kinase, and altered substrate specificity of the viral DNA polymerase (61). The most common mechanism for acyclovir-resistant HSV is the loss of thymidine kinase activity, and these drug-resistant mutants have decreased pathogenicity in animal models (58-61).

We have isolated acyclovir-resistant HSV from 11 AIDS patients with severe and progressive HSV disease who had failed systemic acyclovir therapy (personal observations). All these strains were thymidine-kinase-deficient, but they were clearly the cause of severe and progressive mucocutaneous HSV disease in these AIDS patients and often contributed to eventual death.

We have performed in vitro susceptibility testing of these resistant strains to a variety of antiviral agents. All these strains displayed marked resistance to both acyclovir (ID_{50} = 31.2-402.2 μM) and ganciclovir (DHPG) (ID_{50} = 37.0-428.0 μg/ml), but remained susceptible to both vidarabine (ID_{50} = 3.3-33.3 μg/ml). and foscarnet (ID_{50} = 1.9-23.5 μg/ml). Because both acyclovir and ganciclovir require phosphorylation by viral-induced thymidine kinase for antiviral activity, resistance to these drugs is expected with the loss of thymidine kinase activity (62). Two patients in our series received ganciclovir during their illness with no clinical improvement. By comparison, vidarabine is phosphorylated by cellular enzymes rather than viral thymidine kinase, and foscarnet does not require phosphorylation for antiviral activity; hence, these drugs retain activity against thymidine-kinase-deficient HSV strains (63). Clinical experience with vidarabine and foscarnet in the treatment of acyclovir-resistant HSV is limited, however. One of the patients in our study received vidarabine without clinical improvement. Experience with foscarnet therapy for acyclovir resistant HSV has been encouraging, but to date only seven such patients have been treated with this drug (Astra Pharmaceuticals, personal communication). Routine use of any of these alternative drugs for acyclovir-resistant HSV in AIDS should be viewed cautiously.

H. Management of HSV Infections in AIDS

Mucocutaneous Infection

AIDS patients with recurrent mucocutaneous HSV infections can usually be managed without hospitalization. Herpes infections may not contribute to mortality, but they are painful and should be treated. Oral acyclovir, 200 mg five times daily, should be instituted as soon as possible at the time of diagnosis and should be continued until all external lesions have crusted. Topical acyclovir should not be used unless the patient is unable to tolerate systemic treatment with either oral or intravenous therapy.

Severe of life-threatening mucocutaneous HSV infections should be treated initially with intravenous acyclovir in the hospital. A dosage of 15 mg/kg per day in divided doses (5 mg/kg every 8 hours), with adjustments for renal dysfunction (Table 9), should be used and continued until complete crusting of all lesions has occurred. Patients who require prolonged therapy can be switched to oral acyclovir 200 mg five times daily or 400 mg two to three times daily when they are able to be discharged from the hospital.

Frequently recurring or chronic indolent HSV infections should be treated with oral acyclovir as suppressive therapy. Patients should be started initially on 200 mg of acyclovir three times a day, and the dose can be adjusted as needed based on the patient's clinical response. Patients who continue to develop HSV eruptions while on suppressive therapy may benefit from a higher suppressive dose, since gastrointestinal absorption of the drug may be limited in some patients. A reduction of the suppressive dose can be attempted in patients who demonstrate a good clinical response to the oral regimen.

Topical acyclovir should be reserved for patients who cannot be managed parenterally, as some patients will not be ill enough to require hospitalization for intravenous therapy but will be unable to tolerate or absorb the oral drug due to nausea, vomiting, or diarrhea. Topical acyclovir applied four to five times daily can be used in this instance, but beneficial effects will be less than in patients who receive either oral or intravenous medication.

HSV Encephalitis

Treatment of HSV encephalitis in AIDS should be instituted as soon as possible when the diagnosis is suspected. All patients should undergo diagnostic brain biopsy to confirm the diagnosis, since many other CNS infections can mimic the clinical presentation of HSV encephalitis. Acyclovir 30 mg/kg per day in divided doses (10 mg/kg every 8 hours) with adjustments for renal dysfunction (Table 10) is the therapy of choice. An alternative regimen of vidarabine 15 mg/kg per day is less effective than acyclovir but is superior to no treatment (46,47,54). Therapy should be continued for a minimum of 10 days, but can be prolonged if necessary.

Treatment Failure

Persistent ulcerative HSV infection in the face of standard doses of intravenous or oral acyclovir should raise the suspicion of acyclovir-resistant HSV. Virus isolates suspected to be acyclovir-resistant should be tested for in vitro susceptibility by a well-established reference laboratory. If acyclovir resistance is documented, the drug should be discontinued and alternative antiviral therapy (e.g., vidarabine or foscarnet) should be considered. Serial virus cultures and drug susceptibility studies should be obtained to detect possible reversion to acyclovir-susceptible virus.

Local Care of External Lesions

Local care of cutaneous and mucosal lesions in the AIDS patients is important for patient comfort and the prevention of secondary infection. External HSV-infected areas should be kept clean and dry when possible. Gentle cleansing with mild soap and water should be used for perianal lesions and for other areas subject to frequent contamination. Extensive lesions with large areas of tissue necrosis can be gently debrided by "wet-to-dry" dressing changes.

Palliative Measures

Pain and discomfort due to mucocutaneous HSV lesions can be severe, and analgesics should be administered to the infected patient as needed to minimize discomfort. Acetominophen with codeine is effective for pain control in most patients, but occasional individuals will require the administration of parenteral narcotics. Because codeine can be constipating, care must be taken to keep bowel movements soft, particularly in patients with rectal HSV.

Acknowledgment

Kim S. Erlich is supported by NIH Training Grant 5-T-32-AI07234.

References

1. Hutfield DC. History of herpes genitalis. Br J Vener Dis 1966; 42:263-8.
2. Rogers MF, Morens DM, Stewart JA, et al. National case control study of Kaposi's sarcoma and *Pneumocytis carinii* pneumonia in homosexual men. Part 2. Laboratory results. Ann Intern Med 1983; 99:151-8.
3. Armstrong D, Gold JWM, Dryjanski BJ, et al. Treatment of infections in patients with the acquired immunodeficiency syndrome. Ann Intern Med 1985; 103: 738-43.

4. Nahmias AJ, Josey WE. Herpes simplex viruses 1 and 2. In: Evans A, ed. Viral Infections of Humans: Epidemiology and Control. 2nd ed. New York: Plenum, 1982:351-72.
5. Nerurkar L, Goedert J, Wallen W, Madden D, Sever J. Studv of antiviral antibodies in sera of homosexual men. J Fed Proc 1983; 42:6109.
6. Meyers JD, Fluornoy N, Thomas ED. Infection with herpes simplex virus and cell-mediated immunity after marrow transplant. J Infect Dis 1980; 142:338-46.
7. Nahmias AJ, Roizman B. Infection with herpes simplex viruses 1 and 2. N Engl J Med 1973; 289:667-74, 719-25, 781-9.
8. Quinnan GV, Masur H, Rook AH, et al. Herpes virus infections in the acquired immune deficiency syndrome. JAMA 1984; 252:72-7.
9. Reeves WC, Corey L, Adams HG, Vontver LA, Holmes KK. Risk of recurrence after first episodes of genital herpes: Relation to HSV type and antibody response. N Engl J Med 1981; 305:315-9.
10. Quinn TC, Corey L, Chaffee RG, Schuffler MD, Brancato FP, Holmes KK. The etiology of anorectal infections in homosexual men. Am J Med 1981; 71:395-406.
11. Goodell SE, Quinn TC, Mkrtichian E, Schuffler MD, Holmes KK, Corey L. Herpes simplex virus in homosexual men: Clinical, sigmoidoscopic and histopathologic features. N Engl J Med 1983; 308:868-71.
12. Baringer JR, Swoveland P. Recovery of herpes simplex virus from human trigeminal ganglions. N Engl J Med 1972; 88:648-50.
12a. Dix RD, Mills J. Experimental mouse models of herpes simplex virus infection. In: Sande MM, Zak O, eds. Experimental Models in Antimicrobial Chemotherapy. Vol. 2. New York: Academic Press, 1986:219-57.
13. Corey L, Adams HG, Brown ZA, Holmes KK. Genital herpes simplex virus infections: Clinical manifestations, course, and complications. Ann Intern Med 1983; 98:958-72.
14. Spruance SL, Overall JC, Kern ER, et al. The natural history of recurrent herpes simplex labialis: Implications for antiviral therapy. N Engl J Med 1977; 297:69-75.
15. Glezen WP, Fernald GW, Lohr JA. Acute respiratory disease of university students with special reference to the etiologic role of herpesvirus hominis. Am J Epidemiol 1975; 101:111-21.
16. Straus SE, Smith HA, Brickman C, de Miranda P, McClaren C, Kenney RE. Acyclovir for chronic mucocutaneous herpes simplex virus infection in immunosuppressed patients. Ann Intern Med 1982; 96:270-7.
17. Siegel FP, Lopez C, Hammer GS, et al. Severe acquired immunodeficiency in male homosexuals, manifested by chronic perianal ulcerative herpes simplex lesions. N Engl J Med 1981; 305:1439-44.
18. Chapel T, Brown WJ, Jeffries C, Stewart JA. The microbiological flora of penile ulcerations. J Infect Dis 1978; 137:50-7.
19. Centers for Disease Control. Update on acquired immunodeficiency syndrome (AIDS). MMWR 1982; 31:507-14.
20. Nahmias AJ, Whitley RJ, Visintine AN, et al. Herpes simplex virus type 2 encephalitis: Laboratory evaluations and their diagnostic significance. J Infect Dis 1982; 146:829-36.

21. Dix RD, Waitzman DM, Follansbee S, et al. Herpes simplex virus type 2 encephalitis in two homosexual men with persistent lymphadenopathy. Ann Neurol 1985; 17:203-6.
22. Dix RD, Bredeson DE, Davis RL, Milk J. Herpesvirus neurologic diseases associated with AIDS: Recovery of viruses from CNS tissues, peripheral nerve and CSF (abstract). International Conference on AIDS, Atlanta, 1985:M-82.
23. Corey L, Holmes KK. Genital herpes simplex virus infections: Current concepts in diagnosis, therapy, and prevention. Ann Intern Med 1983; 98:973-83.
24. Brown ST, Jaffee HW, Zaidi A, et al. Sensitivity and specificity of diagnostic tests for genital infections with herpesvirus hominis. Sex Transm Dis 1979; 6:10-3.
25. Moseley RC, Corey L, Benjamin D, Winter C, Remington ML. Comparison of viral isolation, direct immunofluorescence, and indirect immunoperoxidase techniques for detection of genital herpes simplex virus infection. J Clin Microbiol 1981; 13:913-8.
26. Yeager AS, Moris JE, Prober CG. Storage and transport of cultures for herpes simplex virus, type 2. Am J Clin Pathol 1979; 72:977-9.
27. Buchman TG, Roizman B, Adam G, Stover BH. Restriction endonuclease fingerprinting of herpes simplex virus DNA: A novel epidemiological tool applied to a nosocomial outbreak. J Infect Dis 1978; 138:488-98.
28. McClurg H, Seth P, Rawls WE. Relative concentrations in human sera of antibodies to cross-reacting and specific antigens of herpes simlex virus types 1 and 2. Am J Epidemiol 1976; 104:192-201.
29. Davis LE, Johnson RT. An explanation for the localization of herpes simplex encephalitis. Ann Neurol 1979; 5:2-5.
30. Whitley RJ, Soong SJ, Dolin R, et al. Adenine arabinoside therapy of biopsy proved herpes simplex encephalitis: National Institute of Allergy and Infectious Diseases collaborative antiviral study. N Engl J Med 1977; 297:289-94.
31. Dix RD, Bredeson DE, Erlich KS, Mills J. Recovery of herpes viruses from cerebrospinal fluid of immunodeficient homosexual men. Ann Neurol 1985; 18: 611-4.
32. Whitley JR, Soong Sj, Linneman C, et al. Herpes simplex encephalitis: Clinical assessment. JAMA 1982; 247:317-20.
33. Hevron JE. Herpes simplex virus type 2 meningitis. Obstet Gynecol 1977; 49: 622-4.
34. Heller M, Dix RD, Baringer JR, Schachter J, Conte JE. Herpetic proctitis and meningitis: Recovery of two strains of herpes simplex virus type 1 from cerebrospinal fluid. J Infect Dis 1982; 146:584-8.
35. Klastersky J, Cappel R, Snoeck JM, Flament J, Thiry L. Ascending myelitis in association with herpes simplex virus. N Engl J Med 1972; 287:182-4.
36. Steel JG, Dix RD, Baringer JR. Isolation of herpes simplex virus type 1 in recurrent (Mollaret) meningitis. Ann Neurol 1982; 11:17-21.
37. Wade JC, Newton B, McLaren C, Flournoy N, Keeney RE, Meyers JD. Intravenous acyclovir to treat mucocutaneous herpes simplex virus infection after marrow transplantation. Ann Intern Med 1982; 96:265-9.
38. Mitchell CD, Gentry SR, Boen JR, Bean B, Groth KE, Balfour HH Jr. Acyclovir therapy for mucocutaneous herpes simplex infections in immunocompromised patients. Lancet 1981; 1:1389-94.

39. Shepp DH, Newton BA, Dandliker PS, Flournoy N, Meyers JD. Oral acyclovir therapy for mucocutaneous herpes simplex virus infections in immunocompromised marrow transplant recipients. Ann Intern Med 1985; 102:783-5.
40. Saral R, Burns WH, Laskin OL, Santos GW, Lietman PS. Acyclovir prophylaxis of herpes simplex virus infections. N Engl J Med 1981; 305:63-7.
41. Saral R, Ambinder RF, Burns WH, et al. Acyclovir prophylaxis against herpes simplex virus infection in patients with leukemia. Ann Intern Med 1983; 99: 773-6.
42. Gluckman E, Devergie A, Melo R, et al. Prophylaxis of herpes infections after bone marrow transplantation by oral acyclovir. Lancet 1983; 2:706-8.
43. Wade JC, Newton B, Flournoy N, Meyers JD. Oral acyclovir for prevention of herpes simplex virus reactivation after marrow transplantation. Ann Intern Med 1984; 100:823-8.
44. Straus SE, Seidlin M, Takiff H, Jacobs D, Bowen D, Smith HA. Oral acyclovir to suppress recurring herpes simplex virus infections in immunodeficient patients. Ann Intern Med 1984; 100:522-4.
45. Corey L, Fife KH, Benedeti JK, et al. Intravenous acyclovir for the treatment of primary genital herpes. Ann Intern Med 1983; 98:914-21.
46. Whitley RJ, Alford CA, Hirsch MS, et al. Vidarabine versus acyclovir therapy in herpes simplex encephalitis. N Engl J Med 1986; 314:144-9.
47. Skoldenberg B, Alestig K, Burman L, et al. Acyclovir versus vidarabine in herpes simplex encephalitis. Lancet 1984; 2:707-11.
48. Bryson YJ, Dillon M, Lovett M, et al. Treatment of first episodes of genital herpes simplex virus infection with oral acyclovir. N Engl J Med 1983; 308:916-21.
49. Reichman RC, Badger GJ, Mertz GJ, et al. Treatment of recurrent genital herpes simplex infections with oral acyclovir. JAMA 1984; 251:2103-7.
50. Straus SE, Takiff JE, Mindell S, et al. Suppression of frequently recurring genital herpes. N Engl J Med 1984; 310:1545-50.
51. Douglas JM, Critchlow C, Benedetti J, et al. Double blind study of oral acyclovir for suppression of recurrences of genital herpes simplex virus infection. N Engl J Med 1984; 310:1551-6.
52. Corey L, Nahmias AJ, Guinan ME, Benedetti JK, Critchlow CW, Holmes KK. A trial of topical acyclovir in genital herpes simplex virus infections. N Engl J Med 1982; 306:1313-9.
53. Whitley RJ, Levin M, Barton N, et al. Infections caused by herpes simplex virus in the immunocompromised host: Natural history and topical acyclovir therapy. J Infect Dis 1984; 150:323-9.
54. Whitley RJ, Soong SJ, Dolin R, et al. Adenine arabinoside therapy of biopsy proved herpes simplex encephalitis: National Institute of Allergy and Infectious Diseases collaborative antiviral study. N Engl J Med 1977; 297:289-94.
55. Whitley RJ, Nahmias AJ, Soong SJ, et al. Vidarabine therapy of neonatal herpes simplex virus infection. Pediatrics 1980; 666:495-501.
56. Whitley RJ, Spruance S, Hayden FJ, et al. Vidarabine therapy for mucocutaneous herpes simplex virus infections in the immunocompromised host. J Infect Dis 1984; 149:1-8.
57. Crumpacker CS, Schnipper LE, Marlowe SI, Kowalsky PN, Hershey BJ, Levin MJ. Resistance to antiviral drugs of herpes simplex virus isolated from a patient treated with acyclovir. N Engl J Med 1982; 306:343-6.

58. Schnipper LE, Crumpacker CS, Marlowe SI, Lowalsky P, Hershey BJ, Levin MJ. Drug resistant herpes simplex virus in vitro and after acyclovir treatment in an immunocompromised patient. Am J Med 1982; 73:387-92.
59. Field HJ, Darby G. Pathogenicity in mice of strains of herpes simplex virus which are resistant to acyclovir in vitro and in vivo. Antimicrob Agent Chemother 1980; 17:209-16.
60. Field HJ. Development of clinical resistance to acyclovir in herpes simplex virus-infected mice receiving oral therapy. Antimicrob Agent Chemother 1982; 21: 744-52.
61. Dorsky DI, Crumpacker CS. Drugs five years later: acyclovir. Ann Intern Med 1987; 107:859-74.
62. Smee DF, Bochme R, Chernow M, Binko BP, Matthews. Intracellular metabolism and enzymatic phosphorylation of 9-(1,3-dihydroxy-2-propoxymethyl) guanine and acyclovir in herpes simplex virus-infected and uninfected cells. Biochem Pharmacol 1985; 34:1049-56.
63. Larder BA, Darby G. Susceptibility to other antiherpes drugs of pathogenic variants of herpes simplex virus selected for resistance to acyclovir. Antimicrob Agent Chemother 1986; 29:894-8.

III. Epstein-Barr Virus

Evelyne T. Lennette *Virolab, Inc., Berkeley, California*

A. Introduction

During the early search for the etiology of AIDS, Epstein-Barr virus (EBV) was frequently proposed as a possible causal agent. This notion was soon dispelled by the discovery of the human immunodeficiency virus (HIV) and its close association with AIDS and ARC. Moreover, there are now reports of EBV-seronegative AIDS cases among neonates and young children with hemophilia (1). Although EBV is no longer considered a causative agent of AIDS, its possible role as a cofactor in the disease and its contribution to the wide array of possible complications in AIDS patients are not yet understood. However, it is clear that EBV does affect AIDS patients clinically. It is an opportunistic herpesvirus, capable of inducing serious secondary malignancies and hitherto unknown lesions. EBV's well recognized B lymphotropism and its tumorigenic potential confer to the virus a more complicated and interactive role with the effects of HIV infections. To understand the situation in the AIDS patients, it is necessary to examine EBV's action in the normal host.

B. EBV Transmission and Pathogenesis

EBV, a human herpesvirus, was first detected in tumors of patients with Burkitt's lymphoma, a common childhood malignancy in Africa (3). The close association of this malignancy with well-defined geographic and climatic conditions led Burkitt to postulate an infectious etiology for this tumor. Although the precise role of EBV in Burkitt's lymphoma is still undetermined, we now know EBV to be the causal agent of infectious mononucleosis (3). It has a worldwide distribution and is probably transmitted to more than 95% of the world's adults through salivary exchange. Although most often silent, primary EBV infections can be associated with infectious mononucleosis—a self-limiting lymphoproliferative illness involving spleen, liver, and lymphoid tissues (3). In vivo, EBV infects both the epithelium of the orapharynx and B lymphocytes. Replication of the virus at the former site serves as reservoir for intermittent, low-level viral shedding (4,5). Infected B lymphocytes are transformed and endowed with permanent growth potential (6). Transformation of the lymphoid tissues, in turn, always results in the integration of EBV DNA in the cellular chromosomes, producing a persistent, latent carrier state both in vitro and in vivo (7,8). Many copies of viral DNA also remain present in an unintegrated plasmid state. During the latent infection, expression of EBV antigens continues both on the membrane and in the nucleus. As a result, EBV antibodies in the patient (neutralizing, antiviral capsid, and anti-EB nuclear antigen) are maintained for life at remarkably stable levels, indicating tight regulation of the virus and its expression by immune defenses. The mechanisms by which this equilibrium is maintained are unknown. At present, they can only be surmised from the clinical complications observed in patients with various immunosuppressive conditions—of which patients with AIDS undoubtedly represent the most extreme cases.

Intermittent reactivations leading to transient viral shedding are not uncommon, even in the normal healthy person. The frequency of these reactivations increases with immunosuppressive conditions, including infections by other agents, as well as malignancies, chemotherapies, and inherited immune dysfunctions (9).

The majority of EBV-reactivated infections are asymptomatic. However, recent reports have implicated EBV in chronic illnesses in two categories of patients. The first include rare individuals whose primary infectious mononucleosis illnesses were followed by a series of protracted, serious complications involving multiple organs. In these patients, EBV infections appear to be the precipitating factor, and immune deficiencies are suspected to contribute to the disease development (10). EBV has also been suggested as a possible etiological agent in a second group of patients, mostly young adults and middle-aged patients, whose illnesses were characterized by low-grade fever, chronic fatigue, and in some cases recurrent lymphadenopathy (11, 12). While the serologic findings in many of these patients were compatible with EBV reactivations, the causative link between the patients' illnesses and EBV reactivity is still tenuous at best.

C. Host Defenses Against EBV Infections

One hallmark of infectious mononucleosis is the prominent lymphocytosis during the acute phase of illness. This polyclonal B cell activation is associated with a significant increase in serum levels of all classes of immunoglobulins. Antibodies are specifically directed against EBV antigens, as well as non-EBV antigens of yet-to-be-determined specificities (13-15). Antibodies against the latter antigens include the Paul-Bunnell heterophile antibodies, autoantibodies such as antiplatelet, antineutrophil, antinuclear, and rheumatoid factor. The most striking change during lymphocytosis, however, is in the number of T lymphocytes, including the characteristic atypical lymphocytes. The majority of the T cells during the lymphocytosis have been shown to bear a suppressor phenotype (T8. Leu 2) (16). In addition to their cytotoxic and suppressive properties against EBV-infected cells, these activated T cells inhibit lymphocyte proliferation and immunoglobulin production by B lymphocytes; they therefore presumably stop the lymphoproliferative process of infectious mononucleosis (17).

During the acute phase of primary infections, whether associated with infectious mononucleosis or asymptomatic, the majority of patients show characteristic antibody responses against a number of EBV-specific antigens (13). Laboratory diagnosis of EBV infection relies on the demonstration of serum antibodies to EB viral capsid antigen (VCA), early antigen diffuse (EA/D) and restricted (EA/R) components, and nuclear antigen (EBNA). Both IgM and IgG anti-VCA antibodies appear within 2 weeks of onset, but IgM-VCA antibodies disappear within 4 weeks whereas IgG-VCA antibodies are maintained for life and can be used as a reliable marker for immunity. Anti-EBNA antibodies, in contrast, do not appear until the second to third month after onset and also are maintained for life. During active primary infections, anti-EA/D or EA/R antibodies are present transiently for several months in the majority of patients. Anti-EA antibodies are also detected in patients with EBV reactivations, and can persist for years in patients with chronic underlying conditions.

D. EBV Infections in Immunocompromised Hosts

Primary EBV infections of an immunocompromised patients can result in many possible outcomes, depending on the patient's genetic makeup and degree of immune dysfunction. For example, in patients with Hodgkins' disease and in transplant recipients, primary EBV infections are not particularly severe clinically, although their humoral responses are delayed and protracted (18). In contrast, X-linked lymphoproliferative syndrome (XLP) is a disorder involving both T- and B-cell immune functions, which predisposes the majority of the patients to fatal EBV primary infections (19,20). This syndrome is characterized by uncontrolled infiltration of the liver, spleen, and other lymphoid organs by cytotoxic T cells, leading to necrosis of the organs. In addition, many of the patients are hypoglobulinemic and develop only a limited spectrum of the expected EBV antibodies; some patients have no detectable humoral response. In many ways the syndrome resembles a graft-versus-host reaction.

In immunosuppressed patients, it is difficult to assess clinically the effects of EBV reactivations independently from the patients' underlying illnesses and associated therapies. In general, there have not been reports of clinical manifestations attributable to these reactivations in patients with recognized immunosuppression. Allograft recipients with both congenital and secondary immunodeficiencies undergo reactivation with high frequency, as determined by viral shedding in the saliva and presence of EBV antibodies (21,22). Their antibody profiles characteristically exhibit abnormally high levels of anti-VCA and anti-EA/D antibodies. At the same time, their anti-EBNA titers are often below the geometic mean observed in normal controls. The decrease in anti-EBNA antibodies can be correlated with a general decrease in T-cell functions, as measured by delayed hypersensitivity reactions and in vitro lymphocytic response to a battery of mitogens (23). Similar serologic findings are seen in patients with inherited T-cell immunodeficient disorders such as ataxia-telangectasia and Wiskott-Aldrich syndrome (9).

E. EBV and AIDS

To date, nearly all of the adult ARC and AIDS patients tested have had exposure to EBV prior to their HIV infections. While there have been pediatric AIDS patients who are EBV-negative, their number is small and more time is needed to evaluate the effects of EBV infections in these patients. It remains to be seen whether primary EBV infections would induce clinical manifestations as severe as those observed with other known immunodeficiencies such as XLP.

Not surprisingly, patients with ARC and AIDS whose T-cell function is compromised undergo EBV reactivations readily. Their serologic profiles show increased IgG titers to both VCA and EA-D. In 107 male homosexual patients with AIDS and 99 with ARC seen in the San Francisco area, the geometric mean titer of IgG-VCA was four times that observed for healthy controls (Table 12). IgA anti-VCA titers may be present at low to moderate

Table 12 Distribution of EBV Antibodies in AIDS and ARC Patients

Clinical state	No. of subjects	Geometric mean titers		
		VCA IgG[a]	EA-D[b]	EBNA[c]
AIDS	107	1724.3	66.2	90.5
ARC	99	1144.4	22.7	128.3
Healthy male controls	66	418.5	16.7	208.4

[a]Viral capsid antigen.
[b]Epstein-Barr virus early diffuse-type antigen.
[c]Epstein-Barr virus nuclear antigen.
Figures derived from reciprocal of end-dilution of sera.

titers in some of the patients. The significance of the latter antibodies is undetermined. As is the case with EBV reactivations in other patients, IgM antibodies specific for EBV antigens do not recur in these patients. Interestingly, the frequency of EBV reactivations as measured by the presence of anti-EA does not increase with the progression of ARC to AIDS. Similar fractions of both patient categories (34 and 37%, respectively) show detectable titers to EA, compared to 13% in controls. However, the geometric mean anti-EA/D titer was three times higher in AIDS compared to ARC patients and healthy controls. It is noteworthy that antibodies to the diffuse and not restricted early antigen are found. Anti-EA/D antibodies are usually present in patients with lymph-node involvement. As in other patients with T-cell anergy, anti-EBNA titers in HIV-infected patients show a declining trend as the disease progresses. With AIDS patients, the geometric mean titer of anti-EBNA was 90.5, compared to 128.3 observed in ARC patients and 208.4 in normal healthy controls (Table 12).

The rate of EBV shedding observed in ARC and AIDS patients is similar to that found in all other categories of immunosuppressed patients (18, 21,24,25). Transforming EB virus can be recovered from 60-85% of the patients tested. In addition to the increased viral shedding in the saliva, there appears to be a slight increase in the number of EBV-transformed B lymphocytes in the peripheral blood of these patients (26). While the circulating EBV-positive B cells show a statistically significant increase (6-10-fold above normal), it is moderate compared to that (1000-fold) observed in infectious mononucleosis (27).

So far, there is little evidence to suggest that EBV is involved in the marked lymphadenopathy characteristic of ARC patients. Lymph-node biopsies showing diffuse hyperplasia in the majority of ARC patients have not yielded EBNA-positive cells (24). With nucleic acid hybridization, a more sensitive procedure, EBV-genome-positive cells were shown to be present in four of six lymph nodes studied (28). However, this result is also consistent with that described in a normal seropositive individual (29).

F. EBV-Associated Malignancies

EBV is closely associated with Burkitt's lymphoma and undifferentiated nasopharyngeal carcinoma (NPC). EBV appears to be a necessary but not a sufficient factor in the etiologies of these two malignancies. A predisposing genetic background is believed to be necessary for NPC, while environmental factors appear to account for the time and space clustering of Burkitt's lymphoma in Africa and the U.S. (30,31). In both of these malignancies, EBV genomes and antigen expression (primarily EBNA) can be easily demonstrated in the tumor cells. While Burkitt's lymphoma is lymphoid and NPC is of epithelial origin, both tumors are monoclonal. Extensive chromosomal analyses of Burkitt's lymphoma tumors show reciprocal chromosomal translocations involving chromosomes 8 and 14 (32,33). No information is available on NPC cells because they are not cultivable at present.

The most striking similarity among patients with severe primary or secondary immunodeficiencies and HIV-infected patients is their increased risk of developing lymphoproliferative diseases and neoplasms of B-cell origin. In the immunodeficiencies unrelated to HIV, the risk is estimated to range from 100 times higher in allograft recipients compared with an age-matched control population to 1000-fold in patients with congenital immunodeficiencies. Many of the hyperplastic and neoplastic growths in patients with and without HIV infections were shown to be positive for both EB antigens and genomes (34,37).

Although the role of EBV in AIDS-associated B-cell lymphoma is still under investigation, the number of reports of EBV-associated neoplasms is increasing steadily (35-37). In several cases of Burkitt's-like lymphoma in AIDS patients, EBNA was readily detected in the tumors, as was the characteristic chromosomal t(8;14) and t(8;22) reciprocal translocations found in African Burkitt's lymphoma (38,39). Yet, in contrast to the pediatric African Burkitt's lymphoma cases, neither anti-VCA nor anti-EA/R was elevated in the AIDS patients with Burkitt's lymphoma. The difference in the humoral response is probably a reflection of the smaller tumor burden, its distribution in the latter patients, and/or a difference in the degree of the patients' immunodeficiency.

G. EBV-Associated Oral Hairy Leukoplakia in Patients at Risk for AIDS

A flat, poorly demarcated, painless tongue lesion, described as oral hairy leukoplakia, has been reported among homosexual men, many of whom

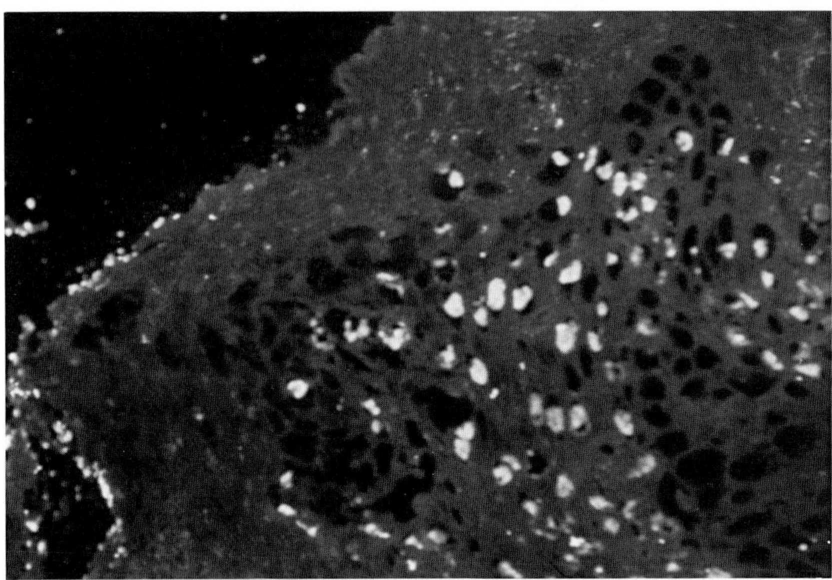

Figure 5 Cryosection of oral leukoplakial biopsy stained with anti-EBV VCA-positive human serum in the anticomplement indirect immunofluorescence assay (13). Note the presence of viral antigens in the prickle-cell and koilocytotic-cell layers.

subsequently developed AIDS (40). Cryostat sections of lesions from nearly all the patients studied contained epithelial cells expressing high levels of EBV-induced antigens, including VCA, EA/D, and EA/R (Figure 5). The cells showed intact herpeslike viruses by electron microscopy, while DNA hybridization studies revealed an average of more than 200 EBV genome copies per cell. Unlike in B-lymphoid tissues, EB virus in the infected epithelium undergoes productive replication, as indicated by the presence of morphologically complete virions by electron microscopy and linear virion DNA by nucleic acid hybridization (41). The EBV-infected cells were associated only with biopsies of the involved lesion. Normal mucosal tissues collected from the same patients at the same time were EBV-negative by all tests. In this hitherto undescribed epithelial lesion, EBV appears to replicate more efficiently than it does in B lymphocytes. In the latter cells, EBV infections generally result in transformation without subsequent viral replication.

H. Interactions Between HIV and EBV

There are suggestions, both in vitro and in vivo, that EBV may interact with HIV, at least at the level of B lymphocytes. In vitro, a continuous EBV-negative B lymphoid line (BJAB) was found to be susceptible to HIV only after the cells were infected with EBV (42). This observation and others (43) suggest that prior EBV infection may facilitate subsequent HIV superinfection of B lymphocytes, perhaps by induction of appropriate receptors for HIV. The occurrence of dual EBV/HIV infections in peripheral B lymphocytes has not been reported. Almost all B-lymphocyte lines established from the peripheral blood of HIV-positive donors are EBV-positive and do not show coinfection with HIV (28).

The interaction(s) between EBV and HIV may not be necessarily direct since EBV affects the humoral limb and HIV the cellular limb of immunity. With respect to EBV infections, the T-suppressor cells are necessary to maintain the equilibrium between latency and activation. Regulated, intermittent reactivations apparently are responsible for the lifelong, stable humoral response. Therefore, perturbations of T-suppressor cells resulting from HIV infections could lead to enhanced EBV replication. As the T-cell population diminishes, the effects of EBV-induced B-cell activity becomes more pronounced. The latter probably include the hyperimmunoglobulinemia, hyperplasia, and some of the autoimmune disorders observed in the ARC/AIDS patients. In the final stage of T-cell depression, B-cell dysregulation may lead to lymphoproliferative growth and, most prominently, to EBV-associated tumors.

References

1. Cowan MJ, Hellman D, Chudwin D, Wara DW, Chang RS, Ammann AJ. Maternal transmission of acquired immune deficiency syndrome. Pediatrics 1984; 73: 382-6.
2. Epstein MA, Achong BG, Barr YM. Virus particles in cultured lymphoblasts from Burkitt's lymphoma. Lancet 1964; 1:702-3.
3. Henle G, Henle W. The virus as the etiologic agent of infectious mononucleosis. In: Epstein MA, Achong BG, eds. The Epstein-Barr Virus. New York: Springer, 1979:297-307.
4. Sixbey JW, Nedrud JG, Raab-Traub N, Hanes RA, Pagano JS. Epstein-Barr virus replication in oropharyngeal epithelial cells. N Engl J Med 1984; 310:1225-30.
5. Gerber P, Nonoyama M, Lucas, Perlin E, Goldstein LI. Oral excretion of Epstein-Barr virus by healthy subjects and patients with infectious mononucleosis. Lancet 1972; 2:988-9.
6. Pope JH. Transformation by the virus in vitro. In: Epstein MA, Achong BG, eds. The Epstein-Barr Virus. New York: Springer, 1979:205-23.
7. zur Hausen H, Diehl V, Wolf H, Schulte-Holthausen H, Schneider U. Occurrence of Epstein-Barr virus genomes in human lymphoblastic cell lines. Nature New Biol 1973; 237:189-90.
8. Nonoyama M, Pagano JS. Homology between Epstein-Barr virus DNA and viral DNA from Burkitt's lymphoma and nasopharyngeal carcinoma determined by DNA-DNA reassociation kinetics. Nature 1973; 242:44-7.

9. Henle W, Henle G. Consequences of persistent Epstein-Barr virus infections. In: Essex M, Todaro H, zur Hausen H, eds. Viruses in Naturally Occuring Cancers. Cold Spring Harbor Conference on Cell Proliferation. Vol. 7. Cold Spring Harbor Laboratory, 1980:3-9.
10. Schooley RT, Carey RW, Miller G, Henle W, Eastman R, Mark EJ, Kenyon K, Wheeler EO, Rubin R. Chronic Epstein-Barr virus infection associated with fever and interstitial pneumonitis: Clinical and serologic features and response to anti-viral chemotherapy. Ann Intern Med 1986; 104:636-43.
11. Jones JF, Ray CG, Minnich LL, Hicks MJ, Kibler R, Lucas DO. Evidence for Epstein-Barr infection in patients with persistent unexplained illnesses: Elevated anti-early antigen antibodies. Ann Intern Med 1985; 102:1-7.
12. Straus SE, Tosato G, Armstrong G, Lawley T, Preble OT, Henle W, Davey R, Pearson G, Epstein J, Brus I, Blaese RM. Persisting illness and fatigue in adults with evidence of Epstein-Barr virus infection. Ann Intern Med 1985; 102:7-16.
13. Henle W, Henle G, Horwitz CA. Epstein-Barr virus specific diagnostic tests in infectious mononucleosis. Hum Pathol 1974; 5:551-65.
14. Paul JR, Bunnell WW. The presence of heterophile antibodies in infectious mononucleosis. Am J Med Sci 1932; 183:80-104.
15. Carter RL. Antibody formation in infectious mononucleosis. II. Other 19S antibodies and false-positive serology. Br J Haematol 1966; 12:268-75.
16. Tosato G, Magrath I, Koski I, Dooley N, Blaese M. Activation of suppressor T cells during Epstein-Barr virus-induced infectious mononucleosis. N Engl J Med 1979; 301:1133.
17. Rickinson AB, Crawford D, Epstein MA. Inhibition of the in vitro outgrowth of Epstein-Barr virus-transformed lymphocytes by thymus-dependent lymphocytes from infectious mononucleosis patients. Clin Exp Immunol 1977; 28:72-9.
18. Lange B, Arbeter A, Hewetson J, Henle W. Longtitudinal study of Epstein-Barr virus antibody titers and excretion in pediatric patients with Hodgkin's disease. Int J Cancer 1978; 22:521-7.
19. Bar RS, Delor CJ, Clausen KP, Hurtubise P, Henle W, Hewetson J. Fatal infectious mononucleosis in a family. N Engl J Med 1974; 290:363-7.
20. Purtilo DT, Szymanski I, Bhawan J, Yang JPS, Hutt LM, Boto W, DeNicola L, Maier R, Thorley-Lawson D. Epstein-Barr virus infections in the X-linked recessive lymphoproliferative syndrome. Lancet 1978; 1:798-801.
21. Chang RS, Lewis JP, Reynolds RD, Sullivan MJ, Neuman J. Oropharyngeal excretion of Epstein-Barr virus by patients with lymphoproliferative disorders and renal homografts. Ann Intern Med 1978; 88:34-40.
22. Henle W, Henle G. Epstein-Barr virus-specific serology in immunologically compromised individuals. Cancer Res 1981; 41:4222-5.
23. Johansson B, Holm G, Mellstedt H, Henle W, Henle G, Soderberg G, Klein G, Killander D. Epstein-Barr virus (EBV)-associated antibody patterns in relation to the deficiency of cell-mediated immunity in patients with Hodgkin's disease (HD). In: de The G, et al., ed. Oncogenesis and Herpesvirus. II. Lyons: International Agency for Research on Cancer, 1975:237.
24. Crawford DH, Willard I, Leiscu I, Wara DW. Epstein-Barr (EB) virus infection in homosexual men in London. Br J Vener Dis 1984; 60:258.

25. Cheeseman SH, Henle W, Rubin RH, Tolkoff-Rubin NE, Cosimi B, Cantell K, Winkle S, Herrin JT, Black P, Russell P, Hirsch MS. Epstein-Barr virus infection in renal transplants. Ann Intern Med 1980; 93:39-42.
26. Birx DL, Redfield RR, Tosato G. Defective regulation of Epstein-Barr virus infection in patients with acquired immunodeficiency syndrome (AIDS) or AIDS-related disorders. N Engl J Med 1986; 314:874-8.
27. Rocchi G, deFelic A, Ragona G, Heiviz A. Quantitative evaluation of Epstein-Barr virus infected mononuclear peripheral blood leukocytes in infectious mononucleosis. N Engl J Med 1977; 296:132-4.
28. Purtilo DT, Kipscomb, Krueger G, Sonnabend J, Casareale D, Volsky DJ. Role of Epstein-Barr virus in acquired immune deficiency syndrome. Adv Exp Med Biol 1985; 187:53-65.
29. Nilsson K, Klein G, Henle W, Henle G. The establishment of lymphoblastoid lines from adult and foetal human lymphoid tissue and its dependence on EBV. Int J Cancer 1971; 8:443-50.
30. Henle W, Henle G. Epstein-Barr virus and human malignancies. Cancer 1974; 34:1368-74.
31. Klein G. The Epstein-Barr virus and neoplasia. N Engl J Med 1975; 292:1353-7.
32. Manalov G, Manalova Y. Marker band in one chromosome 14 from Burkitt's lymphoma. Nature 1972; 237:33-4.
33. Zech L, Haglund U, Nilsson K, Klein G. Characteristic chromosomal abnormalities in biopsies and lymphoid cell lines from patients with Burkitt and non-Burkitt lymphomas. Int J Cancer 1976; 17:47-56.
34. Hanto DW, Frizzera G, Gajl-Pezalska KJ, Simmons RL. Epstein-Barr virus, immunodeficiency and B cell lymphoproliferation. Transplantation 1985; 39: 461-72.
35. Ziegler JL, Beckstead JA, Volberding PA, et al. Non-Hodgkin's lymphoma in 90 homosexual men: relation to generalized lymphadenopathy and the acquired immunodeficiency syndrome. N Engl J Med 1984; 311:565-70.
36. Cheeseman SH, Gang DL. A 40 month old girl with the acquired immunodeficiency syndrome and spinal cord compression. N Engl J Med 1986; 314:629-40.
37. Ziegler JL, Drew WL, Miner RC, et al. Outbreak of Burkitt's-like lymphoma in homosexual men. Lancet 1982; 2:631-3.
38. Chaganti RSK, Jhanwar SC, Arlin Z, Mertelsmann R, Clarkson BD. Specific translocations characterized Burkitt's-like lymphoma of homosexual men with the acquired immunodeficiency syndrome. Blood 1983; 61:1265-8.
39. Magrath I, Erickson J, Whang-Peng J, Sieverts H, Armstrong G, Benjamin D, Triche T, Alabaster O, Croce CM. Synthesis of kappa light chains by cell lines containing an 8;22 chromosomal translocation derived from a male homosexual with Burkitt's lymphoma. Science 1983; 222:1094-8.
40. Greenspan D, Greenspan JS, Conant M, Petersen V, Silverman S Jr, deSouza Y. Oral "hairy" leucoplakia in male homosexuals: evidence of association with both papillomavirus and a herpes-group virus. Lancet 1984; 2:831-4.
41. Greenspan JS, Greenspan D, Lennette ET, Abrams DI, Conant MA, Petersen V, Freese UK. Replication of Epstein-Barr virus within the epithelial cells of oral "hairy" leukoplakia and AIDS-associated lesion. N Engl J Med 1985; 313: 1564-71.

42. Montagnier L, Gruest J, Chamaret S, Dauguet C, Axler C, Guetard D, Nugeyere MT, Barre-Sinoussi F, Chermann JC, Klatzmann D, Gluckman JC. Adaptation of lymphadenopathy associated virus (LAV) to replication in EBV-transformed B lymphoblastoid cell lines. Science 19843; 225:63-6.
43. Levy JA, Shimabukeno J, McHugh T, Casavant C, Stites D, Oshiro L. AIDS-associated retrovirus (ARV) can productively infect other cells besides human T helper cells. Virology 1985; 147:441-8.

IV. AIDS and Hepatitis B Virus Infection

Girish N. Vyas *School of Medicine, University of California, San Francisco, California*

Hepatitis B virus (HBV) is a 3200-bp DNA virus that replicates through reverse transcription of a full-length RNA template of the minus strand viral DNA (1). The genome is the smallest known human DNA virus. Its minus strand is used for transcription and translation of the gene products necessary for viral replication and functions. A chronic carrier state for HBV is estimated to affect 200 million persons in the world who have a 25% chance of suffering from chronic liver diseases. The risk of hepatocellular carcinoma is 200 times greater among the carriers of HBV as compared with normal persons in the same geographic environment. While perinatal transmission of HBV from the carrier mothers to their newborn babies leads to a chronic carrier state in virtually all infected babies, HBV infection in adults leads to persistent infection in 10% of the infected persons. The HBV carrier state leads to a spectrum of liver diseases, including liver cancer. However, the large-scale availability of the hepatitis B surface antigen (HBsAg) as a vaccine against HBV infection has raised an unprecedented opportunity to interrupt the perinatal transmission, avoid the resultant chronic carrier state, and ultimately prevent the hepatocellular carcinoma associated with chronic HBV infection.

Because HBV DNA is transmitted by occult microcontamination with infected serum, the routes of transmission include perinatal, parenteral, and sexual modes. Homosexually active men have a prevalence of seropositivity over 80%, and 7-10% become chronic carriers. Although HBV infection is not immunosuppressive per se, as the cytomegalovirus infection is, the immunosuppression can lead to active HBV replication in homosexual men infected with the human immunodeficiency virus (HIV). Because HIV is transmitted in a manner analogous to HBV—i.e., sexually, perinatally, and by transfusion of blood and blood products—several investigators have hypothe-

Table 13 "Sensitivity" (%) of Test Combinations in Association with AIDS and Lymphadenopathy

	Th/Ts[a]		Anti-HBc[b]	β-2-M[c]	CIC[d]	α-1-Th[e]
Th/Ts		AIDS	96	95	100	98
Anti-HBc	90	ARC		98	97	96
β-2-M	86		92		100	84
CIC	72		100	72		100
α-1-Th	88		93	73	73	

[a]T-helper and -suppressor cells.
[b]Hepatitis B core antibodies.
[c]Beta-2 microglobulins.
[d]Orthomonoclonal anti-C1q binding assay for detection of circulating immune complexes (CIC).
[e]Alpha-1-thymosin.
Source: Data from Centers for Disease Control. Reprinted from Ref. 6.

sized an etiological role of HBV as a cofactor in AIDS, ARC, and Kaposi's sarcoma (2-6). The serologic association of anti-HBc (see Table 13) with markers of HIV infection is most significant and greater than 92%.

The hypothesis of HBV as a cofactor gained support from observations of persistent noncytopathic infection of normal lymphoid elements of blood with either HIV (7) or HBV (8-11) and concurrent infection with HBV and HIV in long-term cultures of T cells of patients with AIDS or ARC (12). These observations are supported by the fact that HBV DNA is consistently found in the peripheral blood mononuclear cells of patients with AIDS/ARC (13,14). The report of Laure et al. (12) includes two patients with AIDS in whom all serologic markers for HBV infection were negative, yet HBV DNA was detectable in bone marrow, semen, and lymph nodes as well as peripheral blood lymphocytes. Using in situ nucleic acid hybridization analysis of HIV-infected T cells, one of us (GNV) has failed to confirm the occurrence of HBV DNA in cells containing HIV RNA (unpublished observations).

In a study from Copenhagen, 33 consecutive male homosexual HBsAg carriers were followed for a period ranging from 4 to 109 months (15). While anti-HIV was detectable in eight patients, 23 remained persistently antibody negative. At the end of the follow-up, six patients had lymphadenopathy and two of the six developed AIDS. Although HBV DNA in the serum was persistently detectable in seven anti-HIV-positive persons, only 15 of the 28 had persistent HBV DNA in the serum. Thus, it appeared that HBV DNA was more readily detectable in anti-HIV-positive persons than in anti-HIV-negative persons. This finding probably reflects the immunocompromised state of anti-HIV-positive persons that can lead to persistent HBV expression.

Whether or not HBV is shown to be an etiological cofactor in AIDS affecting homosexual men, the epidemiological association of HBV and HIV may give the former a role in the pathogenesis of transfusion-related cases. Among the reported cases of AIDS, 3% had none of the recognized risk factors, and among them 28% had received blood components within 5 years of the onset of illness (6). Because of an 88% prevalence of anti-HBc in homosexual men as opposed to 3% in heterosexual men, blood containing anti-HBc was excluded from transfusion in San Francisco beginning in 1984 (see Chapter 5). No direct evidence is available as to whether such a practice has actually resulted in a reduction of transfusion-associated AIDS, but several current studies may provide the data in the foreseeable future. We have found that 40-60% of the anti-HIV-containing units of blood excluded from transfusion are reactive for anti-HBc. Thus, we feel satisfied with the unprecedented action of anti-HBc screening introduced in San Francisco at a time when no serologic test was available for HIV screening of donor blood.

The major challenge to the safety of blood transfusion is the long-term morbidity and mortality of posttransfusion hepatitis, due predominantly to the undefined viral agents termed non-A, non-B viruses. Inevitably, some of the so-called non-A, non-B agents may be the genetic variants termed HBV-like (1). The exclusion of blood containing anti-HBc is expected to reduce posttransfusion hepatitis caused by transmission of HBV, HBV-like, delta, and non-A, non-B agents. Hepatitis A virus (HAV) does not produce chronic infection and viremia is short-lived, so it is rarely transmitted through transfusion.

In summary, the hypothesis of HBV as a cofactor in the etiology of AIDS/ARC due to HIV infection has gained considerable strength from the published reports (12-15); however, the conclusive etiological proof of this seroepidemiological association remains to be obtained by molecular virological methods. Because homosexual men protected against HBV infection by vaccination have been known to be infected by HIV and to consequently suffer from AIDS, the evidence for HBV as a cofactor is controversial at best and deserves further study.

Acknowledgment

This work was supported by National Institutes of Health grant PO1 HL 36589.

References

1. Vyas GN. Blum HE. Hepatitis B virus infection—Current concepts of chronicity and immunity. West J Med 1984; 140:754-62.
2. Ravenholt RT. Role of hepatitis B virus in acquired immune deficiency syndrome. Lancet 1983; 2:885-6.
3. McDonald MI, Hamilton JD, Durack DT. Hepatitis B surface antigen could harbour the infectious agent of AIDS. Lancet 1983; 2:882-4.

4. Wright T, Friedman S, Altman D. Hepatitis B virus implicated in the pathogenesis of Kaposi's sarcoma in homosexual men. Gastroenterology 1983; 84:1402.
5. Siddiqui A. Hepatitis B virus DNA in Kaposi's sarcoma. Proc Natl Acad Sci USA 1983; 80:4861-4.
6. Anderson RE, Winkelstein W Jr, Blum HE, Vyas GN. Hepatitis B virus infection in the acquired immune deficiency syndrome (AIDS). In: Vyas GN, Dienstag JL, Hoofnagle JH, eds. Viral Hepatitis and Liver Disease. Orlando: Grune and Stratton, 1984:339-43.
7. Hoxie JA, Haggarty BS, Rackowski JL, Pillsbury N, Levy JA. Persistent noncytopathic infection of normal human T lymphocytes with AIDS-associated retrovirus. Science 1983; 229:1400-2.
8. Lie-Injo LE, Balasegaram M, Lopez CG, Herrera AR. Hepatitis B viral DNA in liver and white blood cells of patients with hepatoma. DNA 1983; 2:229-306.
9. Blum HE, Stowring L, Figus A, Montgomery CK, Haase AT, Vyas GN. Detection of HBV DNA in hepatocytes, bile duct epithelium and vascular elements by in situ hybridization. Proc Natl Acad Sci USA 1983; 80:6685-8.
10. Blum HE, Figus A, Haase AT, Vyas GN. Laboratory diagnosis of hepatitis B virus infection by nucleic acid hybridization analyses and immunohistologic detection of gene products. 18th Congress, Joint IABS/WHO Symposium on Standardization and Control of Biologicals Produced by Recombinant DNA Technology, Geneva, Switzerland, 1983. Develop Biol Standard 1985; 59:125-39.
11. Romet-Lemonne JL, McLane MF, Elfassi E, Hazeltine WA, Azocar J, Essex M. Hepatitis B virus infection in cultured human lymphoblastoid cells. Science 1983; 221:667-9.
12. Laure F, Zagury D, Saimot AG, Gallo RC, Hahn BH, Brechot C. Hepatitis B virus DNA sequences in lymphoid cells from patients with AIDS and AIDS-related complex. Science 1985; 229:561-3.
13. Noonan CA, Yoffe B, Mansell PWA, Metnick JL, Hollinger FB. Extrachromosomal sequences of hepatitis B virus DNA in peripheral blood mononuclear cells of acquired immune deficiency syndrome patients. Prod Natl Acad Sci USA 1986; 83:5698-702.
14. Laure F, Chatenoid L, Pasquenelli C, Gazengel C, Beaurain G, Torchet MF, Zagury D, Bach JF, Brechot C. Frequent lymphocyte infection by hepatitis B virus in hemophiliacs. Brit J Haemat 1987; 181-5.
15. Krogsgaard K, Lindhardt BO, Nielsen JO, Anderson P, Kryger P, Aldershuile J, Gerstoft J, Pedersen C. The influence of HTLV-III infection of the natural history of hepatitis B virus infection in male homosexual HBsAg carriers. Hepatology 1987; 7:37-41.

20

Developing Comprehensive Care Systems for Individuals with HIV Infection

Gayling Gee*

Cancer Research Institute
School of Medicine
University of California
and San Francisco General Hospital
San Francisco, California

I. Introduction

In well-publicized reports, the Centers for Disease Control (CDC) have estimated that between 1 and 2 million people have been exposed to human immunodeficiency virus (HIV), the causative agent of acquired immunodeficiency syndrome (AIDS). Of those individuals, from 5 to 20% may develop symptoms and progress to actual AIDS (1). The projected number of AIDS cases by the year 1991 is 270,000 (2). Many hospitals in such major metropolitan areas as New York City, San Francisco, and Los Angeles have seen their average inpatient AIDS census double from year to year. A similar situation is occurring in many smaller cities and towns as hospitals begin to admit their first AIDS patients. Despite such widely disseminated information, communities may not be fully aware of the scope of the problem until a "critical mass" of actual

---

**Current affiliation*: San Francisco General Hospital and School of Nursing, University of California, San Francisco, California.

cases suddenly overwhelms its resources. Thus, it is highly advantageous to plan for AIDS care. A city that fails to do so jeopardizes the health and well-being of all its residents—both those who are infected and those who may potentially be infected.

In May 1986, the CDC revealed a new classification system for HIV-associated infections and neoplasms that reflects the growing knowledge about the natural history of the virus (3). The clinical entity called AIDS is now known to be the end-stage manifestation of HIV disease; early disease manifestations include acute infection, asymptomatic carrier states, generalized lymphadenopathy, and constitutional and neurological symptoms—specific events subsequent to the actual viral insult.

The broad, clinical spectrum of HIV infection defined by the CDC may be conceptualized as a continuum, with transitory virus-induced symptoms at one extreme and terminal opportunistic infection at the other. The course of the infection varies from individual to individual; it does not progress over time in a linear fashion from wellness to illness to death. The initial insult with HIV may produce mildly acute, transitory viral symptoms (see Chapter 8). When these symptoms resolve, the only remaining sign of infection may be a positive HIV antibody test that, in actuality, confers no immunity to the development of AIDS.

As a group, persons with HIV infection will experience some level of illness, but the majority will feel clinically well. Within a time span of 2 months to 5 years, new symptomatology may develop. As the infection progresses first to AIDS-related complex (ARC) and then to AIDS, infected persons will experience increasing illness and debilitation, and few will ever feel completely well again. The course of illness averages 18 to 24 months and is characterized by a roller-coaster pattern of wellness and illness. In time, multiple episodes of acute illnesses with recurrent symptoms, relentless disease progression, and overwhelming infection occur, resulting ultimately in death. Patients along the entire spectrum of HIV infection require medical evaluation and treatment, as well as extensive nursing care. The catastrophic nature of the disease, and the epidemic proportions of infection, pose a major challenge to the medical system for the provision of services.

Education and social service interventions play a crucial role in this spectrum of clinical disease. An individual may have a history of risk behaviors for developing HIV infection, such as intravenous drug use or sexual contact with someone with existing infection. Whether this person is even aware that such behavior places him or her at risk may depend on the kind of public information or education that is available. If the level of awareness about risk of infection can be raised, perhaps modification of habits or lifestyle can minimize the risk and therefore transmission of disease.

Once aware of the possibility of infection, the individual, whether symptomatic or asymptomatic, may desire screening or evaluation for AIDS. Symptomatic patients may have either pulmonary, infectious disease, oncological, or neurological problems, or any combination of these. Obtaining services can be a problem if the person wishes to maintain confidentiality, if the medical system is not easily accessible, or if its personnel lack the knowledge and experience necessary for proper advice, evaluation, and treatment. Misdiagnosis and inappropriate treatments are possibilities in facilities unfamiliar with AIDS. Inappropriate labeling of persons who are HIV-antibody-seropositive as having AIDS can endanger the employment and insurance status of these individuals, as well as their personal relationships.

Once AIDS or ARC has been diagnosed, follow-up patient care is essential. The frequency of hospitalization and clinical follow-up increases as the disease progresses, requiring more and more nursing and social service intervention. Coordination of treatment approaches becomes more complex when the goal becomes maintaining the patient at home for terminal care. Moreover, providing care to the patient with the ''dual diagnoses'' of AIDS and substance abuse is especially taxing for the staff members involved in the case.

This conceptual framework of HIV infection as a spectrum of clinical presentations is central to the development of comprehensive care systems. It encourages health planners and physicians, nurses, and hospital administrators to focus not only on those individuals who have frank disease, but also on those who require care for symptoms and clinical events occurring well before the development of CDC-defined AIDS. A disease of such medical complexity and multiplicity of patient needs can be managed only by a systems approach.

The clinical spectrum of HIV infection, therefore, has implications as to the types of services needed in a community threatened by AIDS (see Figure 1). The development of a continuum of services for HIV infection and AIDS is essential for alleviating the burden on the health-care system created by this disease. Such services include: community and professional education about HIV infection and AIDS, screening and diagnostic services for symptomatic or asymptomatic people at risk for AIDS, treatment and follow-up care for the chronic illnesses related to AIDS and ARC, supportive and restorative care for acute AIDS-related illnesses, and palliative and terminal care for end-stage disease. Corresponding care sites for the provision of these services include: community AIDS projects, ambulatory-care clinics, acute-care facilities, and home-care and hospice agencies. A comprehensive, community-wide approach to the AIDS epidemic can be used to develop this continuum of health-care services.

The following discussion will focus on a description of these four models of health-care delivery, with particular emphasis on the outpatient model of

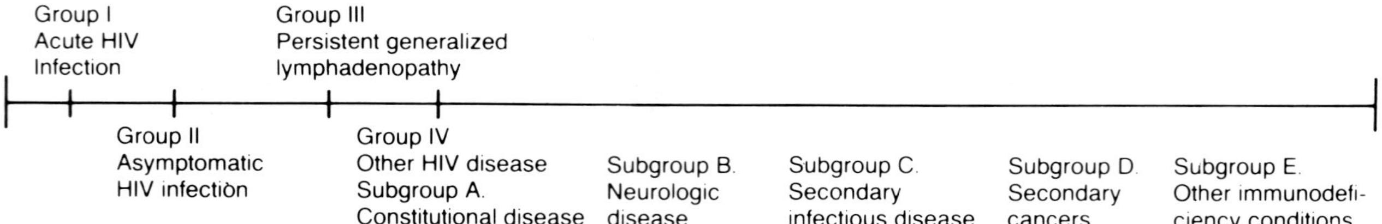

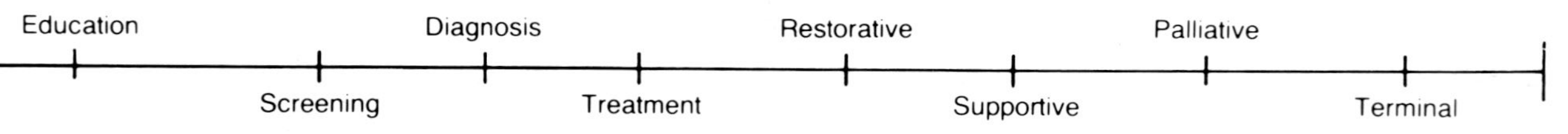

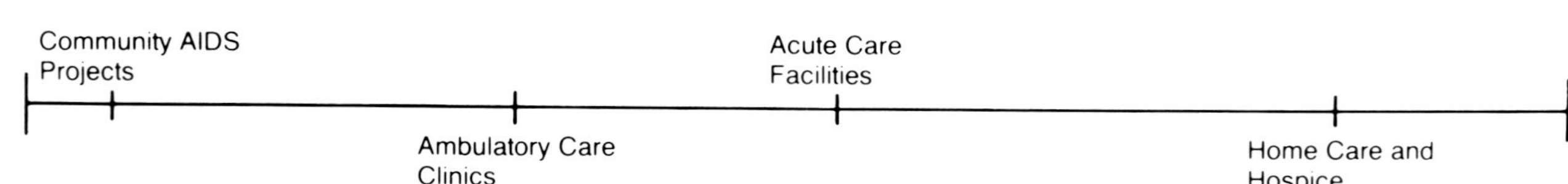

Figure 1 Clinical care requirements of HIV-infected individuals

care. Lastly, common issues and problems encountered in establishing and operating such units will be discussed, with suggestions for possible solutions.

II. Community AIDS Projects

Community AIDS projects can be instrumental in providing the educational outreach that is so vital to the dissemination of accurate information about HIV and AIDS, on both community and professional levels (see Table 1). With the lack of an effective treatment or vaccine for HIV infection, prevention becomes the most critical element in disease control. The target populations include people at risk for HIV infection and asymptomatic carriers. Since high-risk activities for contracting HIV have been identified, education and outreach to sexually active, and soon-to-be sexually active, individuals or to intravenous-drug-using populations may be effective in changing risk-taking behaviors and reducing the incidence of infection. Once aware of their risk behaviors or suspicious symptomatology, certain individuals may then seek referral for assistance or support in altering their behaviors or lifestyles, or for medical evaluation of symptoms.

Coordinated community education programs can do much to demystify AIDS and quell fear and hysteria. By addressing issues of contagion and homophobia and providing information on preventive measures and risk reduction for AIDS, the community hostility and rejection of AIDS patients and their care-givers may be reduced. Occasionally, community members will express negative feelings toward AIDS patients and reaction to their presence may be strong. However, a firm, consistent message from community agencies, backed by strong physician support, will alleviate fear. AIDS has never been just a "gay disease," but many people hold to this misconception and ignore the possibility that the disease may spread to their own communities. As AIDS begins to move into the heterosexual and non-intravenous-drug-using populations, open, frank discussions become imperative so that all may become aware of the risks of infection.

AIDS projects can also coordinate the publication and dissemination of appropriate, patient-oriented educational pamphlets, leaflets, and videotapes about AIDS. Outreach activities may involve community groups such as schools, parent-teacher organizations, youth and church groups, political and government agencies, labor unions, and private business organizations.

Professional education programs can also be coordinated by local AIDS projects in cooperation with the medical, nursing, and counseling staffs of community hospitals familiar with AIDS care issues. Appropriate targets for outreach might include medical and nursing organizations, psychiatric and mental health agencies, substance abuse and gay health organizations, hospitals and skilled nursing facilities, and other public health agencies.

Table 1 Key Responsibilities of Community AIDS projects

1. Providing community education for AIDS awareness and prevention
Pamphlets, brochures
Public service announcements, billboards
Telephone hotlines, referral networks
Speakers bureau, community forums
2. Coordinating professional activities and education
Speakers bureau, continuing education classes
Task force development
Fund-raising, research
3. Providing direct services for persons with AIDS
Individual counseling
Support groups or "buddy system"
Social service referrals
Financial assistance
Emergency and long-term housing
Volunteer support for practical or home services
Legal assistance
Transportation

Services provided by community AIDS projects are not restricted to educational programs. Patient advocacy for quality care and representation in antidiscriminatory issues are other roles of community agencies. Across the nation, AIDS projects are also involved in patient counseling services: support groups for patients, families, the "worried well," and health-care providers; financial assistance; emergency and long-term housing; legal aid; transportation; volunteer home services; telephone hotlines; and a "buddy system" for people with AIDS (4,5).

Community involvement is an integral part of the development of AIDS care systems. Without the support of a knowledgeable and compassionate community, the health-care provider will find the provision of quality health care to an AIDS patient to be an insurmountable task.

III. Ambulatory-Care Clinics

Ambulatory care sites are appropriate places to provide screening services to people at risk for HIV infection and diagnostic evaluation for people with persistent generalized lymphadenopathy (PGL) syndrome or other symptoms of HIV disease. The development of screening protocols, decision-making about the use of the HIV antibody test, cutaneous testing for anergy and other immunological laboratory tests, and the development of a referral process are initial considerations.

In any community, individuals who engage in high-risk activities for transmission of HIV, regardless of whether they are symptomatic, will be likely candidates for screening. Depending on the population at risk, various types of agencies can serve as appropriate screening sites. A venereal disease clinic could target the sexually active population. Substance abuse programs may also be appropriate sites for screening. Community health centers, women's clinics, gay health clinics, or hospital-based clinics are also possible sites for initial evaluation for AIDS.

A. HIV Antibody Testing

HIV antibody testing as a screening tool remains controversial. While the accuracy of the enzyme-linked immunosorbent assay (ELISA) and Western blot tests for antibody have been demonstrated, fears of violation of patient confidentiality and misinterpretation or misuse of the test results have been major concerns (6-9) and may have contributed greatly to its limited use. Nevertheless, the alarming rise in numbers of HIV infections and AIDS cases has prompted health officials to recommend greater use of serologic testing (10). In order to ensure appropriate utilization of the antibody test (see Table 2) and proper allocation of resources, ambulatory-care sites need to consider two major issues: first, what the role of their agency is in the AIDS epidemic and second, who the target populations are.

The Agency's Role

Is it the agency's goal to be primarily an alternative test site where free or low-cost and anonymous or confidential testing are done for purposes of screening and prevention? If this is the primary role of the center, then this function can be handled by phlebotomy and specially trained counseling or nursing staff, and the agency will rely heavily on its outreach and educational capabilities to accomplish its goal. Careful counseling should be offered to clarify what the test does and does not mean. Informed consent for antibody testing is usually required, but this procedure varies from state to state. Patients should also be advised whether the test result becomes a permanent part of their medical record.

If the serologic test is positive, careful assessment of the patient's emotional response is essential to determine if crisis intervention or mental-health referral is indicated. Education about ways to prevent exposure to others, such as decreasing the number of sexual and intravenous drug encounters, informing others of their antibody status, practicing protective or "safe" sex, and avoiding pregnancy, should be an integral part of the program. A referral network to a medical facility should be established for symptomatic seropositive individuals requiring further care. If the serologic test is negative,

Table 2 Recommendations for Use of HIV Antibody Test

Purpose	Appropriate	Not appropriate
Prevention	For voluntary and confidential testing programs that include informed consent and counseling in groups with high prevalence of infection	For mandatory mass screening programs without informed consent or counseling in groups with low prevalence of infection
	For screening blood and blood products	
Diagnosis	To confirm AIDS diagnosis in high-risk individuals with uncommon manifestation of AIDS- vs. non-AIDS-related infection or neoplasm	As sole diagnostic indicator of AIDS or ARC
	To confirm AIDS diagnosis in persons with no clear history of high-risk behavior vs. non-AIDS-related infection or neoplasm	Not necessary or indicated for confirmation of AIDS or ARC diagnosis in individuals who have CDC-defined manifestations of AIDS or ARC
	To confirm ARC diagnosis in persons with uncommon chronic medical problems typical of AIDS- vs. non-AIDS-related infection or neoplasm	
Research	To collect epidemiological data	
	To determine appropriate seropositives for antiviral or immunomodulator drug studies or therapy	
Infection control		Not known to be a useful tool for infection-control purposes

the same sort of counseling can be done to assist the patient in reducing his or her own risk of exposure to the virus. Additionally, repeat antibody testing within 1 to 6 months may be indicated for those with a negative result and known HIV exposure occurring less than 1 month before the initial antibody test.

If, instead, the agency chooses to be primarily a diagnostic and treatment center for AIDS, then the guidelines for the use of serologic testing should be based on the following considerations:

1. An HIV antibody test result is not required in 99% of all cases defined as AIDS by the CDC (11).

2. Generally, the test serves no diagnostic purpose in determining AIDS or in influencing treatment decisions, except in the following infrequent cases:
   a. To establish a diagnosis of AIDS in a high-risk individual with an uncommon manifestation of AIDS
   b. To establish a diagnosis of AIDS in persons with no clear history of high-risk behavior
   c. To establish a diagnosis of ARC in persons with unusual chronic medical problems, especially if there is no clear history of high-risk behavior (12)
3. Serious psychosocial consequences can accompany a positive antibody test result if the patient is not made to understand the meaning of the test or if proper systems to insure confidentiality or anonymity have not been established. Primarily because of this issue, the role of antibody testing should be carefully considered by every agency before it establishes its policy.
4. The antibody test will be used increasingly in epidemiological and clinical research trials, especially to identify ARC patients for antiviral and immunomodulator drug therapies.
5. The antibody test is not an infection-control tool; infection-control guidelines should not be based on antibody test results.

An agency that chooses to provide diagnostic and treatment services will, of course, require nursing, medical, and psychosocial staff. Ideally, it should be hospital-based to ensure easy access to diagnostic services, as well as acute-care beds for its patients. Finally, whatever administrative decisions are made as to the appropriate use of the antibody test, it is important for every agency to have this test available for all its patients.

Target Population

Despite a 99% sensitivity and specificity, the ELISA test produces an unacceptably high number of false-positive results in certain populations (6,27,28). When the ELISA test is used in groups with a high incidence of HIV infection, such as sexually active gay men, intravenous drug users, or hemophiliacs, it has a high positive predictive value; that is, the positive test results are reliably positive. When the ELISA test is used in groups with a low incidence of infection, such as members of the military or monogamous, non-intravenous-drug-using heterosexual men and women, it has a low positive predictive value; that is, the positive test results are unreliable and may be false-positives. ELISA testing also has a very high negative predictive value regardless of the incidence of HIV in the population. Therefore, the assay reliably predicts negative antibody test results in all persons screened. The overall implications for use of HIV antibody testing are that:

1. The test has serious problems when used in a mandatory mass-screening campaign in groups with a low prevalence of infection because of its unreliability in predicting positives.
2. The diagnostic value of the antibody test is questionable in the same groups.
3. However, the test *can* play a major role in the prevention or control of HIV infection when used in screening programs that include risk-reduction counseling and follow-up care to those populations with a high prevalence of infection.

B. Other Services

Screening protocols for HIV infection should include detailed histories of chief complaints, AIDS-related symptoms, illnesses, and related risk factors (see Table 3), and an AIDS-specific physical examination (see Table 4). Based on the severity or suspiciousness of symptoms, further evaluation may be indicated. If the agency lacks the resources to do extensive laboratory testing, a referral process to a hospital or hospital-based clinic should be established to facilitate diagnostic evaluation. Laboratory and other diagnostic procedures may then be ordered depending on presenting symptoms (see Tables 5 and 6).

Table 3 AIDS Screening History

Chief complaint/history of present illness	Previous history
Fatigue	Sexual orientation/years active/multiple partners/high-risk sexual activity
Fever, chills, night sweats	Intravenous drug usage
Adenopathy	Transfusions in last 5 years
Anorexia	Known AIDS exposure
Weight loss	Previous sexually transmitted disease
Respiratory	Gonorrhea—body site, when, treatment
Cough, shortness of breath, dyspnea on exertion	Syphilis—stage, treatment, last serology
Gastrointestinal	Condylomata accuminata—site, treatment, when
Diarrhea, bloating, gas, thrush	Intestinal parasites—when, treatment, last parasitology stool exam
Dermatological	Hepatitis—when, type, hepatitis B serologic status if known
Herpes simplex, herpes zoster, tinea, suspicious lesions	History of herpes simplex zoster (shingles)
Neurological	Alcohol/tobacco/recreational drugs
Headache, change in mental status, paralysis, weakness, stiff neck, seizures	Present medications
	Allergies
	Chronic illness
	Major surgery
	Other significant medical/health history

Source: Ref. 21.

Table 4 AIDS Screening Physical Examination

Physical examination	Markers of suspicion	Possible indication
Eyes	Cotton-wool exudate	PCP-associated
	Diffuse hemorrhage, exudates	Cytomegalovirus retinitis
Oral	Thrush (*Candida albicans*)	Immune deficiency
	Hairy leukoplakia on tongue	Immune deficiency
	Red to purple palate/ mucosal lesions	Intraoral Kaposi's sarcoma
Neck	Lymphadenopathy	Diffuse PGL, Kaposi's sarcoma in lymph nodes
Axillae/epitrochlear areas	Lymphadenopathy	Diffuse PGL, Kaposi's sarcoma in lymph nodes
Lungs	Dry cough elicited by deep breathing, rales	PCP
Abdomen	Hepatomegaly	Hepatitis
	Splenomegaly	ITP, PGL
	Masses, tenderness	PGL, diarrhea
Groin	Lymphadenopathy, inguinal and femoral sites	Diffuse PGL, Kaposi's sarcoma in lymph nodes
Rectal	Red to purple perianal lesions	Kaposi's sarcoma
	Condylomata	Papillmovirus, syphilis
	Ulcers	Herpes simplex, syphilis
	Candida	Immunodeficiency
Skin	Red to purple lesions	Kaposi's sarcoma
	Seborrheic dermatitis	PCP-associated
	Herpes zoster (shingles), including old scarring	Immune deficiency
	Tinea	
	Molluscum	Immune deficiency
Extremities	Edema	Lymphatic duct blockage by Kaposi's sarcoma lesions
	Red to purple lesions	Kaposi's sarcoma
Neurological	Decreased intellectual acuity	Cryptococcus
	Parathesias	Toxoplasmosis
	Extremity pains	CNS lymphoma
	Weakness, paralysis	PML
	Retinal abnormalities	Cytomegalovirus
		M. avium
		Subacute encephalitis

CNS, central nervous system; ITP, idiopathic thrombocytopenia purpura; PCP, *Pneumocystis carinii* pneumonia; PGL, persistent generalized lymphadenopathy syndrome; PML, progressive multifocal leukoencephalopathy.
Source: Ref. 21.

Table 5 Laboratory Data for AIDS Screening

Lab evaluation	Markers of suspicion	Possible indication
CBC, differential	Leukocytopenia (<4000)	Immune deficiency
	Lymphocytopenia	Immune deficiency
	Decreased RBC, hematocrit, hemoglobin	Anemias associated with chronic disease
Platelet count	Dramatic thrombocytopenia (<50K)	ITP, probably AIDS-related
	Mild thrombocytopenia (80-120K)	Frequently seen in immune deficiency
Erythrocyte sedimentation rate	Elevation	Elevated with PCP or other opportunistic infection (usually normal in PGL and Kaposi's sarcoma)
SGOT, SGPT	Elevation	Hepatitis
LDH	Elevation	May be elevated in PCP
Alkaline phosphatase	Elevation	Intra-abdominal adenopathy with obstruction
Serum cholesterol, iron	Decrease	Frequently depleted in early chronic disease with wasting
VDRL	Positivity	Syphilis
Hepatitis B surface antigen (HB_sAg)	Positivity	Acute hepatitis or carrier status
Hepatitis B surface or core antibodies (HB_sAb, HB_cAb)	Positivity	Acute hepatitis or carrier status
Herpesvirus culture (skin ulcerations)	Positive for virus	Herpes simplex; persistent or severe cases (>1 mo) are diagnostic of AIDS
Cytomegalovirus blood culture	Positive for cytomegalovirus	Cytomegalovirus infection; disseminated cases are diagnostic of AIDS
Chest x-ray	Diffuse interstitial infiltrates Usually bilateral	PCP
Stool exam for ova and parasites	Ameobiasis, giardiasis	Persistent case despite treatment may indicate immune deficiency
Stool culture	Shigella, Salmonella, Campylobacter	Treatable infections
Stool exam for cryptosporidiosis	Positivity	Cryptosporidiosis: cases >1 mo are diagnostic of AIDS

CBC, complete blood count; ITP, idiopathic thrombocytopenia purpura; LDH, lactic dehydrogenase; PCP, *Pneumocystis carinii* pneumonia; PGL, persistent generalized lymphadenopathy syndrome; RBC, red blood cells; VDRL, syphilis serology test.
Source: Ref. 21.

Table 6 AIDS Evaluation by Organ System

Organ system	Basic evaluation	Secondary evaluation	Extensive evaluation (M.D. consultation)	Possible diagnosis
Pulmonary	CBC, diff, plt, ESR SMAC Chest x-ray	Pulmonary function tests Gallium scan	Sputum induction Transbronchial biopsy	PCP Cytomegalovirus pneumonia Kaposi's sarcoma in the lung Other opportunistic infections
Gastrointestinal	CBC, diff, plt, ESR SMAC Stool culture Stool parasitology and Crypto-sporidium exam	Oropharyngeal candida culture Pharyngeal gonorrhea culture Rectal gonorrhea culture Rectal HSV culture HB_sAg, HB_sAb, HB_cAb	Colonoscopy Endoscopy Barium studies	Candidiasis Herpes simplex Cytomegalovirus colitis *M. avium* Cryptosporidium *Isospora belli* Kaposi's sarcoma in gastrointestinal system
Genitourinary	CBC, diff, plt, ESR SMAC, urinalysis, C&S	VDRL Urethral gonorrhea culture	KUB	Syphilis Gonorrhea
Cutaneous	Herpes culture VDRL	Dark-field exam	Biopsy	Kaposi's sarcoma Herpes simplex Syphilis
Neurological	Mental status exam Neurological exam	Cryptococcal antigen Toxoplasmosis titer	CT scan Lumbar puncture	Cryptococcus Toxoplasmosis Cytomegalovirus PML *M. avium* CNS lymphoma Subacute encephalitis *M. tuberculosis*
Systemic (fever)	CBC, diff, plt, ESR SMAC Stool culture O & P × 3 Chest x-ray	Blood cultures	Bone marrow biopsy and culture AFB blood culture Viral blood culture Lymph-node biopsy	*M. avium* Cytomegalovirus Toxoplasmosis PCP Cryptococcus Herpes simplex PML Candidiasis

AFB, acid-fast bacillus; CBC, complete blood count; C&S, culture and sensitivity; CT, computed tomography; diff, differential; ESR, erythrocyte sedimentation rate; HSV, herpes simplex virus; KUB, kidney, ureter, bladder x-ray; O & P, ova and parasite; PCP, *Pneumocystis carinii* pneumonia; plt, platelets; PML, progressive multifocal leukoencephalopathy; SMAC, chemistry panel; VDRL, syphilis serology test.
Source: Ref. 21.

Treatment and follow-up care may also be provided in an ambulatory-care location. For AIDS cases, these options might include establishing a regular clinic schedule for providing primary AIDS care and an "intravenous infusion center" or "day treatment center" for the administration of both standard and investigational drugs, blood and blood products, and hydration fluids. The need for medical monitoring and treatment visits will vary from patient to patient, ranging from once every 2 to 3 months for ARC patients to weekly or daily for more debilitated AIDS patients. Hospital-based clinics are most ideally suited for the provision of primary-care services. Access to radiology, clinical laboratories, nuclear medicine, pulmonary labs, and other departments is a necessity for evaluating AIDS.

Clinic nursing staff are able to develop expertise in triaging patient problems over the phone or when the patient is a "drop-in." Laboratory tests and x-rays can be ordered immediately to facilitate the evaluation. Emergency-room visits can be reduced when an AIDS clinic has such resources available for patients. Outpatient intravenous infusion centers offer patients the option of therapy without requiring hospitalization. Utilization of such services reduces overall medical-care costs by decreasing the number of hospital days.

Patients requiring hospitalization can be admitted through the clinic. Discharged patients can easily be given follow-up clinic appointments. Continuity of care is greatly facilitated by this process, especially if there are a dedicated AIDS clinic and an AIDS inpatient unit that work together (see Table 7).

IV. Acute-Care Facilities

Hospitalization occurs with increasing frequency for those patients with opportinistic infections, and those with the neurological, pulmonary, and gastrointestinal complications of HIV disease. Patients in the early stages of AIDS, with a single opportunistic infection, may require a level of nursing care similar to that of any other hospitalized patient on a general ward. As the disease progresses, greater patient demands are noted (13). This result is related to increased diagnostic and laboratory testing, complex drug regimens with toxic reactions, and respiratory-care needs. Personal-care requirements are intensified because of problems with chronic diarrhea, fevers and night sweats, fatigue, debilitation, and neurological dysfunction affecting motor skills and mental status.

Dedicated AIDS inpatient units can effectively manage such problems by 1) developing nursing expertise in assessment and management, 2) becoming knowledgeable about treatment regimens and monitoring toxicity,

Table 7 Benefits of Dedicated AIDS Units

1. Development of nursing clinical expertise
Facilitates medical care
Rapid identification of medical and emotional needs
Up-to-date knowledge base, educational support
2. Medical and nursing care centralized
Team efforts concentrated
More effective patient management
More efficient discharge planning
3. Counseling staff on site
Immediate crisis intervention and support
Social service intervention
Grief and bereavement counseling
4. Improved quality of care
Comprehensive, coordinated
Sensitive, holistic
Integrated with community services

and 3) determining adequate staffing levels based on accurate assessment of nursing-care requirements. When a dedicated inpatient unit is not feasible because of a low AIDS census, a multidisciplinary AIDS team can be created to make rounds on AIDS patients scattered throughout the hospital. This group would assess patient needs, coordinate approaches for their care, and provide the necessary inservice training for other hospital staff.

Early discharge planning can be an effective means of coordinating nursing services for the patient at home and of shortening hospital days. Family, volunteer, and home nursing support systems can meet with discharge planning staff to make appropriate care decisions and assignments. Placement in an extended care facility is always difficult; many agencies are unwilling to take AIDS patients. Unfortunately, for some patients without home supports, such as intravenous drug users, extended hospitalization may be required if such facilities are unavailable. This problem remains serious and unresolved in many metropolitan areas, and can increase the inappropriate use of acute-care facilities for AIDS patients.

With progressing AIDS debilitation, a patient's decision of whether to receive life-sustaining measures or experimental drug treatment frequently becomes an issue. The onset of neurological changes in many patients with resultant dementia of varying degrees often makes it essential for staff to address such issues earlier in the disease process. Although there are some exceptions, most patients are willing to discuss these issues if they are approached in a sensitive, appropriate manner. In California, there is a legal document—the Durable Power of Attorney for Health Care—that allows the patient to designate an individual to make medical decisions in case the patient becomes incompetent. Other documents, such as a "living will" and "directive of physicians," have been used for the same purpose (8).

V. Home Care and Hospice Services

The relentless progression of HIV disease results in increasing debilitation of the patient despite treatment and resolution of acute infectious episodes. Once an acutely ill hospitalized patient becomes medically stabilized, discharge and placement becomes a principal concern of the health-care team. In communities where home nursing services are available for people with AIDS or ARC, hospital stays are shortened, and the patient is afforded the opportunity to receive care in the familiar surroundings of home. Hospice services, when available, offer even more intensive home-care involvement, including greater availability of nursing hours, on-call nursing services, social service support, and home attendant care time (4,16).

Long-term, nonacute nursing care focusing on specific needs becomes the patient's major necessity. The constitutional symptoms of fevers, fatigue, weight loss, and diarrhea; the neurological manifestations of dementia, neuropathy, and seizure activity; and the nutritional management and drug therapy administration are major issues that challenge the home-care nurse. Each of these clinical problems requires ongoing assessment and intervention. As the patient becomes increasingly debilitated, terminal care issues predominate. Staff and family support become critical as the patient faces the decision whether to die at home or in the hospital. In the home, frequent monitoring of pain and symptoms places great responsibility on the hospice nurse's clinical assessment and judgement skills. Medication administration, physician consultation, and supervision of home-care attendants are other aspects of the nurse's role in coordinating care. Grief and bereavement counseling and support groups are required by staff and family alike, especially when working with the dying AIDS patient.

The home support team should include nurses, social workers, attendants, and physician consultants. Because the needs of terminally ill homebound AIDS patients are so great, the agency may want to foster the development of a volunteer staff to further assist patients in the home. This group could provide practical support—for example, by shopping for food, doing errands, and escorting patients—and, in so doing, extend the capabilities of the health-care team.

VI. Multidisciplinary Care

A multidisciplinary approach has been found by practitioners experienced in working with AIDS to be the most effective and efficient means for meeting patient as well as staff needs (15-17). This approach centralizes services among a group of providers or within a physical location, or both, and allows for the development of clinical expertise and clinical research in AIDS. It facilitates referrals and coordination of services, and allocates the responsibilities of care through the inclusion of various medical subspecialists, nurses, psychiatrists, social workers, and counselors. A multidisciplinary team is best equipped to meet not only the physical but also the emotional and spiritual needs of the person with AIDS. The models of care previously described, including ambulatory-care clinics, acute-care facilities, and home-care and hospice agencies, are particularly effective when operated under the aegis of such a multidisciplinary team.

VII. Model for Ambulatory Care

Ward 86 of San Francisco General Hospital opened in January 1983 as an outpatient medical clinic specializing in the care of the AIDS patient (5,15,

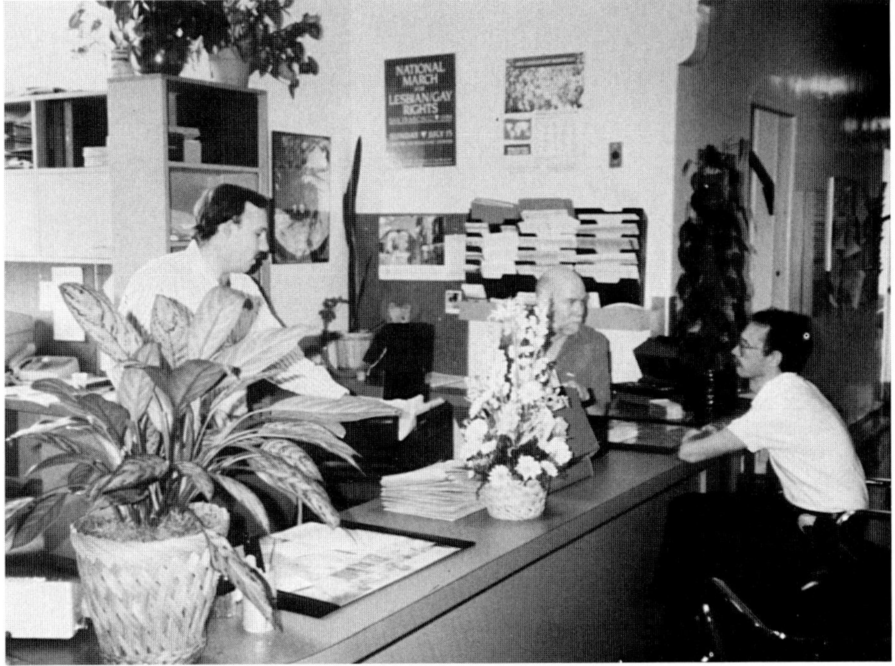

Figure 2 Registration desk at the Ward 86 AIDS Clinic. The AIDS Clinic offers multidisciplinary services to people with AIDS, including medical, nursing, and psychosocial support services.

18-20). This clinic has evolved over a 4-year period to provide a spectrum of services to its ARC and AIDS patients, including AIDS screening services, comprehensive medical evaluation and diagnosis, and treatment and follow-up care. Additional services include a comprehensive psychosocial support system. Clinical research is also an integral part of clinical operations. Ward 86 has now become a national and international model for AIDS care. (See Figure 2.)

A. The Clinic Schedule

The Ward 86 clinic schedule includes seven half-day clinics (see Figure 3). General AIDS Clinics are held on Mondays, with both oncology and infectious disease physicians in attendance. On Tuesday mornings, the AIDS Clinic focuses on ARC care issues. Wednesday and Thursday mornings, clinics are staffed solely by nurse practitioners, first, to see AIDS patients who are on clinical trials for research-related physical examinations and second, to evaluate self-referred patients in the Nursing Screening Clinic for AIDS. The Thursday-afternoon AIDS/Opportunistic Infection (OI) Clinic is staffed by infectious disease physicians. The focus is, of course, AIDS-related infections, and the most debilitated Ward 86 patients are seen in this clinic. The Friday-morning AIDS/Kaposi's sarcoma (KS) Clinic is run by oncologists; its primary focus is to manage KS, lymphomas, and other AIDS-related malignancies. Besides these clinics, registered nursing staff administer treatments daily, Monday through Friday. Some treatment protocols call for daily intravenous medication, while others require weekly intravenous chemotherapy or oral drug dispensing.

Evening and weekend medical coverage for nonhospitalized clinic patients is provided by the Ward 86 clinic physician staff, whose members are

WARD 86 CLINIC SCHEDULE

	MON	TUES	WEDS	THURS	FRI
AM	AIDS	AIDS/ARC	AIDS/NP CLINIC	AIDS/NP SCRNING	AIDS/KS
PM	AIDS			AIDS/OI	

Figure 3 Schedule of Ward 86 AIDS Clinic. NP Clinic = clinic for physical examinations only; NP scrning = nurse-practitioner-staffed screening clinic for AIDS and HIV infection; OI = opportunistic infection clinic; KS = Kaposi's sarcoma clinic.

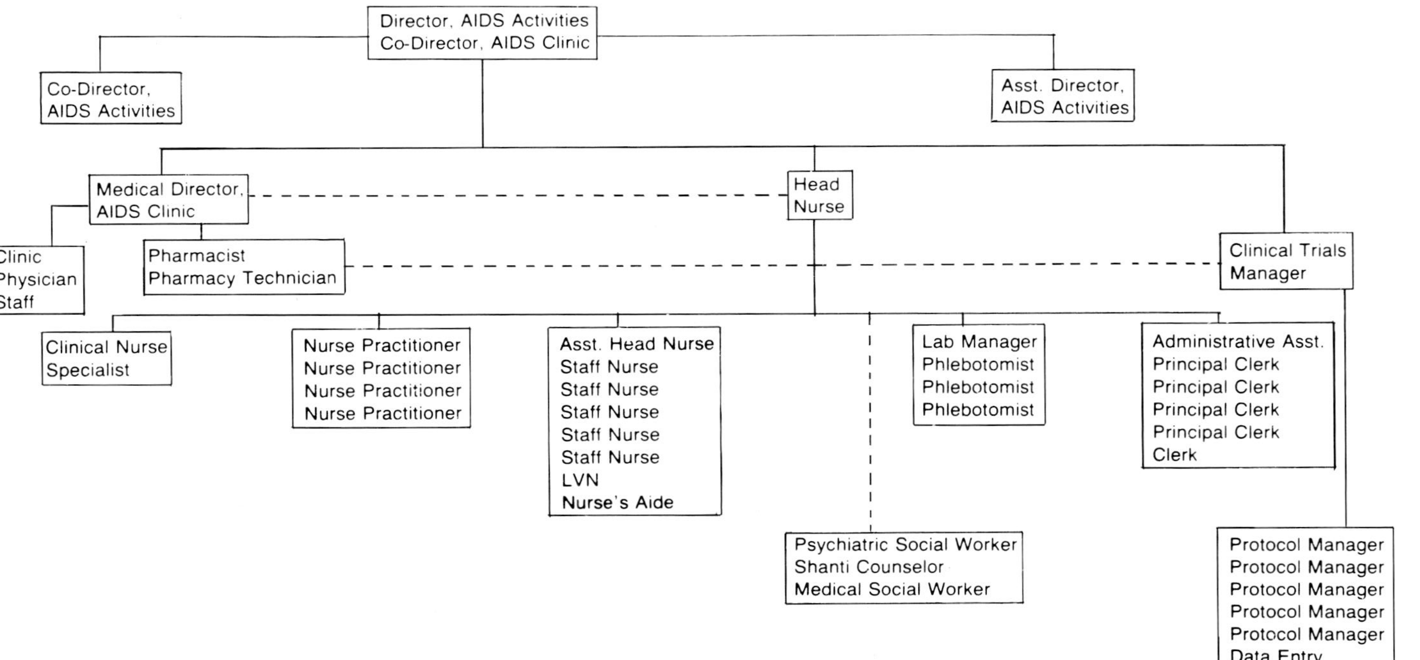

Figure 4 Ward 86 AIDS Clinic organizational chart.

assigned to a rotating on-call schedule. (Nurse practitioner staff are not assigned to on-call duties.) A physician's answering service forwards urgent medical calls from clinic patients to the on-call physician for triage. Patients with acute or life-threatening symptoms are referred to the hospital's Emergency Department, with the on-call physician phoning to alert the triage nurse and the medical staff as to the patient's condition and estimated time of arrival. For problems that are determined to be medically nonacute, patients are referred back to clinic on the following day as a "drop-in" for evaluation or to their primary-care provider at the earliest available appointment. Since all hospitalized AIDS patients are cared for by the house staff, members of the clinic on-call staff are not paged for inpatient consultation.

In 1983, Ward 86 had 3500 AIDS-related patient visits; in 1984 there were 7900; in 1985, 11,600. In 1986 and 1987, over 14,000 and 18,000 patient visits, respectively, were recorded. The clinic census has expanded exponentially as the epidemic has grown.

B. Clinic Staff Roles and Responsibilities

The Ward 86 clinic staff has also grown rapidly with the epidemic, from one physician and one nurse to the team shown in Figure 4. Fifteen oncology and infectious disease attending physicians and fellows now handle the daily scheduled AIDS Clinics. In addition to the medical staff, there is one head nurse, one assistant head nurse, four nurse practitioners, four registered nurses, one licensed vocational nurse, and one nurse's aide. A senior lab assistant and three phlebotomists draw blood, collect and bank research specimens, operate a cell counter, and maintain the clinic-based satellite laboratory. (See Figures 5, 6.) The clerical support staff maintains a clinic chart system to facilitate chart review and research data collection, and registers and schedules appointments for clinic patients. A clinical pharmacist and pharmacy technician are responsible for the handling and dispensing of all investigational as well as approved drugs administered in the clinics. A clinical trials supervisor and protocol and data-entry staff are involved in investigational study implementation and data collection. Staff functions are summarized in Table 8, and services offered by the clinic are summarized in Table 9.

Physicians

The physicians on the AIDS team, in addition to providing direct outpatient care, have general medical and medical specialty inpatient consult duties as well. (One physician serves as the inpatient AIDS consult service.) Each has attending responsibilities for at least two AIDS Clinics during the week and rotating weekend on-call duties, and they also conduct clinical research trials.

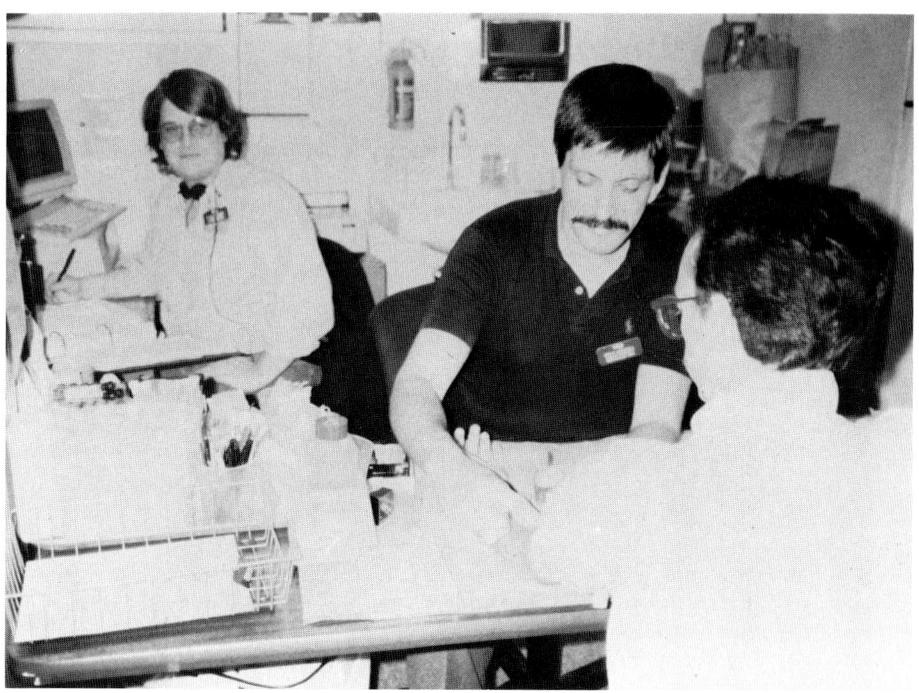

Figure 5 Phlebotomy services. On-site clinic laboratory testing facilitates dose adjustments for chemotherapy administration.

Nurse Practitioners

In order to expand the primary care capabilities of Ward 86, nurse practitioner (NP) process protocols have been developed for AIDS evaluation (see Tables 3-6) (21). The protocols employed include a very specific AIDS history and physical examination format. The NP can order screening and other diagnostic blood or stool tests, x-rays, pulmonary function tests, cultures, or skin biopsies based on specific findings. Referrals to other clinics for such specialties as dermatology, oral surgery, ophthalmology, or neurology are also covered by these protocols. Using process protocols, nurse practitioners can perform about 90% of the workup required in the screening evaluation of any patient with suspected signs of HIV infection. Special nurse clinics have been established for the purpose of screening for AIDS. The Ward 86 Nurse Screening Clinic for AIDS was specifically designed for individuals coming to the clinic for the first time, either fearing infection with HIV or with definite symptoms of disease. Individuals screened in this clinic have been both self-referred and physician-referred. If an individual

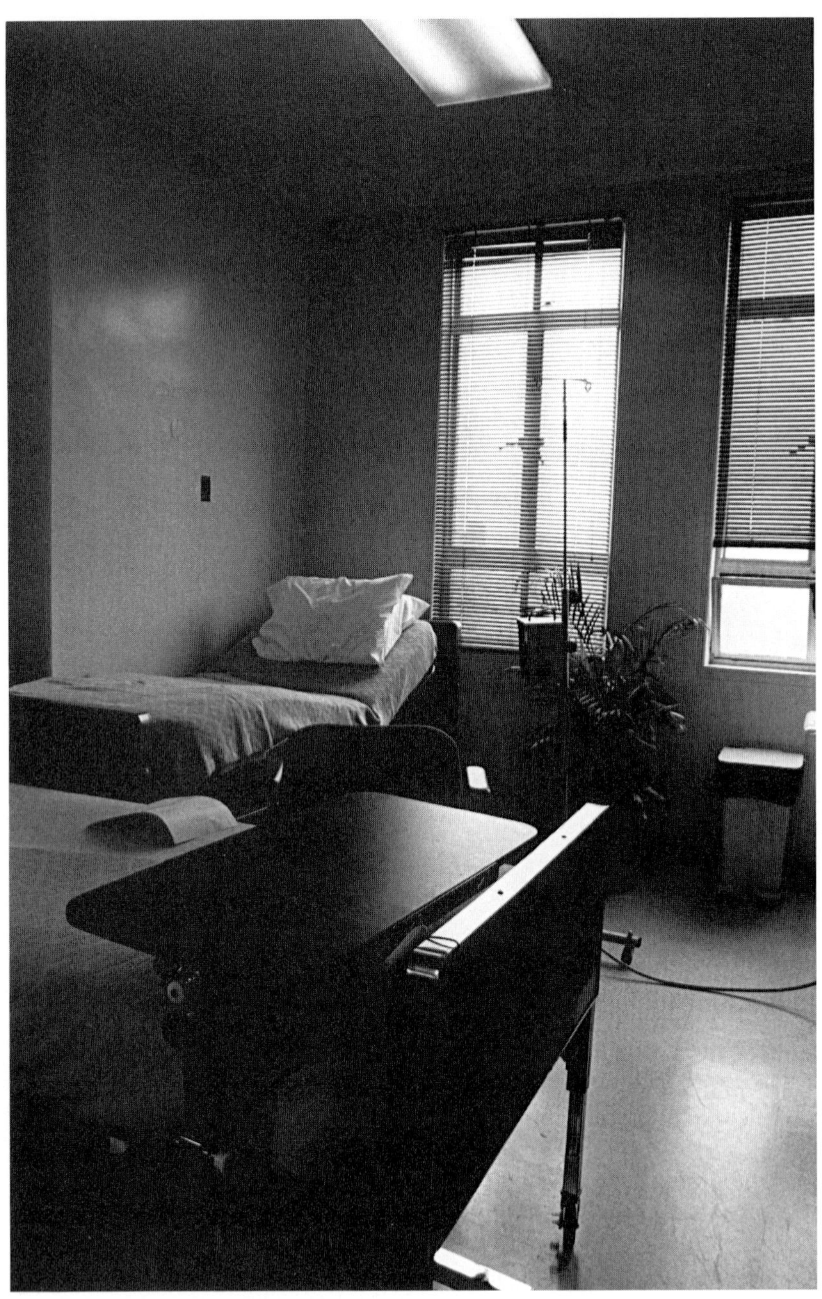

Figure 6 Intravenous infusion room. An outpatient infusion center allows clinic staff to administer both standard and investigational drugs, blood and blood products, and hydration fluids to reduce the number of hospital days. (Photo copyright Susan Schwartzenberg.)

Table 8 Ward 86 AIDS Clinic: Staff Fucntions

Physician staff
Primary care—outpatient
Consultation—inpatient and outpatient
Research, teaching
Nurse practitioners
Primary care—outpatient
Screening Clinic
Research
Nursing staff
Clinic coordination, triage
Administration of chemotherapy, investigationals, blood products
Patient referrals
Research
Pharmacist
Drug consultation
Prescription Refill Clinic
Research, pharmacokinetics
Clinical trials manager
Coordination of all study activities
Data gathering, monitoring, protocol administration
Psychiatric social worker
Crisis intervention
In-depth counseling
Medical social worker
Concrete needs
Social service referrals
Shanti counselor
Crisis counseling
Bereavement counseling

Table 9 Ward 86 AIDS Clinic: Summary of Services

Primary medical care for AIDS
AIDS consultation services
Nurse Screening Clinic for AIDS
Prescription Refill Clinics
Chemotherapy/investigational drug administration
Outpatient transfusions
Shanti counseling services
Medical social services
Psychiatric counseling services

presents to clinic and is determined by the NP to be asymptomatic and without risk factors for HIV infection, education and counseling about AIDS and its prevention are offered by the NP. If a patient is symptomatic, gives a history of being positive for HIV antibody, or is a member of a high-risk group with a history of possible exposure, screening laboratory tests will be ordered. The patient will then be brought back to an AIDS Clinic attended by a physician, for further evaluation by either an NP or a physician. The symptomatic patient is then incorporated into the clinic system and seen by the same NP or physician provider at each visit.

Because Ward 86 is a diagnostic and treatment center for AIDS, the HIV antibody test is not done on a routine basis in the Nurse Screening Clinic. The guidelines for the use of antibody testing on Ward 86 are as outlined in Section III.A. Both the ELISA and Western blot tests are available and may be ordered for those patients with unusual presentations suggestive of HIV infection. Clinic providers order them only when the test result will influence the diagnosis or the choice of therapy for research purposes, or if the patient insists on having the test done. The majority of AIDS cases seen in the Ward 86 clinic are identified by clinical diagnosis and do not require serologic testing.

The antibody test for screening is offered at "alternative test sites," i.e., the district health centers. This service reduces the burden on Ward 86 of the screening process. The health centers are specially funded and staffed to provide this service, and are able to provide complete anonymity of results. Pre- and posttest counseling and medical and psychiatric referral services are provided to each person undergoing antibody testing, as required by California state law. In addition, physicians and NPs at the health centers have adopted the Ward 86 clinic's nurse screening protocols and have established their own AIDS screening and ARC clinics. When an ARC patient is suspected of developing AIDS, a referral is made to Ward 86 for further evaluation. Because the same forms are employed, the data base is consistent and duplication of effort is avoided.

The NP follows his or her own case load of patients in the various AIDS clinics and works closely with the clinic physicians to provide primary care. NPs must seek physician consultation for more invasive or extensive evaluation, treatment decisions, and hospitalizations. In addition to responsibilities for primary care and AIDS screening care, the NP has a major role in clinical research. Each NP is familiar with the investigational trials approved for clinic implementation. Physical examinations, documentation of side effects, and laboratory review are all responsibilities of the NP. Special clinics have been established where NPs perform required physical exams on those enrolled in studies.

Registered Nurses

The registered nurses (RNs) are responsible for the overall coordination of the AIDS Clinics. After registering, every patient has vital signs taken and blood drawn if necessary, and is placed in an examination room. After the medical appointment, the RN staff will assist with procedures; administer chemotherapy, blood products, or hydration fluids intravenously; schedule appointments for special consultation or diagnostic tests; or make referrals for home-care nursing or psychosocial support. RNs triage all incoming patient phone calls as well as drop-in visits. Patients may also come in and see the nurse for "chemotherapy only" visits or for outpatient transfusions. Nursing staff, including a licensed vocational nurse and health worker, are given assignments as the Triage Nurse (RN only), Vital Signs/Flow Nurse, or Chemotherapy Nurse (RN only). Assignments are rotated so that each RN is familiar with all the roles. (See Figure 7.)

The Pharmacist

The function of the AIDS Clinic is not only to provide primary care but also to perform clinical research. The clinical pharmacist provides drug consultation on new investigational drugs, dispenses oral investigational drugs, takes drug histories, monitors patients for toxicity, and coordinates pharmacokinetic studies. Because most drugs used for the treatment of diseases related to HIV are new, information sheets for both staff and patients are developed for each drug by the pharmacist. Although the pharmacist's primary role is research, he or she also has primary-care responsibilities, which are performed at a Prescription Refill Clinic held twice a week. In this unique model of care, the clinical pharmacist, under medical supervision and guided by process protocols, can see patients who have a stable, nonacute medical problem, take a medication history, and refill a previously ordered medication. Such refills are honored only at the San Francisco General Hospital Pharmacy.

The Clinical Trials Manager

The clinical research trials manager, who is also a registered nurse, oversees the other research component for the clinic. The trials manager's role is to coordinate study activities and to supervise the RN-protocol managers who perform the main data-gathering activities. Institutional review board correspondence for study approval, coordination of data forms, and orientation of staff to new clinical study protocols are additional duties of the trials manager. Data-entry staff are responsible for entering research information into clinic computers.

Psychosocial Support Staff

One of the strengths of the San Francisco General Hospital system of AIDS care has been its psychosocial support staff. Both the outpatient and inpatient wards opened with counseling staff present. Shanti counselors and medical social workers have always been available to provide services. The more recent addition in 1985 of a licensed clinical counselor complemented the existing staff.

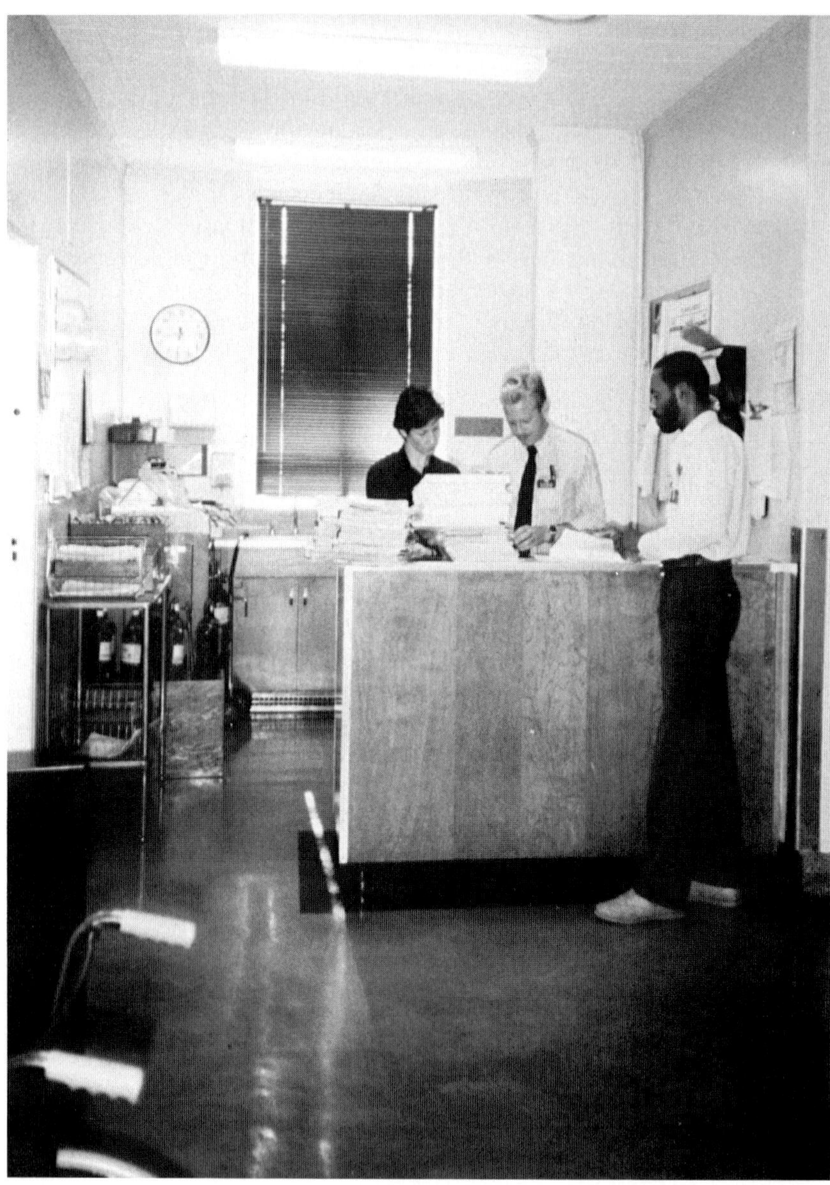

Figure 7 Nursing station. The AIDS Clinic nursing staff triages phone calls and drop-in visits, administers outpatient chemotherapy and transfusions, and coordinates all aspects of AIDS outpatient care.

The Shanti Counselor

The Shanti Project was organized in 1974 as a nonprofit organization to provide free volunteer counseling to people with life-threatening illness (5). Since 1981, Shanti's focus has been the care of the AIDS patient. The Shanti counselor is a specially trained layperson who establishes contact with all new patients and assists those who are newly diagnosed with AIDS or who are in crisis due to a change in their medical status. The counselor is able to provide immediate crisis intervention and a supportive atmosphere for ventilation and normal expressions of fear and anxiety, and can asess the patient for referral to more professional counseling or psychiatric services. Most patients seen in clinic have normal reactions of denial, fear, and anxiety related to their diagnosis. The use of a trained layperson to help these patients is appropriate and allows licensed counseling staff to handle more serious emotional needs. Bereavement counseling is also available for families, lovers, and spouses of AIDS patients.

The Medical Social Worker

HIV infection and its consequences often wreak havoc with a patient's livelihood and lifestyle. A young, active person becomes acutely ill, requiring hospitalization. Subsequent illness and debilitation result in possible layoff from work and loss of income and medical insurance. The medical social worker can assist the patient in applying for Medicaid benefits, disability, emergency housing or placement, home attendant care, and transportation. Addressing these concrete needs is a critical part of discharge planning and is essential for sustaining the patient after hospitalization.

The Licensed Clinical Counselor

While most patients exhibit normal anger and grief reactions related to diagnosis, it is not unusual for some to respond with severe depression or anxiety. The danger of suicide is real (5). When requested by clinic, Shanti, or medical social worker staff, the clinical counselor does an in-depth psychological evaluation to assist the staff in determining the patient's emotional state. Short-term counseling may be offered to the patient. Psychiatric referrals may be initiated if long-term therapy is recommended. Evaluation of suicide ideation and psychiatric emergencies is also done by the clinical counselor. Clinic providers and the counselor share information to rule out the possibility of organic mental syndromes.

VIII. Interagency Cooperation

A. Ward 5A

The nation's first inpatient unit dedicated to AIDS care opened in July 1983 at San Francisco General Hospital (22). (See Figures 8, 9.) The unit, developed

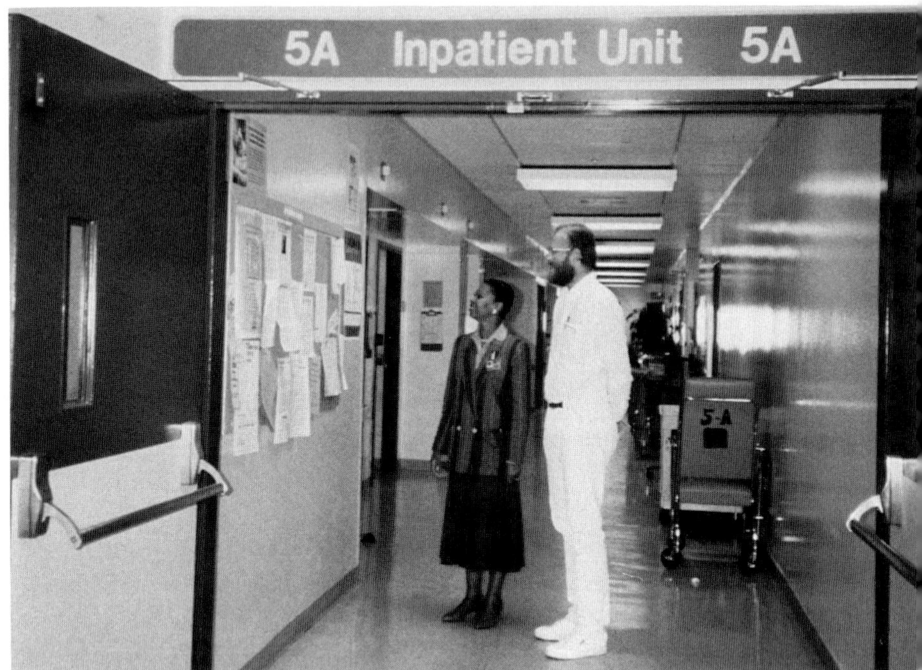

Figure 8 Ward 5A Inpatient AIDS Unit. Ward 5A was the nation's first inpatient unit dedicated to AIDS care, developed in response to the need for coordinated, sensitive AIDS hospital care.

in response to the large number of AIDS patients needing hospitalization, facilitated coordination and standardization of care, infection control, emotional support, and education. The inpatient equivalent to Ward 86, Ward 5A has also become a model unit for AIDS care, providing a high degree of nursing expertise and coordinated psychosocial counseling services. When a Ward 86 Clinic patient requires hospitalization, he or she is admitted to Ward 5A. Upon discharge, the patient is given a return appointment to Ward 86 for follow-up care.

B. The San Francisco AIDS Foundation

The San Francisco AIDS Foundation is a nonprofit organization that opened initially in 1982 with an AIDS telephone hotline. The foundation has grown to provide community and professional education programs to local groups. Ward 86 staff are used as resources, and educational materials are made available to both Wards 86 and 5A for distribution to patients. An AIDS

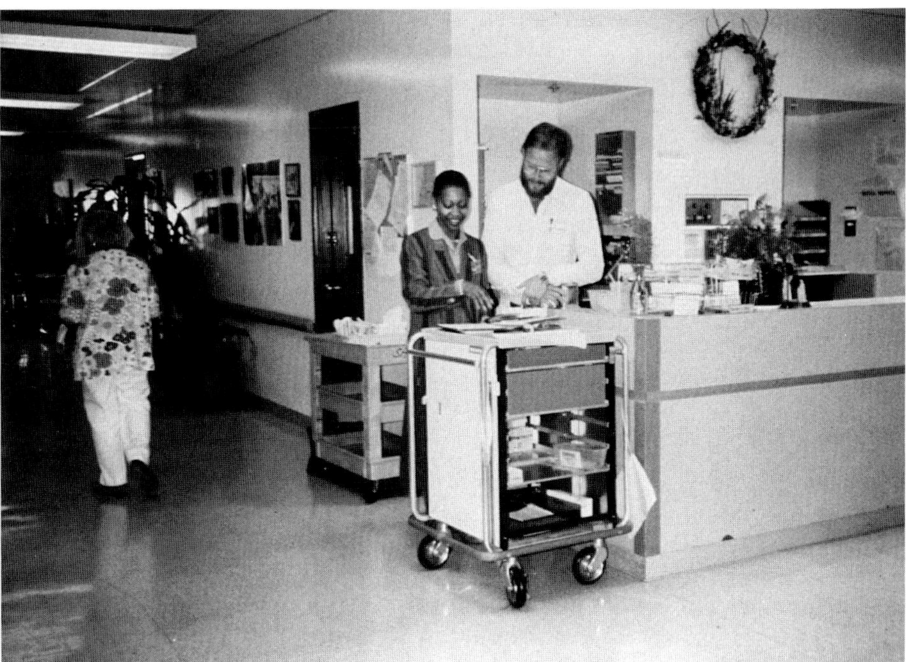

Figure 9 Nursing station at Ward 5A. The physical layout of the inpatient unit is similar to that of any other medical nursing unit; its uniqueness lies in the development of nursing expertise, standardization of care, infection control, and emotional support services for the care of people with AIDS.

telephone hotline is maintained by the foundation staff. Anxious people in need of AIDS information can be referred to the hotline by clinic staff, thereby helping to relieve the latter of time spent on the telephone. Conversely, foundation hotline staff can refer people with suspicious symptoms to the clinic for services. Referrals can also be made to the foundation for limited social service and legal assistance.

C. District Health Centers

Two of San Francisco's five district health centers have established AIDS screening and ARC clinics. Using the same screening format as that of Ward 86, a data base consistent with the Ward 86 patient data base is maintained. Physicians who work at the health center AIDS screening clinics are temporarily assigned to Ward 86 to become acquainted with the staff and services. They accompany clinic providers as they evaluate and treat patients, in order to become familiar with the staff's methods and to learn about the wide range of ARC and AIDS clinical manifestations. Referral from the health centers to the clinic is done with relative ease because of this cooperative relationship between the two agencies.

D. AIDS Home Care and Hospice Services

The AIDS Hospice Program was established by the City of San Francisco in 1984 to facilitate the early discharge and home care of its many AIDS patients (10). Hospice referrals are made at the Ward 5A inpatient AIDS unit at a discharge planning conference. Home care to an average caseload of 55 patients is coordinated by hospice nurses, who call the clinic to report clinical changes, renew medications, or arrange for clinic appointments or hospitalization on Ward 5A.

IX. Coordination of Care

AIDS patients along the entire spectrum of HIV infection are followed at the Ward 86 AIDS Outpatient Clinic. Effective use of all four components of care, including a community AIDS project, ambulatory- and acute-care facilities, ahd home nursing, ensures comprehensive delivery of services (see Figure 10). This coordination is facilitated not only by the referral process but also through several AIDS patient-care conferences. Ward 86 conducts a weekly conference around outpatient medical management issues or on relevant topics of AIDS. Ward 5A has a weekly patient-care conference on inpatient cases and a weekly discharge planning conference. Physicians, nurses, and social workers from the inpatient Ward 5A unit, the Ward 86 AIDS Outpatient Clinic, and community and home-care agencies attend these meetings. The Shanti Project and the AIDS Health Project each has its own weekly patient conferences.

Emotional and physical care are handled by on-site staff at both inpatient and outpatient levels. The philosophy and commitment to quality AIDS care are consistent throughout the system. These models provide multidisciplinary medical and nursing care, as well as mutidisciplinary psychosocial care, and integrate that care with various community agencies.

X. Common Issues in Systems Development

Health-care programs across the nation have begun to face the challenge of treating the person with AIDS (23-26,29-32). Common concerns of administration and staff include staff anxiety, fears of contagion, fears of being labeled an "AIDS facility," and prejudices against certain patient lifestyles. Other concerns that are not initially apparent but that can become major

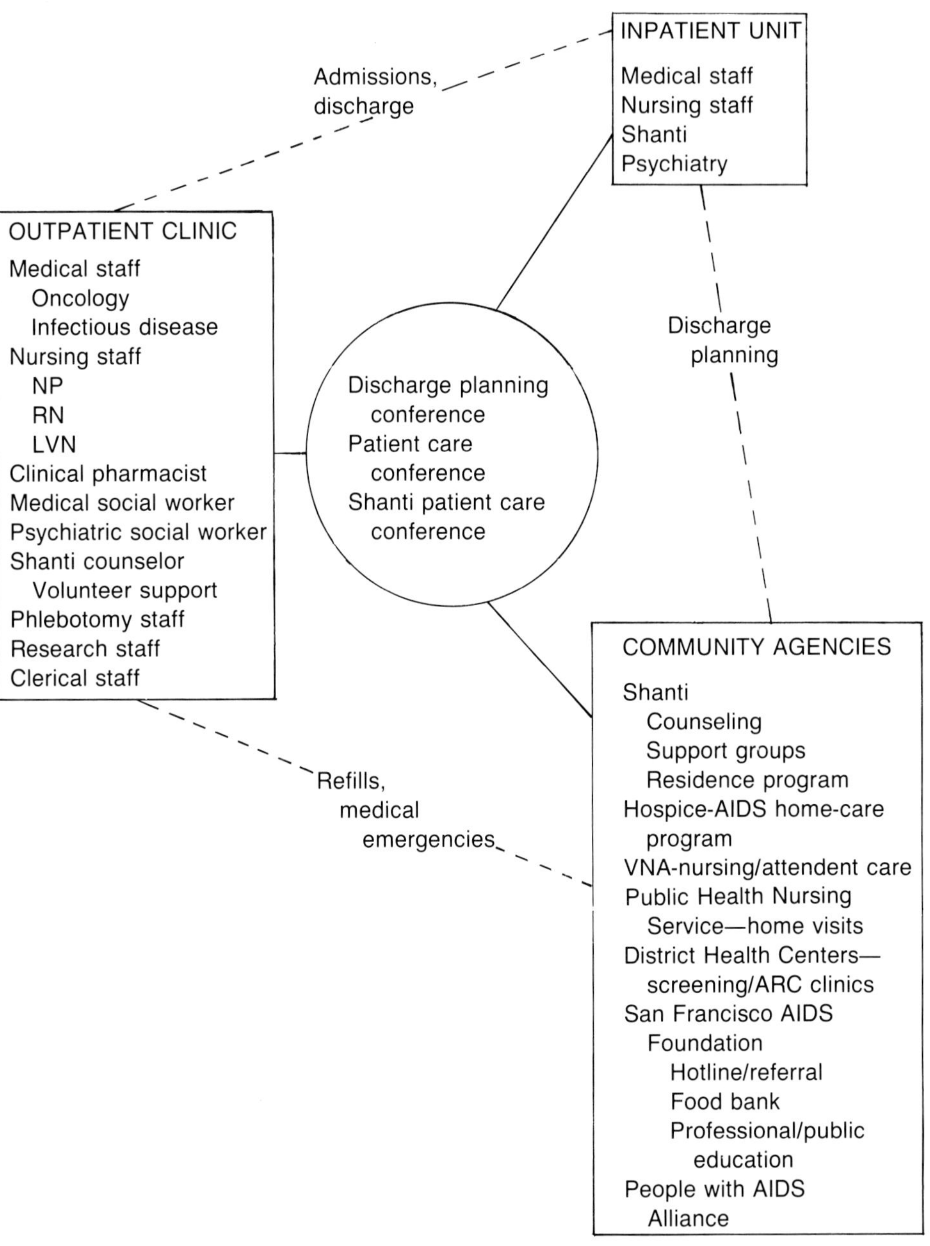

Figure 10 Elements of optimal AIDS care. LVN, licensed vocational nurse; NP, nurse practitioner; RN, registered nurse; VNA, Visiting Nurses Association.

Table 10 Common Problems in Establishing Care Systems for AIDS

Problem	*Possible solution*
Staff anxiety over caring for an AIDS patient	Provide intensive AIDS education classes with periodic updates to all hospital departments, including administration, physician, nursing, pharmacy, housekeeping, dietary, maintenance, etc.
	Initiate staff support groups to discuss issues of homophobia, gay culture, substance abuser, heterosexual spread
	Incorporate AIDS education into standard orientation classes for all departments
Fear of AIDS contagion	Establish written infection control guidelines specifically for AIDS, covering such areas as protective apparel, specimen handling, CPR, outpatients, inpatients, obstetrics, pediatrics, surgery, based on CDC guidelines
	Provide infection-control classes for all hospital departments; incorporate this information into standard orientation agenda
	Establish written employee health policies for needle sticks and other exposures and follow-up care
	Establish firm and consistent administrative philosophy and policy regarding care of AIDS patients, especially refusal to care for AIDS patients
	Establish personnel policies to address employees who have ARC or AIDS
"AIDS hospital" reputation/negative community reaction	Decide on a consistent administrative philosophy of care for AIDS patients and provide ongoing staff support
	Publicly stress the climate of caring and support provided to the patient and the hospital's humanitarian role
	Publicly stress the staff's adherence to proper infection-control guidelines and the lack of contagion to health-care providers
	Participate in community and professional programs about AIDS
	Elicit community support
	Work with staff to promote positive feelings, provide reassurance, and develop sensitivity in caring for AIDS patients and to ensure accurate, nonalarmist media coverage
Breach of confidentiality/intense media coverage	Establish and enforce strict confidentiality guidelines; educate staff as to guidelines and sensitivity to patient's need for privacy

Table 10 (continued)

	Establish philosophy and guidelines for media access to the agency, its staff, and patients
	Communicate regularly with staff so as to be in agreement on issues and statements to the press, to avoid confusion
	Educate hospital staff on how to avoid making inflammatory statements on AIDS-related issues and how to promote a positive image about AIDS
	Use media-relations department to control news media access to patient care areas, insure that written patient consent is obtained for news stories
	Use press conferences judiciously to inform community of relevant issues before they become crisis issues
	Actively work with media to present accurate educational and sensitive news stories about AIDS
	Be aware of media miscommunication or manipulation
Difficulty coordinating AIDS care	Establish a multidisciplinary AIDS team to review all AIDS patients and educate staff on medical, nursing, and psychosocial issues
	Establish regular AIDS patient-care conferences and grand rounds to update staff
	Establish regular AIDS discharge planning conferences that include community and home-care agency participation to insure continuity of care
	Establish a dedicated AIDS clinic or inpatient unit, utilizing multidisciplinary approach to include physicians, nurses, social workers
Staff burnout	Provide formal support group with facilitators
	Encourage informal staff support
	Offer stress-management classes
	Acknowledge staff contributions and achievements
	Provide ongoing administrative support
	Rotate responsibilities where possible

issues include maintaining confidentiality, surviving intense media coverage, managing the complexities of coordinating AIDS care, and preventing staff burnout. Various approaches to these issues have been employed in the San Francisco model as well as other institutions and are summarized in Table 10.

It is encouraging that the establishment and development of Wards 86 and 5A as "centers of clinical excellence" has had a strongly positive community response. The staff's unwavering commitment to quality care and research, patient confidentiality, and patient advocacy has enabled the clinic to weather the social and political storms around the issues of AIDS and HIV infection, and to continually refocus and refine its priorities as the epidemic continues to grow. The value of the Ward 86 program and, indeed, all of the AIDS programs developed in San Francisco can be reflected in the cooperation, contributions, and volunteer support of the surrounding community. What is finally developed in any given community actually depends on the community's specific needs, available help and resources, perceived health threat, and philosophy of health care.

XI. Conclusion

The purpose of this discussion has been fourfold: 1) to broaden the concept of CDC-defined AIDS to include care issues for those people with Group I to III HIV infection, 2) to discuss systems of care as they relate to the clinical spectrum of HIV infection, 3) to describe actual models of care for HIV infection and AIDS, and 4) to discuss common problems related to the development of those systems.

The models of care described here are flexible enough to accommodate most needs. From education to initial screening and evaluation, to diagnosis, treatment, clinical remission, progression, and terminal care, the patient can use the AIDS clinic as its primary care provider. These models of care can be adapted to meet specific community needs.

References

1. Selwyn P. AIDS: what is now known: epidemiology. Hosp Pract 1986; 21:127-64.
2. Koop CE. Surgeon General's report on acquired immune deficiency syndrome. Washington, D.C., 1986.
3. Classification system for human T-lymphotropic virus type III/lymphadenopathy-associated virus infections. MMWR 1986; 35:324-39.
4. Schietinger H. A home care plan for AIDS. Am J Nurs 1986; 86:1021-8.
5. Abrams DI, Dilley JW, Jaxey LM, Volberding PA. Routine care and psychosocial support of the patient with the acquired immunodeficiency syndrome. Med Clin N Am 1986; 70:707-20.
6. Weiss SH, Goedert JJ, Sarhgadharan MG, et al. Screening test for HTLV-III (AIDS agent) antibodies: specificity, sensitivity, and applications. JAMA 1985; 253:221-5.
7. Francis DP, Chin J. The prevention of acquired immunodeficiency syndrome in the United States: an objective strategy for medicine, public health, business, and the community. JAMA 1987; 257:1357-66.
8. Bayer R, Levine C, Wolf SM. HIV antibody screening: an ethical framework for evaluating proposed programs. JAMA 1986; 256:1768-74.

9. Mills M, Wofsy CB, Mills J. Special report: the acquired immunodeficiency syndrome; infection control and public health law. N Engl J Med 1986; 314:931-6.
10. Additional recommendations to reduce sexual and drug abuse related transmission of human T-lymphotropic virus type III/lymphadenopathy-associated virus. MMWR 1986; 35:152-5.
11. Revision of the case definition of acquired immunodeficiency syndrome for national reporting—United States. MMWR 1985; 34:373-5.
12. Jacobson MA. Laboratory evaluation of ARC and AIDS patients. AIDS File 1986; 1:1-2.
13. Jackson MM, Healy SA, Straube RC, McPherson DC, Greenawalt NC. The AIDS epidemic: dilemmas facing nurse managers. Nurs Econ 1986; 4:109-16.
14. Lo B. Durable power of attorney for health care. AIDS File 1986; 1(2):6.
15. Volberding P. The clinical spectrum of the acquired immunodeficiency syndrome: implications for comprehensive patient care. Ann Intern Med 1985; 103: 729-33.
16. Martin JP. The AIDS home care and hospice program, a multidisciplinary approach to caring for persons with AIDS. Am J Hospice Care 1986; 3:35-7.
17. Cote AA, Drusin LM. An interdisciplinary approach to dealing with the problems of AIDS patients at a tertiary medical center. Hosp Tops 1984; 62:28-30.
18. Gee G. Nursing. In: Jones P, ed. Proceedings of the AIDS Conference. Ponteland: Newcastle upon Tyne. Intercept, 1986:131-46.
19. Volberding P, Gee G, Linton B. Psychosocial sensitivity in hospital care: San Francisco General Hospital. In: McKusick L, ed. What to Do About AIDS. Berkeley, CA: University of California Press, 1986:173-83.
20. Gee G. Systems of care: ambulatory care nursing management. In: Cohen PT, Sande MA, Volberding PA, et al., eds. San Francisco General Hospital AIDS Knowledgebase [computer data base]. Boston, MA: Massachusetts Medical Society, 1988.
21. Carr G, Gee G. AIDS and AIDS-related conditions: screening for populations at risk. Nurs Practitioner 1986; 11:25-52.
22. Viele CS, Dodd MJ, Morrison C. Caring for the acquired immune deficiency syndrome patients. Oncol Nurs Forum 1984; 11:56-60.
23. AIDS cited as major administrative concern. Hospitals 1983; 1:45-6.
24. Hospitals stepping up effort to protect staff from AIDS. Am J Nurs 1983; 83: 1468.
25. Is your facility an "AIDS hospital?" Mod Healthcare 1985; 15:5.
26. Wallace C. Hospitals must plan for increase in number of AIDS patients—experts. Mod Healthcare 1985; 15:52-4.
27. Cleary PD, Barry MJ, Mayer KH, Brandt AM, Gostin L, Fineberg HV. Compulsory premarital screening for the HIV. JAMA 1987; 258:1757-62.
28. Elion R. Antibody testing and ambulatory care. J Ambulatory Care Manage 1988; 11:33-8.
29. Pascarelli EF, Holtzworth AS. Developing an ambulatory care program for AIDS patients. J Ambulatory Care Manage 1987; 10:44-55.
30. Andrulis DP, Beers VS. Coordinating hospital and community-based care for AIDS patients. J Ambulatory Care Manage 1988; 11:5-13.

31. Osborn JE. AIDS: The challenge of ambulatory care. J Ambulatory Care Manage 1988; 11:19-26.
32. Schobel DA. Management's responsibility to deal effectively with the risk of HIV exposure for healthcare workers. Nurs Manage 1988; 19:38-45.

21

Conclusions: In Pursuit of an AIDs Virus Vaccine

Maurice R. Hilleman
Merck Institute for Therapeutic Research
West Point, Pennsylvania

I. AIDS and Vaccines

The retroviruses that cause acquired immunodeficiency syndrome (AIDS) belong to the lentivirus subfamily and can be divided into two separable subtypes: human immunodeficiency virus type 1 (HIV-1) and type 2 (HIV-2) Chapters 8, 9). The mounting importance of these viruses, which threaten to cause a "Great Plague" of the present century, makes it imperative that some form of effective prophylactic control be developed. In the past, vaccines have provided the cheapest and simplest means for control of major infectious diseases. It is not surprising, therefore, that vaccine approaches to prevention of AIDS are being vigorously pursued.

Contemporary viral vaccines, listed in Table 1, consist of either attenuated live viruses or nonliving viral preparations. Killed vaccines are made of inactivated whole virus or subunits of virus from a natural or genetically engineered recombinant source. Vaccines present the host with immunological determinants, or epitopes, that are recognized as foreign and induce an immunological response. Some of the epitopes are essential for establishing infection or for survival of the virus, and the immune response against them protects the host.

Table 1 Contemporary Antiviral Vaccines[a]

Kind	Example
Live	Vaccinia
	Poliovirus
	Measles
	Mumps
	Rubella
	Yellow fever
Killed	
Whole virus	Poliovirus
	Influenza
	Rabies
Subunit	
Plasma-derived	Hepatitis B
Recombinant	Hepatitis B

[a]Adenovirus and varicella/zoster vaccines are not yet licensed for general use.

II. Specific Immune Responses to Viruses

The immune system of mammalian species is very complex and imperfect. Yet it does manage to keep most people alive into and past the reproductive age, despite the fact that it can cause harm to the host (e.g., in autoimmunity) as well as bring great benefit (1-3).

Specific immune responses to viral infections, summarized briefly in Table 2, are both humoral and cell-mediated (see Chapter 10).

Humoral antibodies are made by B lymphocytes and are believed to neutralize virus infectivity by a variety of incompletely understood mechanisms that may include: a) blockade of viral attachment to host cell receptors, b) induction of conformational changes in the viral proteins, resulting in epitope alteration or permitting entry of destructive enzymes into the virion, and c) prevention of fusion of virus with the host cell membrane, thereby precluding viral entry and uncoating. Antibodies also destroy infected cells that display virus-encoded antigens on their surface by a process called antibody-dependent cell-mediated cytotoxicity (ADCC). In this process, the antibody-coated cell is recognized by cytotoxic effector cells of the host. Additionally, humoral antibody is regulated by antiidiotype networking, whereby an antibody is produced against the specific antigen binding site (paratope) of the initial antibody (4). This response, in turn, leads to production of antibodies resembling that of the original antigen (antiidiotype). The overall result is a sequence of alternate-generation antibodies resembling, in some respects, the images seen in a hall of mirrors. This phenomenon is believed to provide

Table 2 Specific Immune Responses to Viruses[a]

Immune response	Antigen presentation	Lymphocyte response: Kind of cell	Lymphocyte response: Product	Antiviral action
Humoral	Virus particle or antigens	B cell (B)[b]	Antibody[c]	N (neutralization) ADCC (antibody-dependent cell-mediated cytotoxicity)
Cell-mediated	Virus particle	T suppressor (T_s)[b]	T_s factor	Regulatory (suppress B, T_h, T_c, T_d)
	Macrophage[a] (HLA-restricted)	T helper (T_h)[b]	T_h factor	Regulatory (helps B, T_c, T_d)
	Macrophage[a] (HLA-restricted)	T delayed hypersensitivity (T_d)	Lymphokines, interferon	Inflammation, macrophage activation
	Virus-infected[a] (HLA-restricted)	T cytotoxic (T_c)[b]	—	Immune cytolysis

[a]A simplified overview is presented. T_h and perhaps T_s responses are Class 2 (e.g., HLA-DR) restricted; T_c is Class 1 (e.g., HLA-A.B.C) restricted.
[b]Both immediate response and memory cells are induced, permitting anamnestic recall.
[c]Anti-idiotype antibodies against primary antibodies are immunoregulatory.

for homeostatic regulation of specific antibody production. As noted below, antiidiotype antibody induction has been considered as an approach to vaccines.

Cell-mediated immunity is directed mainly at clearance of virus-infected cells and is brought about by cytotoxic T lymphocytes (T_c) or by the T_d lymphocytes of delayed hypersensitivity. Regulation of the cells of the immune system is the function of T-suppressor (T_s) and T-helper (T_h) lymphocytes (generally identified phenotypically as CD8+ and CD4+ T lymphocytes, respectively) (see Chapter 10). B and T_s lymphocytes respond to antigens on cell-free viruses or in solution. T_h and T_d lymphocytes react with antigenic epitopes usually presented to them by cells of the macrophage series in association with major histocompatibility HLA antigens of the host. T_c cells recognize viral antigens and epitopes on infected host cells in association with HLA antigens. The T_h and T_s cells maintain immunological homeostasis via control of both humoral and cell-mediated immunity. The restriction imposed on T_h, T_d, and T_c cell responses by the HLA antigens of the host prevent their effect from being too broadly responsive and self-destructive.

III. Vaccine Mechanisms

The host responds to viral vaccines and antigens in much the same way as the infected individual responds to ordinary viral exposures in nature. The difference is that the experience with vaccines is brought to bear prior to infection, or shortly following exposure to agents that cause diseases such as rabies and hepatitis B that have long incubation periods. Vaccines prevent infection; they do not cure infections.

Attenuated live virus vaccines, although often causing mild disease, are generally to be preferred because they activate all arms of the immune system and induce both humoral and cell-mediated immunities. Killed vaccines, which induce good humoral response, may give only a weak cell-mediated immune response, if any. The action of humoral antibodies is limited principally to virus neutralization and to ADCC clearance of infected cells. Cell-mediated immunity, by contrast, eliminates virus-infected cells by cytotoxic T cell (T_c) and delayed hypersensitivity (T_d) reactions.

A. Adjuvants and Immunopotentiation

Killed vaccines are sometimes incorporated into immunological adjuvants in order to potentiate immune responses through a) slow antigen release, b) distribution to distal sites, c) elicitation of appropriate cellular responses at sites of microdeposition of antigen, and d) other purported mechansims. Alum adjuvant is acceptable for use in human beings and is employed routinely.

Freund's mineral-oil adjuvants are excessively inflammatory and are used only for animal experimentation. Allison's SAF-1 adjuvant (4), consisting of squalene, pluronic polymer, MDP-T, and antigen, is being tested experimentally in man. An important merit of this adjuvant is that it includes MDP-T, which is a potent stimulator of cell-mediated immune responses. Improved antigen presentation/adjuvant systems such as liposomes and Morein's immunostimulatory complexes (ISCOMS) (6,7) of Quil A glycoside with antigen have shown promise in animal investigations. ISCOMS possess the unique attribute of forming micelles of cagelike structure, having regions that are accessible for hydrophobic interaction with amphipathic polypeptides and glycoproteins extracted from biological membranes. Viral antigens having hydrophobic regions may bind to the micelles, resulting in an increase in their ability to elicit an immune response.

B. Vaccination Procedure

The regimen used for administering nonlive virus vaccines is extremely important in achieving maximal antibody responses with the longest possible duration. Usually, two or three priming doses are given within a period of a few weeks, followed by a rest period of suitable length during which time there is a substantial decline in the level of antibody. Then a booster dose, given 6 months to a year after initiation of immunization, elicits a very rapid and remarkably increased level of antibody, together with maximal induction of memory lymphocytes on which long-term anamnestic sensitization depends.

IV. AIDS Vaccine Considerations

A. Adverse Circumstances

The development of a vaccine against AIDS is hindered by the worst possible confluence of viral and pathogenetic factors that seem to preclude any simple or easy resolution in the foreseeable future. These factors, listed in Table 3, include virus transit between and among hosts by means of virus-infected cells as well as free virus. The RNA genome of the virus, following reverse transcription to DNA, integrates into the DNA of the host cell and can then be passed by cell-to-cell transmission (Chapters 8, 9). The virus is sequestered in the central nervous system beyond the blood-brain barrier and peripheral immune responses (Chapter 15). There are numerous antigenic serotypes (Chapter 8) and the virus impairs the function of or destroys the very cells of the immune system meant to combat it (Chapters 8, 10). Added to this is the absence of any successful lentivirus for any species, and the lack of promise for any experimental HIV vaccine tested to date in challenge studies in chimpanzees (8).

Table 3 Special Problems Involved in Developing an AIDS Vaccine

Transmission of infection by infected cells, as well as free virus
Integration of viral DNA into cell genome
Cell-to-cell transfer of infection
Sequestered infection in the central nervous system
Numerous antigenic subtypes
Impairment or destruction of the immune system
No successful prototype lentivirus vaccine
Failure of experimental AIDS virus vaccines to date

B. Transmission of Infection by Cells

Perhaps the most unusual challenge to an AIDS virus vaccine is the unique transfer of the infection from the donor source by infected cells. Following introduction, the infection can then continue by cell-to-cell contact (Chapter 8). Blockade of free virus transmission would be approached in much the same way as for other viral vaccines. But preventing infected cell transmission would require establishment of effective immune responses against infected cells prior to initial exposure. In effect, this approach would require a vaccine capable of providing the equivalent of "therapeutic" infected cell clearance. Such a capability has not yet been needed for any other vaccine.

C. Antigenic Diversity

Few other viruses show the remarkable antigenic diveristy of serologic types and variants of lentiviruses. There is no example of any successful viral vaccine capable of providing protective coverage against such hypervariable strains as those of HIV, save for influenza and for foot and mouth disease viruses. And, with these agents, the degree of diversity and the numbers of circulating types and variants at any particular time are minuscule and limited by comparison.

The surface glycoproteins of HIV that are encoded by the envelope (*env*) gene consist of both conserved and hypervariable segments (Chapter 9). Conventional wisdom suggests, therefore, that vaccines should be studied that are made of antigens from the conserved regions of gp120 or gp160, especially those that might not be immunodominant and might fail to be recognized in response to natural infection. Whether such antigens would elicit protective antibodies remains to be determined. Some glycoproteins can be immunosuppressive (9).

Another target is the highly conserved attachment site on the viral envelope that interacts with the CD4 receptor of the host cell (Chapter 8). Unfortunately, such sites on viruses may lie within deep canyons (10), clefts, or pockets in the surface antigen topography to which antibodies may not have access, even if they were produced. In addition, formation of antibodies against proteins that are complementary to the CD4 receptor protein may be restricted. It may be necessary for the survival of the virus that it line the rims of the canyons, pockets, or clefts with hypervariable antigens, since antibodies against them might prevent access of receptor to the attachment site through steric hindrance. Nevertheless, peptides that are conserved (some immunosuppressive) have been identified in viral envelope proteins of HIV (11,12) and may be a worthy target for vaccine development.

D. Hepatitis B Vaccine

In view of the problems with the variability of HIV surface antigens, it is reasonable to explore the usefulness for vaccines of nonvariant antigens encoded by the highly conserved *gag* gene. Any antigen, in fact, that might a) find its way onto the surface of the virus and be accessible to antibody or b) appear on the surface of cells infected with the virus should be fair game for vaccine consideration.

The potential usefulness of *gag* gene-encoded antigen in inducing immunity is illustrated with the virus of hepatitis B. This enveloped virus is smaller but roughly similar morphologically to HIV. Its surface antigen, however is only poorly glycosylated and contains immunodominant group *a* antigen epitopes that are totally cross-reactive among virus strains and are highly effective in inducing antibodies that can prevent hepatitis B virus infection (13,14). The presence of circulating antibody against the surface antigen of hepatitis B virus indicates immunity, while neutralizing antibodies against HIV glycoprotein antigens may coexist in serum with infectious virus. It is of importance, in the hepatitis B example, that partial protection against challenge with homologous virus can be achieved by immune responses to core antigen and to its associated *e* antigen epitope (15,16). It appears that core and *e* antigens may be present in the surface membrane of infected hepatocytes and that humoral and cell-mediated immune mechanisms may be present that clear away infected cells. It seems a fair presumption that, were hepatitis B surface antigen as polymorphic as that of HIV, there might now be a protective hepatitis B vaccine composed of core antigen elements rather than surface antigen. The basis for the protective efficacy is not fully elucidated, but this important clue should not be lost in the quest of a vaccine against the AIDS virus.

E. HIV Vaccines (17-23)

It is not the purpose of this overview to discuss the findings in the early attempts to prepare and test experimental HIV vaccines for their ability to prevent infection in chimpanzees. It is worthy of note, however, that all killed surface antigen preparations—whether whole gp120 or gp160 and whether derived from cell-culture-propagated virus or subunits produced by recombinant technology or by chemical synthesis—have failed to date to provide protection. Live virus vectors, such as vaccinia, bearing gene segments encoding HIV surface antigen, also have not shown promise (8). These experiments, which have been limited to homologous virus challenge, have not addressed the problem of surface antigen polymorphism (Chapter 8), nor have they considered the even more important problem of inducing immunity against virus-infected cells. Findings reported at recent meetings have also indicated failure to demonstrate protective efficacy in chimpanzees that were given pooled high-titer HIV immune globulin from infected human beings and subsequently challenged with the virus (F. Prince, personal communication). Also, an HIV-infected chimpanzee with neutralizing antibodies has been superinfected by a nonhomologous HIV (24). Although lacking promise to date, it is important to observe that experimentation is only beginning and that the findings reported in investigations thus far are few in number. It is hoped that future research will include tests of *gag* gene-encoded antigens and approaches with HIV antigens that will induce protective immune responses (see below). Moreover, the experiments should be designed to measure protection against infected cells as well as against free virus on challenge.

V. Concerns for AIDS Virus Vaccines

Once useful antigens or epitopes that elicit protective immunity against HIV infection have been identified, a variety of means to deliver them may be utilized. This could include attenuated live HIV virus, recombinant live viral vectors, whole killed virus propagated in cell culture, or subunit antigens produced by recombinant technology or by chemical synthesis. The most promising approach to an efficacious vaccine, that of an attenuated live virus, is least likely to be acceptable because of the theoretical and real problems of a) mutation, b) reversion to virulence, c) intracellular genetic recombination with or transactivation by indigenous viruses, and d) activation of cellular protooncogenes by "promoter insertion" (18, 25) that cannot be meaningfully assessed outside the human species.

The single most important problem with prospective AIDS vaccines lies, in fact, with safety. So little is known about the immunology and pathogenesis of the disease that perturbation of the immune response pattern through prior vaccination might lead to adverse rather than beneficial effects when the person is subsequently exposed to natural infection. Moreover, the possible harm may not be known until the vaccinated person has been exposed to infection with the virus at some indefinite time period after vaccination—when it is too late.

Concerns for possible adverse effects are not born of fancy or of extreme conservatism in clinical testing. Instead, they are based on adverse reaction experiences with vaccines and infections that were observed in the past.

The focus for concern lies in three areas, listed in Table 4: first, immunopotentiation of disease by vaccines, second, inappropriate immunological responses to vaccines, and third, possible adverse consequences of anti-idiotype networking.

A. Immunoenhancement

There are many epitopes on viral surface antigens. Improper or excessive response to immunodominant nonneutralizing epitopes through vaccination may block access to the critical neutralization sites on the virion and actually enhance rather than protect against infection. Reduction in effectiveness of experimental vaccine against feline leukemia, resulting in an increase in disease, has been reported (18, 26, 27). The many examples of immunoenhancement of both virus-induced and non-virus-induced tumor by vaccines (28-31) are usually interpreted to indicate undesirable antibody responses against tumor cell epitopes that by attachment block immunological detection and prevent destruction of cancer cells by cytotoxic cell-mediated immune mechanisms. Alternatively, nonneutralizing antibodies may help virus entry into cells via endocytosis, most likely mediated by the F_c receptor (32, 33). Recent studies have indicated that these types of enhancing antibodies can be found in HIV-infected individuals and immunized animals (34, 35).

Table 4 Possible Adverse Effects to Be Considered in Tests of AIDS Vaccines in Man

Adverse effect	Example
Immunoenhancement on exposure to virus, subsequent to vaccination	nonneutralizing antibodies Feline leukemia (retroviral) Tumor enhancement by vaccines
Inappropriate immune response to vaccine	Killed and subunit measles vaccines Respiratory syncytial virus Dengue Autoimmunity
Antiidiotypes and blockade of normal cell receptors (conceptual)	Hepatitis B AIDS (autoimmune theory)

B. Inappropriate Immune Responses

Measles The consequences of inappropriate immune responses are illustrated in the example of killed measles vaccine (Figure 1) (36, 37). Children who were given formalin-killed measles vaccine or purified hemagglutinin vaccine in the 1960s developed moderate to severe atypical measles with generalized Arthus-like reactions on vaccination with live measles vaccine or on natural exposure to virus. They had high fevers and developed immune complex disease affecting the lungs and skin. These vaccines were devoid of the fusion factor, or F antigen (destroyed by formalin), that is the basis for sustained immunity against measles. This same mechanism has been used to explain the reactions, sometimes fatal, in infants who received formalin-killed respiratory syncytial virus vaccine and who were later exposed to natural infection with homologous virus (38). In these cases, antibodies to the fusion protein were not produced, so infection by the agent was not prevented. Continual virus replication and spread by cell-to-cell contact in the host led to substantial immune reactions against the virus and virus-infected cells, thereby inducing pathological sequelae.

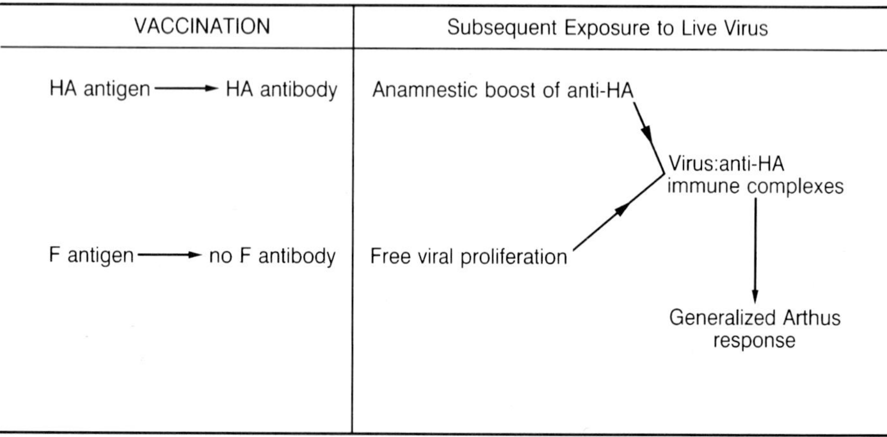

Figure 1 The steps that could lead to adverse reaction in individuals receiving nonliving measles virus vaccine that contained hemaggluttinin (HA) antigen but no fusion protein (F antigen). Immunization does not induce production of antibodies to the F protein, so viral replication and spread by cell-to-cell contact are not prevented. Infection can take place via the F protein, and the continual presence of viral antigens leads to immune complex formation and enhanced immunological reaction against viral proteins. This response can cause a pathological condition.

Dengue

Inappropriate responses also occur with dengue viruses (33), of which there are four distinct serotypes that also share common antigens. Initial infection with dengue virus results in benign febrile disease. Second infection with any heterologous serotype may cause severe hemorrhagic disease, often with shock. This effect is believed to result from the union of virus with nonneutralizing antibody against common antigens that are already present. Resulting complexes of virus and antibody gain ready access to susceptible macrophages via the F_c receptors on these cells. Infection of mononuclear cells is overwhelmingly increased, and possible immune complex disorders are induced as well.

An alternative explanation for the reactions observed in children given formalin-killed respiratory syncytial virus (see above; also, Ref. 38) could be a similar mechanism. Thus, nonneutralizing antibodies of IgG subtype might bind to the virus and facilitate infection in the infected host.

As noted above, potential for inappropriate immune response also exists with the AIDS virus. Besides antibody enhancement of virus infection, some HIV proteins that cross-react with epitopes on natural cellular proteins (e.g., viral envelope and HLA antigen) might induce an autoimmune response following immunization (see Chapter 8).

C. Anti-Idiotype Networking

Hepatitis B

Another example of possible adverse vaccine effects, although only hypothetical, seems disturbingly plausible and is illustrated in Figure 2. The binding of hepatitis B virus to the hepatocyte receptor is currently believed to involve the pre-S1 region of the surface antigen of the virus.

Hellström, et al. (39) reported that persons who convalesced satisfactorily from hepatitis B virus infection had lost their antibodies against pre-S. In contrast, persons who showed persistence of pre-S antibody often went on to develop chronic liver disease. These findings were explained by a failure to reduce production of the pre-S antibody.

Conceivably, these antiviral antibodies could induce antiidiotype antibodies that have the same configurational specificity as the pre-S1 antigen found on the virus. Subsequently, these second antibodies could attach to hepatocyte receptors and thereby cause the autoimmune pathology of the chronic liver disease associated with hepatitis B virus. With this possibility in mind, Hellström et al. (38) suggested that antigens in the pre-S1 region should not be considered suitable for a vaccine. While these observations and interpretations by Hellstöm have been severely criticized (40,41), the hepatitis B virus example does point out a need for caution in developing HIV vaccines.

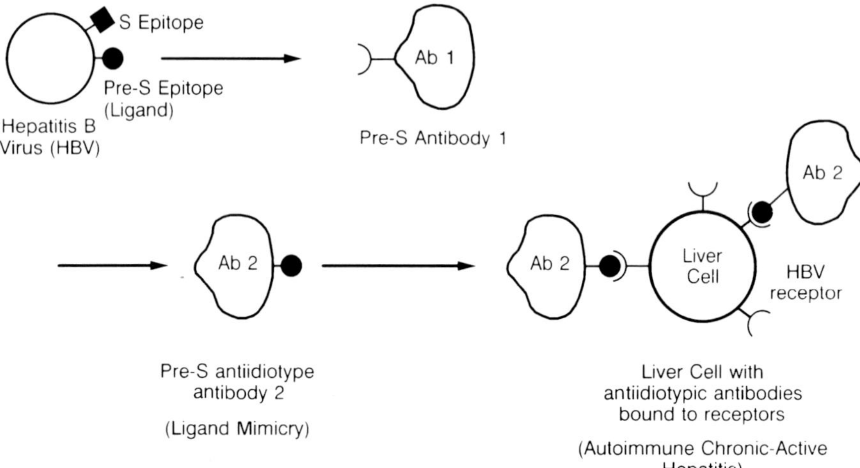

Figure 2 Potential induction of autoimmune chronic hepatitis by an anti-idiotype response. Antibodies are made to the pre-S region of the hepatitis B surface antigen. This antibody (Ab-1) induces production of an anti-idiotype (Ab-2) whose active site resembles the pre-S epitope of the virus. This anti-idiotype might then react with the natural receptor for HBV on a liver cell and induce an autoimmune condition.

To preclude this possibility, the proteins represented in a vaccine should not induce antibodies reacting with ligands on the virus that attach specifically to normal host cell receptors (e.g., CD4 receptor).

It is worthy of note that the plasma-derived and recombinant hepatitis B vaccines currently available in the U.S. do not contain pre-S antigens.

HIV Infection

Several investigators have considered that AIDS may be, in part, an autoimmune disease (see Chapters 8, 10). Ziegler and Stites (42) have suggested that, since a ligand on the viral gp120 mimics an invariant MHC component that normally binds to CD4 receptor on lymphocytes, immune responses to the gp120 ligand would be directed as well against the MHC component and cause dysfunction of the immune system. This hypothesis reinforces the concept that AIDS virus vaccines containing the viral ligand for CD4 receptors (or other viral proteins) should be critically examined, since damaging autoimmune responses might result from their use.

The validity for citing dangers involving antiidiotype and autoimmune reactions in hepatitis B and AIDS remains to be determined. As of now, the principal focus for much of the AIDS vaccine research effort is on whole and subunit gp120 antigens that contain the CD4 ligand. Hopefully, the planned human trials with purified HIV envelope protein will provide answers to the nagging possibility of an adverse effect, so that the development of this otherwise rational approach to a prophylactic immunogen can be pursued without concern.

VI. Chimpanzees and Safety Assessment

The assurance of safety for man is a most important concern in AIDS vaccine development. The chimpanzee is thus far the only primate model for assessing safety and efficacy of prospective vaccines aimed at preventing HIV infection in human beings. Although infected chimpanzees have not yet developed the full-blown AIDS disease, they do become persistently infected with HIV and mount immune responses against it (see Chapter 8). The markers of immune responses and infection following challenge in chimpanzees provide the best available, if not the only, means for judging the protective efficacy and the possible induction of adverse responses to experimental AIDS virus vaccines prior to initiation of human trials. The Macacus monkey model, using the simian immunodeficiency virus (SIV) (43), may be of great value in providing clues and in guiding development of vaccines against HIV. But any HIV vaccine for tests in man needs to first be evaluated in chimpanzee challenge studies.

Chimpanzees are available by the hundreds; the need is for thousands. It must be hoped that every avenue and means for augmenting the chimpanzee supply will be explored, and that unnecessary use of this valuable primate will be avoided. The intensive pursuit of a vaccine against AIDS ought not to be impaired by lack of this important animal resource.

Research on the AIDS virus has progressed well, but, as with other viruses, a vaccine requires many scientific, economic, and political considerations. It took between 10 and 15 years to develop and distribute the vaccines against polio, measles, and rubella. The live mumps virus vaccine took 7 years. HIV has been grown in the laboratory only since 1983. Our hope is that the advanced techniques in virology, cell biology, and molecular biology available today will shorten the interval leading to the development of the AIDS virus vaccine. Nevertheless, as noted in this review, no truly effective vaccine has been developed against a lentivirus, and HIV poses many new and difficult problems in virology that must be surmounted before immunological prevention of this disease can be achieved.

References

1. Mims CA, White DO. Viral Pathogenesis and Immunology. London: Blackwell Scientific Publications, 1984.
2. Dixon FJ, Fisher DW. The Biology of Immunologic Disease. Sunderland, MA; Sinauer Associates, 1983.

3. Paul WE, ed. Fundamental Immunology. New York: Raven Press, 1984.
4. Bona CA, Pernis B. Idiotypic networks. In: Paul WE, ed. Fundamental Immunology. New York: Raven Press, 1984:577-92.
5. Allison AC, Byars NE. An adjuvant formulation that selectively elicits the formation of antibodies of protective isotypes and of cell-mediated immunity. J Immunol Meth 1986; 95:157-68.
6. Morein B, Lövgren K, Höglund S, Sundquist B. The ISCOM: an immunostimulating complex. Immunol Today 1987; 8:333-8.
7. Osterhaus A, Weijer K, Uytdehaag F, et al. Introduction of protective immune response in cats by vaccination with feline leukemia virus ISCOM. J Immunol 1985; 135:591-6.
8. Hu SL, Fultz PN, McClure HM, et al. Effect of immunization with a vaccinia-HIV env recombinant on HIV infection of chimpanzees. Nature 1987; 328:721-3.
9. Muchmore AV, Shifrin S, Decker JM. In vitro evidence that carbohydrate moeties derived from uromodulin, an 85,000 dalton immunosuppressive glycoprotein isolated from human pregnancy urine, are immunosuppressive in the absence of intact protein. J Immunol 19877; 138:2547-53.
10. Luo M, Vriend G, Kamer G, et al. The atomic structure of Mengo virus at 3.0 A resolution. Science 1987; 235:182-91.
11. Cianciolo GJ, Bogerd H, Snyderman R. Human T-cell lymphotropic virus (HTLV) envelope-related peptides inhibit human lymphocyte proliferative responses. Clin Res 1986; 34:492A (abstr.).
12. Ho DD, Kaplan JC, Rackauskas IE, Gurney ME. Second conserved domain of pg120 is important for HIV infectivity and antibody neutralization. Science 1988; 239:1021-3.
13. Hilleman MR, Buynak EB, McAleer WJ, et al. Hepatitis A and hepatitis B vaccines. In: Szmuness W, Alter H, Maynard J, eds. Viral Hepatitis: 1981 International Symposium. Philadelphia: Franklin Institute Press, 1982:385-97.
14. Hilleman MR. Yeast recombinant hepatitis B vaccine. Infection 1987; 15:3-7.
15. Tabor E, Gerety RJ. Possible role of immune responses to hepatitis B core antigen in protection against hepatitis B infections. Lancet 1984: 1:172.
16. Murray K, Bruce SA, Hinnen A, et al. Hepatitis B virus antigens made in microbial cells immunise against viral infection. EMBO J 1984; 3:645-50.
17. Homsy J, Steimer K, Kaslow R. Towards an AIDS vaccine: Challenges and prospects. Immunol Today 1987; 8:193-7.
18. Fischinger PJ, Gallo RC, Bolognesi DP. Toward a vaccine against AIDS: Rationale and current progress. Mt Sinai J Med 1986; 53:639-47.
19. Frazer IH, Mulhall BP. Second international conference on the acquired immune deficiency syndrome. Med J Australia 1986; 145:524-9.
20. Hilleman MR. Perspectives in the quest for a vaccine against AIDS. In: Bolognesi D, ed. Human Retroviruses, Cancer and AIDS: Approaches to Prevention and Therapy. New York: Alan R. Liss, 1988:291-311.
21. Hilleman MR. Hepatitis B and AIDS and the promise for their control by vaccines. Vaccine 1988; 6:175-9.
22. Hilleman MR. Prospects for a vaccine to protect against AIDS. In: Villarejos VM, ed. Viral Hepatitis and Acquired Immunodeficiency Syndrome. San Jose, Costa Rica: Trejos Hermanos, Suc., 1987:53-68.

23. Hilleman MR. New era vaccinology. In: Kohler H, LoVerde PT, eds. Vaccines: New Concepts and Developments. Essex, England: Longman, 1988:391-402.
24. Fultz PN, Srinivasan A, Green C, et al. Superinfection of a chimpanzee with a second strain of human immunodeficiency virus. J Virol 1987; 61:4026-9.
25. Hayward WS, Neel BG, Astrin SM. Activation of a cellular *onc* gene by promoter insertion in ALV-induced lymphoid leukosis. Nature 1981; 290:475-80.
26. Olsen RG, Hoover EA, Schaller JD, et al. Abrogation of resistance to feline oncornavirus disease by immunization with killed feline leukemia virus. Cancer Res 1977; 37:2082-5.
27. Pedersen NC, Johnson L, Birch D, Theilen GH. Possible immunoenhancement of persistent viremia by feline leukemia virus envelope glycoprotein vaccines in challenge-exposure situations where whole inactivated virus vaccines were protective. Vet Immunol Immunopathol 1986; 11:123-48.
28. Kaliss N. Immunological enhancement of tumor homografts in mice. A review. Cancer Res 1958; 18:992-1003.
29. Kaliss N. The elements of immunologic enhancement. A consideration of mechanisms. Ann NY Acad Sci 1962; 101:64-79.
30. Hellström KE, Möller G. Immunological and immunogenetic aspects of tumor transplantation. Prog Allergy 1965; 9:158-245.
31. Goldner H, Girardi AJ, Hilleman MR. Attempts to interrupt virus tumorigenesis by immunization using homologous "Bjorklund-type" antigen. Proc Soc Exper Biol Med 1963; 114:456-67.
32. Dimmock NJ. Initial stages in infection with animal viruses. J Gen Virol 1982; 59:1-22.
33. Halstead SB. Immune enhancement of viral infection. Prog Allergy 1982; 31:301-64.
34. Robinson WE, Jr, Montefiori DC, Mitchell WM. Antibody-dependent enhancement of human immunodeficiency virus type 1 infection. Lancet 1988; 1:790-4.
35. Homsy J, Levy JA. Antibody-dependent enhancement of HIV infection. Lancet 1988; 1:1285-6.
36. Fulginiti VA, Eller JJ, Downie AW, Kempe CH. Altered reactivity to measles virus: Atypical measles in children previously immunized with inactivated measles virus vaccines. J Amer Med Assoc 1967; 202:1075-80.
37. Buser F. Side reaction to measles vaccination suggesting the Arthus phenomenon. N Engl J Med 1967; 277:250-1.
38. Murphy BR, Prince G, Wagner D, et al. The immune response of humans and cotton rats to respiratory syncytial virus (RSV) infection of formalin-inactivated vaccine. Modern approaches to new vaccines including prevention of AIDS. Cold Spring Harbor, NY: Cold Spring Harbor Laboratory, 1986:47 (abstr.).
39. Hellström U, Sylvan S, Kuhns M, Sarin V. Absence of pre-S2 antibodies in natural hepatitis B virus infection. Lancet 1986; 2:899-93.
40. Alberti A, Pontisso P, Fraiese A. Pre-S2 antibodies in hepatitis B. Lancet 1986; 2:1457 (letter).
41. Aihara S, Ise I, Tsuda F, et al. Pre-S2 antibodies in hepatitis B. Lancet 1986; 2:1457-8 (letter).

42. Ziegler JL, Stites DP. Hypothesis: AIDS is an autoimmune disease directed at the immune system and triggered by a lymphotropic retrovirus. Clin Immunol Immunopathol 1986; 41:305-13.
43. Kanki PJ, McLane MF, King NW Jr, Letvin NL, Hunt RD, Sehgal P, Danial MD, Desrosiers RC, Essex M. Serologic identification and characterization of a macaque T-lumphotropic retrovirus closely related to HTLV-III. Science 1985; 228:1199-201.

Index